Pediatric Neurosurgery Board Review

Nir Shimony • George Jallo
Editors

Pediatric Neurosurgery Board Review

A Comprehensive Guide

Springer

Editors
Nir Shimony
St. Jude Children's Research Hospital
Le Bonheur Children's Hospital
Semmes-Murphey Clinic
University of Tennessee Health
Science Center
Johns Hopkins University School
of Medicine
Memphis, TN, USA

George Jallo
David Goldenberg Family
Endowed Chair, Institute for Brain
Protection Sciences, Johns Hopkins
All Children's Hospital
St. Petersburg, FL, USA

ISBN 978-3-031-23686-0 ISBN 978-3-031-23687-7 (eBook)
https://doi.org/10.1007/978-3-031-23687-7

This Springer imprint is published by the registered company Springer Nature Switzerland AG
The registered company address is: Gewerbestrasse 11, 6330 Cham, Switzerland

I dedicate this book to my children. Maxwell, Nicky, and Lexi, for their unconditional love, understanding, and support.

George Jallo

I dedicate this book to my parents; my dear wife, Hila; and my kids, Liya, Darya, and Yahav, who remind me every day all about love and give me the strength to keep on going. To my patients who give me each time the motivation never to stop exploring for better solutions for their health and happiness

Nir Shimony

Foreword

To study the phenomena of disease without books is to sail an uncharted sea, while to study books without patients is not to go to sea at all.—Sir William Osler

It is wholly unlikely that when, in 1929, Harvey Cushing directed his protégé, Franc Ingraham, to staff the neurosurgical cases at Boston Children's Hospital he envisioned that pediatric neurosurgery would become the first official subspecialty of neurological surgery, as it is today. Dr Ingraham, with his junior partner Donald Matson, published *Neurosurgery of Infancy and Childhood*, the first textbook dedicated to pediatric neurosurgery, in 1954. It was not long after that that the European Society of Pediatric Neurosurgery (ESPN), the oldest international society dedicated to the practice of pediatric neurosurgery, held its first meeting in Vienna in 1967. Following this, Kenneth Shulman organized the first meeting of the Joint AANS/CNS Section of Pediatric Neurosurgery meeting in 1969, followed by the first meeting of the International Society for Pediatric Neurosurgery (ISPN) organized by Anthony Raimondi in 1972.

A half century later, pediatric neurosurgery has come into its own on all continents and in most developed countries. Formal pediatric subspecialty fellowships continue to flourish and increasingly require a dedicated year of dedicated pediatric neurosurgical training followed by passage of a Board Examination to permit credentialing.

Having served nine years on the American Board of Pediatric Neurological Surgeons (ABPNS) and now completing 6 years on the American Board of Neurological Surgeons (ABNS), I have often felt that a new textbook dedicated to Board preparation for the subspecialty of pediatric neurosurgery would be timely. In that regard, Jallo and Shimony, two internationally acclaimed pediatric neurosurgeons, have introduced their textbook, *Pediatric Neurosurgery Board Review: A Comprehensive Guide*.

The authors have assembled twenty-one chapters which review all the major topics common to the practice of pediatric neurosurgery. Each chapter is written by an internationally acclaimed author who is a recognized world authority on his given topic. The chapters follow a comprehensive format which includes a historical overview, pathogenesis, comorbidities, clinical diagnosis, medical imaging, current neurosurgical management, and anticipated outcomes. Each chapter is complete with current references for more detailed information should one wish. The chapters are comprehensive and current; the imaging is both sophisticated and legible.

With the scholarly tips and tricks offered in this book, followed by the review questions offered at the end of each chapter, it would be unlikely that any reader would be unprepared for their subspecialty Board examination, be it either a written or an oral examination; furthermore, given the rapid pace at which the field of pediatric neurosurgery is advancing, many more experienced pediatric neurosurgeons may also wish to read this book, as it gives us a comprehensive update of current management strategies for each topic. Given this "Comprehensive Guide," no pediatric neurosurgeon with a copy of this text should any longer find themselves sailing in an uncharted sea!

Memphis, TN, USA Fredrick A. Boop

Preface

In the wake of the twenty-first century, neurosurgery has become a multi-subspecialty field, comprised of complex pathologies across the central and peripheral nervous system, highly dependable upon the knowledge and skill of the surgeon as well as evolving technology and instruments. As a unique field within neurosurgery, pediatric neurosurgery comprises every aspect of the child involving the nervous system. The pediatric neurosurgeon has to diagnose, evaluate, and treat pathologies related to the brain, spinal cord, and peripheral nerves, including the vascular system, congenital malformation, skeletal malformation, trauma, and many more. It is hard to keep up with the growing body of knowledge in all the aspects of pediatric neurosurgery, and pediatric neurosurgeons find themselves in a unique position that demands knowledge, control, and a variety of surgical skills that are not seen in other neurosurgical subspecialties.

Keeping our knowledge up to date is a cumbersome task that is almost impossible without collaboration with our colleagues in the different neurosurgical subspecialties, as well as neurology, neuroradiology, neuropathology, physiatry, and more. Our vast knowledge base as pediatric neurosurgeons, and our attention to the growing child, the parents, and the needs across different age groups, allow us to provide better care for our patients. Pediatric neuro-oncology has evolved as a completely different field in recent years, with much more emphasis on precision-led medicine, with vast advancement regarding molecular with genetic subtyping that must be considered in our decision-making as surgeons. The use of neoadjuvant treatment, second-look surgeries, and targeted therapy, pushing the envelope for better surgical results while avoiding complications such as posterior fossa syndrome, are now embedded in our daily practice. The better implementation of technology in the detection and surgical treatment of intractable epilepsy, such as StereoEEG, minimally invasive techniques such as tubular retractors, or use of LiTT has become the standard of treatment, allowing for much better results in once deemed to be cases of diffuse epilepsy with no surgical cure. The standardization in pediatric neurosurgery practice, such as the implementation of shunt surgery protocol which thrives to achieve minimal to no shunt-related infection or complications, is now gradually becoming a routine. All these changes are a small part of our field's tremendous progress and evolution.

In this book, *Pediatric Neurosurgery Board Review: A Comprehensive Guide*, we intend to bring the reader an international spectrum of knowledge from around the globe. The authors were given considerable flexibility and independence in writing the chapters so that they could share their own experience and knowledge with the reader without any limitations, updating the current knowledge of pediatric neurosurgery, for the neurosurgeon who wishes to stay current or up-to date, for the young neurosurgeon doing their first steps in pediatric neurosurgery, for pediatric neurosurgeons about to take their pediatric neurosurgery board exam, or for the resident trying to better understand topics in this vast field of pediatric neurosurgery. Each chapter is written by world-renowned neurosurgeons, neurologists, neurooncologists, or neuroradiologists, sharing their knowledge and updating the knowledge on the specific topic they master in their daily life. Each chapter also contains review questions and answers.

We are honored to assemble and edit this vast body of work focusing on delivering up-to-date knowledge updates in the field of Pediatric Neurosurgery. We are grateful to our contributors for making this happen relatively quickly!

Memphis, TN, USA Nir Shimony
St. Petersburg, FL, USA George Jallo

Acknowledgments

We would like to thank our colleagues, neurologists, neuro-oncologists, and pediatricians, who are a crucial part of the multidisciplinary team taking care of children suffering from complex neurological conditions. We should also like to deeply acknowledge our mentors, Fred Epstein, Rick Abbott, Jeff Wisoff, Shlomi Constantini, Jonathan Roth, and Zvi Ram, who have encouraged and sparked our interest in pediatric neurosurgery. We also thank our fellows, residents, and medical students for their passion and dedication to medicine. Most of all, we are grateful to our partners who allowed and encouraged us in this endeavor of this book.

We are grateful to Springer editorial and production team members. Their professionalism and guidance enabled us to complete this book.

Contents

Contributors

P. David Adelson Department of Neurosurgery, Rockefeller Neuroscience Institute, College of Medicine, West Virginia University, J. W. Ruby Memorial Hospital and Children's Hospital, Morgantown, WV, USA

Edward S. Ahn Mayo Clinic Department of Neurologic Surgery, Rochester, MN, USA

S. Hassan A. Akbari Division of Pediatric Neurosurgery, Johns Hopkins University School of Medicine, Johns Hopkins All Children's Hospital, St. Petersburg, FL, USA

Allan Belzberg Department of Neurosurgery, Johns Hopkins University School of Medicine, Baltimore, MD, USA

Archis R. Bhandarkar Mayo Clinic Department of Neurologic Surgery Rochester, MN, USA

Cameron Brimley Geisinger Neuroscience Institute, Danville, PA, USA

Department of Neurosurgery, Geisinger Commonwealth School of Medicine, Scranton, PA, USA

Douglas L. Brockmeyer Department of Neurosurgery, University of Utah School of Medicine, Salt Lake City, UT, USA

Oguz Cataltepe Department of Neurological Surgery, University of Massachusetts Chan Medical School and Medical Center, Worcester, MA, USA

Samer Elbabaa Pediatric Neurosurgery, Leon Pediatric Neuroscience Center of Excellence, Arnold Palmer Hospital for Children, Orlando, FL, USA

Michael J. Fisher Division of Oncology, Department of Pediatrics, Children's Hospital of Philadelphia and University of Pennsylvania Perelman School of Medicine, Philadelphia, PA, USA

Joanna E. Gernsback Department of Neurosurgery, University of Oklahoma Health Sciences Center, Oklahoma City, OK, USA

Timothy C. Gooldy Department of Neurosurgery, Barrow Neurological Institute, St. Joseph's Hospital and Medical Center, Phoenix, AZ, USA

Mari Groves Department of Neurosurgery, Johns Hopkins University, Baltimore, MD, USA

John A. Heflin Department of Orthopedic Surgery, University of Utah School of Medicine, Salt Lake City, UT, USA

Andrew M. Hersh Department of Neurosurgery, Johns Hopkins University School of Medicine, Baltimore, MD, USA

David S. Hersh Division of Neurosurgery, Connecticut Children's, Hartford, CT, USA

Department of Surgery, UConn School of Medicine, Farmington, CT, USA

Thierry A.G.M. Huisman Edward B. Singleton Department of Radiology, Texas Children's Hospital, Houston, TX, USA

Christopher Inglese Division of Pediatric Neurology, Johns Hopkins All Children's Hospital, St. Petersburg, FL, USA

Rajiv R. Iyer Department of Neurosurgery, University of Utah School of Medicine, Salt Lake City, UT, USA

George Jallo Department of Neurosurgery, The Johns Hopkins University School of Medicine, Baltimore, MD, USA

Department of Neurosurgery, Johns Hopkins Medicine, Institute for Brain Protection Sciences, Johns Hopkins All Children's Hospital, St. Petersburg, FL, USA

David M Goldenberg Family Endowed Chair, Institute for Brain Protection Sciences, Johns Hopkins All Children's Hospital, St. Petersburg, FL, USA

Andrew Jea Department of Neurosurgery, University of Oklahoma Health Sciences Center, Oklahoma City, OK, USA

Ari D. Kappel Department of Neurosurgery, Boston Children's Hospital, Boston, MA, USA

Harvard Medical School, Boston, MA, USA

Department of Neurosurgery, Brigham and Women's Hospital, Boston, MA, USA

Paul Klimo Jr Division of Pediatric Neurosurgery, Department of Surgery, St. Jude Children's Research Hospital, Memphis, TN, USA

Department of Neurosurgery, The University of Tennessee Health Science Center, Memphis, TN, USA

Department of Neurosurgery, Le Bonheur Children's Hospital, Memphis, TN, USA

Semmes Murphey, Memphis, TN, USA

Chelsea Kotch Division of Oncology, Department of Pediatrics, Children's Hospital of Philadelphia and University of Pennsylvania Perelman School of Medicine, Philadelphia, PA, USA

Nathan K. Leclair School of Medicine, University of Connecticut, Farmington, CT, USA

Daniel Lubelski Department of Neurosurgery, Johns Hopkins University School of Medicine, Baltimore, MD, USA

Avner Meoded Edward B. Singleton Department of Radiology, Texas Children's Hospital, Houston, TX, USA

Andreas Mitsios "National and Kapodistrian" University of Athens, Athens, Greece

Jeffrey Nadel Department of Neurosurgery, University of Utah School of Medicine, Salt Lake City, UT, USA

Rebecca Reynolds Division of Pediatric Neurosurgery, Johns Hopkins All Children's Hospital, St. Petersburg, FL, USA

Division of Pediatric Neurosurgery, Johns Hopkins University School of Medicine, Johns Hopkins All Children's Hospital, St. Petersburg, FL, USA

Casey Ryan Department of Neurosurgery, University of South Florida, Tampa, FL, USA

Alfred P. See Department of Neurosurgery, Boston Children's Hospital, Boston, MA, USA

Harvard Medical School, Boston, MA, USA

Spyros Sgouros "Iaso" Childrens Hospital, Marousi, Greece

"National and Kapodistrian" University of Athens, Athens, Greece

Nir Shimony Department of Neurosurgery, University of Tennessee - Health Science Center, Memphis, TN, USA

Department of Surgery, St. Jude Children's Research Hospital, Memphis, TN, USA

Le Bonheur Neuroscience Institute, Le Bonheur Children's Hospital, Memphis, TN, USA

Department of Neurosurgery, The Johns Hopkins University - School of Medicine, Baltimore, MD, USA

Semmes-Murphey Clinic, Memphis, TN, USA

Edward R. Smith Department of Neurosurgery, Boston Children's Hospital, Boston, MA, USA

Harvard Medical School, Boston, MA, USA

Rita Snyder Baylor College of Medicine, Houston, TX, USA

Jesse A. Stokum Department of Neurosurgery, University of Maryland School of Medicine, Baltimore, MD, USA

U. -W. Thomale Pediatric Neurosurgery, Charité Universitaetsmedizin Berlin, Campus Virchow Klinikum, Berlin, Germany

Howard L. Weiner Neurosurgery, Texas Children's Hospital, Houston, TX, USA

Neurosurgery, Baylor College of Medicine, Houston, TX, USA

1 The Neurological Assessment of Pediatric Patient and the Differences Across Different Age Groups

Rebecca Reynolds and Christopher Inglese

Introduction

The neurologic examination as it is routinely performed today was developed in the late nineteenth century by eminent neurologists, including William Erb, Joseph Babinski, William Gowers, and Jean-Martin Charcot. Their work was compiled by Gordon Holmes into what is known as the modern "neurologic examination" [2]. The neurologic exam varies significantly from infancy into adulthood. Pediatrics is unique in that a patient may not be willing to participate in the exam, which often confounds a clinic appointment or inpatient exam. Objective signs, serial examinations, and a parent's opinion can frequently reveal findings that would otherwise be overlooked in a non-verbal or non-compliant child.

The adage or dictum "make it a game" is essential, and sitting on the floor or on a mat, with a variety of blocks, colored toys, or stuffed animals is far more important and valuable in this setting than the reflex hammer, stethoscope, and other quintessential diagnostic tools traditionally found in the doctor's office. For example, the infant with emerging stranger anxiety may be impossible to seduce with patience, toys, or games. In this case with the child seated on parent's lap and the examiner sitting several feet away may prove to be the best initial approach. Conversely, a teenager may be less willing to participate with parents in the room, and an independent interview solely with the patient may provide additional insight into a clinical problem.

The goal of the neurologic examination is to ascertain whether or not something is truly abnormal on exam and if there is a problem to localize the lesion as central or peripheral. This concept of localization can then be further subcategorized into cortical, subcortical, bulbar, thalamic/basal ganglia, brainstem, spinal cord, peripheral nerve, or muscle. Below are common components of the neurological exam and relevant diagnostic findings within each section.

Helpful Tools

1. Developmental timeline.
2. Pediatric growth charts.
3. Reflex hammer, safety pins, and cotton to test sensation.
4. One hundred twenty-eight or 256 Hz tuning forks for vibration sense and 512 Hz fork for Rinne and Weber testing for hearing loss,

R. Reynolds
Division of Pediatric Neurosurgery, Johns Hopkins All Children's Hospital, St. Petersburg, FL, USA
e-mail: rreyno26@jhmi.edu

C. Inglese (✉)
Division of Pediatric Neurology, Johns Hopkins All Children's Hospital, St. Petersburg, FL, USA
e-mail: cingles2@jhmi.edu

N. Shimony, G. Jallo (eds.), *Pediatric Neurosurgery Board Review*,
https://doi.org/10.1007/978-3-031-23687-7_1

which can be warmed or cooled with water to test cool or warm temperature sensations.
5. Ophthalmoscope for a fundus exam.
6. Visual acuity or Snellen charts. Of note, the "tumbling E chart" is useful in younger children under 5 years old who have not mastered the alphabet.

Components of the Neurological Exam

Vital Signs

Head circumference (OFC) occipital frontal circumference, height, and weight are diagnostic measures that lend insight into a child's overall growth when compared to the standard estimated gestational age-corrected growth curves. The most widely accepted curves are those of the World Health Organization [3]. As long as a child is "following the growth curve," there is typically no cause for concern; however, once a child begins to "cross percentiles" in a particular growth marker, further diagnostic workup should be considered.

The standard vital signs for both children and adults should also be taken into consideration in an age-dependent fashion: heart rate, blood pressure, and respiratory rate. Vital signs can be particularly useful when evaluating the etiology of headaches, syncope versus seizure, and unexplained falls. Below is a table of age-specific vital signs [4].

	Heart rate	Systolic blood pressure	Respiratory rate
Neonate, <1 year old	100–160	60–90	30–60
Toddler, 1–5 years old	90–150	80–120	20–30
5–12 years old	80–120	90–110	15–20
>12 years old	60–100	100–120	12–15

Anterior Fontanelle

The anterior fontanelle serves as an additional vital sign in neonates for the pediatric neurosurgeon. An objective datapoint, the fontanelle, is typically classified in one of three ways: above the bone (full), at the bone (flat), or below the bone (sunken). If the fontanelle is above the bone, then it is further stratified into soft or tense. A tense fontanelle is one that typically needs to be acted upon quickly and is concerning for elevated intracranial pressure. The anteror fontanelle is optimally examined with the child sitting and not crying.

General Appearance [5–8]

The child's general appearance and grossly their level of consciousness are assessed. Important things to note are head shape, cranial sutures, and dysmorphic features. Assessing head shape can provide information about a child at risk for craniosynostosis, hydrocephalus, or other genetic conditions. The cranial sutures can often be palpated in infants and also aid in the diagnosis of elevated intracranial pressure or craniosynostosis. Dysmorphic facial features are often stigmata of an underlying condition when present in multiple locations. Assessing for bruises and the rapport and parent-child relationship can also be particularly useful to monitor for signs of nonaccidental trauma.

Head Shape

- Macrocephaly: large head, >98th percentile on growth curve
- Microcephaly: small head, <3rd percentile on growth curve
- Brachycephaly: head wide, occiput flat, indicative of coronal craniosynostosis
- Scaphocephaly: long and narrow head, indicative of sagittal craniosynostosis
- Plagiocephaly: flattening of one side of the head, positional without craniosynostosis
- Oxycephaly: pointed head, Crouzon's syndrome, pan-suture craniosynostosis
- Acrocephaly: high, tower-like head and prominent vertical forehead
- Trigonocephaly: triangular cranial contour, metopic ridge mid forehead

Cranial Sutures

- Overriding: low or normal intracranial pressure suspected
- Approximated: within normal limits
- Splayed: elevated intracranial pressure suspected

Dysmorphic Features and Associated Conditions

- Single midline incisor: holoprosencephaly
- Hypotelorism: holoprosencephaly
- Hypertelorism: cerebral gigantism, Apert syndrome with craniosynostosis
- Inner epicanthal folds: Zellweger syndrome, Down syndrome, Rubinstein-Taybi syndrome
- Slanted palpebral fissures: Apert syndrome, Down syndrome, DiGeorge syndrome, Miller-Decker syndrome, and peroxisomal disorders
- Low-set ears: Noonan syndrome, Miller-Decker syndrome, Rubenstein-Taybi syndrome
- Brittle hair: Menkes' disease

Mental Status

Mental status can be quantified in many different ways. Qualitatively, patients are often described as awake and alert versus comatose or obtunded, yet there are many in-between statuses of mentation. Commonly used in neurosurgery is the Glasgow Coma Scale (Fig. 1.1) [9], which can be modified for pediatric patients based on their age. A fundamental knowledge of the pediatric developmental trajectories is key to ascertaining whether or not true cognitive or neuromotor delays are present (Figs. 1.2 and 1.3).

		All Ages		
Eyes	4	Spontaneous		
	3	To loud voice		
	2	To pain		
	1	No eye opening		
		Infant	**Toddler**	**School-age**
Verbal	5	Smiles, coos, cries	Appropriate words	Oriented, fluent
	4	Cries	Inappropriate words	Disoriented, fluent
	3	Inconsolable crying	Inconsolable crying	Inappropriate words
	2	Grunts	Grunts	Grunts
	1	No response	No response	No response
		Infant	**Toddler and older**	
Motor	6	Spontaneous	Obeys commands	
	5	Localizes to pain	Localizes to pain	
	4	Withdraws	Withdraws	
	3	Decorticate posture	Decorticate posture	
	2	Decerebrate posture	Decerebrate posture	
	1	No movement	No movement	

Fig. 1.1 Pediatric Glasgow Coma Scale

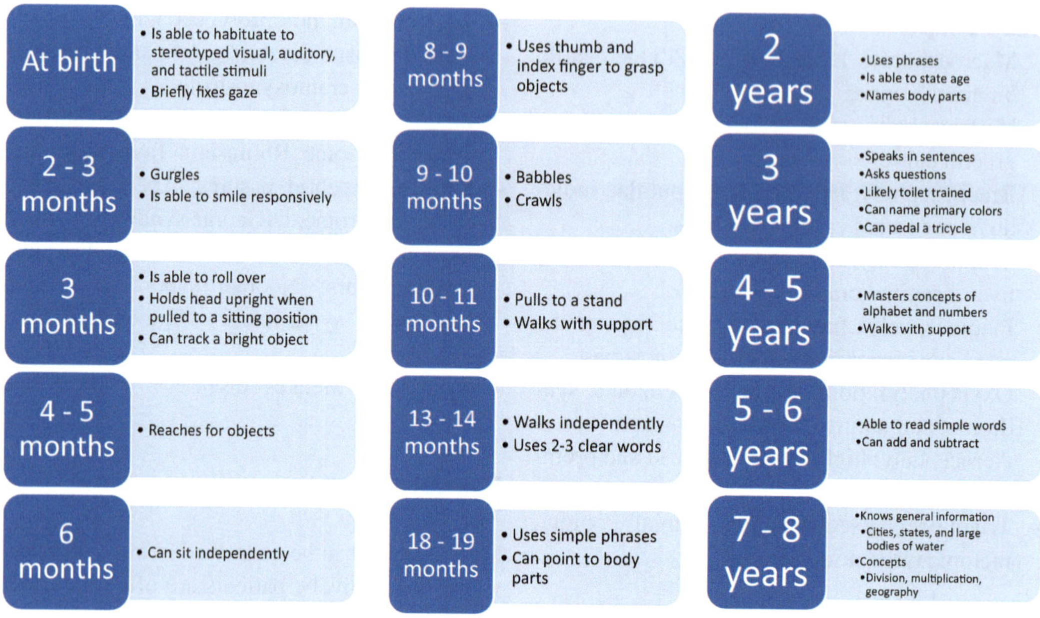

Fig. 1.2 Developmental milestones

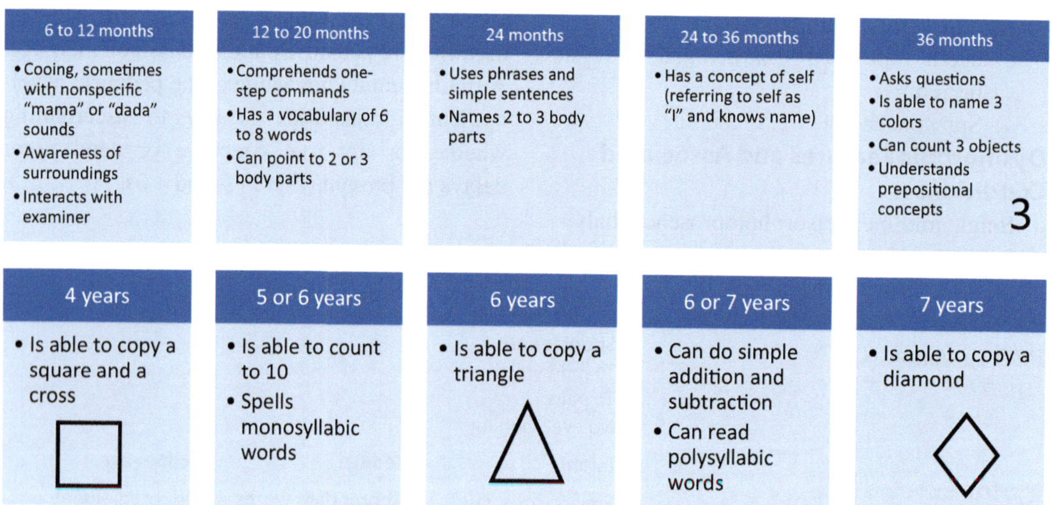

Fig. 1.3 Normal cortical function in children

Cranial Nerves [8]

I. Olfactory nerve: sense of smell

   (a) Infants of diabetic mothers may have decreased olfaction.

II. Optic nerve: vision, afferent pupillary response

   (a) Absent red reflex in retinoblastoma.

III. Oculomotor nerve: extraocular movement, relative afferent pupillary defect or efferent pupillary) response

   (a) Ptosis, miosis, preserved pupillary light reflex in Horner's syndrome, which can be present in brachial plexus palsies.

IV. Trochlear nerve: extraocular movement

V. Trigeminal nerve: facial sensation, afferent corneal reflex

VI. Abducens nerve: extraocular movement

VII. Facial nerve: facial motor function, efferent corneal reflex

 (a) Asymmetric crying facies can be due to traumatic birth delivery with forceps.

VIII. Vestibulocochlear nerve: hearing and balance

 (a) If congenital deafness, consider TORCHes infection (toxoplasma, other, rubella, cytomegalovirus, and herpes simplex virus HIV, syphyllis).

IX. Glossopharyngeal nerve: palate elevation, posterior tongue sensation, afferent gag reflex

X. Vagus nerve: palate elevation, visceral organ function (heart, respiratory, digestion), efferent gag reflex

XI. Spinal accessory nerve: shoulder elevation and head turn

XII. Hypoglossal nerve: tongue movement

Examining children can be challenging and varies based upon a child's age. A full cranial nerve exam can often be completed with a Snellen eye chart (CN II), bright-colored objects (CN III, IV, VI), cotton (CN V), direct observation (CN VII, XI), and providing a snack (CN IX, X, XII).

Motor Exam

The nuances of the motor exam depend on a child's age and can help determine an upper versus lower motor neuron lesion. Asymmetric findings on exam are the most definitive insight that a problem exists in infants and toddlers where it can be difficult to perform a focused motor exam. In older children who can participate in manual motor testing of isolated motor groups, the standard assessment applies with a motor scale from 0 (no movement) to 5 (normal function).

Reflexes

Children are unique in that there are many reflexes beyond stretch tendon responses that are retained throughout adulthood if abnormally persistent. The presence or absence of these primitive reflexes, depending on a child's age, can help diagnose an underlying clinical problem. An outline of these reflexes can be found below and in Fig. 1.4. Common reflexes tested in children and adults are the Babinski reflex and clonus. While there is debate, the Babinski reflex is typically considered pathologic after the age of 1 year old. Asymmetry to the reflexes is considered pathologic at any age. Sustained clonus beyond the age of 2 months old is abnormal.

Standard reflexes commonly tested in comatose children are the pupillary, corneal, and cough/gag reflex. These reflexes can be assessed with a pen light, saline, and endotracheal tube and are a quick assessment of brainstem function, specifically the midbrain (pupillary reflex), pons (corneal reflex), and medulla (gag reflex).

Fig. 1.4 Developmental reflexes

Reflex	Age at Appearance	Description	Age at Resolution
Moro (startle)	34 to 36 weeks post-conceptual age	The infant is held supine in the examiners arms and the examiner then suddenly drops the infant's head slightly. This causes the infant to extend and abduct the arms with palms open and sometimes evokes crying.	5 to 6 months
Trunk incurvation (Galant)	38 to 40 weeks post-conceptual age	While the infant is in a prone position the examiner strokes or taps along the side of the spine eliciting a twitch of the hips toward the side of the stimulus.	1 to 2 months
Asymmetric tonic neck reflex (fencing)	38 to 40 weeks post-conceptual age	While the infant is relaxed and lying a supine position the examiner rotates the head to one side. This causes the infant to extend the leg or arm on the side toward which the head was turned, while flexing the arm on the contralateral side (fencing posture).	3 to 4 months
Rooting	38 to 40 weeks post-conceptual age	The infant turns his or head toward the side of the cheek that is stroked and makes sucking motions.	2 to 3 months
Palmar grasp	38 to 40 weeks post-conceptual age	The infant closes his or her hand around the examiners finger when it is placed in their open palm. The infant tightens the grip if the examiner attempts to withdraw the finger.	5 to 6 months
Plantar grasp	38 to 40 weeks post-conceptual age	The examiner places a finger under the infant's toes causing the infant to flex the toes downward to grasp the finger.	9 to 10 months
Parachute	8 to 9 months of age	The examiner holds the infant upright facing away. The examiner then rotates the infant quickly forward as if falling causing the infant to extend the upper extremities toward the ground as if to break a fall.	Persists throughout life

Primitive Reflexes: Full Description in Fig. 1.4 [5, 10]

- Galant reflex or trunk incurvation: disappears by 2 months of age
- Rooting: disappears by 3 months of age
- Moro reflex or startle reflex: disappears by 6 months of age
- Suck reflex: develops at 32 weeks and is fully developed by 36 weeks
- Palmar grasp (hand): disappears by 6 months of age
- Plantar grasp (foot): disappears by 10 months of age
- Asymmetric tonic neck reflex or "fencing" reflex: disappears by 4 months of age
- Parachute response or "break the fall": develops by 9 months of age and is present lifelong

Tone

Smooth flowing movements that are symmetric are reassuring. Jerky random fast movements and gross asymmetries are not.

- Hypertonia: resistance to passive movement, independent of velocity
- Spasticity: velocity-dependent increase in muscle tone to movement

Gait

Most children learn to walk between 12 and 18 months of age, after which point, gait can begin to be reliably assessed. Other developmental gross motor milestones that can be useful in the interim include prone head extension at 3 months, sitting unsupported by 7 months, and pulling to stand by 10 months. Asking the child to walk tiptoe and on their heels and stand on each leg generally denotes normal power or weakness.

Sensory

The sensory examination is a challenge to derive meaning from under most circumstances in young children. Gross withdrawal from cool temperature or noxious stimuli is relevant in the context of altered mental status, obtundation, or coma. In older children, a good sensory exam that includes light touch, pain/temperature, and vibration can provide meaningful data to isolate spinal cord, nerve root, or peripheral nerve pathology. A Romberg sign is a test of proprioception and posterior column function that can prove to be a useful proxy to assess sensory function in an otherwise unreliable patient.

Cutaneous Exam

A skin exam is not typically held to be a part of the neurological exam, but is particularly useful in young children given the neurocutaneous manifestations of relatively common pediatric neurological conditions. A Wood's lamp assesses for hypomelanotic macules, ash leaf spots, in the context of tuberous sclerosis complex. Neurofibromatosis frequently manifests café au lait spots. Sacral dimples, hairy patches, or other cutaneous manifestations of a tethered spinal cord should be part of a standard neurological exam for an infant. If granted permission and when there is a reasonable index of suspicion of a neurocutaneous syndrome, examining parents may be of benefit.

Brain Death Testing [11, 12]

Brain death testing in adults and children are similar. Clinically, the child must demonstrate the absence of brain activity on physical exam prior to proceeding with the apnea test. In addition to no evidence of cortical function, brain death testing should include non-reactive pupils, absent corneal response, no oculocephalic reflex/vestibular ocular reflexes (doll's eyes reflex), and no cough/gag response to deep suctioning. In the setting of clinical evidence of brain death on physical exam, an apnea test is pursued to assess the respiratory response to hypercarbia. The following criteria must be met:

1. Inspired oxygen increased to 100% (can be via nasal cannula or T-piece).
2. Starting ABG with PCO_2 35–45 mmHg and $PaO_2 > 200$ mmHg.
3. Stable blood pressure.
4. Repeat ABG after 8–10 min should show CO_2 of ≥60 mmHg or more than 20 mmHg above baseline.

Conclusion

Overall, children present a complex, diagnostically separate entity from their adult counterparts. Examining children is often best performed at a distance with the most accurate information obtained by observing their spontaneous actions and interactions with their surroundings [8].

Questions and Answers

1. Which of the following signs and symptoms could be suggestive of raised intracranial pressure in a neonate?

   (a) A full anterior fontanelle in a crying infant
   (b) Frequent unexplained bradycardic events
   (c) Loss of upward gaze
   (d) Abnormal posturing to noxious stimulation
   (e) Absent spontaneous venous pulsations in an otherwise well-appearing child

2. Macrocephaly
Select one or more.

   (a) Is defined as an occipital frontal circumference (OFC) greater than three standard deviations above the age-corrected norm.
   (b) Is diagnostic of elevated intracranial pressure.
   (c) Is less concerning in a child whose parent's OFC was elevated for age.
   (d) Is harder to interpret on a single measurement than on serial measurements over time.
   (e) Is synonymous with megalocephaly.

3. Primary craniosynostosis
Choose one or more.

   (a) Can be associated with an asymmetrical ridge along the affected cranial suture line.
   (b) Is likely to be associated with normal head shape and microcephaly.
   (c) May be mimicked by overriding sutures.
   (d) May result from atrophy after hypoxic ischemic encephalopathy.
   (e) Affecting the sagittal suture at a young age is likely to need surgical intervention.

4. Brain tumors in infancy
Choose one or more.

   (a) Usually present with focal or lateralized findings.
   (b) Present more commonly with seizures than in adolescence.
   (c) Are more often supratentorial than infratentorial.
   (d) Are low-grade in around 40% of children.
   (e) Are more promptly diagnosed than brain tumors in older children.
   (f) Usually present with endocrinopathies, visual symptoms, and failure to thrive.

5. When should one consider inflicted or nonaccidental traumatic brain injury?

   (a) If the injuries seem out of proportion to the provided mechanism or circumstances.
   (b) If there are injuries or evidence of trauma to the scalp, skin, long bones, ribs, viscera, and retinal hemorrhages.
   (c) If the child cries excessively or is described as colicky.

(d) If parents are isolated, exhausted, and without support.
(e) If the provided history is variable.

6. A 15-month-old child presents to clinic with his mother who states that he is non-verbal, is unable to sit independently, and has difficulty picking things up with his hands. On examination, you note an open fontanelle, dysconjugate gaze, and a left pupil that does not constrict when light is shined at it. A head CT is obtained that demonstrates bilateral extra-axial fluid collections with septations and fluid layering. The most likely diagnosis is:

   (a) Brain tumor
   (b) Benign extra-axial fluid collections of infancy
   (c) Hydrocephalus
   (d) Nonaccidental trauma

7. A 16-year-old mid-adolescent woman sustained a severe traumatic brain injury during a competitive downhill ski race. She remains intubated post injury day 7 but has well-controlled intracranial pressure since hospital day 4. Imaging shows a minimal stable right tentorial subdural hematoma on CT scan but no other acute intracranial pathology. MRI was consistent with diffuse axonal injury. She has episodic tachycardia, diaphoresis, fever, and extensor limb posturing. She has had continuous video EEG which has not shown ictal correlates with her spells. She is on maximal levetiracetam and fosphenytoin, and she has a fosphenytoin level at trough of 20. She has left interictal epileptiform discharges. Her paroxysmal events are rarely spontaneously evident and typically occur during neurologic examinations and suctioning. She is on appropriate anti-infectives, but no source of fever has been determined by infectious disease subspecialist. The best explanation for her paroxysmal episodes is.

   1. Focal autonomic seizures undetected by scalp EEG.
   2. Mass effect from subdural hemorrhage.
   3. Paroxysmal sympathetic hyperactivity.
   4. Behavioral reactions to pain and anxiety and ICU delirium.
   5. Neuroleptic malignant syndrome.

8. A 14-year-old presents with headache worse while sitting, relieved while supine, and photophobia. He was in a motor vehicle collision 5 days prior during which he was not seat belted and forcibly struck the dashboard sustaining transient loss of consciousness and facial trauma and a broken nose. He perceived the injury as minor. In addition to postural headache, he complained of postnasal drip causing sore throat, a metallic taste in his mouth, inability to smell his favorite foods, and worsening of his seasonal allergic rhinitis. He felt that it was unusual however that his nose was dripping from one nostril only. He was uncomfortable but with a normal examination otherwise with moderate headache. He was very tall and thin and had long spiderlike fingers.

Choose one or more correct answers.

   1. He has metallic taste due to overuse of antihistamines.
   2. Allergies and antihistamines can affect the sense of smell.
   3. His rhinorrhea may be due to facial trauma.
   4. Individuals with Marfan's and other connective tissue diseases are at risk for CSF leaks.
   5. He has low-pressure headache and needs an urgent blood patch.
   6. Leaning forward and collecting fluid from his nose may help diagnose CSF leak versus rhinitis from allergies.
   7. Imaging, ENT evaluation, and neurosurgical consultation are all appropriate.

Answers

1. b, c, d
2. a, c, d
3. a, c, e
4. d, e
5. All of the above
6. d
7. 3
8. 2, 3, 4, 6, 7

References

1. Pappworth M. A primer of medicine. 4th ed. London: Butterworths; 1978.
2. Boes CJ. History of neurologic examination books. Proc (Bayl Univ Med Cent). 2015;28(2):172–9.
3. Organization WH. Child growth standards. https://www.who.int/tools/child-growth-standards/standards. Accessed 12 Aug 2022.
4. Sepanski RJ, Godambe SA, Zaritsky AL. Pediatric vital sign distribution derived from a multi-centered emergency department database. Front Pediatr. 2018;6:66.
5. Fenichel GM. Neurological examination of the newborn. Brain Dev. 1993;15(6):403–10.
6. Volpe J. Volpe's neurology of the newborn. 6th ed. Philadelphia: Elsevier; 2017.
7. Sarnat HB, Sarnat MS. Neonatal encephalopathy following fetal distress. A clinical and electroencephalographic study. Arch Neurol. 1976;33(10):696–705.
8. Aicardi J. Diseases of the nervous system in childhood. 3rd ed. London: Mac Keith Press; 2009.
9. Jain S, Iverson LM. Glasgow Coma Scale. StatPearls Publishing. StatPearls Web site. https://www.ncbi.nlm.nih.gov/books/NBK513298/. Published 2022. Updated 21 June 2022. Accessed 12 Aug 2022.
10. Amiel-Tison C. Neurological evaluation of the maturity of newborn infants. Arch Dis Child. 1968;43(227):89–93.
11. Sims K. Handbook of pediatric neurology. 1st ed. LWW; 2013.
12. Aboubakr M, Yousaf M, Alameda G. Brain death criteria. StatPearls Publishing. https://www.ncbi.nlm.nih.gov/books/NBK545144/. Published 2021. Updated 27 Dec 2021. Accessed 12 Aug 2022.

Additional Suggested Readings and Resources

Cioni G, Mercuri E. Neurological assessment in the first two years of life. 1st ed. Mac Keith Press; 2008.

Forsyth R, Newton R. Pediatric neurology. 1st ed. Oxford University Press; 2007.

Maria B. Current management in child neurology. 4th ed. PMPH USA; 2008.

Larson P, Steensaas S. PediNeurologic exam: a neurodevelopmental approach. https://neurologicexam.med.utah.edu/pediatric/html/home_exam.html. Updated May 2020. Accessed 12 Aug 2022.

Ricci D, Romeo DM, Haataja L, et al. Neurological examination of preterm infants at term equivalent age. Early Hum Dev. 2008;84(11):751–61.

2 The Changes of the Nervous System from Fetal Stages to Early Adulthood, as Seen in Different Imaging Modalities

Avner Meoded and Thierry A. G. M. Huisman

Introduction

The embryology of the fetal brain is a complex, eloquent process that begins in the embryonic period, conception through the eighth week of gestation. During gestation, the brain shows a sequential development of transient laminar compartments, from the center to the periphery: the proliferative zone (ventricular and subventricular zone), the intermediate zone (future white matter [WM]), the subplate zone, the cortical plate (future gray mater [GM]), and the marginal zone. Neural proliferation and migration are predominant during the first trimester of pregnancy, while axon and dendrite growth and proliferation occur mainly during the second and third trimester of gestation. Subsequently, prolonged maturation phenomena are observed, with synaptogenesis and pruning mechanisms, myelination, and neurochemical maturation being the most influential [1].

At the macroscopic level, brain growth is intense in the last trimester of pregnancy and the first two postnatal years, with a significant increase in GM and WM volumes.

This goes with an increasing complexity of the brain morphology and the formation of gyri, primary, secondary, and tertiary sulci from 20, 32, and 40 weeks of gestational age (GA), respectively [1].

Prenatal and postnatal ultrasound and MRI are the modalities of choice for evaluating the developing brain and spine. CT plays an important role in evaluation of developmental skull base and craniocervical junction abnormalities. Advanced MR imaging techniques including diffusion tensor imaging hold a great value in understanding the more detailed normal and abnormal developing brain [1, 2].

In this chapter we will describe the developmental and maturational changes of the central nervous system (CNS) from fetal stages to early adulthood, as seen by different imaging modalities, and discuss and present the normal gyration, sulcation, and myelination of the fetal and pediatric brain through different neuroimaging modalities.

Diagnostic Imaging Modalities for the Study of the Developing and Maturing Brain

Modern neuroimaging modalities such as ultrasound (US), CT, and MRI have significantly advanced our understanding of pediatric CNS development. Here we briefly discuss the technical aspects of each of these modalities.

A. Meoded (✉) · T. A. G. M. Huisman
Edward B. Singleton Department of Radiology, Texas Children's Hospital, Houston, TX, USA
e-mail: axmeoded@texaschildrens.org; huisman@texaschildrens.org

N. Shimony, G. Jallo (eds.), *Pediatric Neurosurgery Board Review*,
https://doi.org/10.1007/978-3-031-23687-7_2

Brain Ultrasound

Ultrasound is nearly always the first study of choice in fetus and neonates, as it is noninvasive, inexpensive, and portable (can be performed at the bedside) [3]. There is no risk of radiation and sedation is not required.

Measurements of brain structures with ultrasound and MRI are nearly identical [4]. Ultrasonography of the neonatal brain should always be performed using multiple transducers, taking advantage of variable frequencies. When the brain is analyzed via the anterior and posterior fontanelles and the temporal, mastoid, and occipital synchondroses, all regions of the brain (central and peripheral) can be seen appropriately. Optimal depiction of brain morphology is possible if images are acquired in the sagittal, parasagittal, coronal, and axial planes. Both static and real-time images should be evaluated.

Finally, major arteries and veins should be assessed by Doppler techniques, looking for peak systolic velocities, end diastolic velocities, and subsequent calculation of resistive indices of the various branches of the circle of Willis.

Brain CT

CT still plays an important role in evaluation of developmental skull base and craniocervical junction abnormalities and pediatric CNS trauma.

Radiation dose is always a consideration in pediatric radiology, as younger patients have a greater chance of long-term radiation-associated sequelae [5–7].

The increasing utilization of CT over the past decade among the entire US population, including pediatric patients, and the variability in scan parameters for CT [8] have resulted in an increased focus on the need to consider alternative modalities first. When CT is deemed indicated/necessary, the radiologist must take advantage of any available dose reduction technique [9]. The indications for the study and scan parameters should be weighed together. CT studies should always be performed with the lowest possible dose that allows for a diagnostic quality scan.

Because the newborn brain has a very high-water content, proper window/leveling of the CT scan is essential for optimal analysis of brain abnormalities.

Anatomical Brain MRI

Qualitative and quantitative MR has significantly advanced our understanding of brain changes during development. MRI plays an important role in the delineation and characterization of the CNS anatomy, especially during the early years, particularly the period from birth to 2 years of age, which represent the most dynamic and important phase of postnatal brain development in humans [10].

Essential planes/sequences include a sagittal, T1-weighted sequence which should be performed on all patients to assess important midline structures such as the corpus callosum, pituitary gland, hypothalamus, and cerebellar vermis. Secondly, axial T2-weighted images should be acquired in all patients. Depending on the indication and suspected findings, various additional anatomical imaging planes and imaging sequences must be considered including susceptibility-weighted imaging (SWI).

Fetal MRI

Fetal ultrafast MRI is the study of choice when prenatal sonography demonstrates abnormal findings [11, 12].

Standard protocol includes a series of ultrafast T2-weighted ssFSE or HASTE images, echo-planar gradient-echo, T1-weighted images. The ultrafast T2-weighted images are acquired in less than 1 s, reducing the likelihood of fetal motion during image acquisition. With increasing gestational age and engagement of the fetal head in the pelvis, the amount of motion is decreased, and the quality of the studies improves.

Advanced Brain MR

Diffusion-weighted imaging (DWI) and diffusion tensor imaging (DTI) are unique imaging techniques that provides highly specific and sensitive qualitative and quantitative information of the white matter (WM) ultrastructure [13]. It is a noninvasive and non-contrast-enhanced method. By sampling the three-dimensional shape, direction, and magnitude of the water diffusion/mobility within the brain, DWI/DTI generates unique tissue contrasts that can be used to study the WM organization of the CNS. Its application allows to study the normal and abnormal brain development including connectivity, for various pediatric CNS disorders, such as congenital malformations, stroke, tumors, infections, trauma, and neurometabolic/neurodegenerative diseases [14, 15].

Imaging of the Brain During Development

Neuroimaging allows assessment of many aspects of brain maturation, including anatomical, physiological, and functional changes during development.

Sulcation and gyration patterns can be evaluated with all modalities. In addition, MRI provides sensitive assessment of the maturation of gray and white matter myelination.

Imaging of the Fetus and Preterm Brain

The imaging modality being used determines which features of brain development can be evaluated. Through the anterior fontanelle, ultrasound shows morphological/maturational changes of the gyri and sulci nearly as well as MRI. MRI adds excellent assessment of the white matter myelination, sulcation, and chemical maturation. As CT requires the use of ionizing radiation and does not provide any information that cannot be obtained by ultrasound and MR, it is rarely recommended for non-urgent fetal or neonatal brain imaging.

Ultrasound

Complete evaluation of the fetal CNS requires scanning in axial, coronal, and sagittal planes (Figs. 2.1, 2.2, 2.3, 2.4, 2.5, 2.6, 2.7, 2.8, and 2.9). These planes should be ideally performed transvaginally since this approach typically provides the better image resolution [16, 17].

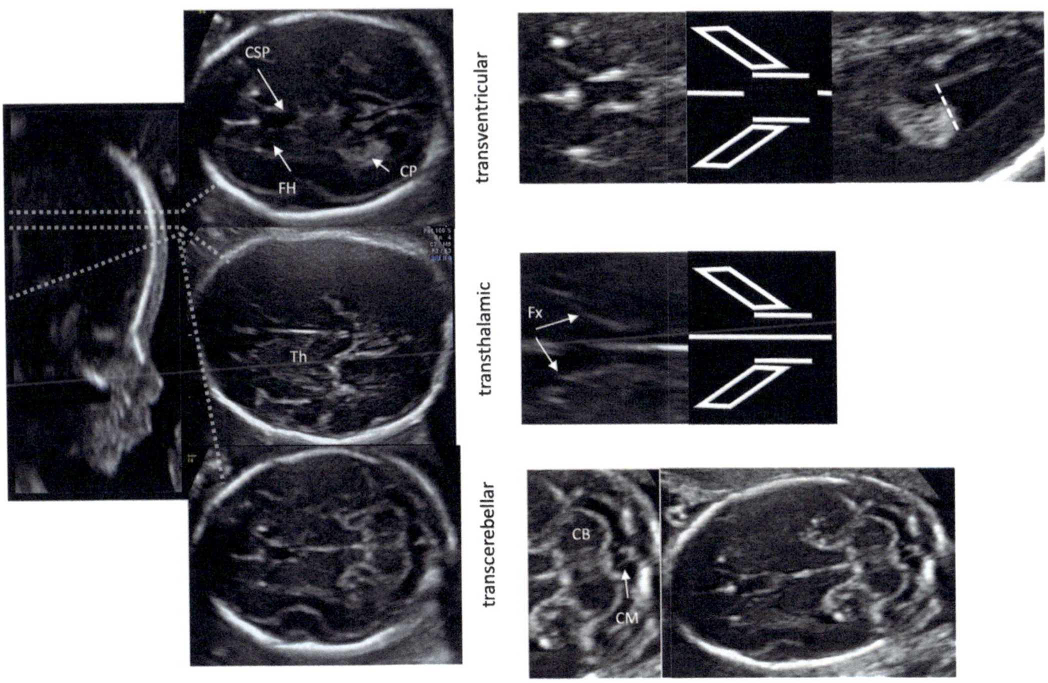

Fig. 2.1 Late second/third trimester images. Axial planes obtained by transabdominal ultrasound are essential for examination of CNS included in screening. Important structures are shown on the transventricular, transthalamic, and transcerebellar planes

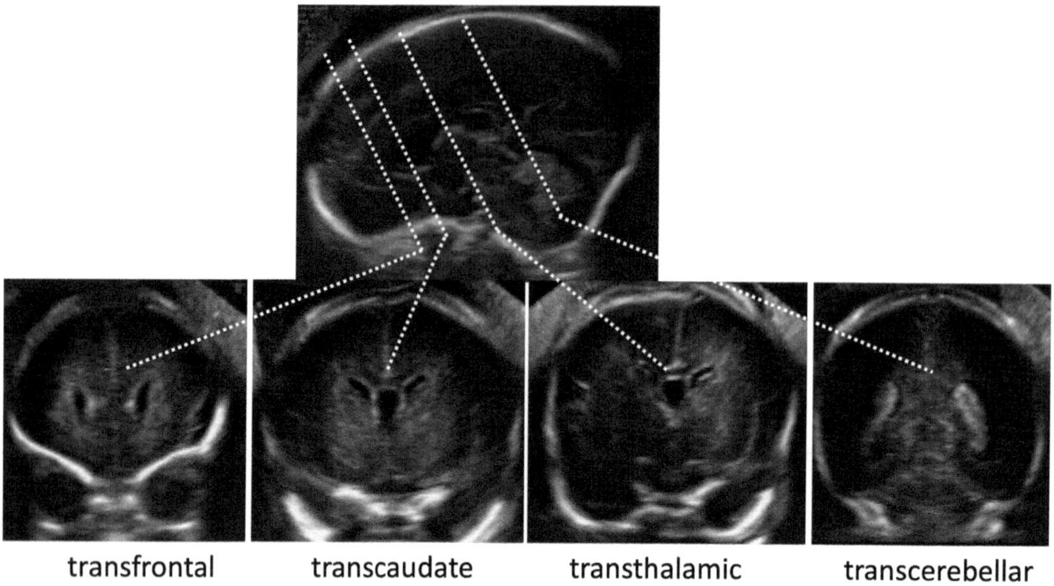

Fig. 2.2 Four planes can be seen: transfrontal, transcaudate, transthalamic, and transcerebellar that allow to evaluate specific structures

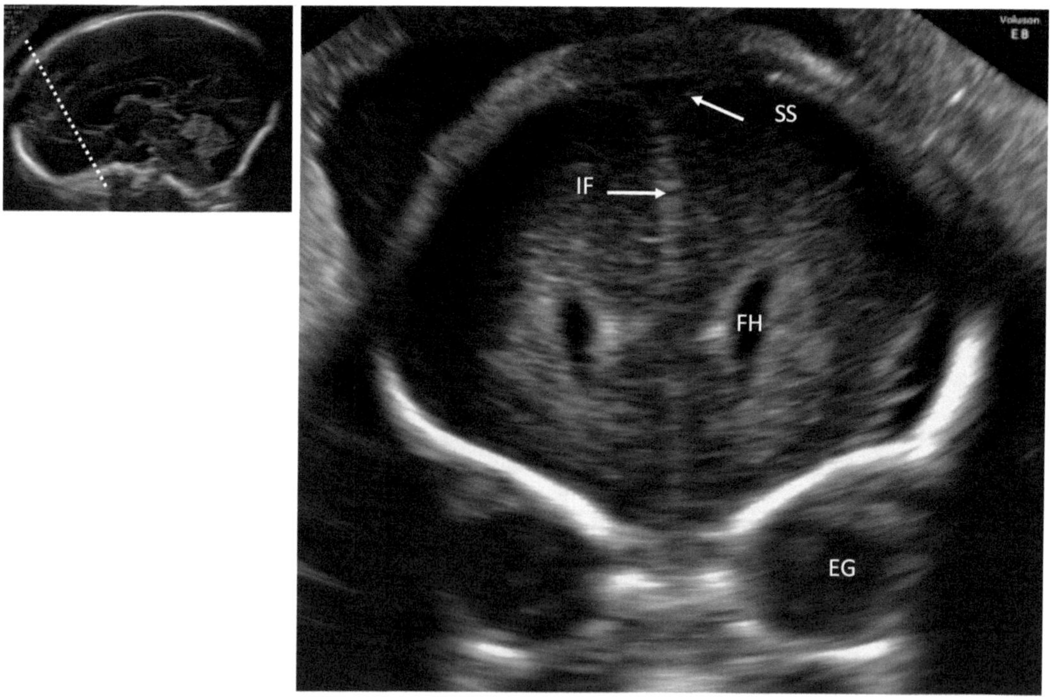

Fig. 2.3 Here, we can identify midline interhemispheric fissure, the anterior horns of the lateral ventricles, and the orbits. The plane is rostral to the genu of the corpus callosum, and this explains the presence of an uninterrupted interhemispheric fissure

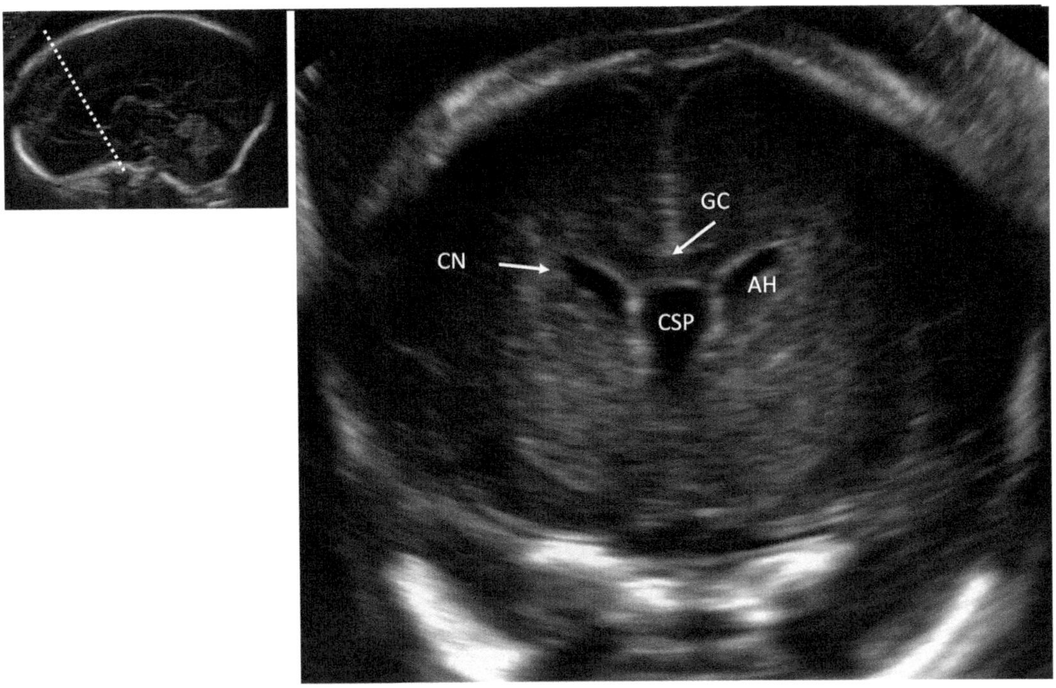

Fig. 2.4 In this plane we can identify the genu or anterior portion of the corpus callosum that interrupts the continuity of the interhemispheric fissure. We also identify the cavum septum pellucidum inferior to the corpus callosum, the anterior horns of the lateral ventricles, and the caudate nuclei

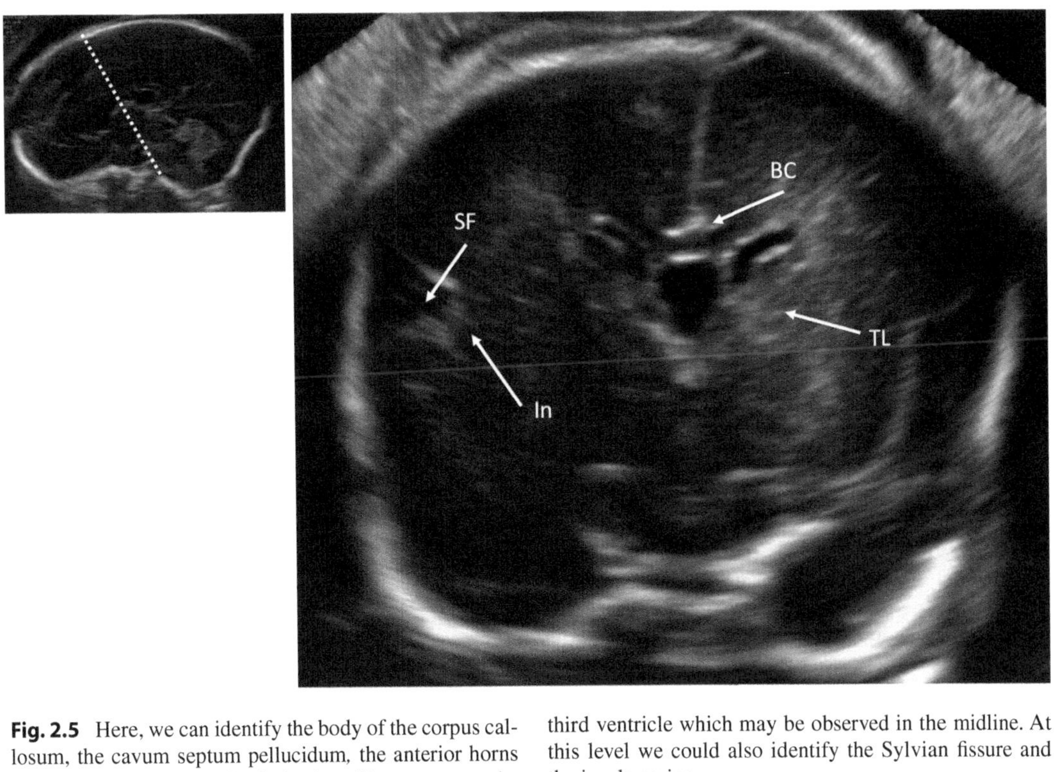

Fig. 2.5 Here, we can identify the body of the corpus callosum, the cavum septum pellucidum, the anterior horns of the lateral ventricles, the thalami, and in some cases the third ventricle which may be observed in the midline. At this level we could also identify the Sylvian fissure and the insula region

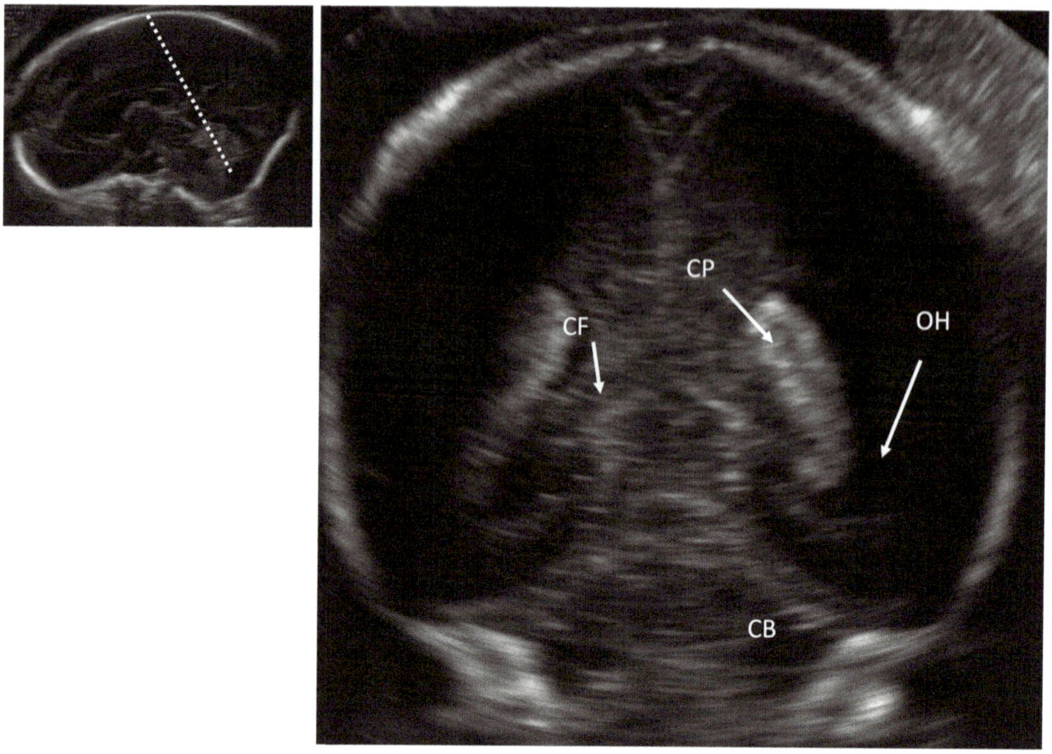

Fig. 2.6 We can identify the occipital horns of the lateral ventricles, cerebellar hemispheres, vermis, and tentorium

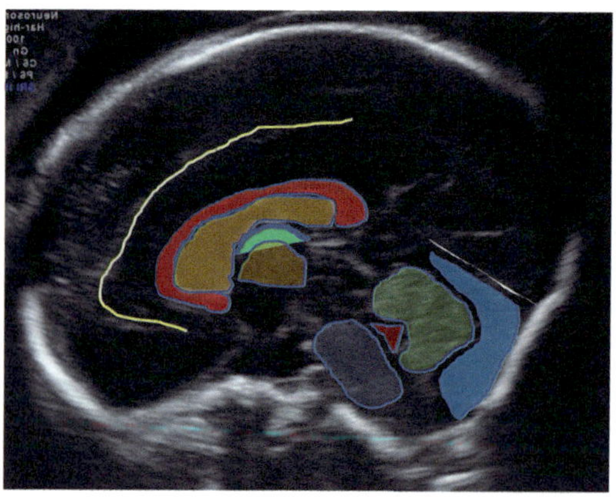

Fig. 2.7 The midsagittal plane is very useful to assess midline structures including. The corpus callosum: red. Cingulate fissure that runs parallel to CC: yellow. Cavum of septum pellucidum and cavum vergae that appear as an anechogenic structures below the CC: orange. The fornix that appears as a hyperechogenic structure below the cavum septum pellucidum: green. The third ventricle, located below the fornix: gold. The fourth ventricle, with his characteristic triangle or beak shape: dark red. The pons, located in front of the cerebellum: gray. The vermis that appears as hyperechogenic structure: light green. The cisterna magna, the anechogenic space behind vermis: blue. The tentorium which is the membrane that constitutes the upper limit of posterior fossa: white

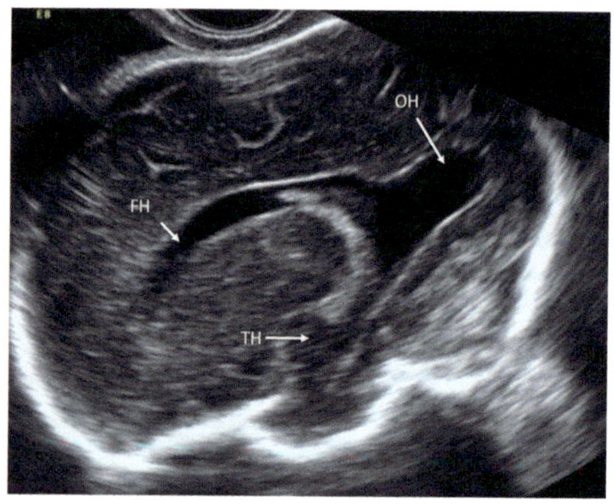

Fig. 2.8 The parasagittal plane is very useful to assess morphology and content of the lateral ventricles identifying frontal, temporal, and occipital horn together and also periventricular areas

The following measurements represent an integral part of sonographic screening for CNS malformations: atrial width and transverse cerebellar diameter.

Axial planes obtained by transabdominal ultrasound are the basis for routine examination of CNS included screening. In these planes we should pay special attention to specific brain areas in order to rule out some of the most important CNS abnormalities.

In the transventricular plane (Figs. 2.1, 2.2, 2.3, 2.4, 2.5, 2.6, 2.7, and 2.8), we should carefully examine two structures: first, the cavum of septum pellucidum that appears as a fluid-filled cavity between two thin parallel lines located in the midline between the anterior horns. These appear as two comma-shaped fluid-filled structures in a divergent direction. Identification of normal CSP allows us to discard some severe abnormalities such as agenesis of the corpus callosum or septo-optic dysplasia. The second region is the posterior horns of the lateral ventricles at the level of the atrium. At this level we should measure the atrium at the level of the glomus of the choroid plexus, since the presence of an enlarged lateral ventricle is the most sensitive sign of abnormal development of CNS.

In the transthalamic plane (Figs. 2.1, 2.2, 2.3, 2.4, 2.5, 2.6, 2.7, and 2.8), one will identify the columns of the fornix that appear as three thin parallel lines. It is very important to differentiate this structure from CSP, because in some cases the columns of the fornix can be mistaken as the CSP leading to confusions, especially with ACC.

In the transcerebellar plane (Figs. 2.1, 2.2, 2.3, 2.4, 2.5, 2.6, 2.7, and 2.8), one will explore the structures contained in the posterior fossa: cerebellum, vermis, and cisterna magna including its measurements.

MRI

The fetal sulci appear in an orderly sequence: the phylogenetically older sulci appear first, and the more recently acquired sulci appear later [2, 18]. The principal sulci and gyri form the characteristic pattern of the human cortex that can be identified in the full-term infant (Table 2.1) (Figs. 2.9 and 2.10). The Sylvian fissure, the earliest fetal sulcus, is usually present when the fetus is imaged in the fourth gestational month. The next sulci to appear are the calcarine, parieto-occipital, and cingulate sulci during the fifth month (by 20–22 weeks); the rolandic (central), interparietal, and superior temporal sulci that appear toward the end of the sixth month (by 25 weeks); and the precentral, postcentral, superior frontal, and middle temporal sulci that appear during the seventh gestational month (24–28 weeks) [19] (Figs. 2.9 and 2.10).

Table 2.1 Chronology of sulcation as seen on MR imaging

	Gestational age (week)
Interhemispheric fissure	22–23
Callosal sulcus	22–23
Parieto-occipital fissure	22–23
Hippocampal fissure	22–23
Cingular sulcus	24–25
Calcarine fissure	24–25
Marginal sulcus	27
Central sulcus	27
Precentral sulcus	27
Superior temporal sulcus (posterior part)	27
Intraparietal sulcus	28
Postcentral sulcus	28
Superior frontal sulcus	29
Inferior frontal sulcus	29
Superior temporal sulcus (anterior part)	32
Inferior temporal sulcus	33
Occipitotemporal sulcus	33
Insular sulci	34
Secondary occipital sulci	34

Sulcation, myelination, and corpus callosum development tend to be delayed in prematurely born neonates compared to fetuses of the same postconceptual age.

Practical standard for normal development of gyri and sulci in preterm and term neonates has been previously published. The gyral maturity is determined by measurements of the width of the gyri and depth and arborization of the sulci. The stage of gyral development is then assigned based upon the degree of gyral maturity in seven different regions of the brain [20].

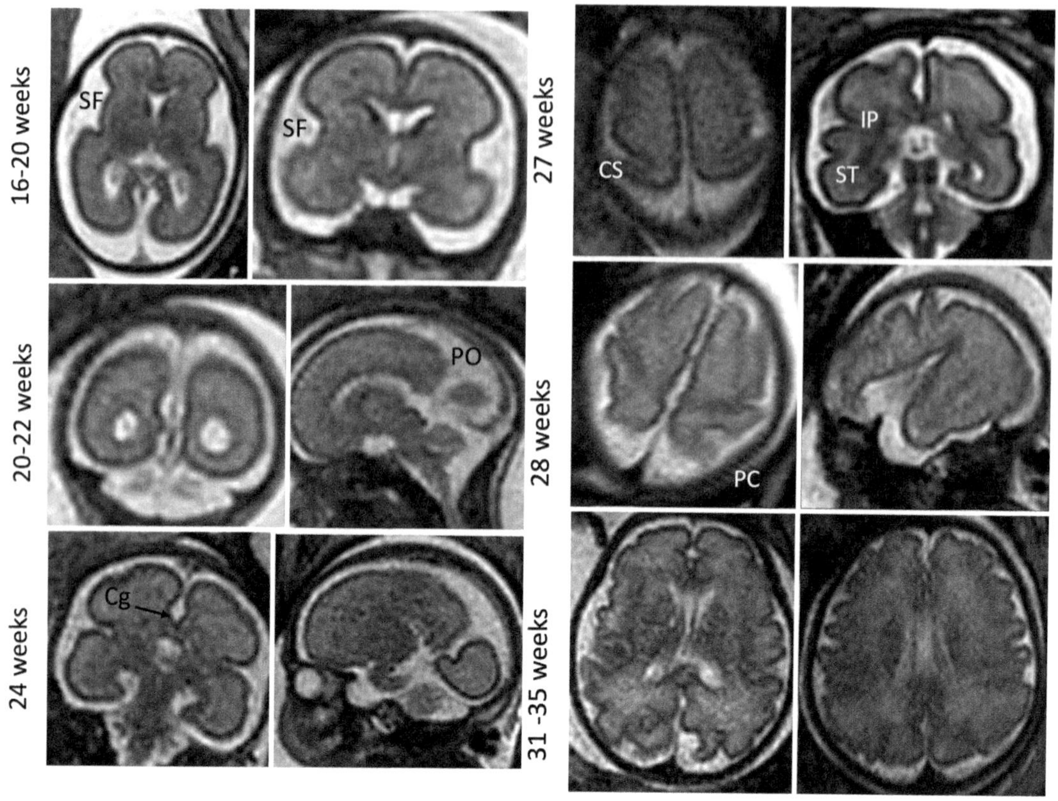

Figs. 2.9 and 2.10 Depiction of major sulci development of the brain for each gestational week from 16 to 35 weeks of gestation. *SF* Sylvian fissure, *PO* parieto-occipital sulcus, *Cg* cingulate sulcus, *CS* central sulcus, *IP* intraparietal sulcus, *ST* superior temporal sulcus, *PC* postcentral sulcus. Beyond 30 weeks, secondary and tertiary sulcus can be depicted

Finally, it appears that sulcal development may appear earlier in utero than ex utero when comparing pre- and postnatal imaging [21–24].

Prior to 24 weeks of gestation, the brain is essentially agyric with the exception of the wide, vertically oriented Sylvian fissures (Figs. 2.9 and 2.10). Between the germinal zones and the cortex, MRI also shows a layer of intermediate signal intensity, separated from the more peripheral cerebral cortex and more central germinal matrix which has been identified as the intermediate zone or the developing fetal white matter [25].

Immediately peripheral to the intermediate zone and deep to the cerebral cortex is a region of relative T1 hypointensity/T2 hyperintensity, which is likely to be the subplate, the region where thalamocortical afferent axons accumulate and "wait" before entering the cortical plate to establish definitive synapses [25–27]. The lateral ventricles and the cisterns around the brainstem and cerebellum are visible and more prominent at this age than in the mature infant.

Between 24 and 30 weeks, the cerebral cortex shows the development of shallow rolandic (central), calcarine, pericallosal/callosomarginal, interparietal, and superior temporal sulci (Figs. 2.9 and 2.10). Myelination is seen in some brainstem structures during this period, including the median longitudinal fasciculus (MLF), the lateral lemnisci, the medial lemnisci, and the superior and inferior cerebellar peduncles [28]. The basal ganglia and thalami are better seen at this age on MRI and have intensity similar to the cerebral cortex on both T1W and T2W imaging (Figs. 2.9 and 2.10). The ventrolateral nucleus of the thalamus becomes T2 hypointense compared to the remainder of the thalamus by about 25 weeks and is T1 hyperintense by 27–28 weeks, likely due to hypercellularity and possibly to early myelination. The lateral ventricles, particularly the trigones and occipital horns, are less prominent at this age than at 22–23 weeks, probably secondary to both growth of the cerebral white matter and development of the calcarine sulci.

By the 32th week, an increased number of gyri and shallow sulci become visible in the cerebral cortex of prematurely born neonates (Figs. 2.9 and 2.10). The Sylvian fissures retain their immature appearance, although some development of the opercula can be detected. The cavum septum pellucidum and cavum vergae are prominent and will remain so throughout the first 40 postconceptual weeks.

Between 34 and 36 weeks, the cerebral cortex has further thickened, and more sulci have developed. Little change occurs in the signal intensity of the white matter between 32 and 36 postconceptional weeks [29]. On T1-weighted MR, the posterior limb of the internal capsule remains hypointense as compared to the lentiform nucleus. On T2-weighted images, the posterior limb of the internal capsule remains entirely hyperintense compared with surrounding structures.

By 38–40 weeks, the brain approaches a normal adult sulcal pattern.

Normal Postnatal Brain Development

Development of the postnatal brain on MRI consists primarily of changes in signal intensity secondary to the process of myelination and progressing white matter packing. Myelination of the brain begins during the fifth fetal month with the myelination of the cranial nerves and continues throughout the first two decades of life. In general, the myelination progresses from caudal to rostral, from dorsal to ventral, and from central to peripheral. The brainstem, therefore, myelinates prior to the cerebellum and basal ganglia, and the cerebellum and basal ganglia myelinate prior to the cerebral hemispheres. Another generalization is that, within any particular portion of the brain, the posterior region tends to myelinate first.

Neonatal MRI Brain Development

In general, changes in white matter maturation are best seen on T1-weighted images during the first 6–8 months of life and on the long echo time T2-weighted images between the ages of 6 and 18 months. Progression of myelination of both the brainstem and cerebellum seems to be more sensitively assessed on T2-weighted images [30–32]. Myelination milestones can be evaluated by the changes in the T1 and T2 relaxation times of the brain tissue (Table 2.2).

Although visually apparent signal changes of the white matter seem to be complete by about the age of 2 years, measurements of relaxation rates have shown that T1 shortening of white matter and gray matter continues into adolescence, probably secondary to continued myelination and consequent diminution of brain water [33].

Table 2.2 Myelination milestones evaluated by the changes in the T1 and T2 relaxation times of the brain tissue

Age (months)	T1 (signal)	T2 (signal)
Newborn	Medulla ↑ Dorsal pons↑ MCP↑ ICP and SCP ↑ midbrain↑ VL thalamus↑ PLIC↑ Perirolandic ↑ Optic nerves, tracts, and radiations↑	Medulla ↓ dorsal pons ↓ midbrain ↓ Perirolandic ↓ ICP and SCP ↓ VL thalamus ↓
2	Deep cerebellar WM↑ ALIC↑	MCP ↓ PLIC ↓ Perirolandic↓ Optic tracts↓
4	Entire cerebellum↑ CC (splenium) ↑	Optic radiations↓ Calcarine fissure ↓
6	CC (entire) ↑	CC (splenium) ↓ Ventral pons ↓
8	Subcortical U-fiber occipital ↑	ALIC ↓ CC (entire) ↓
12	Subcortical U-fibers frontal and temporal↑ Brain achieves adult appearance on T1	Deep WM cerebellum↓ Early occipital subcortical U-fibers ↓ Temporal central WM↓
18	No significant change	Subcortical U-fiber occipital poles↓ Entire posterior fossa↓
24	No significant change	Subcortical U-fiber frontal and temporal poles↓

ALIC anterior limb of internal capsule, *CC* corpus callosum, *MCP* middle cerebellar peduncle, *ICP* inferior cerebellar peduncle, *SCP* superior cerebellar peduncle, *VL* ventrolateral, *WM* white matter

Myelination Milestones as Depicted by MRI

The ages at which the changes of myelination appear on T1- and T2-weighted MR images, as well as normal MRI milestones for myelination of the brain, have previously been described [34, 35] (Table 2.1). During the first 6 months of life, T1-weighted images are most useful for assessing normal brain maturation. The splenium of the corpus callosum should be of moderately high signal intensity by the fourth month, and the genu of the corpus callosum should be of high signal intensity by age 6 months (Figs. 2.11, 2.12, 2.13, 2.14, 2.15, 2.16, and 2.17). By approximately 8 months of age, advanced myelination can be seen with the exception that some of the most subcortical white matter fibers (association fibers in the anterior frontal and anterior temporal lobes) have not yet acquired high signal intensity. After age 6 months, T2-weighted images are more useful in the assessment of normal brain maturation. On T2-weighted images, the splenium of the corpus callosum should be of low signal intensity by 6 months of age, the genu of the corpus callosum by 8 months of age, and the anterior limb of the internal capsule by 11 months of age. The deep frontal white matter should be of low signal intensity by age 14 months. With the exception of the subcortical white matter, the entire brain should have an adult appearance by 18 months, and the subcortical white matter should be mature by about 30 months.

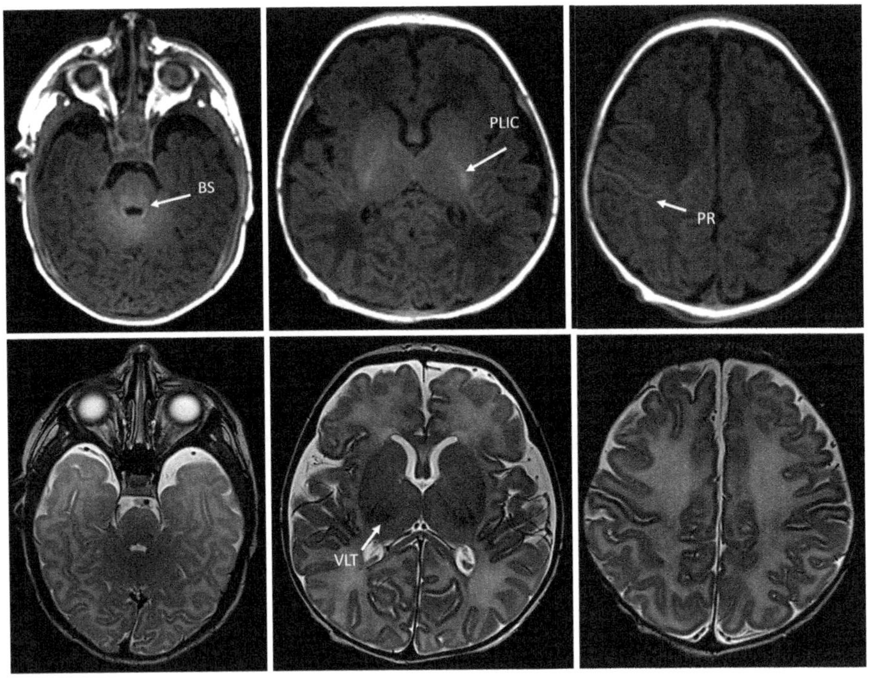

Fig. 2.11 Myelination pattern can be valuated using T1W and T2W imaging. T1W hyperintensity develops first before T2W hypointensity appears. The myelination process continues by 3–4 years of life. In general, normal myelination progresses from inferior to superior, from posterior to anterior, and from central to peripheral. Figure newborn: Similar signal on both T1 and T2 wi. Dorsal brainstem VL thalamus, dorsal posterior limb internal capsule, corticospinal tract, and perirolandic cortices

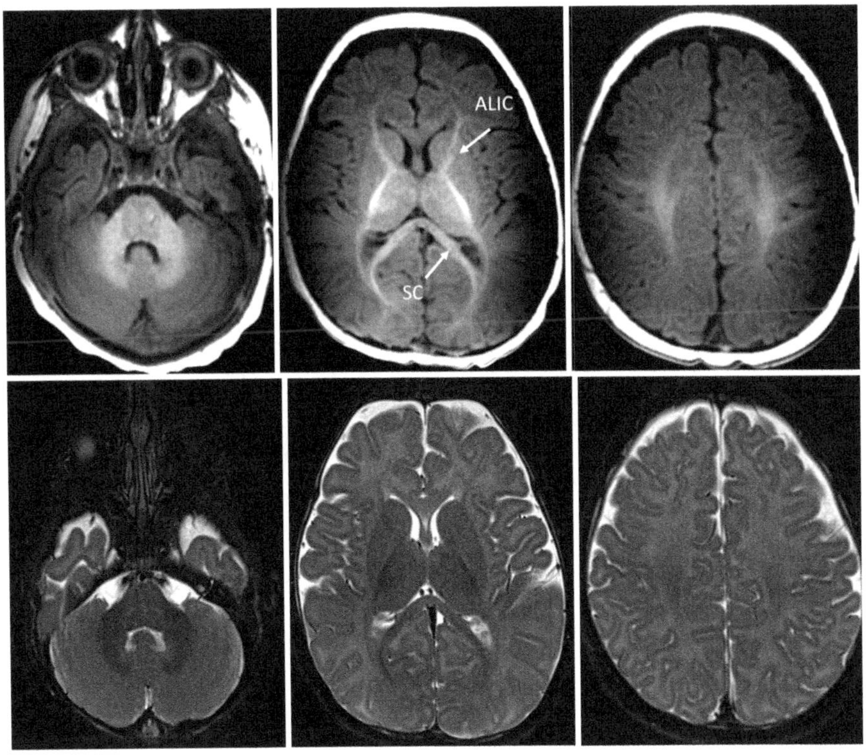

Fig. 2.12 (4 months) Anterior limb internal capsule and splenium of corpus callosum myelinate

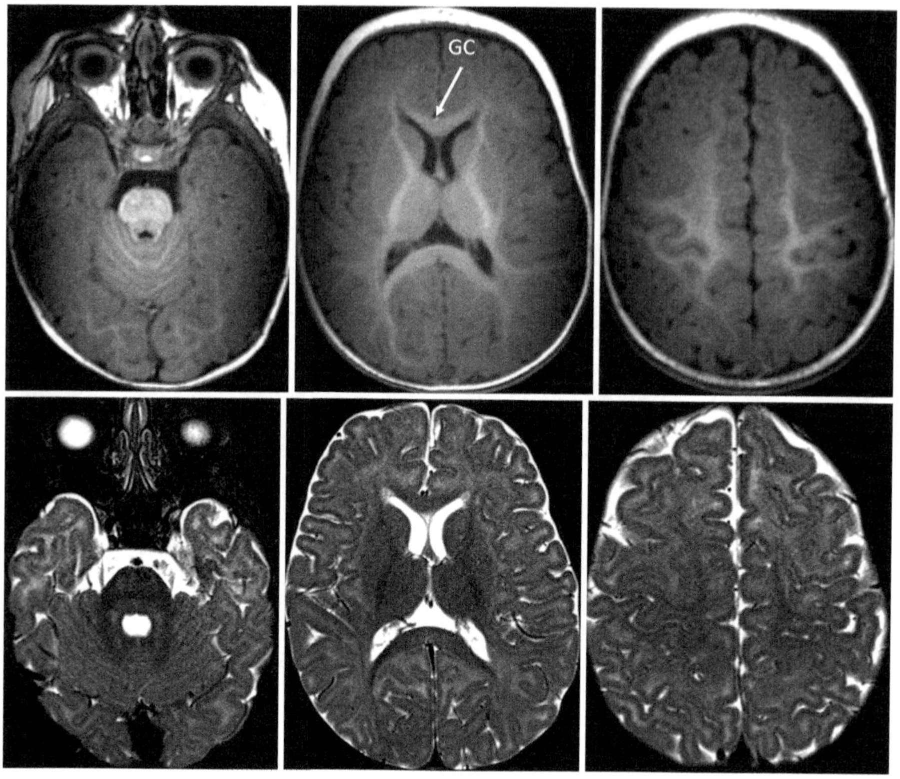

Fig. 2.13 (6 months) T1, genu of corpus callosum myelinates. T2, splenium of corpus callosum myelinates

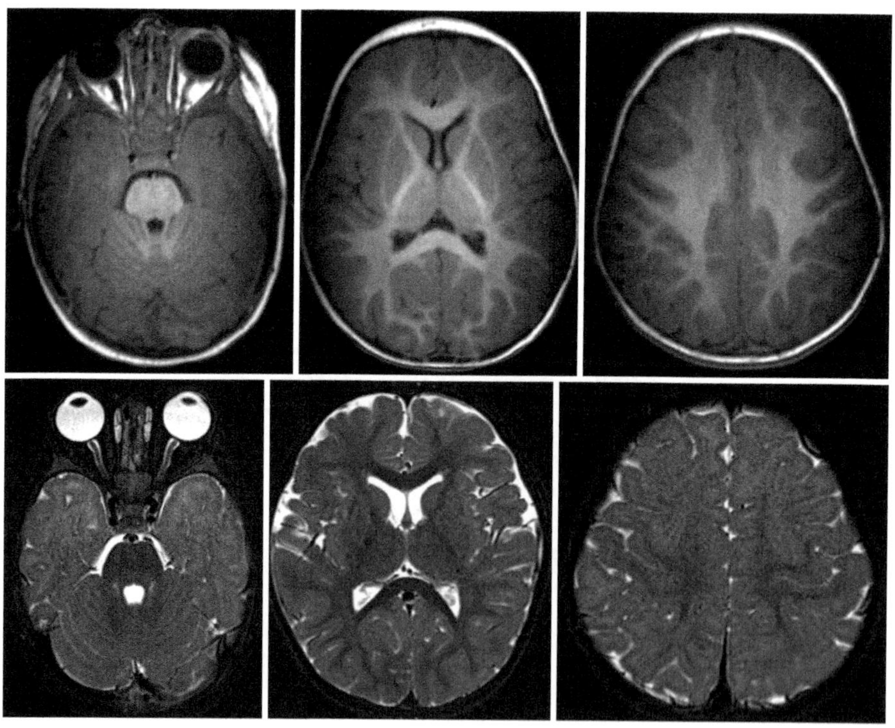

Fig. 2.14 (9 months) T1, additional white matter myelination except for the major association cortico-cortical fibers. T2, genu of the corpus callosum and anterior limb internal capsule myelinate

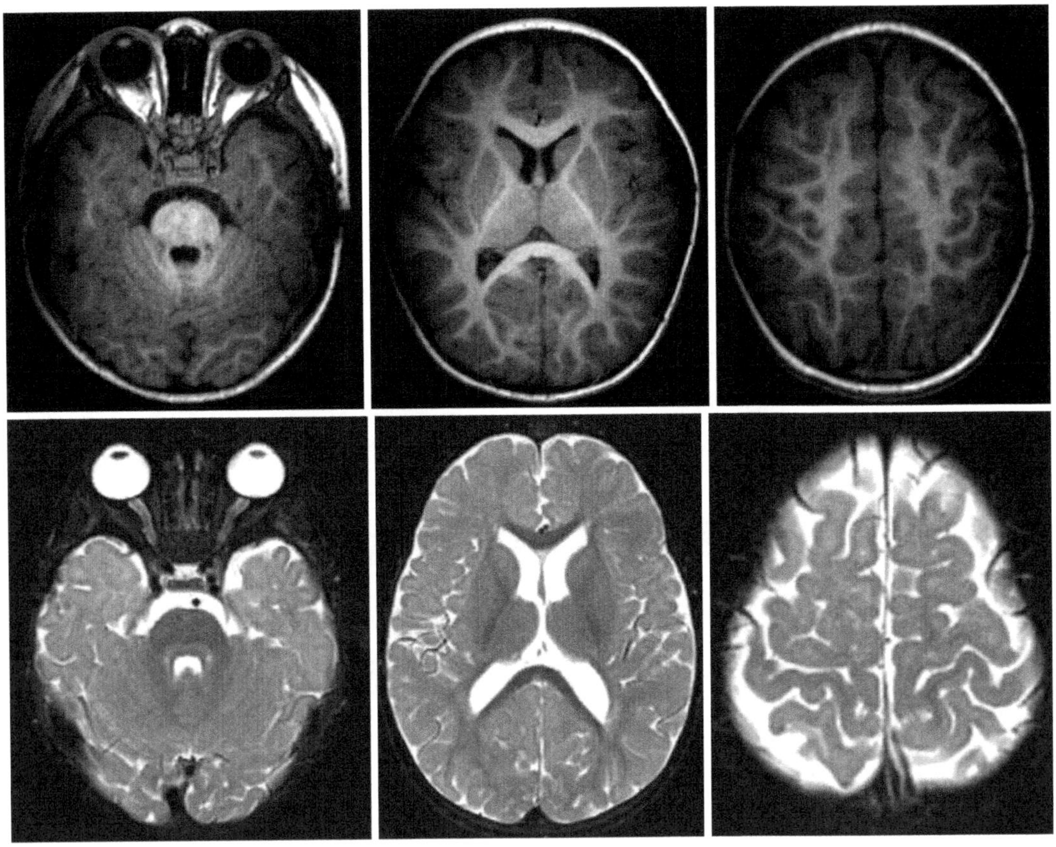

Fig. 2.15 (12 months) T1, complete myelination. T2, occipital subcortical white matter myelinates

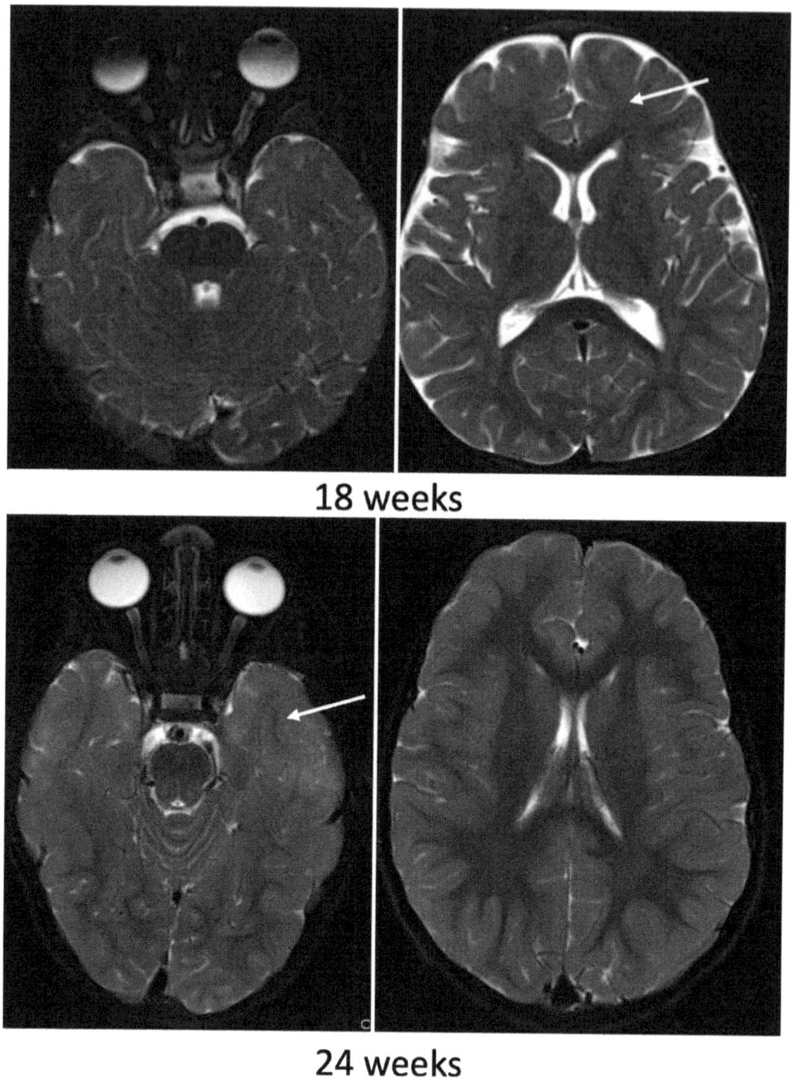

Fig. 2.16 (18 months) Frontal subcortical white matter myelinates. (24 months) T1, complete myelination. T2, complete except for terminal zones in the periatrial white matter and anterior temporal subcortical white matter

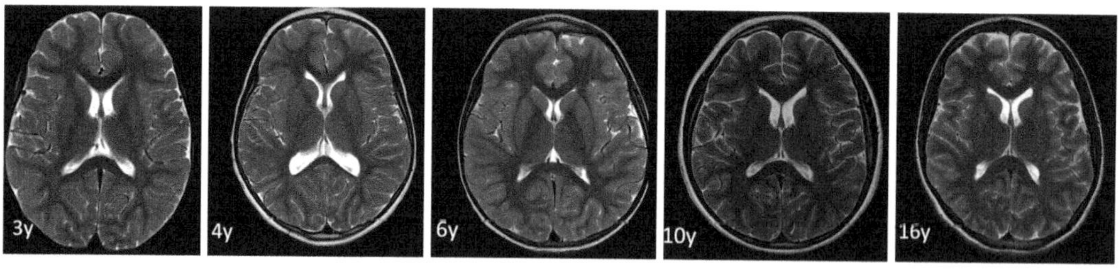

Fig. 2.17 (3–16 years) Myelination is complete with better depiction of cortico-cortical association fibers in older children

Diffusion Tensor Imaging and Tractography

Diffusion tensor imaging (DTI) allows to study the three-dimensional shape and direction of water diffusion/mobility by adding diffusion gradients along multiple orthogonal directions in space. When the complete tensor of the diffusion is measured, the degree of anisotropic diffusion can be calculated (fractional anisotropy, FA) [13, 36]. The degree of anisotropic diffusion can also be represented by two-dimensional FA map (Fig. 2.18).

FA values vary between 0 (maximal isotropic diffusion) and 1 (maximal anisotropic diffusion). High FA values are typically found along fiber tracts (e.g., corticospinal tracts [CSTs], corpus callosum). Measurement of the entire diffusion tensor also provides information about the principal direction of water diffusion/mobility within the brain. Consequently, the FA maps can be color coded. By convention, regions with a predominant left to right diffusion are color coded in red, and regions with a superior-inferior diffusion direction are color coded in blue, whereas anterior-posterior diffusion is color coded in green. The intensity of the color coding relates to the magnitude of anisotropic diffusion, respectively, the FA value which is predominantly determined by progressing white matter tract

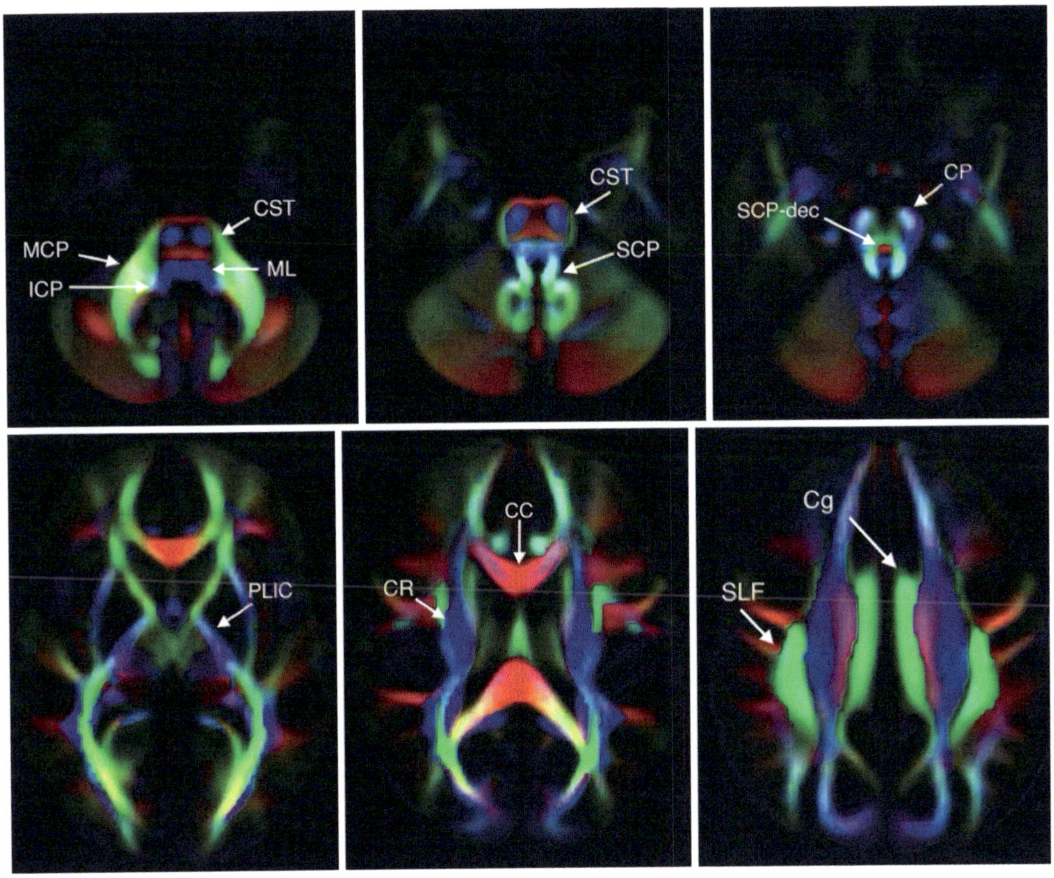

Fig. 2.18 Axial DEC maps showing normal tracts of a 4-year-old boy. *CC* corpus callosum, *Cg* cingulate, *CR* corona radiata, *CST* corticospinal tract, *MCP* middle cerebellar peduncle, *ML* medial lemniscus, *PLIC* posterior limb of internal capsule, *SCP-dec* superior cerebellar peduncle decussation, *SCP* superior cerebellar peduncle, *SLF* superior longitudinal fasciculus

myelination and packing (Fig. 2.18). Finally, with advanced algorithms, one can reconstruct the course of fiber tracts within the brain in three dimensions (fiber tractography, FT). The resulting FT allows to study the internal neuroarchitecture of the normal and pathologic brain noninvasively and may provide insights in the development of the various connections (white matter tracts) between functional systems [36, 37]. Fiber tracking and DTI add important information for the study of normal and anomalous white matter tracts, both in development and in aging. DTI has been previously used to measure maturational changes separately in the pyramidal tract, somatosensory radiations, and visual pathways of premature newborns [38, 39].

FA increases with age as indicated by increasing intensity on gray scale maps and changing color on DEC maps in different regions especially in "cross roads" areas. The thickness of corpus callosum and corticospinal tracts is seen to gradually progress with age. In addition, more branching cortico-cortical association fibers are noted in older children (Fig. 2.19).

A fiber tractography study of the corpus callosum in 315 normal volunteers of ages 5–59 years showed that peak FA values were reached in the third decade of life, whereas the minimum isotropic diffusivity values were reached somewhat later, often during the fourth decade of life [40]. Importantly, the corticospinal tract showed evidence of particularly early and rapid maturation, whereas the dorsal and ventral cingulum bundles showed more protracted development compared to the other tracts examined which matches functionally observed clinical development.

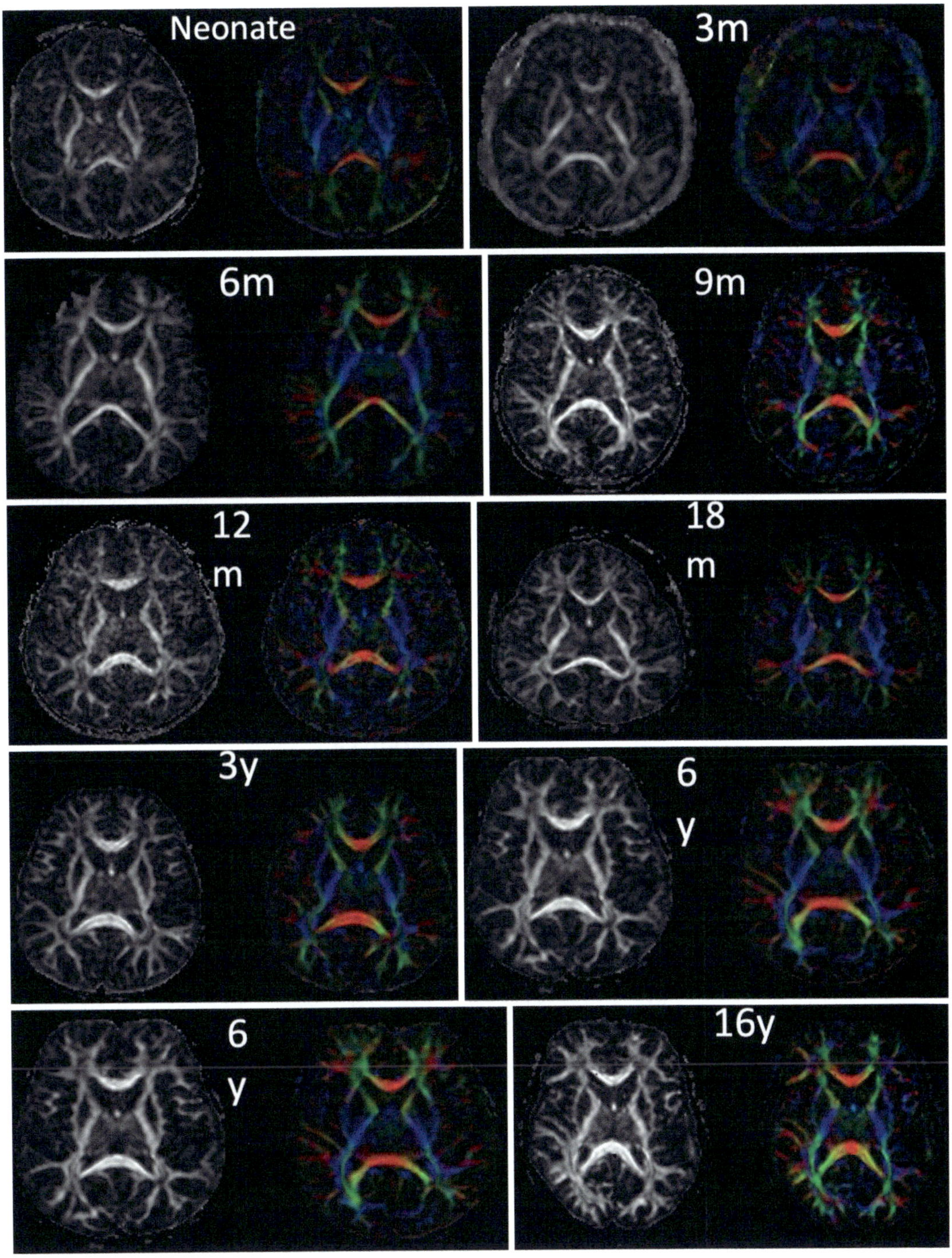

Fig. 2.19 Axial DEC and FA maps during normal development. Directionally encoded fractional green indicates those white matter (WM) tracts oriented anterior to posterior. Red indicates WM tracts oriented in a transverse direction. Blue indicates WM tracts oriented in the superior-inferior direction. Notice the increasing FA with age progression as indicated by increasing color in different regions especially in "cross roads" areas. The thickness of corpus callosum and corticospinal tracts is seen to gradually progress with age. In addition, more branching cortico-cortical association fibers are noted in older children

Review Questions

1. The corpus callosum develops:
   (a) From anterior to posterior
   (b) From posterior to anterior
   (c) From right to left
   (d) Simultaneous growth in different locations
2. On fetal US, what is the plane best showing the cavum septum pellucidum?
   (a) Transcaudate
   (b) Transthalamic
   (c) Transcerebellar
   (d) Transfrontal
3. At what age the posterior brain stem myelination can be appreciated on MRI?
   (a) 12 months
   (b) 3 months
   (c) 6 months
   (d) At birth
4. What is the large red structure seen on midsagittal DEC map derived from DTI?
   (a) Superior longitudinal fasciculus
   (b) Corticospinal tract
   (c) Cingulum
   (d) Corpus callosum
5. A 30-year-old pregnant patient was referred for postnatal MRI after a mid-trimester screening US demonstrated ventriculomegaly and colpocephaly. Postnatal MRI showed the absence of the corpus callosum and presence of the bundle of Probst running along the lateral ventricular walls. Name the associated morphological changes one can appreciate on MRI in patients with corpus callosum agenesis:
   (a) No inversion of the cingulate gyrus
   (b) High-riding third ventricle
   (c) Parallel course of the lateral ventricles
   (d) All of the above
6. A 3-year-old male was seen at the clinic for developmental delay. The patient underwent brain MRI exam which showed diffuse mild T2 hyperintensity of the supratentorial white matter, resulting in blurred gray-white matter interface, consistent with hypomyelination. There was unchanged myelination pattern not appropriately progressed for the patient's corrected gestational age on two successive brain MRI scans carried out at least 1 month apart. What are the white matter fibers considered to be the last to myelinate in the human brain?
   (a) Corpus callosum
   (b) Superior longitudinal fasciculus
   (c) Subcortical association fibers in the frontal and temporal poles
   (d) Corticospinal tracts

Answers

1. (a)
2. (a)
3. (d)
4. (d)
5. (d)
6. (c)

References

1. Stiles J, Jernigan TL. The basics of brain development. Neuropsychol Rev. 2010;20:327–48. https://doi.org/10.1007/s11065-010-9148-4.
2. Garel C, Chantrel E, Brisse H, et al. Fetal cerebral cortex: normal gestational landmarks identified using prenatal MR imaging. AJNR Am J Neuroradiol. 2001;22:184–9.
3. Orman G, Benson JE, Kweldam CF, et al. Neonatal head ultrasonography today: a powerful imaging tool! J Neuroimaging. 2015;25:31–55. https://doi.org/10.1111/jon.12108.
4. Leijser LM, Srinivasan L, Rutherford MA, et al. Structural linear measurements in the newborn brain: accuracy of cranial ultrasound compared to MRI. Pediatr Radiol. 2007;37:640–8. https://doi.org/10.1007/s00247-007-0485-2.
5. Hall EJ. Lessons we have learned from our children: cancer risks from diagnostic radiology. Pediatr Radiol. 2002;32:700–6. https://doi.org/10.1007/s00247-002-0774-8.
6. Berrington de González A, Mahesh M, Kim K-P, et al. Projected cancer risks from computed tomo-

graphic scans performed in the United States in 2007. Arch Intern Med. 2009;169:2071–7. https://doi.org/10.1001/archinternmed.2009.440.
7. James Barkovich A, Raybaud C. Pediatric neuroimaging. 6th ed; 2018.
8. King MA, Kanal KM, Relyea-Chew A, et al. Radiation exposure from pediatric head CT: a bi-institutional study. Pediatr Radiol. 2009;39:1059–65. https://doi.org/10.1007/s00247-009-1327-1.
9. Smith AB, Dillon WP, Gould R, Wintermark M. Radiation dose-reduction strategies for neuroradiology CT protocols. AJNR Am J Neuroradiol. 2007;28:1628–32. https://doi.org/10.3174/ajnr.A0814.
10. Knickmeyer RC, Gouttard S, Kang C, et al. A structural MRI study of human brain development from birth to 2 years. J Neurosci. 2008;28:12176–82. https://doi.org/10.1523/JNEUROSCI.3479-08.2008.
11. Glenn OA, Barkovich AJ. Magnetic resonance imaging of the fetal brain and spine: an increasingly important tool in prenatal diagnosis, part 1. AJNR Am J Neuroradiol. 2006;27:1604–11.
12. Glenn OA, Barkovich J. Magnetic resonance imaging of the fetal brain and spine: an increasingly important tool in prenatal diagnosis: part 2. AJNR Am J Neuroradiol. 2006;27:1807–14.
13. Meoded A, Orman G, Huisman TAGM. Diffusion weighted and diffusion tensor MRI in pediatric neuroimaging including connectomics: principles and applications. Semin Pediatr Neurol. 2020;33:100797. https://doi.org/10.1016/j.spen.2020.100797.
14. Meoded A, Poretti A, Mori S, Zhang J. Diffusion tensor imaging. In: Reference module in neuroscience and biobehavioral psychology. 2017. p. 1–11.
15. Poretti A, Meoded A, Huisman T. Maturation of the brainstem and cerebellar white matter tracts from the neonatal period to adolescence: a diffusion tensor imaging study. Neuropediatrics. 2013;44:PS21_1043. https://doi.org/10.1055/s-0033-1337861.
16. International Society of Ultrasound in Obstetrics & Gynecology Education Committee. Sonographic examination of the fetal central nervous system: guidelines for performing the "basic examination" and the "fetal neurosonogram". Ultrasound Obstet Gynecol. 2007;29:109–16. https://doi.org/10.1002/uog.3909.
17. Cohen-Sacher B, Lerman-Sagie T, Lev D, Malinger G. Sonographic developmental milestones of the fetal cerebral cortex: a longitudinal study. Ultrasound Obstet Gynecol. 2006;27:494–502. https://doi.org/10.1002/uog.2757.
18. Chi JG, Dooling EC, Gilles FH. Gyral development of the human brain. Ann Neurol. 1977;1:86–93. https://doi.org/10.1002/ana.410010109.
19. Norman MG. Normal and abnormal development of the human nervous system. Ronald J. Lemire, John D. Loeser, Richard W. Leech, Ellsworth C. Alvord Jr. Harper and Row, Hagerstown, Maryland, 1975, 237 pp. + ix. Teratology. 1976;14:359. https://doi.org/10.1002/tera.1420140312.
20. van der Knaap MS, van Wezel-Meijler G, Barth PG, et al. Normal gyration and sulcation in preterm and term neonates: appearance on MR images. Radiology. 1996;200:389–96. https://doi.org/10.1148/radiology.200.2.8685331.
21. Hill J, Dierker D, Neil J, et al. A surface-based analysis of hemispheric asymmetries and folding of cerebral cortex in term-born human infants. J Neurosci. 2010;30:2268–76. https://doi.org/10.1523/JNEUROSCI.4682-09.2010.
22. Girard N, Raybaud C, Poncet M. In vivo MR study of brain maturation in normal fetuses. AJNR Am J Neuroradiol. 1995;16:407–13.
23. Levine D, Barnes PD. Cortical maturation in normal and abnormal fetuses as assessed with prenatal MR imaging. Radiology. 1999;210:751–8. https://doi.org/10.1148/radiology.210.3.r99mr47751.
24. Chung R, Kasprian G, Brugger PC, Prayer D. The current state and future of fetal imaging. Clin Perinatol. 2009;36:685–99. https://doi.org/10.1016/j.clp.2009.07.004.
25. Kostović I, Judas M, Rados M, Hrabac P. Laminar organization of the human fetal cerebrum revealed by histochemical markers and magnetic resonance imaging. Cereb Cortex. 2002;12:536–44. https://doi.org/10.1093/cercor/12.5.536.
26. Allendoerfer KL, Shatz CJ. The subplate, a transient neocortical structure: its role in the development of connections between thalamus and cortex. Annu Rev Neurosci. 1994;17:185–218. https://doi.org/10.1146/annurev.ne.17.030194.001153.
27. Kostovic I, Rakic P. Developmental history of the transient subplate zone in the visual and somatosensory cortex of the macaque monkey and human brain. J Comp Neurol. 1990;297:441–70. https://doi.org/10.1002/cne.902970309.
28. Counsell SJ, Maalouf EF, Fletcher AM, et al. MR imaging assessment of myelination in the very preterm brain. AJNR Am J Neuroradiol. 2002;23:872–81.
29. Sie LT, van der Knaap MS, van Wezel-Meijler G, Valk J. MRI assessment of myelination of motor and sensory pathways in the brain of preterm and term-born infants. Neuropediatrics. 1997;28:97–105. https://doi.org/10.1055/s-2007-973680.
30. Martin E, Krassnitzer S, Kaelin P, Boesch C. MR imaging of the brainstem: normal postnatal development. Neuroradiology. 1991;33:391–5. https://doi.org/10.1007/BF00598609.
31. van der Knaap MS, Valk J. MR imaging of the various stages of normal myelination during the first year of life. Neuroradiology. 1990;31:459–70. https://doi.org/10.1007/BF00340123.
32. Barkovich AJ. MR of the normal neonatal brain: assessment of deep structures. AJNR Am J Neuroradiol. 1998;19:1397–403.

33. Steen RG, Ogg RJ, Reddick WE, Kingsley PB. Age-related changes in the pediatric brain: quantitative MR evidence of maturational changes during adolescence. AJNR Am J Neuroradiol. 1997;18:819–28.
34. Barkovich AJ, Kjos BO, Jackson DE, Norman D. Normal maturation of the neonatal and infant brain: MR imaging at 1.5 T. Radiology. 1988;166:173–80. https://doi.org/10.1148/radiology.166.1.3336675.
35. Welker K, Patton A. Assessment of normal myelination with magnetic resonance imaging. Semin Neurol. 2012;32:015–28. https://doi.org/10.1055/s-0032-1306382.
36. Chokshi FH, Poretti A, Meoded A, Huisman TAGM. Normal and abnormal development of the cerebellum and brainstem as depicted by diffusion tensor imaging. Semin Ultrasound CT MR. 2011;32:539–54. https://doi.org/10.1053/j.sult.2011.06.005.
37. Conturo TE, Lori NF, Cull TS, et al. Tracking neuronal fiber pathways in the living human brain. Proc Natl Acad Sci U S A. 1999;96:10422–7. https://doi.org/10.1073/pnas.96.18.10422.
38. Berman JI, Mukherjee P, Partridge SC, et al. Quantitative diffusion tensor MRI fiber tractography of sensorimotor white matter development in premature infants. NeuroImage. 2005;27:862–71. https://doi.org/10.1016/j.neuroimage.2005.05.018.
39. Berman JI, Glass HC, Miller SP, et al. Quantitative fiber tracking analysis of the optic radiation correlated with visual performance in premature newborns. AJNR Am J Neuroradiol. 2009;30:120–4. https://doi.org/10.3174/ajnr.A1304.
40. Lebel C, Caverhill-Godkewitsch S, Beaulieu C. Age-related regional variations of the corpus callosum identified by diffusion tensor tractography. NeuroImage. 2010;52:20–31. https://doi.org/10.1016/j.neuroimage.2010.03.072.

Hydrocephalus and Surgical Solutions for It

3

U.-W. Thomale

Pathophysiology

Cerebrospinal fluid (CSF) flow remains to be only partially understood. Recent knowledge subdivides different forces and pathways, which are involved in CSF flow and are prone to contribute to pathophysiological disturbance which may lead to hydrocephalus [1–4]. Former theories of unidirectional CSF flow from the location of production—mainly the choroid plexus—via the ventricles toward the external CSF spaces and the spinal canal and CSF resorption at the location of Pacchioni granulations have further been elaborated [5]. In general, there are seven factors that need to be classified to understand the complexity of CSF dynamics: pulsatility, CSF production, major CSF pathways, minor CSF pathways, CSF resorption, venous outflow, and respiration [6] (Table 3.1).

Pathophysiological disturbances may occur in all these seven stages. The arterial *pulsation* generated by the heart beat is directly transferred through arterials and arterioles into the intracranial space and the CSF. If elasticity or compliance is impaired, the peaks in pulsatility may cause imbalance of CSF flow and enlargement of CSF spaces. This is typically seen in normal-pressure hydrocephalus (NPH) or at least in parts in arrested hydrocephalus in the pediatric population [7]. The *production of CSF* is considered to take place by ultrafiltration of the blood within the arterioles and capillary bed as being present in the choroid plexus and the microvasculature in the brain tissue. Choroid plexus papilloma is associated with hydrocephalus due to CSF overproduction [8]. *Major CSF pathways* are the four ventricles and its connections such as the foramen of Monro, the Sylvian aqueduct, and the outlets of the fourth ventricle (foramen of Luschka and foramen of Magendie) as well as the external CSF spaces such as the cisterns, the subarachnoid space, and the spinal canal. Any blockage is causing imbalance of CSF flow and may lead to proximal CSF overload. Any occlusion of these major CSF pathways will lead to non-communicating hydrocephalus [9, 10]. *Minor CSF pathway* activity includes the transependymal and transtissue CSF flow throughout the interstitial spaces and the so-called Virchow-Robin spaces, supported by aquaporin channels [11]. Additionally, micro-movements of CSF along the ependymal wall are supported by cilial structures [12]. In congenital hydrocephalus microstructural changes on the basis of genetic alterations may lead to impairment of CSF flow throughout the brain. *CSF resorption* has large capacities and is represented by tissue and ependymal capillaries and venules, Pacchioni granulations, and nerve

U.-W. Thomale (✉)
Pediatric Neurosurgery, Charité Universitaetsmedizin Berlin, Campus Virchow Klinikum, Berlin, Germany
e-mail: uthomale@charite.de; ulrich-wilhelm.thomale@charite.de

N. Shimony, G. Jallo (eds.), *Pediatric Neurosurgery Board Review*,
https://doi.org/10.1007/978-3-031-23687-7_3

Table 3.1 Overview of contributing pathophysiological factor, type of hydrocephalus, anatomical correlates, and hydrocephalus entities leading to different subtypes of CSF circulation disturbances

Contributing factor	Type of HC	Anatomical correlates	HC entities
Pulsatility	Communicating	Hemodynamics, arterials	NPH, arrested hydrocephalus
CSF production		Arterioles, capillaries, choroid plexus	Choroid plexus papilloma
Major CSF pathways	Non-communicating	Ventricles, FM, SAq, 4thVOL, cisterns, SAS, SC	Aqueduct stenosis/ obstructuion, Blake's pouch
Minor CSF pathways	Communicating	VRS, aquaporin, cilia	Congenital HC, PHH PIH
CSF resorption		Venules, capillaries, PG, lymphatics	PHH, PIH
Venous outflow		Veins, sinus, right heart	Subarachnomegaly, IIH
Respiration		Respiratory cycle, spinal epidural venes	*Not specified*

HC hydrocephalus, *CSF* cerebrospinal fluid, *FM* foramen Monro, *SAq* Sylvian aqueduct, *4thVOL* fourth ventricular outlet, *SAS* subarachnoid space, *SC* spinal canal, *VRS* Virchow-Robin spaces, *PG* Pacchioni granulations, *NPH* normal-pressure hydrocephalus, *PHH* post-hemorrhagic hydrocephalus, *PIH* post-infectious hydrocephalus, *IIH* idiopathic intracranial hypertension

root excavations as well as lymphatic drainages [13]. Post-hemorrhagic and post-infectious alterations are considered to reduce the CSF resorption capacity leading to global CSF blockage. Similarly, *venous congestion*, which may be caused by stenosis of major venous structures at the sinus or skull base level, venous thrombosis, or right-sided heart failure, lead to high venous pressure, which blocks the resorption of CSF in venule system and may lead to subarachnomegaly in infancy [14] or idiopathic intracranial hypertension in children, adolescents, or younger adults [15]. Finally *respiration*, which enables the spinal upward movement of CSF from the spinal canal via the epidural venous system, also called the "venous pump," may additionally contribute to CSF flow disturbances but remains the least understood mechanism until today [16].

Different pathophysiologic conditions, which are linked to hydrocephalus development, may include one or more of these mechanisms leading to CSF flow disturbances, and each may have different importance in the individual case (Fig. 3.1) [6].

Diagnostics

Hydrocephalus dynamics in the neonate are measured by fontanelle status, head circumference changes not matching percentile growth patterns, ultrasonographic proven ventricular enlargement, and possible impairment of flow patterns in Doppler sonography with reduced end-diastolic flow and increased resistance index [17]. Clinical symptoms such as irritability, lethargy, vomiting, or opisthotonic posture may also be present but may be difficult to interpret due to other comorbidities. In the infant age, macrocephaly and sunset phenomenon with downward gaze are age-specific disturbances. In older children and adolescence, typically clinical signs of increased intracranial pressure may be present with headaches, nausea vomiting, and impaired consciousness as acute signs of deterioration. Neurological symptoms may include cranial nerve disturbances specifically oculomotor symptoms or gait disturbances but would also depend on the underlying cause of hydrocephalus. In severely acute cases, the Cushing triad may develop with bradycardia hypertension and breathing depression. Chronic cases may also show additional symptoms similar to the elderly such as urinary dysfunction or new cognitive disturbances. Diagnostic measures will be fundoscopy for evaluation of a papilledema, which may be objectified by optic coherence tomography (OCT) or transorbital ultrasound.

Image acquisition tools other than sonography, which may only be applicable in the open

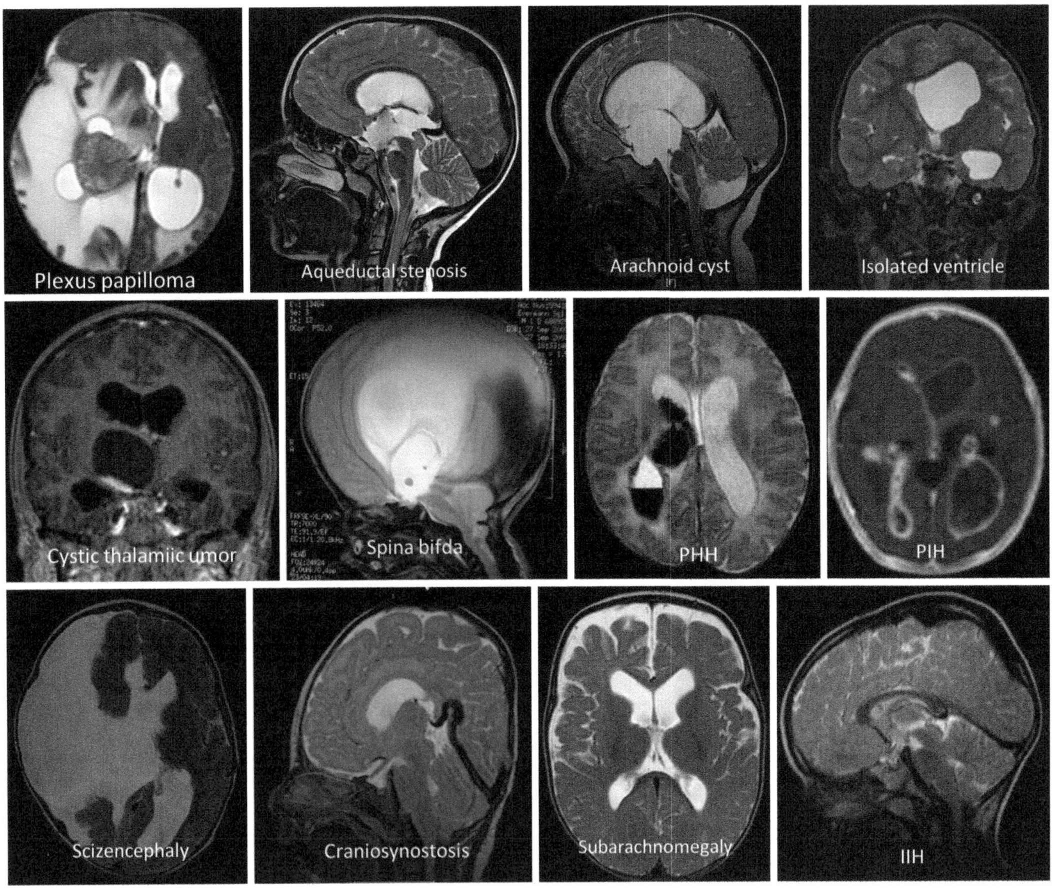

Fig. 3.1 Hydrocephalus is not a solitary disease but rather a consequence of an underlying cause. The possible causes are heterogeneous, and they will influence the type of treatment and prognosis. Representative examples are given of typical underlying diseases, which will need frequently additional treatment for hydrocephalus. (*PHH* post-hemorrhagic hydrocephalus, *PIH* post-infectious hydrocephalus, *IIH* idiopathic intracranial hypertension)

fontanelle, are evaluation of ventricular width and identification of a possible underlying cause. Computer tomography has the advantage of relatively good availability, but the big disadvantage of radiation exposure may be reserved for emergency circumstances whenever alternatives are available. Magnetic resonance imaging has the disadvantage of longer duration and higher costs but the advantage of delivering images with high-resolution quality in which underlying causes for the hydrocephalus can be better identified, since multiple modalities of image sequences such as high contrast T2 images, flow studies and cine sequences are available. In shunted patients x-ray of the shunt and sonography of the abdomen should be applied in addition to evaluation of shunt functionality [18, 19] (Fig. 3.2).

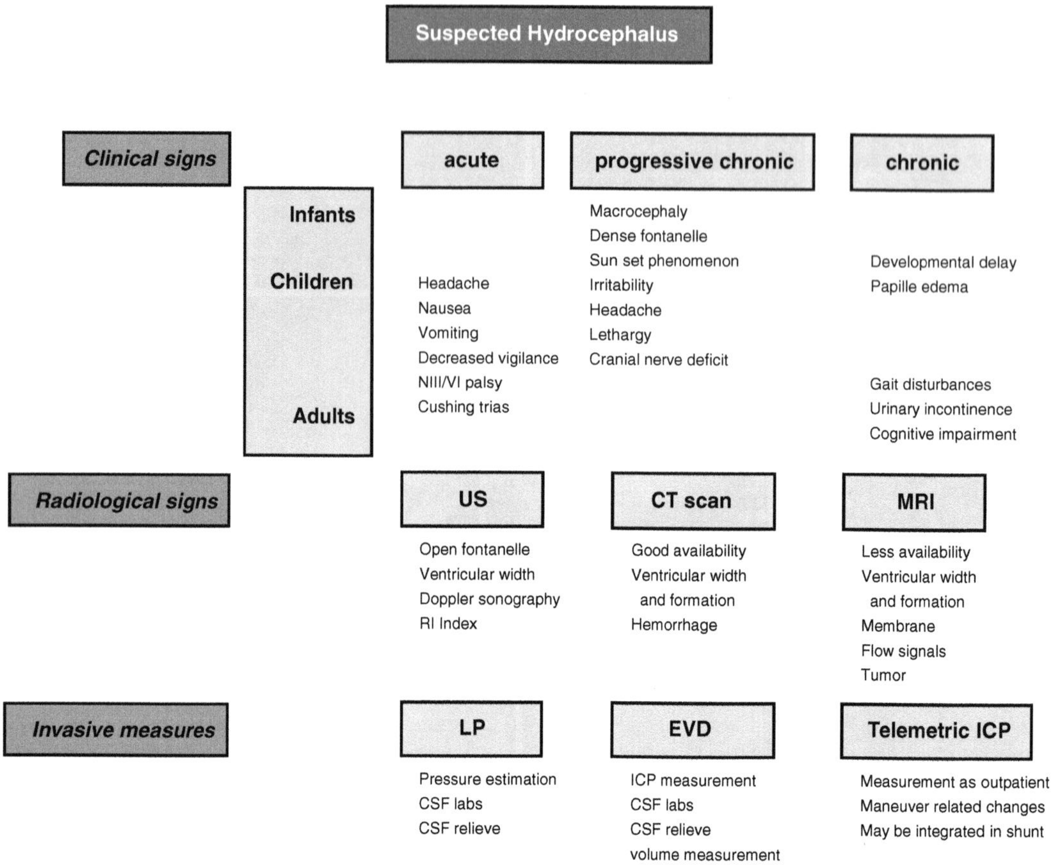

Fig. 3.2 Diagnostic tools for hydrocephalus are divided in clinical evaluation, imaging, and invasive measures. The combination of imaging and clinical symptomatology is usually sufficient to define the diagnosis and draw therapeutic conclusions. Ultrasonography is preferably in infants with open fontanelle for principle diagnosis and follow-up. Magnetic resonance imaging (MRI) is clearly advantageous compared to computer tomography due to high resolution and CSF pathology-associated multimodal sequence to better define the correct diagnosis but involves more efforts and higher costs. Clinical symptoms are related to acuteness of development as well as the age at diagnosis. In chronic conditions when imaging shows clear signs of CSF circulation disturbances but clinical signs are difficult to interpret, invasive methods such as lumbar puncture or external ventricular drain may be indicated, which enable not only pressure measurements but also diagnostic conclusions after CSF volume reduction. Obviously LP is less invasive but also less reliable in pressure measurements. Telemetric ICP monitoring is the future perspective of integrated measurement unit into the shunt system to objectify the shunt-dependent patient with intracranial pressure measurements in different body positions

Neonatal IVH with Hydrocephalus

Intraventricular hemorrhage is observed predominantly in the premature neonate and may lead to hydrocephalus in about 9.3% of all cases. If ventricles become dilated, the rate of shunt dependency is reported to be 38% [20]. If temporary measures become necessary for CSF relieve such as lumbar puncture, implanting of a ventricular access device (VAD), a ventriculosubgaleal shunt (VSGS), or external ventricular drainage (EVD), the rate of shunt dependency is calculated at higher rates of more than 80% [20]. In general, IVH itself does not represent indication for surgical intervention but the consecutive occurrence of hydrocephalus. While the primary damage is caused by the hemorrhage itself and the fragile condition of prematurity, secondary damage may occur with brain compression and shear forces due to enlargement of ventricles. In addition, possible treatment complications and comorbidities will contribute to long-term developmental impairment [21, 22]. Since the degradation of blood is associated with biochemical process like oxidative stress, inflammatory response, and excitotoxicity and might harm brain development by itself, evacuation of the blood particles from the ventricular system is more discussed [23]. Drainage and irrigation together with fibrinolytic activity as suggested in the DRIFT protocol or neuroendoscopic lavage are recent surgical approaches to effectively externalize blood products from the ventricular system and interrupt secondary mechanisms of brain injury [24–27]. A less invasive approach is early and repetitive puncture of a ventricular access device [28]. IVH leading to CSF circulation disturbances results in post-hemorrhagic hydrocephalus (PHH); however different pathophysiological mechanisms will lead to hydrocephalus. One main factor will be protein overload, which may lead to structural ependymal and tissue changes impairing the resorption of CSF into the capillary and venule vasculature. Inflammatory changes may also lead to occlusion of the Sylvian aqueduct or the outlets of the fourth ventricle resulting in non-communicating hydrocephalus. Additionally severe structural damage of the brain will lead to changes in brain tissue elasticity and may impair the pulsatility balance, as well as minor CSF pathways may be disrupted. Thus in the individual case, it is necessary to carefully analyze the pathological changes in order to stratify the best possible therapy.

Infection and Hydrocephalus

Primary infection of the CNS due to meningitis or encephalitis as well as a secondary infection after surgical intervention or septic germ dissemination may lead to CSF circulation disturbances and post-infectious hydrocephalus [29–32]. Pathophysiological considerations are similar to post-hemorrhagic hydrocephalus, but the individual factor will have a different impact in the individual case. If severe infections are associated with the ventricular system, ventriculitis and multiloculated hydrocephalus may develop, which is more often seen in neonates or infants. In these cases early endoscopic treatment by applying neuroendoscopic lavage to clear the ventricular CSF from germs and debris for more effective systemic antibiotic therapy will reduce the re-infection and later shunt revision rate [33]. In multicompartmentalized hydrocephalus navigated endoscopy is necessary to apply for fenestrating of isolated but CSF producing compartments and may be combined with catheter placement in order to simplify a shunt system which is necessary to implant in the vast majority of cases [34, 35]. Detailed information about originating germs and antibiotic treatment protocols will be covered in another chapter.

Myelomeningocele

Spinal dysraphism most often present in myelomeningocele (MMC) as open spina bifida defects is associated with hydrocephalus. The mechanism of CSF circulation disturbance is primarily the hindbrain herniation and associated anatomical alterations of the posterior fossa leading to CSF outflow obstruction and venous congestion. In addition, congenital CNS malformation may lead to major or minor CSF pathway alterations as well. It was shown that intrauterine closure of the MMC defect stops CSF loss at the open dysraphism defect with less exaggerated hindbrain herniation [36–38]. Shunt dependency in these children can significantly be diminished. After postnatal MMC repair, shunt dependency normally is reported at about 85%. Some concepts have tried to diminish shunt rate down to 52% by accepting gradual macrocephaly; however, it is unclear how far this will influence neurodevelopmental potential [39]. Therapy is performed normally by shunting. Hereby it seems to be of importance to avoid overdrainage and taper the CSF diversion drainage to keep up the regular head circumference growth pattern in order to keep anatomical balance especially in the posterior fossa where hindbrain herniation may otherwise lead to critical compression. More recent concepts have applied endoscopic ventriculocisternostomy (ETV) and choroid plexus cauterization (CPC) in order to successfully reduce the shunt rate in MMC patients [40–43]. This concept targets to avoid shunt complications in the future course of these patients; however it is not clear in how far neurodevelopmental potential is affected by ETV CPC compared to shunting. Other concepts have shown that later circumstances of shunt failure may offer possibilities to apply ETV at an older age; thus shunt treatment may only be planned as temporary solution until ETV becomes feasible [43].

Other Congenital Hydrocephalus

A plethora of other congenital CNS malformations are associated with hydrocephalus. Arachnoid cysts of different locations may occlude CSF major pathways by expansion into the third ventricle (suprasellar AC) or compression of the Sylvian aqueduct (lamina quadrigemina AC) or the fourth ventricle (posterior fossa AC). Blake's pouch with its outward expansion of the tela choroidea in the cisterna magna is a classical non-communicating hydrocephalus with obstruction of the fourth ventricular outlets [44–46]. Dandy-Walker malformation with vermian dystrophy, torcular elevation, and enlargement of the cisterna magna is associated with a communicating type of hydrocephalus [47]. The pathophysiological reason might be the combination of minor CSF pathway alterations and venous congestion. In contrast, congenital aqueductal stenosis will classically lead to triventricular hydrocephalus proximal to the occluded Sylvian aqueduct, which represents the communication blockage for CSF from internal to external CSF spaces typically visualized by the outward bulging membranes of the third ventricle such as the lamina terminalis and the floor of the third ventricle indicating the respective pressure gradient. Chiari type I malformation is rarely associated with hydrocephalus; however it may be causing venous congestion or fourth ventricular outflow obstruction [48]. Similarly, craniosynostosis and hydrocephalus are associated especially with syndromic cases in which venous congestion may play a major role sometimes together with constriction of the posterior fossa occluding the major CFS pathways [49–51]. The so-called benign macrocephaly also known as subarachnomegaly is classically caused by venous outflow obstruction alone and is considered to be the idiopathic intracranial hypertension (pseudotumor cerebri) of the infancy [14].

CNS Tumors and Hydrocephalus

Hydrocephalus, e.g., in pediatric brain tumors, is a common condition in about 57% of cases [52]. Choroid plexus tumors represent an unusual condition since an overproduction of CSF is observed in some of these tumors [8]. Most other tumors will cause a major CSF pathway obstruction. In those the primary therapy will always aim for tumor removal to free those pathways sometimes supported by temporary measures such as ETV or EVD [53–55]. Pineal region tumors usually are treated first by combined biopsy and ETV to identify the tumor and define the best possible therapeutic options according to the histopathological diagnosis [54, 56, 57]. Some intrinsic tumors of the mesencephalon also known as tectal plate tumors are only treated by ETV and MRI follow-up observation without the need of biopsy [58–60]. In contrast metastatic disease may lead to the communicating type of hydrocephalus associated with CSF resorption impairment, similar to possible postoperative hemorrhage or infection which may also lead to hydrocephalic complications [61–63].

Therapy

The treatment strategy is directed by the underlying disease, which causes hydrocephalus. The primary aim is always to eliminate the primary cause and thereby solve the CSF flow pathology as well. That would account for tumor removal or arachnoid cyst fenestration. If that is not feasible, direct treatment options for hydrocephalus come into play. Hereby, the pathophysiological

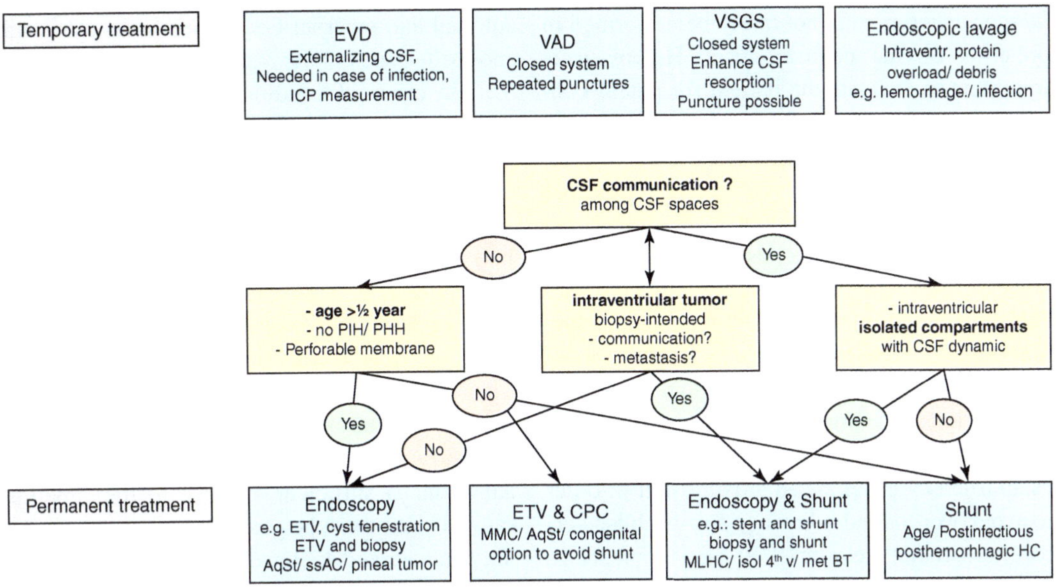

Fig. 3.3 Therapeutic algorithm for hydrocephalus. Temporary treatment options are used in neonates under a body weight of 2 kg. Specifically EVD might predominantly be used in infectious conditions or to monitor ICP together with diverting CSF in neurological unstable patients. Permanent treatment options include the CSF diverting shunt in the majority of cases. Neuroendoscopy however has become essential in the treatment of pediatric hydrocephalus either to reduce the shunt rate, to reduce possible shunt complications or even to simplify the shunt in complex cases

consideration must be taken if non-communicating versus communicating hydrocephalus is present. Generally, in non-communicating hydrocephalus, endoscopy plays the primary role of treatment to reestablish CSF flow and communication by, e.g., membrane fenestration. For communicating hydrocephalus the CSF diversion by shunt implantation is the main treatment option. If communicating hydrocephalus is present but isolated compartments need to be fenestrated or be connected to the shunt system, endoscopy will be combined with shunt implantation. Neuroendoscopic lavage has become an additional treatment option to clear the ventricles from blood products or infectious material in order to reduce shunt dependency and reduce later shunt complications if shunt dependency will still develop. Basically, in the very young-aged patients with a body weight of less than 2 kg, temporary measures are indicated before shunt implantation becomes safely feasible. Additional factors such as anatomical variation, age, the need for biopsy, or CSF protein overload must be taken into consideration before decision-making. These decisions should be taken wisely on an individual-case basis and with sufficient experience in order to reduce surgery-associated complication rates, which is one of the main goals in hydrocephalus treatment especially in pediatric patients (Fig. 3.3) [5, 6, 64, 65].

Temporary Measures

Temporary treatment measures are usually used in the neonatal age. The *ventricular assist device (VAD)* is a reservoir positioned subcutaneously on the bone connected to a ventricular catheter. This may be punctured regularly, e.g., by 10 mL/kg body weight per day, in order to establish repetitive CSF volume reduction [28, 66]. A *ventriculosubgalleal shunt (VSGS)* is similar to the VAD but with an additional outlet into a pocket to establish a subcutaneous CSF collection [21, 67, 68]. This is supposed to enhance CSF resorption capacity and may also be punctured repeatedly. A *lumbar puncture* may not rarely be performed in preterms by the neonatologists. Hereby it is important to evaluate the patient for patent CSF communication; otherwise a pressure gradient will be reinforced [21, 28]. The *external ventricular drainage (EVD)* will continuously divert the ventricular CSF externally into a tube connected and collecting reservoir adjusted by height resistance. In the neonate it may additionally help externalize debris from the CSF outside the system [66, 67]. However, EVD may be more prone to infectious complications and should be avoided in immunocompromised individuals. Additionally the handling on the ward must be established by experienced nursing staff in order to avoid over- or underdrainage and establish correct intracranial pressure (ICP) measurements. In older children EVD should be restricted to infectious conditions, to patients with impaired conscious state to enable ICP measurements in parallel to CSF drainage, and as temporary measure in, e.g., posterior fossa tumor patients with severe hydrocephalus to stabilize CSF pressure condition before major interventions [52, 69]. Temporary measures are usually conditions to decide for permanent treatment necessity along the way. For neonates the precondition for shunt implantation will be a sufficient body weight of 2 kg, a threshold of CSF protein load not higher than 2 g/L, and almost normal white cell counts with normalized inflammatory serum marker.

Endoscopy

The use of neuroendoscopy has become an essential treatment option for hydrocephalus especially in the pediatric age group [70]. Many different variations of techniques are applied for effective therapy.

Endoscopic third ventriculocisternostomy (ETV) is maybe the widest spread technique to enable an alternative CSF pathway from the internal spaces, the third ventricle, to the external CSF spaces, the prepontine cistern, by perforating the floor of the third ventricle. The indication for ETV is typically the non-communicating type of hydrocephalus in which the pathways between internal and external CSF spaces are obstructed most often seen in the aqueductal stenosis [9, 71, 72]. In classical condition, a pressure gradient can be observed at the membranes of the third ventricle such as the floor, the lamina terminalis, or the pineal recess. The surgical technique includes the entry point at a frontal paramedian burr hole, which should be calculated individually per patient. This calculation can be done by defining the trajectory between the floors of the third ventricle toward the foramen of Monro. This trajectory should be elongated toward the convexity of the skull. This would define the optimal entry in the sagittal plane, while in the coronal plane, a sufficient distance to the superior sagittal sinus must be guaranteed, however, staying paramedian which would usually be 2 cm lateral to the midline [73]. The introduction of the straight endoscope toward the lateral ventricle can be performed by a freehand technique in large ventricles and by any kind of guidance in moderate or small ventricles. In the lateral ventricle, the foramen of Monro is identified, and the endoscope is progressed into the third ventricle. With the correct entry point, the floor will be in the straight view. Following a blunt perforation in front of the basilar artery and behind the clivus, a Fogarty catheter or a Decq forceps is used to perform an enlargement of the perforation. The size of the opening should preferably reach 5 mm in diameter, and the free prepontine cistern with the naked basilary artery should be visualized [74, 75].

To estimate the sustainable result, the ETV success score (ETVSS) was introduced by Kulkarni et al. [76]. Hereby the age of the patient, the diagnosis, and the preexistence of a shunt are used to calculate the score which correlates positively with a revision-free survival. Age is the most important factor in the ETVSS, which was also investigated in many different studies (Table 3.2). The International Infant Hydrocephalus Study was able to define the age of 6 months as cutoff since the rate of revision-free survival did not differ from a shunted patient in a pure aqueductal stenosis in older infants [75, 77, 78]. Thus, it becomes more and more accepted to perform a VP shunt before the age of 6 months

Table 3.2 ETV success score (ETVSS) as introduced by Kulkarni et al. (JNS Peds 6, 2010). *MMC* myelomeningocele, *IVH* intraventricular hemorrhage

Score	Age	Etiology	Previous shunt
0	<1 months	Post-infectious	Previous shunt
10	1 to <6 months		No shunt
20		MMC, IVH, non-tectal brain tumor	
30	6 months to <1 year	Aqueductal stenosis, tectal tumor	
40	1 to <10 years		
50	≥10 years		

and an ETV in older infants accordingly. Possible complications for the ETV surgery include CSF fistula, infection, hemorrhage, hygroma, oculomotor deficit, endocrine disturbances, and shunt dependency [79]. In ETV failure at long term a reETV may be considered, while a shunt implantation is rather indicated if an early failure occurs. It was also reported that in very rare cases sudden death is observed in the long-term follow-up [80, 81]. It is suspected that these are related to sudden closure of the stoma and may correlate with small stoma perforation at the time of surgery. Thus, a patient treated with ETV should be in continuous follow-up and may have regular imaging at least every 2 years preferably with MRI to visualize the flow void at the floor of the third ventricle as sign of a patent communication between internal and external CSF spaces. The fundamental question if ETV is better than a shunt even in non-communicating hydrocephalus is still unanswered. The reason to perform the ETV is to avoid the shunt dependency and avoid long-term complications which are observed with shunt systems [77, 82]. However, since in ETV patients the ventricles are remaining large and in shunt patients the ventricles are becoming rather small, it still needs further investigation in how far long-term neurocognitive outcome is affected by either technique [74, 78].

In addition, ETV and choroid plexus coagulation (ETV-CPC) aims to enhance the communication between internal and external CSF spaces together with reducing the CSF production. It was introduced to decrease the rate of shunt dependency as a possible treatment in pediatric hydrocephalus. As the technique was started in Africa by Benjamin Warf due to the lack of implantable shunt hardware, it was observed that shunt independence could be achieved with decent success relatively independent from the type of hydrocephalus [42, 83, 84]. Later studies from the USA showed successful treatment specifically in patients with aqueductal stenosis, myelomeningocele, and other non-post-hemorrhagic hydrocephalus cases [85]. The surgical technique was elaborated over the years and is usually performed by a flexible endoscope, thereby being able to cauterize all portions of the choroid plexus in the lateral ventricles, including the temporal horns after performing an additional ETV [40]. In an African prospective randomized trial, ETV-CPC versus shunting in infant post-infectious hydrocephalus showed non-significant differences of revision-free survival (ETV-CPC 65% versus shunting 76%) between the groups and no significant differences in neurocognitive outcome at 12 months of follow-up [41]. Critical views on ETV-CPC are debating about the role of the choroid plexus for the brain tissue intergity, the risk of the intervention and possible complications affecting relevant cerebral structures and thereby possibly limiting the potential of long-term cognitive neurodevelopmental outcome. The fundamental question is how harmful the technique of ETV-CPC is for long term compared to a shunt dependency coming with possible recurrent maintanance over a life span.

In patients with CNS tumors and secondary hydrocephalus, an ETV together with a biopsy is indicated if the tumor is causing non-communicating hydrocephalus and may not be operable with justifiable risk before knowing the diagnosis [56, 57]. A common example is the pineal region tumor, which will block the Sylvian aqueduct and will cause hydrocephalus in a high rate of patients. The histological diagnosis will decide about the need of initial surgery or if adjuvant therapy should be used as treatment only or before indicating for surgery. The technique of performing ETV and biopsy may usually done by a preplanned trajectory via one burr hole in order to reach both targets at the floor of the third ventricle and the tumor in the posterior portion of the third ventricle [86]. Navigated planning and execution are strongly recommended while using a rigid endoscope. A flexible endoscope specifically helps to better target for tumor biopsy [56]. The success rate is usually high in these patients, and a shunt treatment should be avoided.

Intracranial cysts may cause hydrocephalus typically if they are located in the midline (suprasellar, lamina quadrigemina cysts), in the posterior fossa, or if they are extremely large [45, 46]. In these patients endoscopic or microsurgical cyst fenestration is the first choice of treatment. This is especially true since arachnoid cysts are not primarily a hydrocephalic condition but isolated CSF compartments, which can be resolved if communication is reestablished between the cyst and regular CSF spaces. If an arachnoid cyst is causing hydrocephalus, indication for surgery is clearly given. Since the anatomical conditions are individual and the point of fenestration as well as the optimal entry point will be heterogeneous, the intervention especially when performed endoscopically should preferably be done by neuronavigated guidance [87]. Outcome of navigated cyst fenestration is advantageous for cyst as well as for hydrocephalus treatment [44, 46]. However, a certain rate of patients will still become shunt dependent which seems to be more likely for infants.

A relatively new treatment technique was introduced as neuroendoscopic lavage (NEL) for post-hemorrhagic as well as for post-infectious hydrocephalus in its early stage in order to clear protein, cell, and germ-polluted CSF from the ventricular compartments [26, 88]. An endoscope with at least two channels for irrigation and passive outflow is used to target mainly the supratentorial ventricles via a frontal lateralized entry point and clear both lateral ventricles after performing a septostomy as well as the third ventricle. Warm Ringer solution irrigation can be introduced in the ventricular system through one channel of the endoscope, and another channel will enable passive outflow to avoid increased ICP changes by volume imbalance. If blood clots or debris should be externalized, they can be aspirated by a syringe connected to a tube via the outflow channel to apply short controlled suction directly on the clots. Thereby, soft and loose debris can easily and effectively be externalized step by step. When used in IVH and hydrocephalus, NEL has shown to reduce shunt rate, infection rate, and multiloculated hydrocephalus in various single-center retrospective studies [26, 89–92]. Additionally it was reported to reduce the amount of shunt complications within 12 months after NEL if a shunt was indicated. In ventriculitis and hydrocephalus, the published experience for NEL showed a significant decrease in multiloculated hydrocephalus and lower shunt revision rates and reinfection rates in the follow-up of these patients [33, 93]. It remains debatable, especially for the treatment of IVH and hydrocephalus in premature babies if NEL is justified as more aggressive approach compared to other surgical techniques like VAD, EVD, or VSGS. Further studies are needed in which NEL will be investigated on a multicenter basis to verify its safety and efficacy.

Shunt

The CSF diversion from the ventricular system into another body cavity, most often the peritoneum, by a CSF shunt system has become the most often used hydrocephalus treatment since its introduction in the 1960s. It accounts still for about 80% of all patients suffering from hydrocephalus. Historically seen the CSF shunt therapy is one of the most successful treatments in Neurosurgery since the mortality and high morbidity rate of hydrocephalus was way above 80% before its introduction [94–97]. Nevertheless, it remains to be the "unloved child" of Neurosurgery because of the seemingly unrewarding surgical technique and high rates of possible complications. The main challenge of this surgery is thus not its performance but to avoid shunt-associated complications in short and long term [98]. Therefore, a fundamental understanding of the disadvantages and the possible problems as well as offering long-term solutions is warranted to apply a decent quality of treatment. From the pathophysiological perspective, however, a shunt system is a rather unphysiological solution, since the CSF, which is normally produced and resorbed mainly with the intracranial space, will be diverted in another body cavity at a different height level. Since hydrostatic and differential pressure forces are acting on water columns within the tubing system of a shunt, the drainage activity depends on the factors body position, activity, height, diameter of tubing, and the valve system [99]. Moreover, the heterogeneous conditions of the underlying disease will result in different CSF draining volume requirements. These factors need to be taken into account when choosing the shunt system for long-term treatment abilities.

The ventriculoperitoneal shunt (VPS) is considered to be the primary option and most often used shunt system for hydrocephalus [100]. The shunt system basically consists of three parts, the ventricular catheter, a reservoir, and the subcutaneous tubing to the valve, the valve, and the distal subcutaneous catheter leading into the peritoneum. A ventricular catheter may be placed frontally or parieto-occipitally [101]. Recent literature has shown non-significant advantage for the frontal placement, but it remains under debate which location is the preferable one [102]. The correct positioning of the ventricular catheter will be enhanced by navigation, guided technique, or intraoperative ultrasound [103–106]. The valve system is inserted into the shunt to avoid under- or overdrainage of CSF. The distal catheter may be placed via a paraumbilical or substernal incision into the peritoneum. A sufficient length (30–40 cm) should be inserted in order to enable growth-related elongation of the system in small children [107].

Since shunt surgery is known to be linked to a plethora of complications such as infection, malpositioning, occlusion, and dislocation, a defined protocol should be applied to minimize the risk for surgery-associated failures [108–111]. The described protocol specifically addresses infection avoidance and includes various factors for reducing shunt infection rate [112, 113]. These factors include an experienced surgeon present,

Table 3.3 Possible VP shunt complications. *PC* proximal catheter, *DC* distal catheter

Complication	Clinical signs	Reason	Strategy of avoidance
Infection	Fever, skin irritation/reddening, swelling, infectious serum and CSF parameters, peritoneal pseudocyst (chronic)	Surgical, sepsis	Strict antiseptic protocol compliance, antibiotic-impregnated catheters, vancomycin bath for implants (500 mg/250 mL)
CSF fistula/ collection	Wound rupture/fluid collection	Surgical, shunt underdrainage	Sealing of burr hole entry, reduce shunt resistance, rule out kinking, malpositioning
Malpositioning of PC	Underdrainage, shunt failure	Surgical	Guided placement (guide, navigation, ultrasound)
Malpositioning of DC	Underdrainage, CSF collection	Surgical	Guided placement (laparoscopic ultrasound)
Catheter obstruction	Underdrainage	Malpositioning, overdrainage	Guided placement or increased resistance of shunt valve
Valve obstruction	Underdrainage	CSF protein overload	EVD, neuroendoscopic lavage, valve selection
Valve malfunction	Adjustment failure	Obstruction, magnetic influence	Valve selection
Shunt rupture	Underdrainage	Calcification, fixation failure, short length to burr hole	Barium strip catheters or add initial length in proximal subcutaneous catheter length
Overdrainage	Headaches nausea, lethargy after activity or in the evening, reduced head circumference, slit ventricles, calvarial thickening	Valve selection	Increase resistance of valve system, add overdrainage protection
Underdrainage	Headaches, nausea, lethargy in the morning, dense fontanelle, increased head circumference	Obstruction, rupture, malpositioning	Rule out any shunt malfunctioning, decrease shunt valve resistance

single-shot antibiotics 30 min before incision, sufficient skin cleaning and disinfection of the surgical field, the use of double cloves, limited traffic in the OR, limited handling of implants, and the use of vancomycin bath (500 mg/250 mL) for the implants or antibiotic-impregnated catheters for the shunt system [30, 31, 113–115]. An overview of shunt complications are given in Table 3.3.

For the selection of the valve for the patient, no proven guideline or sufficient evidence data exist. The last prospective randomized trial on valve system dated from the early 1990s and did not show any differences among the three tested types in terms of revision-free survival [116–118]. This study is often mentioned to argue that every valve has the same abilities, which is still unproven. It remains however true that the majority of valves on the market have never been tested in prospective randomized trials [119]. Thus it is at least important for the neurosurgeon in charge to have sufficient understanding on what kind technical characteristics are offered by the valve used in the patient, respectively. In the various amounts of valve which are offered on the market, the following functionalities may be selected [120]: differential pressure setting being fixed or adjustable, flow control abilities, anti-hydrostatic units (anti-siphon, gravity assistance), and magnetic interference of the valve system. Many valves offered on the market are fixed differential pressure valves, such as low-, medium-, high-pressure valves. Flow regulation of the valve is often a misinterpreted term since almost all valves include differential pressure functionalities; however the Delta and the Orbis-Sigma valves are offering some flow regulation being still in relation to differential pressure changes. Those kinds of fixed pressure valves need to be selected wisely in order to fit the needs for long term in the individual patient. Taken into considerations that especially pediatric patients are undergoing different stages of development with altering anatomy of the head, changing activity, and growth, it seems reasonable to use adjustable valve to adapt the shunt system in accordance to the changing circumstances over time. However, different studies have shown that adjustable valves may be non-different or even inferior in terms of revision-free survival compared to fixed-pressure valves [121, 122]. However more important outcome parameters of symptomatology or neurodevelopment have never been investigated on a solid scientific level. For adjustable valves it is important to know if the valve has magnetic resistance functionality for the performance of MR imaging (Certas Plus, proGAV, Polaris). Some other valves not offering MRI resistance have shown unintended adjustments during MR imaging or exposure to domestic magnets [123]. Some studies showed functional failure after placed in a high-field MR scanner. Anti-hydrostatic units were included in different valve systems in order to balance possible overdrainage in the upright position due to the different level of CSF cavity of the cranial space compared to the peritoneum causing hydrostatic force (shunt assistant, anti-siphon device, siphon guard, gravity compensating accessory, SiphonX, Delta Chamber) [124]. An overview of valves is given in Table 3.4.

Alternative solutions to the VPS become necessary especially when the resorption capacity is impaired in the peritoneum, e.g., after peritonitis. The first alternative is ventriculo-arterial shunt (VAS). In this system the distal catheter is placed mostly by Seldinger technique into the right atrium of the heart [71, 125, 126]. Possible complications include hemorrhage, pneumothorax, and malpositioning during placement and thrombotic occlusion, sepsis, and shunt nephritis. Other alternatives include the ventriculo-pleural shunt in which the resorptive capacity is lower compared to peritoneal or arterial shunt system but does still show decent functionality [127, 128]. Other anatomical locations such as gall bladder, uretral, and ileal cavities to divert the CSF have been used in historic reports successfully as well in limited numbers [129, 130]. In general, it might be stated that if the complication rate and the revision rate are kept to be low, the likelihood that any unusual alternative for CSF shunting other than peritoneum, atrium, or pleural becomes necessary can rather be limited.

The follow-up of a shunt-dependent patient is important to monitor for adequate development

Table 3.4 Overview of shunt valves on the market. *ODP* overdrainage protection, *MR* magnetic resistance, *NV* neonatal version, *DP* differential pressure, *NA* not applicable

Name	Company	Description	ODP	MR	NV	Options
Fixed differential pressure valves						
Delta valve	Medtronic	Diaphragm	Delta chamber	NA	+	0.5/1.0/1.5/2.0
CSF flow control	Medtronic	Diaphragm	–	NA	+	Low-low/low/medium/high
Burr hole DP valve	Medtronic	Diaphragm	–	NA	–	0.5/1.0/1.5/2.0
Essential	Integra	Diaphragm	–	NA	–	Low/medium/high
Codman Hakim precision	Integra	Ball in cone	+/– Siphon guard	NA	+	Very-low/low medium/high/very-high
Sophy mini SM1	Sophysa	Ball in cone	–	NA	NA	Low/medium/high
CRx valve	Sophysa	Proximal meters	–	NA	–	20/45/70/100/135
miniNAV	Miethke	Ball in cone	–	NA	NA	0/5/10/15 cmH_2O
paediGAV	Miethke	Ball in cone	Shunt assistant (15/20 cmH_2O)	NA	NA	5/10 cmH_2O
GAV	Miethke	Ball in cone	Shunt assistant (20/25 cmH_2O)	NA	NA	4/9 cmH_2O
Chhabra shunt	Surgiwear	Proximal slits	–	NA	–	Low/medium/high
Orbis-Sigma II (OSV II)	Integra	DP flow regulation	–	NA	–	Self-regulating: 18–30 mL/h
Low flow	Integra	DP flow regulation	–	NA	NA	Self-regulating: 8–17 mL/h
Adjustable valves						
Codman Hakim	Integra	Ball in cone	+/– Siphon guard	–	+	18 steps (3–20 cmH_2O)
Certas Plus	Integra	Ball in cone	+/– Siphon guard	+	+	7 steps 8th 40 cmH_2O ("virtual off")
Strata II	Medtronic	Ball in cone	+/– Delta chamber	–	+	5 steps (1.5–20 cmH_2O)
Strata NSC	Medtronic	Ball in cone	–	–	+	5 steps (1.5–20 cmH_2O)
Polaris	Sophysa	Ball in cone	+/– SiphonX	+	–	5 steps; four versions (10–140/30–200/50–300/80–400 mmH_2O)
Mini SM8	Sophysa	Ball in cone	–	–	NA	8 steps; four versions (10–140/30–200/50–300/80–400 mmH_2O)
proGAV 2.0	Miethke	Ball in cone	Shunt assistant (15/20/25/30 cmH_2O)	+	–	21 steps (0–20 cmH_2O)
Adjustable gravitational valves						
proSA	Miethke	Ball in cone	0–40 cmH_2O	+	+	No DP unit
M.blue	Miethke	Ball in cone	0–40 cmH_2O	+	+	DP 0/5/10/15 cmH_2O
M.blue plus	Miethke	Ball in cone	0–40 cmH_2O	+	+	Adjustable DP 0–20 cmH_2O

Adapted from Cornejo et Elbabaa, 2021

and identify possible factors for the risk of shunt failures [72, 131–134]. A once-a-year outpatient appointment with cranial imaging at least every second year seems to be a reasonable follow up regimen for the shunt-dependent pediatric patient. Relevant developmental parameters are head circumference, clinical symptom evaluation typically seen for high or low ICP, evaluation of the subcutaneous shunt path and imaging based evaluation of ventricular width, or exclusion of secondary hygroma [109, 110, 135]. In general, in the pediatric-shunted patient, the risk of overdrainage in the functioning shunt is higher compared to underdrainage. However, primary overdrainage might lead to slit ventricles and secondary ventricular catheter occlusion, which in turn might also lead to underdrainage [99, 136–138]. Especially in those patients, it is important to clear the ventricular catheter and increase the valve resistance possibly adding anti-hydrostatic functionality in the valve to avoid future recurrence of proximal catheter occlusion [139]. Long term changes of CSF overdrainage are calvarial thickening, enlargement of the pneumatized sinuses, secondary microcephaly or Chiari malformation, which should be counteracted from early on. For future perspective intracranial pressure measurement, which is integrated into the shunt system, will have relevant implication to better objectify the follow-up treatment of shunt-dependent patients with telemetric technical solutions [140].

Endoscopy in Combination with Shunt

In patients with indication for shunt implantation or who already have a shunt received, neuroendoscopy may be necessary to facilitate communication between isolated CSF compartments such as in multiloculated hydrocephalus or isolated ventricles or to decrease protein CSF levels to reduce the risk of future occlusions. Therefore, the neuroendoscopy has become an essential tool not only as treatment alone but in combination with shunt systems to reduce complications and to simplify the shunt system, for better follow-up control.

Most isolated ventricles result from post-infectious or post-hemorrhagic conditions. In isolated lateral ventricles, a septostomy can relatively simply lead to balanced CSF pressure relations [141–143]. In isolated fourth ventricle in which the Sylvian aqueduct as well as the outlets of the fourth ventricle are occluded, different treatment options exist. An additional catheter placement via a suboccipital burr hole might be connected to the shunt system via a y connector. This represents the risk that the catheter might become relatively too long when the fourth ventricle collapses and thereby might lead to brainstem injury when the tip punctures the midline structures. Alternatively, an aqueductal stent might be placed endoscopically to be connected directly to the shunt system [144–147]. If this is performed through a frontal entry point, it becomes important to plan the entry in the alignment trajectory of the Sylvian aqueduct not to injure the mesencephalic structures [73]. The catheter would include proximal perforation holes which are able to drain the lateral and third ventricles as well and is preferably connected to the burr hole reservoir of the shunt [145, 147]. Navigation planning is essential for this procedure. In multiloculated hydrocephalus which is often a result of a ventriculitis in the neonate, multiple isolated CSF compartments develop which will all need CSF diversion and will result in the difficulty to treat this complex hydrocephalic condition [34, 35, 148, 149]. In those cases the goal is to implant one simplified shunt with not more than two catheters in order to drain all cysts connected via the catheters following sufficient endoscopic fenestrations. Navigated planning and execution of the neuroendoscopic procedure are essential. Some authors have also reported that intraoperative ultrasound imaging can help perform the procedure. The optimal entry points must be preoperatively defined in order to reach most likely all cysts during one procedure. However, especially if the inflammatory process has not become inactive, additional cyst development might occur warranting multiple interventions to control the complex condition.

In the context of post-hemorrhagic or post-infectious conditions, neuroendoscopic lavage can be performed in direct combination of shunt implantation [150]. Neuroendoscopic lavage has shown to significantly reduce CSF protein levels [33]. Thus, in cases of post-infectious or post-hemorrhagic hydrocephalus when only protein levels or erythrocytes remain to be high but infectious signs are normalized and debris are already resolved or externalized NEL might facilitate earlier shunt implantation. This might reduce additional waiting time periods for these parameters to normalize in which brain is exposed to continuous intracranial pressure increase and might thus further be harmed.

Summary

Hydrocephalus is a complex disease with multiple possible underlying causes and heterogeneous pathophysiological mechanisms leading to CSF circulation disturbances. The fact that in pediatric patients anatomical changes over time as well as changes in behavior lead to altering conditions affecting shunt drainage in the individual patient add to the complexity of long term follow up. As treatment options temporary treatment is allocated mainly to the neonatal age. EVD becomes additionally relevant in treating infectious conditions or monitoring ICP while draining CSF for pressure relief. Permanent treatment options are endoscopy alone in non-communicating type of hydrocephalus or shunting in communicating hydrocephalus. ETV-CPC might lead to reduction of shunt dependency in selected cases, while neuroendoscopic lavage may additionally lead to reduced rate of multiloculated hydrocephalus and infectious complications in post-hemorrhagic and post-infectious conditions. Shunt procedures are challenging in terms of avoiding complications in the long run. CSF draining characteristics of the shunt should be monitored over time by following on clinical symptoms and head circumference measures and evaluating ventricular width. In complex hydrocephalus the combination of endoscopy together with shunt implantation might lead to simplified shunt systems with lower complication rates. Profound knowledge and decent experience are essential to treat this complex disease with adequate quality for a long-term improved outcome.

Questions

1. What factor is not associated with the ETV success score
   (a) Age
   (b) Etiology of hydrocephalus
   (c) Presence of shunt
   (d) # of shunt malfunction
2. What type of valve showed the best revision-free survival
   (a) Non-programmable
   (b) Differential pressure
   (c) None
   (d) flow regulated
3. Isolated or loculated hydrocephalus is a result of?
   (a) Infection
   (b) Hemorrhagic
   (c) Neither
   (d) Both

Answers

1. (d)
2. (c)
3. (d)

References

1. Di Rocco C, McLone DG, Shimoji T, Raimondi AJ. Continuous intraventricular cerebrospinal fluid pressure recording in hydrocephalic children during wakefulness and sleep. J Neurosurg. 1975;42:683–9.
2. Greitz D. The hydrodynamic hypothesis versus the bulk flow hypothesis. Neurosurg Rev. 2004;27:299–300.
3. Oi S. Classification of hydrocephalus: critical analysis of classification categories and advantages of "Multi-categorical Hydrocephalus Classification" (Mc HC). Childs Nerv Syst. 2011;27:1523–33.
4. Rekate HL. A consensus on the classification of hydrocephalus: its utility in the assessment of abnormalities of cerebrospinal fluid dynamics. Childs Nerv Syst. 2011;27:1535–41.
5. Tully HM, Dobyns WB. Infantile hydrocephalus: a review of epidemiology, classification and causes. Eur J Med Genet. 2014;57:359–68.
6. Thomale UW. Integrated understanding of hydrocephalus—a practical approach for a complex disease. Childs Nerv Syst. 2021;37:3313–24.
7. Greitz D. Paradigm shift in hydrocephalus research in legacy of Dandy's pioneering work: rationale for third ventriculostomy in communicating hydrocephalus. Childs Nerv Syst. 2007;23:487–9.
8. Bettegowda C, Adogwa O, Mehta V, Chaichana KL, Weingart J, Carson BS, Jallo GI, Ahn ES. Treatment of choroid plexus tumors: a 20-year single institutional experience. J Neurosurg Pediatr. 2012;10:398–405.
9. Cinalli G, Spennato P, Nastro A, Aliberti F, Trischitta V, Ruggiero C, Mirone G, Cianciulli E. Hydrocephalus in aqueductal stenosis. Childs Nerv Syst. 2011;27:1621–42.
10. Al-Hakim S, Schaumann A, Tietze A, Schulz M, Thomale UW. Endoscopic third ventriculostomy in children with third ventricular pressure gradient and open ventricular outlets on MRI. Childs Nerv Syst. 2019;35:2319–26.

11. de Laurentis C, Cristaldi P, Arighi A, Cavandoli C, Trezza A, Sganzerla EP, Giussani CG, Di Cristofori A. Role of aquaporins in hydrocephalus: what do we know and where do we stand? A systematic review. J Neurol. 2021;268:4078–94.
12. Sakamoto K, Nakajima M, Kawamura K, Nakamura E, Tada N, Kondo A, Arai H, Miyajima M. Ependymal ciliary motion and their role in congenital hydrocephalus. Childs Nerv Syst. 2021;37:3355–64.
13. Oreskovic D, Rados M, Klarica M. New concepts of cerebrospinal fluid physiology and development of hydrocephalus. Pediatr Neurosurg. 2017;52:417–25.
14. Cinalli G, di Martino G, Russo C, Mazio F, Nastro A, Mirone G, Ruggiero C, Aliberti F, Cascone D, Covelli E, Spennato P. Dural venous sinus anatomy in children with external hydrocephalus: analysis of a series of 97 patients. Childs Nerv Syst. 2021;37:3021–32.
15. Sunderland GJ, Jenkinson MD, Conroy EJ, Gamble C, Mallucci CL. Neurosurgical CSF diversion in idiopathic intracranial hypertension: a narrative review. Life (Basel). 2021;11:393.
16. Ludwig HC, Bock HC, Gartner J, Schiller S, Frahm J, Dreha-Kulaczewski S. Hydrocephalus revisited: new insights into dynamics of neurofluids on macro- and microscales. Neuropediatrics. 2021;52:233–41.
17. Sandhu PK, Banker H, Cohen HL. Neurosonography assessment, protocols, and interpretation. Treasure Island: StatPearls; 2022.
18. Krishnan P, Raybaud C, Palasamudram S, Shroff M. Neuroimaging in pediatric hydrocephalus. Indian J Pediatr. 2019;86:952–60.
19. Raybaud C. MR assessment of pediatric hydrocephalus: a road map. Childs Nerv Syst. 2016;32:19–41.
20. Christian EA, Jin DL, Attenello F, Wen T, Cen S, Mack WJ, Krieger MD, McComb JG. Trends in hospitalization of preterm infants with intraventricular hemorrhage and hydrocephalus in the United States, 2000-2010. J Neurosurg Pediatr. 2016;17:260–9.
21. Christian EA, Melamed EF, Peck E, Krieger MD, McComb JG. Surgical management of hydrocephalus secondary to intraventricular hemorrhage in the preterm infant. J Neurosurg Pediatr. 2016;17:278–84.
22. Mukerji A, Shah V, Shah PS. Periventricular/intraventricular hemorrhage and neurodevelopmental outcomes: a meta-analysis. Pediatrics. 2015;136:1132–43.
23. Ballabh P, de Vries LS. White matter injury in infants with intraventricular haemorrhage: mechanisms and therapies. Nat Rev Neurol. 2021;17:199–214.
24. Luyt K, Jary S, Lea C, Young GJ, Odd D, Miller H, Kmita G, Williams C, Blair PS, Fernandez AM, Hollingworth W, Morgan M, Smith-Collins A, Thai NJ, Walker-Cox S, Aquilina K, Pople I, Whitelaw A. Ten-year follow-up of a randomised trial of drainage, irrigation and fibrinolytic therapy (DRIFT) in infants with post-haemorrhagic ventricular dilatation. Health Technol Assess. 2019;23:1–116.
25. Whitelaw A, Jary S, Kmita G, Wroblewska J, Musialik-Swietlinska E, Mandera M, Hunt L, Carter M, Pople I. Randomized trial of drainage, irrigation and fibrinolytic therapy for premature infants with posthemorrhagic ventricular dilatation: developmental outcome at 2 years. Pediatrics. 2010;125:e852–8.
26. Schulz M, Buhrer C, Pohl-Schickinger A, Haberl H, Thomale UW. Neuroendoscopic lavage for the treatment of intraventricular hemorrhage and hydrocephalus in neonates. J Neurosurg Pediatr. 2014;13:626–35.
27. Thomale UW, Cinalli G, Kulkarni AV, Al-Hakim S, Roth J, Schaumann A, Buhrer C, Cavalheiro S, Sgouros S, Constantini S, Bock HC. TROPHY registry study design: a prospective, international multicenter study for the surgical treatment of posthemorrhagic hydrocephalus in neonates. Childs Nerv Syst. 2019;35:613–9.
28. de Vries LS, Liem KD, van Dijk K, Smit BJ, Sie L, Rademaker KJ, Gavilanes AW, Dutch Working Group of Neonatal Neurology. Early versus late treatment of posthaemorrhagic ventricular dilatation: results of a retrospective study from five neonatal intensive care units in The Netherlands. Acta Paediatr. 2002;91:212–7.
29. de Jonge RC, van Furth AM, Wassenaar M, Gemke RJ, Terwee CB. Predicting sequelae and death after bacterial meningitis in childhood: a systematic review of prognostic studies. BMC Infect Dis. 2010;10:232.
30. Mallucci CL, Jenkinson MD, Conroy EJ, Hartley JC, Brown M, Dalton J, Kearns T, Moitt T, Griffiths MJ, Culeddu G, Solomon T, Hughes D, Gamble C, BASICS Study Collaborators. Antibiotic or silver versus standard ventriculoperitoneal shunts (BASICS): a multicentre, single-blinded, randomised trial and economic evaluation. Lancet. 2019;394:1530–9.
31. van Lindert EJ, Bilsen MV, Flier MV, Kolwijck E, Delye H, Oever JT. Topical vancomycin reduces the cerebrospinal fluid shunt infection rate: a retrospective cohort study. PLoS One. 2018;13:e0190249.
32. Zainel A, Mitchell H, Sadarangani M. Bacterial meningitis in children: neurological complications, associated risk factors, and prevention. Microorganisms. 2021;9:535.
33. Gaderer C, Schaumann A, Schulz M, Thomale UW. Neuroendoscopic lavage for the treatment of CSF infection with hydrocephalus in children. Childs Nerv Syst. 2018;34:1893–903.
34. Spennato P, Cinalli G, Ruggiero C, Aliberti F, Trischitta V, Cianciulli E, Maggi G. Neuroendoscopic treatment of multiloculated hydrocephalus in children. J Neurosurg. 2007;106:29–35.
35. Schulz M, Bohner G, Knaus H, Haberl H, Thomale UW. Navigated endoscopic surgery for multiloculated hydrocephalus in children. J Neurosurg Pediatr. 2010;5:434–42.

36. Adzick NS. Fetal surgery for spina bifida: past, present, future. Semin Pediatr Surg. 2013;22:10–7.
37. Adzick NS, Thom EA, Spong CY, Brock JW 3rd, Burrows PK, Johnson MP, Howell LJ, Farrell JA, Dabrowiak ME, Sutton LN, Gupta N, Tulipan NB, D'Alton ME, Farmer DL, Investigators M. A randomized trial of prenatal versus postnatal repair of myelomeningocele. N Engl J Med. 2011;364:993–1004.
38. Elbabaa SK, Gildehaus AM, Pierson MJ, Albers JA, Vlastos EJ. First 60 fetal in-utero myelomeningocele repairs at Saint Louis Fetal Care Institute in the post-MOMS trial era: hydrocephalus treatment outcomes (endoscopic third ventriculostomy versus ventriculo-peritoneal shunt). Childs Nerv Syst. 2017;33:1157–68.
39. Chakraborty A, Crimmins D, Hayward R, Thompson D. Toward reducing shunt placement rates in patients with myelomeningocele. J Neurosurg Pediatr. 2008;1:361–5.
40. Coulter IC, Dewan MC, Tailor J, Ibrahim GM, Kulkarni AV. Endoscopic third ventriculostomy and choroid plexus cauterization (ETV/CPC) for hydrocephalus of infancy: a technical review. Childs Nerv Syst. 2021;37:3509–19.
41. Kulkarni AV, Riva-Cambrin J, Rozzelle CJ, Naftel RP, Alvey JS, Reeder RW, Holubkov R, Browd SR, Cochrane DD, Limbrick DD, Simon TD, Tamber M, Wellons JC, Whitehead WE, Kestle JRW. Endoscopic third ventriculostomy and choroid plexus cauterization in infant hydrocephalus: a prospective study by the Hydrocephalus Clinical Research Network. J Neurosurg Pediatr. 2018;21:214–23.
42. Kulkarni AV, Schiff SJ, Mbabazi-Kabachelor E, Mugamba J, Ssenyonga P, Donnelly R, Levenbach J, Monga V, Peterson M, MacDonald M, Cherukuri V, Warf BC. Endoscopic treatment versus shunting for infant hydrocephalus in Uganda. N Engl J Med. 2017;377:2456–64.
43. Tamburrini G, Frassanito P, Iakovaki K, Pignotti F, Rendeli C, Murolo D, Di Rocco C. Myelomeningocele: the management of the associated hydrocephalus. Childs Nerv Syst. 2013;29:1569–79.
44. Amelot A, Beccaria K, Blauwblomme T, Bourgeois M, Paternoster G, Cuny ML, Zerah M, Sainte-Rose C, Puget S. Microsurgical, endoscopic, and shunt management of pediatric temporosylvian arachnoid cysts: a comparative study. J Neurosurg Pediatr. 2019;23:749–57.
45. Andre A, Zerah M, Roujeau T, Brunelle F, Blauwblomme T, Puget S, Bourgeois M, Sainte-Rose C, Ville Y, Di Rocco F. Suprasellar arachnoid cysts: toward a new simple classification based on prognosis and treatment modality. Neurosurgery. 2016;78:370–9; discussion 379–80.
46. Schulz M, Oezkan Y, Schaumann A, Sieg M, Tietze A, Thomale UW. Surgical management of intracranial arachnoid cysts in pediatric patients: radiological and clinical outcome. J Neurosurg Pediatr. 2021;28:1–11.
47. Yengo-Kahn AM, Wellons JC, Hankinson TC, Hauptman JS, Jackson EM, Jensen H, Krieger MD, Kulkarni AV, Limbrick DD, McDonald PJ, Naftel RP, Pindrik JA, Pollack IF, Reeder R, Riva-Cambrin J, Rozzelle CJ, Tamber MS, Whitehead WE, Kestle JRW, Hydrocephalus Clinical Research Network. Treatment strategies for hydrocephalus related to Dandy-Walker syndrome: evaluating procedure selection and success within the Hydrocephalus Clinical Research Network. J Neurosurg Pediatr. 2021;1–9.
48. Bartoli A, Soleman J, Berger A, Wisoff JH, Hidalgo ET, Mangano FT, Keating RF, Thomale UW, Boop F, Roth J, Constantini S. Treatment options for hydrocephalus following foramen magnum decompression for Chiari I malformation: a multicenter study. Neurosurgery. 2020;86:500–8.
49. Bonfield CM, Shannon CN, Reeder RW, Browd S, Drake J, Hauptman JS, Kulkarni AV, Limbrick DD, McDonald PJ, Naftel R, Pollack IF, Riva-Cambrin J, Rozzelle C, Tamber MS, Whitehead WE, Kestle JRW, Wellons JC, Hydrocephalus Clinical Research Network. Hydrocephalus treatment in patients with craniosynostosis: an analysis from the Hydrocephalus Clinical Research Network prospective registry. Neurosurg Focus. 2021;50:E11.
50. Coll G, El Ouadih Y, Abed Rabbo F, Jecko V, Sakka L, Di Rocco F. Hydrocephalus and Chiari malformation pathophysiology in FGFR2-related faciocraniosynostosis: a review. Neurochirurgie. 2019;65:264–8.
51. Di Rocco F, Juca CE, Arnaud E, Renier D, Sainte-Rose C. The role of endoscopic third ventriculostomy in the treatment of hydrocephalus associated with faciocraniosynostosis. J Neurosurg Pediatr. 2010;6:17–22.
52. Wong TT, Liang ML, Chen HH, Chang FC. Hydrocephalus with brain tumors in children. Childs Nerv Syst. 2011;27:1723–34.
53. Di Rocco F, Juca CE, Zerah M, Sainte-Rose C. Endoscopic third ventriculostomy and posterior fossa tumors. World Neurosurg. 2013;79:S18.e15–9.
54. Ray P, Jallo GI, Kim RY, Kim BS, Wilson S, Kothbauer K, Abbott R. Endoscopic third ventriculostomy for tumor-related hydrocephalus in a pediatric population. Neurosurg Focus. 2005;19:E8.
55. Sherrod BA, Iyer RR, Kestle JRW. Endoscopic third ventriculostomy for pediatric tumor-associated hydrocephalus. Neurosurg Focus. 2020;48:E5.
56. Roth J, Constantini S. Combined rigid and flexible endoscopy for tumors in the posterior third ventricle. J Neurosurg. 2015;122:1341–6.
57. Schulz M, Afshar-Bakshloo M, Koch A, Capper D, Driever PH, Tietze A, Grun A, Thomale UW. Management of pineal region tumors in a pediatric case series. Neurosurg Rev. 2021;44:1417–27.

58. Mohme M, Fritzsche FS, Mende KC, Matschke J, Lobel U, Kammler G, Westphal M, Emami P, Martens T. Tectal gliomas: assessment of malignant progression, clinical management, and quality of life in a supposedly benign neoplasm. Neurosurg Focus. 2018;44:E15.
59. Niknejad HR, Frederickx M, Salaets E, Lemiere J, Lagae L, Van Calenbergh F. Long-term outcomes of patients with hydrocephalus secondary to tectal plate glioma versus idiopathic aqueductal stenosis: results from a single center. Pediatr Neurosurg. 2021;56:317–27.
60. Roth J, Chaichana KL, Jallo G, Mirone G, Cinalli G, Constantini S. True aqueductal tumors: a unique entity. Acta Neurochir (Wien). 2015;157:169–77.
61. Donahue B, Allen J, Siffert J, Rosovsky M, Pinto R. Patterns of recurrence in brain stem gliomas: evidence for craniospinal dissemination. Int J Radiat Oncol Biol Phys. 1998;40:677–80.
62. Schiff D, Kline C, Meltzer H, Auger J. Palliative ventriculoperitoneal shunt in a pediatric patient with recurrent metastatic medulloblastoma. J Palliat Med. 2009;12:391–3.
63. Won SY, Dubinski D, Behmanesh B, Bernstock JD, Seifert V, Konczalla J, Tritt S, Senft C, Gessler F. Management of hydrocephalus after resection of posterior fossa lesions in pediatric and adult patients-predictors for development of hydrocephalus. Neurosurg Rev. 2020;43:1143–50.
64. Bauer DF, Baird LC, Klimo P, Mazzola CA, Nikas DC, Tamber MS, Flannery AM. Congress of neurological surgeons systematic review and evidence-based guidelines on the treatment of pediatric hydrocephalus: update of the 2014 guidelines. Neurosurgery. 2020;87:1071–5.
65. Rekate HL. The pediatric neurosurgical patient: the challenge of growing up. Semin Pediatr Neurol. 2009;16:2–8.
66. Thomale UW, Auer C, Spennato P, Schaumann A, Behrens P, Gorelyshev S, Bogoslovskaia E, Shulaev A, Kabanian A, Seliverstov A, Alexeev A, Ozgural O, Kahilogullari G, Schuhmann M, Jimenez-Guerra R, Wittayanakorn N, Sukharev A, Marquez-Rivas J, Linsler S, Damaty AE, Vacek P, Lovha M, Guzman R, Stricker S, Beez T, Wiegand C, Azab M, Buis D, Saez M, Fleck S, Dziugan C, Ferreira A, Radovnicky T, Buhrer C, Lam S, Sgouros S, Roth J, Constantini S, Cavalheiro S, Cinalli G, Kulkarni AV, Bock HC. TROPHY registry—status report. Childs Nerv Syst. 2021;37:3549–54.
67. Badhiwala JH, Hong CJ, Nassiri F, Hong BY, Riva-Cambrin J, Kulkarni AV. Treatment of posthemorrhagic ventricular dilation in preterm infants: a systematic review and meta-analysis of outcomes and complications. J Neurosurg Pediatr. 2015;16:545–55.
68. Blauwblomme T, Di Rocco F, Bourgeois M, Beccaria K, Paternoster G, Verchere-Montmayeur J, Sainte-Rose C, Zerah M, Puget S. Subdural to subgaleal shunts: alternative treatment in infants with nonaccidental traumatic brain injury? J Neurosurg Pediatr. 2015;15:306–9.
69. Walker CT, Stone JJ, Jacobson M, Phillips V, Silberstein HJ. Indications for pediatric external ventricular drain placement and risk factors for conversion to a ventriculoperitoneal shunt. Pediatr Neurosurg. 2012;48:342–7.
70. Jallo GI, Kothbauer KF, Abbott IR. Endoscopic third ventriculostomy. Neurosurg Focus. 2005;19:E11.
71. Beuriat PA, Puget S, Cinalli G, Blauwblomme T, Beccaria K, Zerah M, Sainte-Rose C. Hydrocephalus treatment in children: long-term outcome in 975 consecutive patients. J Neurosurg Pediatr. 2017;20:10–8.
72. Coulter IC, Kulkarni AV, Sgouros S, Constantini S, International Infant Hydrocephalus Study Investigators, Constantini S, Sgouros S, Kulkarni AV, Leitner Y, Kestle JR, Cochrane DD, Choux M, Gjerris F, Sherer A, Akalan N, Bilginer B, Navarro R, Vujotic L, Haberl H, Thomale UW, Zuccaro G, Jaimovitch R, Frim D, Loftis L, Swift DM, Robertson B, Gargan L, Bognar L, Novak L, Cseke G, Cama A, Ravegnani GM, Preuss M, Schroeder HW, Fritsch M, Baldauf J, Mandera M, Luszawski J, Skorupka P, Mallucci C, Williams D, Zakrzewski K, Nowoslawska E, Srivastava C, Mahapatra AK, Kumar R, Sahu RN, Melikian AG, Korshunov A, Galstyan A, Suri A, Gupta D, Grotenhuis JA, van Lindert EJ, da Costa Val JA, Di Rocco C, Tamburrini G, Zymberg ST, Cavalheiro S, Jie M, Feng J, Friedman O, Rajmohamed N, Roszkowski M, Barszcz S, Jallo G, Pincus DW, Richter B, Mehdorn HM, Schultka S, de Ribaupierre S, Thompson D, Gatscher S, Wagner W, Koch D, Cipri S, Zaccone C, McDonald P. Cranial and ventricular size following shunting or endoscopic third ventriculostomy (ETV) in infants with aqueductal stenosis: further insights from the International Infant Hydrocephalus Study (IIHS). Childs Nerv Syst. 2020;36:1407–14.
73. Knaus H, Abbushi A, Hoffmann KT, Schwarz K, Haberl H, Thomale UW. Measurements of burr-hole localization for endoscopic procedures in the third ventricle in children. Childs Nerv Syst. 2009;25:293–9.
74. Kulkarni AV, Riva-Cambrin J, Holubkov R, Browd SR, Cochrane DD, Drake JM, Limbrick DD, Rozzelle CJ, Simon TD, Tamber MS, Wellons JC 3rd, Whitehead WE, Kestle JR, Hydrocephalus Clinical Research Network. Endoscopic third ventriculostomy in children: prospective, multicenter results from the Hydrocephalus Clinical Research Network. J Neurosurg Pediatr. 2016;18:423–9.
75. Kulkarni AV, Sgouros S, Constantini S, International Infant Hydrocephalus Study Investigators. Outcome of treatment after failed endoscopic third ventriculostomy (ETV) in infants with aqueductal stenosis: results from the International Infant Hydrocephalus Study (IIHS). Childs Nerv Syst. 2017;33:747–52.
76. Kulkarni AV, Riva-Cambrin J, Browd SR. Use of the ETV Success Score to explain the variation in reported endoscopic third ventriculos-

tomy success rates among published case series of childhood hydrocephalus. J Neurosurg Pediatr. 2011;7:143–6.
77. Kulkarni AV, Sgouros S, Constantini S, Investigators I. International Infant Hydrocephalus Study: initial results of a prospective, multicenter comparison of endoscopic third ventriculostomy (ETV) and shunt for infant hydrocephalus. Childs Nerv Syst. 2016;32:1039–48.
78. Kulkarni AV, Sgouros S, Leitner Y, Constantini S, International Infant Hydrocephalus Study Investigators. International Infant Hydrocephalus Study (IIHS): 5-year health outcome results of a prospective, multicenter comparison of endoscopic third ventriculostomy (ETV) and shunt for infant hydrocephalus. Childs Nerv Syst. 2018;34:2391–7.
79. Bouras T, Sgouros S. Complications of endoscopic third ventriculostomy. J Neurosurg Pediatr. 2011;7:643–9.
80. Javadpour M, May P, Mallucci C. Sudden death secondary to delayed closure of endoscopic third ventriculostomy. Br J Neurosurg. 2003;17:266–9.
81. Lipina R, Palecek T, Reguli S, Kovarova M. Death in consequence of late failure of endoscopic third ventriculostomy. Childs Nerv Syst. 2007;23:815–9.
82. Kulkarni AV, Drake JM, Kestle JR, Mallucci CL, Sgouros S, Constantini S, Canadian Pediatric Neurosurgery Study Group. Predicting who will benefit from endoscopic third ventriculostomy compared with shunt insertion in childhood hydrocephalus using the ETV Success Score. J Neurosurg Pediatr. 2010;6:310–5.
83. Warf BC. Comparison of endoscopic third ventriculostomy alone and combined with choroid plexus cauterization in infants younger than 1 year of age: a prospective study in 550 African children. J Neurosurg. 2005;103:475–81.
84. Warf BC. Hydrocephalus in Uganda: the predominance of infectious origin and primary management with endoscopic third ventriculostomy. J Neurosurg. 2005;102:1–15.
85. Riva-Cambrin J, Kestle JRW, Rozzelle CJ, Naftel RP, Alvey JS, Reeder RW, Holubkov R, Browd SR, Cochrane DD, Limbrick DD, Shannon CN, Simon TD, Tamber MS, Wellons JC, Whitehead WE, Kulkarni AV, Hydrocephalus Clinical Research Network. Predictors of success for combined endoscopic third ventriculostomy and choroid plexus cauterization in a North American setting: a Hydrocephalus Clinical Research Network study. J Neurosurg Pediatr. 2019;24:128–38.
86. Knaus H, Matthias S, Koch A, Thomale UW. Single burr hole endoscopic biopsy with third ventriculostomy-measurements and computer-assisted planning. Childs Nerv Syst. 2011;27:1233–41.
87. Finger T, Schaumann A, Schulz M, Thomale UW. Augmented reality in intraventricular neuroendoscopy. Acta Neurochir (Wien). 2017;159:1033–41.
88. d'Arcangues C, Schulz M, Buhrer C, Thome U, Krause M, Thomale UW. Extended experience with neuroendoscopic lavage for posthemorrhagic hydrocephalus in neonates. World Neurosurg. 2018;116:e217–24.
89. Etus V, Kahilogullari G, Karabagli H, Unlu A. Early endoscopic ventricular irrigation for the treatment of neonatal posthemorrhagic hydrocephalus: a feasible treatment option or not? A multicenter study. Turk Neurosurg. 2018;28:137–41.
90. Frassanito P, Serrao F, Gallini F, Bianchi F, Massimi L, Vento G, Tamburrini G. Ventriculosubgaleal shunt and neuroendoscopic lavage: refining the treatment algorithm of neonatal post-hemorrhagic hydrocephalus. Childs Nerv Syst. 2021;37:3531–40.
91. Honeyman SI, Boukas A, Jayamohan J, Magdum S. Neuroendoscopic lavage for the management of neonatal post-haemorrhagic hydrocephalus: a retrospective series. Childs Nerv Syst. 2022;38:115–21.
92. Tirado-Caballero J, Herreria-Franco J, Rivero-Garvia M, Moreno-Madueno G, Mayorga-Buiza MJ, Marquez-Rivas J. Technical nuances in neuroendoscopic lavage for germinal matrix hemorrhage in preterm infants: twenty tips and pearls after more than one hundred procedures. Pediatr Neurosurg. 2021;56:392–400.
93. Ochoa A, Arganaraz R, Mantese B. Neuroendoscopic lavage for the treatment of pyogenic ventriculitis in children: personal series and review of the literature. Childs Nerv Syst. 2021;38(3):597–604.
94. Boockvar JA, Loudon W, Sutton LN. Development of the Spitz-Holter valve in Philadelphia. J Neurosurg. 2001;95:145–7.
95. Carrington KW. Ventriculo-venous shunt using the Holter valve as a treatment of hydrocephalus. J Mich State Med Soc. 1959;58:373–376 passim.
96. Cushing H, Sladen FJ. Obstructive hydrocephalus following cerebrospinal meningitis, with intraventricular injection of Antimeningitis Serum (Flexner). J Exp Med. 1908;10:548–56.
97. Dandy WE. The operative treatment of communicating hydrocephalus. Ann Surg. 1938;108:194–202.
98. Rekate HL. Shunt revision: complications and their prevention. Pediatr Neurosurg. 1991;17:155–62.
99. Gutowski P, Golz L, Rot S, Lemcke J, Thomale UW. Gravitational shunt valves in hydrocephalus to challenge the sequelae of over-drainage. Expert Rev Med Devices. 2020;17:1155–68.
100. Drake JM, Kestle JR, Tuli S. CSF shunts 50 years on—past, present and future. Childs Nerv Syst. 2000;16:800–4.
101. Whitehead WE, Riva-Cambrin J, Wellons JC 3rd, Kulkarni AV, Browd S, Limbrick D, Rozzelle C, Tamber MS, Simon TD, Shannon CN, Holubkov R, Oakes WJ, Luerssen TG, Walker ML, Drake JM, Kestle JR, Hydrocephalus Clinical Research Network. Factors associated with ventricular

catheter movement and inaccurate catheter location: post hoc analysis of the hydrocephalus clinical research network ultrasound-guided shunt placement study. J Neurosurg Pediatr. 2014;14:173–8.
102. Whitehead WE, Riva-Cambrin J, Wellons JC, Kulkarni AV, Limbrick DD, Wall VL, Rozzelle CJ, Hankinson TC, McDonald PJ, Krieger MD, Pollack IF, Tamber MS, Pindrik J, Hauptman JS, Naftel RP, Shannon CN, Chu J, Jackson EM, Browd SR, Simon TD, Holubkov R, Reeder RW, Jensen H, Koschnitzky JE, Gross P, Drake JM, Kestle JRW. Anterior versus posterior entry site for ventriculoperitoneal shunt insertion: a randomized controlled trial by the Hydrocephalus Clinical Research Network. J Neurosurg Pediatr. 2021;1–11.
103. Hayhurst C, Beems T, Jenkinson MD, Byrne P, Clark S, Kandasamy J, Goodden J, Nandoe Tewarie RD, Mallucci CL. Effect of electromagnetic-navigated shunt placement on failure rates: a prospective multicenter study. J Neurosurg. 2010;113:1273–8.
104. Thomale UW, Knitter T, Schaumann A, Ahmadi SA, Ziegler P, Schulz M, Miethke C. Smartphone-assisted guide for the placement of ventricular catheters. Childs Nerv Syst. 2013;29:131–9.
105. Thomale UW, Schaumann A, Stockhammer F, Giese H, Schuster D, Kastner S, Ahmadi AS, Polemikos M, Bock HC, Golz L, Lemcke J, Hermann E, Schuhmann MU, Beez T, Fritsch M, Orakcioglu B, Vajkoczy P, Rohde V, Bohner G. GAVCA study: randomized, multicenter trial to evaluate the quality of ventricular catheter placement with a mobile health assisted guidance technique. Neurosurgery. 2018;83:252–62.
106. Whitehead WE, Riva-Cambrin J, Wellons JC 3rd, Kulkarni AV, Holubkov R, Illner A, Oakes WJ, Luerssen TG, Walker ML, Drake JM, Kestle JR, Hydrocephalus Clinical Research Network. No significant improvement in the rate of accurate ventricular catheter location using ultrasound-guided CSF shunt insertion: a prospective, controlled study by the Hydrocephalus Clinical Research Network. J Neurosurg Pediatr. 2013;12:565–74.
107. Kestle JR. Shunt insertion. J Neurosurg. 2013;119:64.
108. Oi S, Matsumoto S. Hydrocephalus in premature infants. Characteristics and therapeutic problems. Childs Nerv Syst. 1989;5:76–82.
109. Browd SR, Gottfried ON, Ragel BT, Kestle JR. Failure of cerebrospinal fluid shunts: part II: overdrainage, loculation, and abdominal complications. Pediatr Neurol. 2006;34:171–6.
110. Browd SR, Ragel BT, Gottfried ON, Kestle JR. Failure of cerebrospinal fluid shunts: part I: obstruction and mechanical failure. Pediatr Neurol. 2006;34:83–92.
111. Kestle JR. Shunt malfunction. J Neurosurg. 2010;113:1270–1; discussion 1271–2.
112. Kestle JR, Riva-Cambrin J, Wellons JC 3rd, Kulkarni AV, Whitehead WE, Walker ML, Oakes WJ, Drake JM, Luerssen TG, Simon TD, Holubkov R, Hydrocephalus Clinical Research Network. A standardized protocol to reduce cerebrospinal fluid shunt infection: the Hydrocephalus Clinical Research Network Quality Improvement Initiative. J Neurosurg Pediatr. 2011;8:22–9.
113. Kestle JR, Holubkov R, Douglas Cochrane D, Kulkarni AV, Limbrick DD Jr, Luerssen TG, Jerry Oakes W, Riva-Cambrin J, Rozzelle C, Simon TD, Walker ML, Wellons JC 3rd, Browd SR, Drake JM, Shannon CN, Tamber MS, Whitehead WE, Hydrocephalus Clinical Research Network. A new Hydrocephalus Clinical Research Network protocol to reduce cerebrospinal fluid shunt infection. J Neurosurg Pediatr. 2016;17:391–6.
114. Riva-Cambrin J, Kestle JR, Holubkov R, Butler J, Kulkarni AV, Drake J, Whitehead WE, Wellons JC 3rd, Shannon CN, Tamber MS, Limbrick DD Jr, Rozzelle C, Browd SR, Simon TD, Hydrocephalus Clinical Research Network. Risk factors for shunt malfunction in pediatric hydrocephalus: a multicenter prospective cohort study. J Neurosurg Pediatr. 2016;17:382–90.
115. Sciubba DM, Noggle JC, Carson BS, Jallo GI. Antibiotic-impregnated shunt catheters for the treatment of infantile hydrocephalus. Pediatr Neurosurg. 2008;44:91–6.
116. Drake JM, Kestle JR, Milner R, Cinalli G, Boop F, Piatt J Jr, Haines S, Schiff SJ, Cochrane DD, Steinbok P, MacNeil N. Randomized trial of cerebrospinal fluid shunt valve design in pediatric hydrocephalus. Neurosurgery. 1998;43:294–303; discussion 303–5.
117. Drake JM, Kestle JT. Determining the best cerebrospinal fluid shunt valve design: the pediatric valve design trial. Neurosurgery. 1998;43:1259–60.
118. Kestle J, Drake J, Milner R, Sainte-Rose C, Cinalli G, Boop F, Piatt J, Haines S, Schiff S, Cochrane D, Steinbok P, MacNeil N. Long-term follow-up data from the Shunt Design Trial. Pediatr Neurosurg. 2000;33:230–6.
119. Kestle JRW, Riva-Cambrin J. Prospective multicenter studies in pediatric hydrocephalus. J Neurosurg Pediatr. 2019;23:135–41.
120. Fernandez Cornejo VJ, Elbabaa SK. Shunt technology for infants and a lifetime. Childs Nerv Syst. 2021;37:3475–84.
121. Hatlen TJ, Shurtleff DB, Loeser JD, Ojemann JG, Avellino AM, Ellenbogen RG. Nonprogrammable and programmable cerebrospinal fluid shunt valves: a 5-year study. J Neurosurg Pediatr. 2012;9:462–7.
122. Pollack IF, Albright AL, Adelson PD. A randomized, controlled study of a programmable shunt valve versus a conventional valve for patients with hydrocephalus. Hakim-Medos Investigator Group. Neurosurgery. 1999;45:1399–408; discussion 1408–11.
123. Czosnyka M, Czosnyka Z, Pickard JD. Programmable Shunt Assistant tested in Cambridge shunt evaluation laboratory. Acta Neurochir Suppl. 2012;113:71–6.
124. Kimura T, Schulz M, Shimoji K, Miyajima M, Arai H, Thomale UW. In vitro performance of the fixed

and adjustable gravity-assisted unit with and without motion-evidence of motion-induced flow. Acta Neurochir (Wien). 2016;158:2011–8.
125. Myles LM, Neil-Dwyer G. Ventriculo-atrial shunt insertion: pressure monitoring as an aid to accurate placement. Br J Neurosurg. 2000;14:462–3.
126. Segura-Hernandez A, Hakim F, Ramon JF, Jimenez-Hakim E, Mejia-Cordovez JA, Quintero-Rueda D, Araque-Puello Y, Pedraza-Ciro C, Leal-Isaza JP, Mendoza-Mantilla J, Robles V, Gonzalez M, Jaramillo-Velasquez D, Gomez DF. Ventriculo-atrial shunt. Comparison of an ultrasound-guided peel-away technique versus conventional technique in the management of normal pressure hydrocephalus: a retrospective cohort. Surg Neurol Int. 2021;12:531.
127. Baro V, Leon FF, Sartori L, Denaro L. Ultrasound-guided percutaneous ventriculopleural shunt placement: a minimally invasive technique. Childs Nerv Syst. 2020;36:617–20.
128. Christian EA, Quezada JJ, Melamed EF, Lai C, McComb JG. Ventriculopleural shunts in a pediatric population: a review of 170 consecutive patients. J Neurosurg Pediatr. 2021;28:450–7.
129. Girotti ME, Singh RR, Rodgers BM. The ventriculo-gallbladder shunt in the treatment of refractory hydrocephalus: a review of the current literature. Am Surg. 2009;75:734–7.
130. Pancucci G, Plaza-Ramirez E, Driller C, Miranda-Lloret P, Botella-Asuncion C. Laparoscopy-assisted placement of a ventriculobiliary shunt: a technical note. Childs Nerv Syst. 2019;35:1397–400.
131. Bock HC, Kanzler M, Thomale UW, Ludwig HC. Implementing a digital real-time Hydrocephalus and Shunt Registry to evaluate contemporary pattern of care and surgical outcome in pediatric hydrocephalus. Childs Nerv Syst. 2018;34:457–64.
132. Gebert AF, Schulz M, Haberl H, Thomale UW. Adjustments in gravitational valves for the treatment of childhood hydrocephalus—a retrospective survey. Childs Nerv Syst. 2013;29:2019–25.
133. Gebert AF, Schulz M, Schwarz K, Thomale UW. Long-term survival rates of gravity-assisted, adjustable differential pressure valves in infants with hydrocephalus. J Neurosurg Pediatr. 2016;17:544–51.
134. Vinchon M, Rekate H, Kulkarni AV. Pediatric hydrocephalus outcomes: a review. Fluids Barriers CNS. 2012;9:18.
135. Nilsson D, Svensson J, Korkmaz BA, Nelvig H, Tisell M. Decreased head circumference in shunt-treated compared with healthy children. J Neurosurg Pediatr. 2013;12:483–90.
136. Faulhauer K, Schmitz P. Overdrainage phenomena in shunt treated hydrocephalus. Acta Neurochir (Wien). 1978;45:89–101.
137. Pudenz RH, Foltz EL. Hydrocephalus: overdrainage by ventricular shunts. A review and recommendations. Surg Neurol. 1991;35:200–12.
138. Rekate HL. Shunt-related headaches: the slit ventricle syndromes. Childs Nerv Syst. 2008;24:423–30.
139. Alavi S, Schulz M, Schaumann A, Schwarz K, Thomale UW. Valve exchange towards an adjustable differential pressure valve with gravitational unit, clinical outcome of a single-center study. Childs Nerv Syst. 2017;33:759–65.
140. Pennacchietti V, Prinz V, Schaumann A, Finger T, Schulz M, Thomale UW. Single center experiences with telemetric intracranial pressure measurements in patients with CSF circulation disturbances. Acta Neurochir (Wien). 2020;162:2487–97.
141. Fritsch MJ, Kienke S, Manwaring KH, Mehdorn HM. Endoscopic aqueductoplasty and interventriculostomy for the treatment of isolated fourth ventricle in children. Neurosurgery. 2004;55:372–7; discussion 377–9.
142. Huang JY, Chiu NC, Liang ML, Chen HJ, Lin YJ, Ho CS. Application of sonography in the diagnosis and follow-up of trapped temporal horn of lateral ventricle: two case reports. J Med Ultrasound. 2019;27:154–7.
143. Krahenbuhl AK, Baldauf J, Gaab MR, Schroeder HW. Endoscopic temporal ventriculocisternostomy: an option for the treatment of trapped temporal horns. J Neurosurg Pediatr. 2013;11:568–74.
144. Antes S, Salah M, Linsler S, Tschan CA, Breuskin D, Oertel J. Aqueductal stenting with an intra-catheter endoscope—a technical note. Childs Nerv Syst. 2016;32:359–63.
145. Cinalli G, Spennato P, Savarese L, Ruggiero C, Aliberti F, Cuomo L, Cianciulli E, Maggi G. Endoscopic aqueductoplasty and placement of a stent in the cerebral aqueduct in the management of isolated fourth ventricle in children. J Neurosurg. 2006;104:21–7.
146. Guida L, Beccaria K, Benichi S, Chivet A, de Saint Denis T, James S, Paternoster G, Zerah M, Puget S, Blauwblomme T. Endoscopic aqueductal stenting in the management of pediatric hydrocephalus. J Neurosurg Pediatr. 2020;26:1–7.
147. Schulz M, Goelz L, Spors B, Haberl H, Thomale UW. Endoscopic treatment of isolated fourth ventricle: clinical and radiological outcome. Neurosurgery. 2012;70:847–58; discussion 858–9.
148. El-Ghandour NM. Endoscopic cyst fenestration in the treatment of multiloculated hydrocephalus in children. J Neurosurg Pediatr. 2008;1:217–22.
149. Sandberg DI, McComb JG, Krieger MD. Craniotomy for fenestration of multiloculated hydrocephalus in pediatric patients. Neurosurgery. 2005;57:100–6; discussion 100–6.
150. Schaumann A, Buhrer C, Schulz M, Thomale UW. Neuroendoscopic surgery in neonates—indication and results over a 10-year practice. Childs Nerv Syst. 2021;37:3541–8.

Management of Arachnoid Cysts

4

Spyros Sgouros and Andreas Mitsios

Introduction

Arachnoid cysts are cystic malformations of the arachnoid layer containing cerebrospinal fluid (CSF). The collection of fluid develops within the arachnoid membrane secondary to splitting or duplication of the structural layer.

They have an estimated prevalence of 0.2–2.6% [1, 2, 34, 39, 50]. A recent large study of 11,738 brain MR scans of patients aged 18 years and under revealed the presence of an arachnoid cyst in 309 individuals, a prevalence of 2.6%, with a male preponderance [1]. Another study of 1235 adults over the age of 70 demonstrated prevalence of 2.3% [39]. Arachnoid cysts are nowadays detected more often, as neuroimaging is used more frequently. Commonly, they are discovered as incidental findings at scans performed for other reasons [1].

They may present at any age, but about 60–80% are usually discovered in children before the age of 3–4 years. They are more common in boys than girls, and more often there is a left-sided preponderance. Arachnoid cysts can be seen in the spinal subarachnoid space as well but in much lesser frequency in comparison to the brain.

The occurrence of cysts in neonates, the antenatal diagnosis with modern imaging, the anatomic relationship to the cisterns, and the association with other developmental anomalies support the theory that arachnoid cysts are congenital lesions, developmental in origin and not acquired from other pathological conditions. Cystic formations resembling arachnoid cysts can form in the subarachnoid space following haemorrhage or infection, but these are by-product of arachnoid adhesions and scar tissue formation; hence they are different pathology to the true congenital arachnoid cysts.

Intracranial Arachnoid Cysts

The most common locations are the middle cranial fossa (42%, temporal, Sylvian fissure, the most frequent location; Fig. 4.1a–d), the posterior fossa (24%, midline (Fig. 4.2a) or laterally (Fig. 4.2b–d)), suprasellar region (10%; Fig. 4.3), quadrigeminal cistern (7%; Fig. 4.4), interhemispheric (7%; Fig. 4.5) and other less common locations such as intraventricular and choroidal fissure (Fig. 4.6), prepontine (Fig. 4.7), intrasellar or over the convexity of the hemisphere (Fig. 4.8). Rarely they are seen intraparenchymally. A small proportion of patients, up to 8%, may have multi-

S. Sgouros (✉)
"Iaso" Childrens Hospital, Marousi, Greece

"National and Kapodistrian" University of Athens, Athens, Greece
e-mail: ssgouros@iaso.gr

A. Mitsios
"National and Kapodistrian" University of Athens, Athens, Greece
e-mail: amitsios@iaso.gr

N. Shimony, G. Jallo (eds.), *Pediatric Neurosurgery Board Review*,
https://doi.org/10.1007/978-3-031-23687-7_4

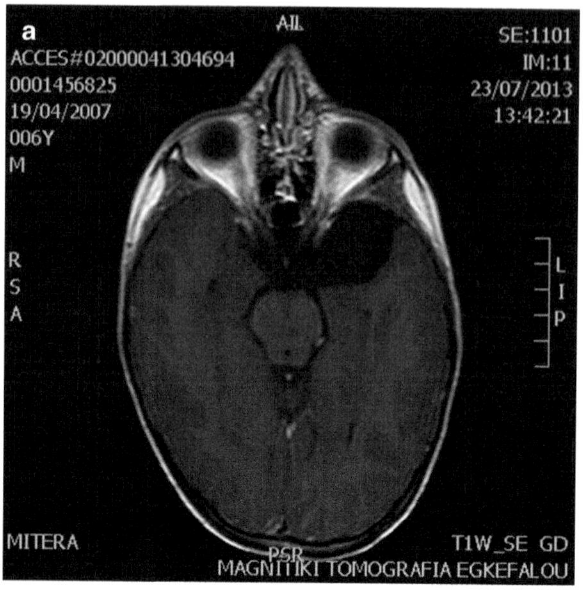

Fig. 4.1 Middle fossa arachnoid cysts. (**a**) Galassi type I: T1-weighted MR scan image of a 6-year-old boy who complained of intermittent headaches. A spindle-shaped arachnoid cyst is seen at the anterior aspect of the left middle cranial fossa, not causing deformation of the overlying temporal bone. He was not offered any treatment as it was considered that his symptoms were not caused by the cyst. His symptoms settled. (**b**) Galassi type II that required surgical treatment: T1-weighted MR scan image of a 5½-year-old boy who presented in 2019 with symptoms of raised intracranial pressure (headaches, intermittent vomiting, papilledema). A quadrangular-shaped arachnoid cyst is seen in the left middle cranial fossa, causing outward deformation and bowing of the overlying temporal bone. He was treated with endoscopic fenestration of the cyst. His symptoms resolved postoperatively. He remains very well 2 years on with no sign of cyst size recurrent increase in follow-up radiological surveillance. In the endoscopic views, seen through the cyst wall are the optic nerve and the carotid artery (top left). The fenestration was performed by pulling the cyst wall with the grabbing forceps and enlarged with balloon dilatation. (**c**) Galassi type III: T2-weighted MR scan images of a 3-month-old boy who presented in 2017 with macrocrania, tense anterior fontanelle and vomiting. There is a large arachnoid cyst in the left middle cranial fossa, extending over the convexity of the hemisphere, causing midline shift and deformation of the overlying cranial bones. He was treated with endoscopic fenestration of the cyst. This had to be re-done a month later but again did not succeed to control the situation. A cyst-peritoneal shunt was inserted, but this later had to be removed because of a subdural haematoma. Eventually endoscopy was re-done, and the child remains well to date. (**d**) Galassi type II that ruptured: T2-weighted MR scan images of a 6-year and 10-month-old boy who in 2014 had head injury while playing basketball; he was hit on the head by the ball unsuspecting. He developed headaches and vomiting after the injury. There is an arachnoid cyst in the right middle cranial fossa, Galassi type II, which has ruptured and formed a subdural hygroma over the convexity of the cerebral hemisphere. He was treated with endoscopic fenestration. Upon dural opening xantho-chromatic subdural fluid under pressure was drained. The fenestration was performed in the region of the carotid cistern. The perforation of the cyst wall was created with the monopolar diathermy electrode used as a blunt probe (no cautery was used) and enlarged with balloon dilatation and scissors. His symptoms settled postoperatively. On subsequent imaging the subdural hygroma had disappeared, and the cyst decreased in size. Seven years on, he remains well and developed normally

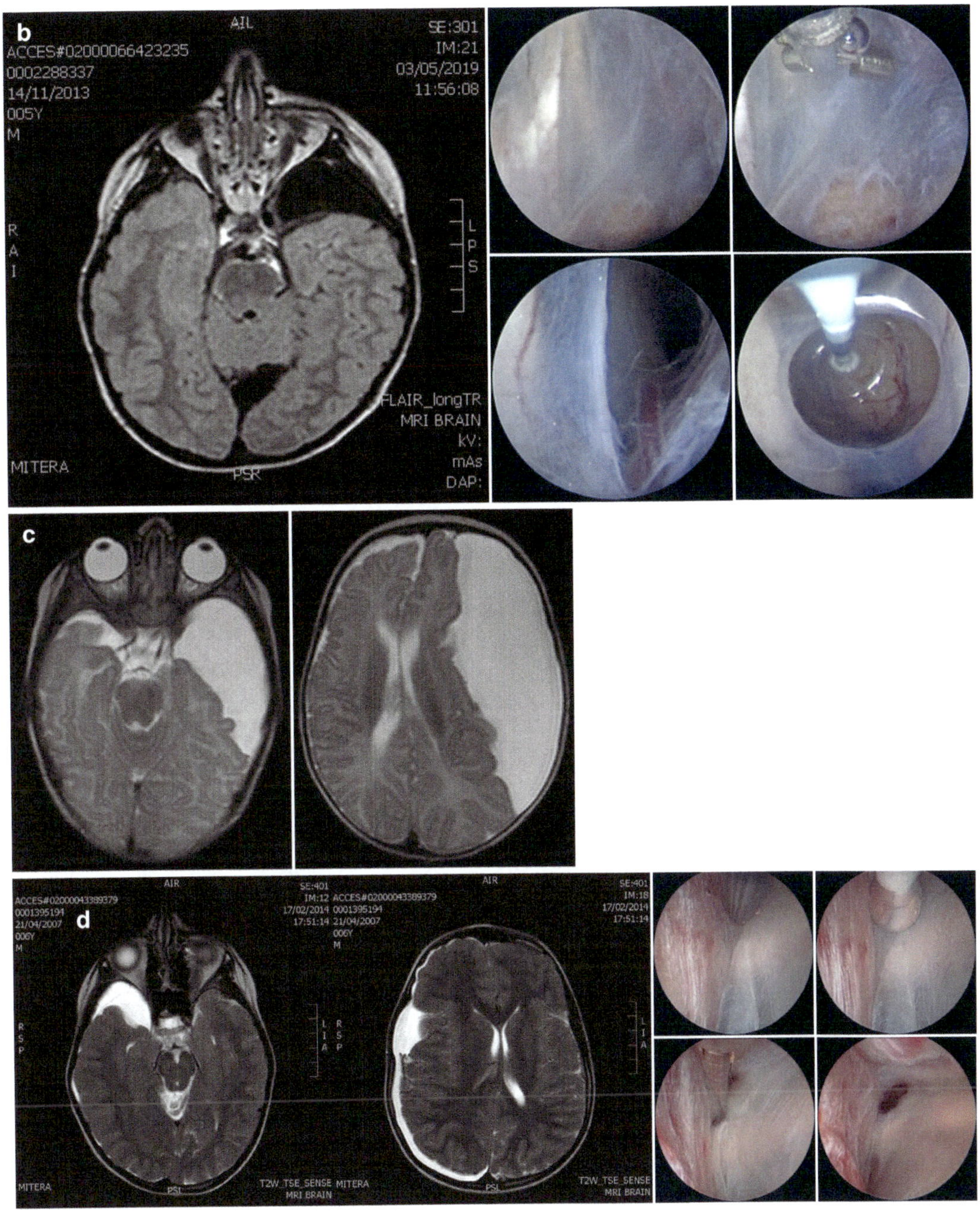

Fig. 4.1 (continued)

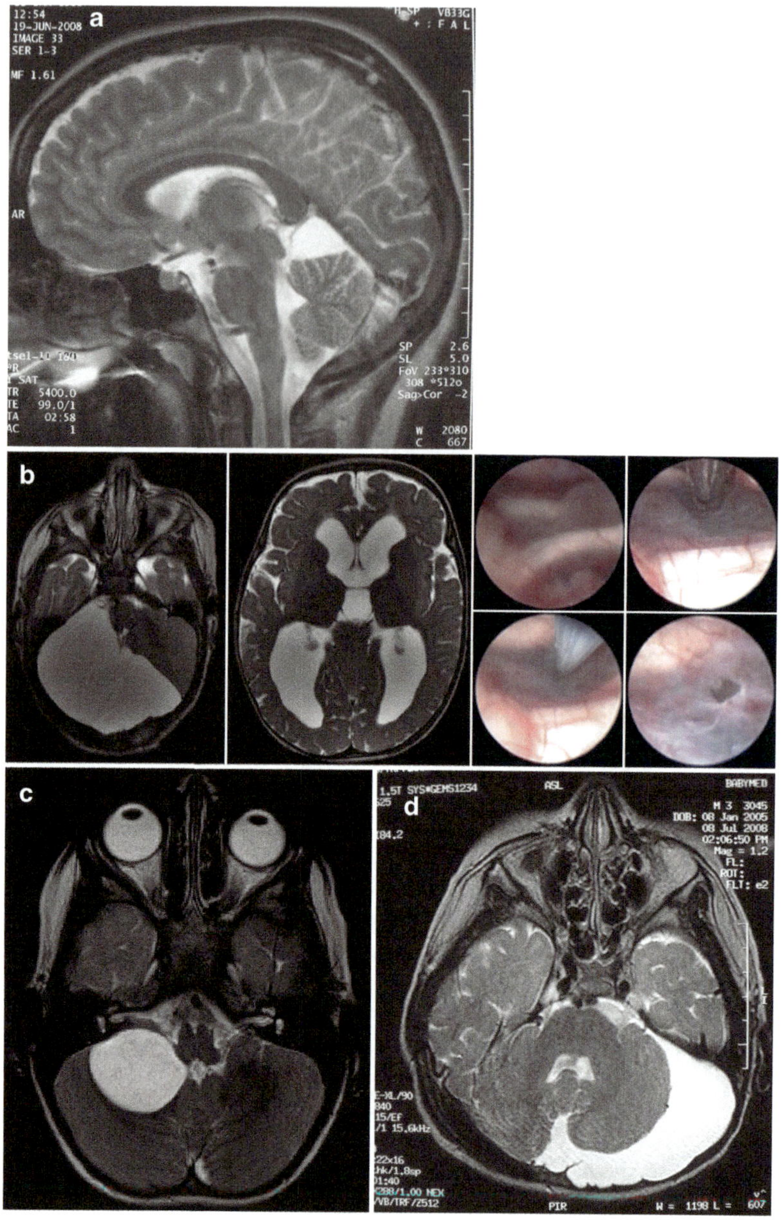

Fig. 4.2 Posterior fossa arachnoid cysts. (**a**) T2-weighted MR scan of an 18-year-old female who was complaining of intermittent headaches. There is a cystic formation containing CSF in the posterior fossa overlying the vermis. It was considered that the cyst was not responsible for her symptoms; hence no treatment was undertaken. Her symptoms settled. (**b**) T2-weighted axial MR scan images of a 6-month-old boy who presented in 2012 with macrocrania, vomiting and tense anterior fontanelle. There is a large arachnoid cyst in the region of the right cerebello-pontine angle, causing compression of the fourth ventricle and hydrocephalus. He was treated surgically with endoscopic fenestration of the wall of the cyst in the region of the seventh/eighth nerve complex. Two separate perforations were made with the monopolar diathermy lead used as a blunt probe and were enlarged with the grasping forceps used as a dilator. No additional treatment was needed for the hydrocephalus as it settled postoperatively. (**c**) T2-weighted axial MR scan image of a 2-year-old boy who presented in 2009 with intermittent unsteady gait. There is an arachnoid cyst in the region of the right cerebello-pontine angle causing indentation on the cerebellar hemisphere. A decision was taken to initially observe the child and reserve surgical treatment if the symptoms deteriorated. He settled and developed normally. He has not required surgical treatment so far. (**d**) T2-weighted axial MR scan image of a 3½-year-old boy who presented with two fainting episodes. There is a retrocerebellar arachnoid cyst on the left which has caused expansion of the overlying occipital bone. He developed no other symptoms, and no treatment was deemed necessary. He developed well

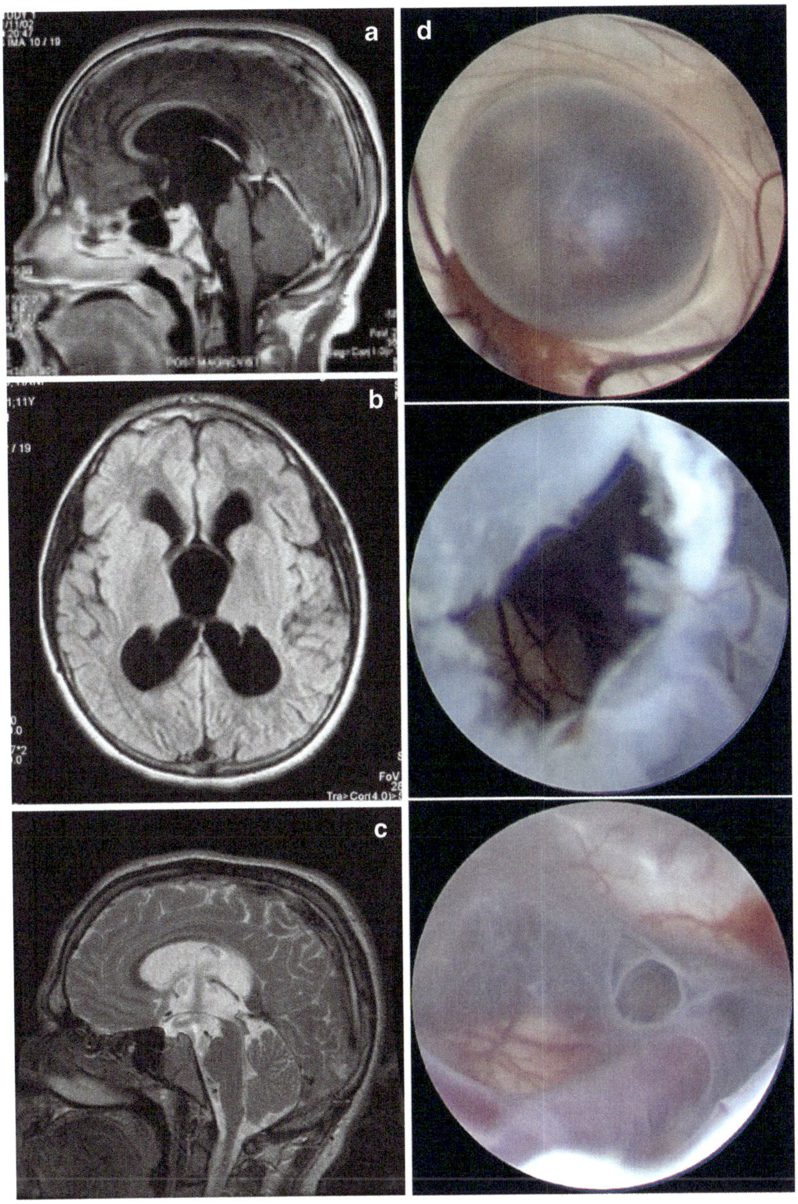

Fig. 4.3 Suprasellar arachnoid cyst. (**a**) T1-weighted sagittal MR scan of an 11-year-old boy who presented in 2002 with headaches, papilledema and stunted growth associated with low growth hormone levels. There is a suprasellar arachnoid cyst causing hydrocephalus. (**b**) Axial image showing the "mickey mouse" appearance that the enlarged lateral ventricles create with the suprasellar cyst. An endoscopic fenestration was performed. He was treated with endoscopic fenestration, mainly for relief of hydrocephalus. (**c**) Postoperative sagittal MR scan showing the flow void of the CSF flow through the cystocisternostomy. The pituitary dysfunction did not recover. (**d**) Endoscopic views during fenestration of suprasellar cyst (patient different to the one of images **a**–**c**). (Top) The endoscope is in the right lateral ventricle. The dome of the cyst is shown through foramen of Monro. The choroid plexus inferiorly, the septal vein to the left and the thalamo-striate vein to the right. (Middle) The fenestration has been performed using the monopolar diathermy cautery. (Bottom) A fenestration has been performed on the inferior wall of the cyst, adjacent to the basilar artery, in effect acting as the third ventriculostomy. The arachnoid membrane on the wall of the basilar artery was seen acting as a filling valve mechanism

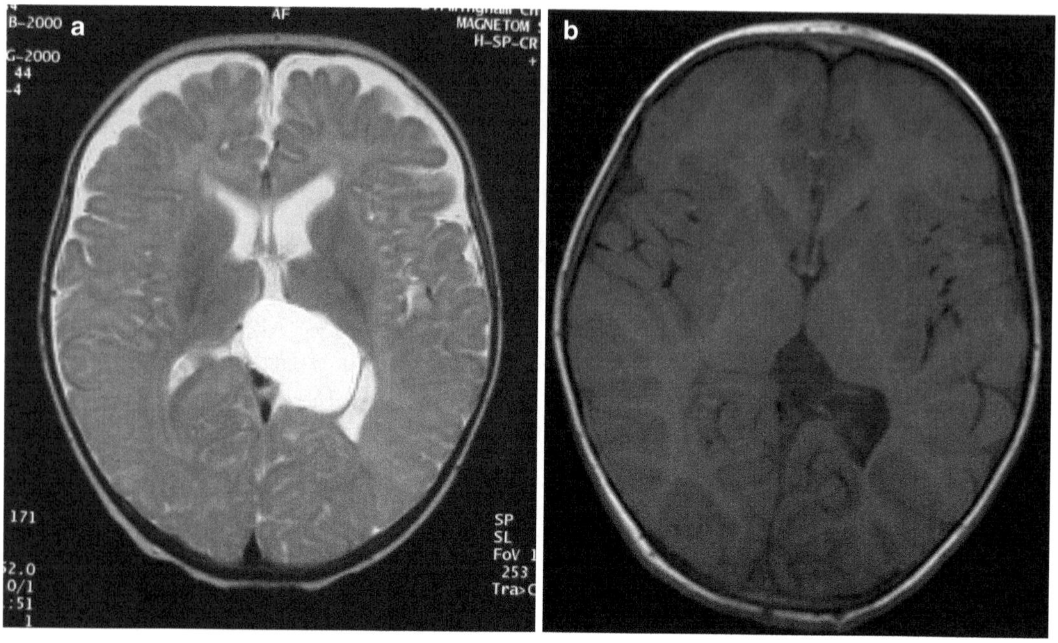

Fig. 4.4 Quadrigeminal cistern arachnoid cyst. (**a**) T2-weighted MR scan of a 6-month-old boy who presented in 2000 with Parinaud syndrome. There is an arachnoid cyst in the quadrigeminal cistern region, causing pressure in the tectal plate and mild ventricular dilatation. A craniotomy and a microsurgical excision of the cyst were performed through a posterior interhemispheric approach. At that time, in year 2000, endoscopic treatment of arachnoid cysts was at an early stage, and the surgeon did not feel comfortable to access that location endoscopically. The clinical signs of Parinaud syndrome settled in the first week postoperatively. (**b**) T1-weighted MR scan performed 12 months postoperatively. The cyst has not reformed and the ventricular system is normal. The child developed normally

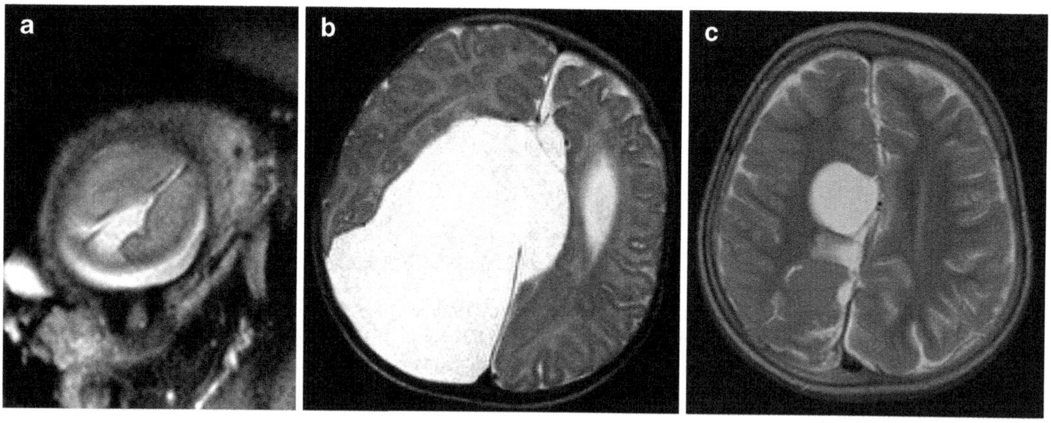

Fig. 4.5 Interhemispheric arachnoid cyst. (**a**) Antenatal MR scan of a foetus with an interhemispheric cyst. A CSF-filled cystic structure is seen adjacent to the falx, displacing the overlying hemisphere. (**b**) Postnatal MR scan, T2-weighted sequence of the baby boy at the age of 3 months, when the baby had developed macrocrania and tense anterior fontanelle. The interhemispheric cyst has increased in size, causing midline shift and causing contralateral ventricular dilatation. An endoscopic fenestration of the cyst to the lateral ventricle was carried out. A month later a ventriculo-peritoneal shunt was inserted to treat the persisting hydrocephalus. (**c**) T2-weighted axial MR scan of the child at the age of 5 years, performed as follow-up. The child was developing well. There is a small residual cyst adjacent to the falx

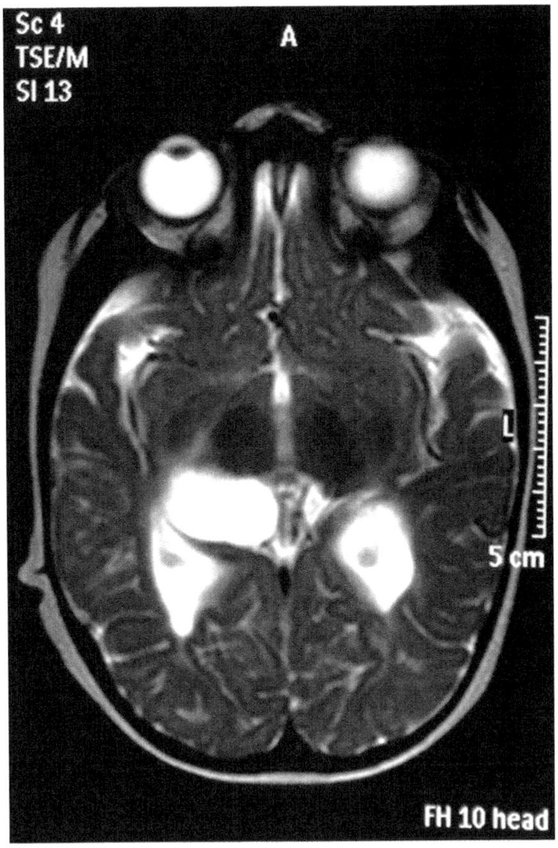

Fig. 4.6 Choroidal fissure arachnoid cyst. T2-weighted MR scan sequence of a 16-month-old boy who presented in 2010 with symptoms of raised intracranial pressure and sixth nerve palsy. There is an arachnoid cyst in the region of the right posterior choroidal fissure. He was subjected to an endoscopic fenestration of the cyst through the atrium of the right lateral ventricle. The sixth nerve palsy settled completely. He has developed to a completely normal 11-year-old boy

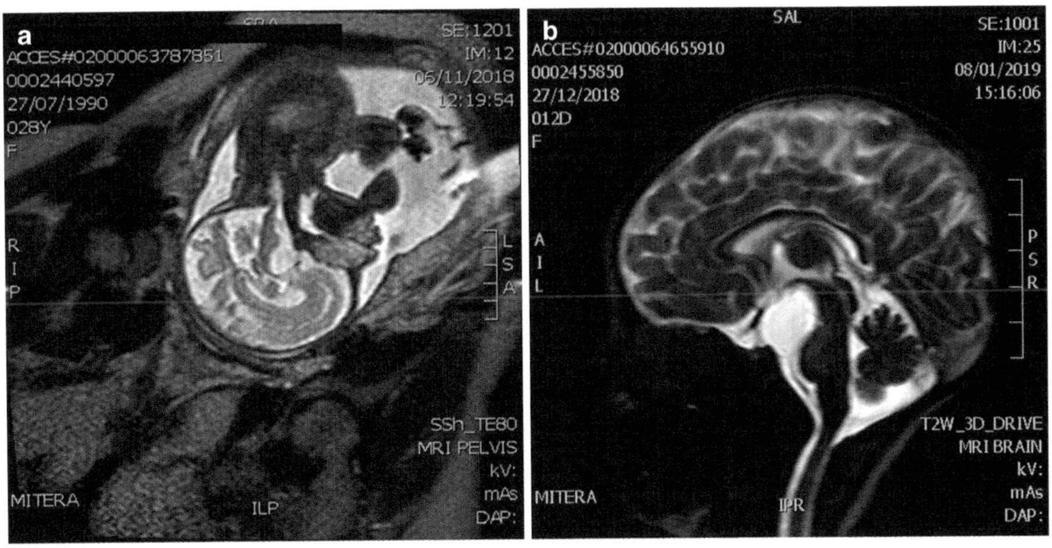

Fig. 4.7 Prepontine arachnoid cyst. (**a**) Antenatal MR scan of a 28-year-old pregnant lady, carrying a foetus found on US scan to have an intracranial cystic lesion. This was further investigated with MR scan. The sagittal projection shows a round lesion in the prepontine cistern with characteristics of an arachnoid cyst. (**b**) Postnatal MR scan, T2-weighted sequence of the baby boy, performed at the 12th day of life. There is a cystic lesion in the prepontine cistern, with well-defined walls, and contents with signal that of CSF. The cyst is in contact with the basilar artery and the anterior surface of the brain stem. The child was asymptomatic and has remained asymptomatic so far. On two subsequent MR scan examinations performed in the first 2 years of life, the cyst has not changed in size. He is developing well, and no treatment has been performed so far

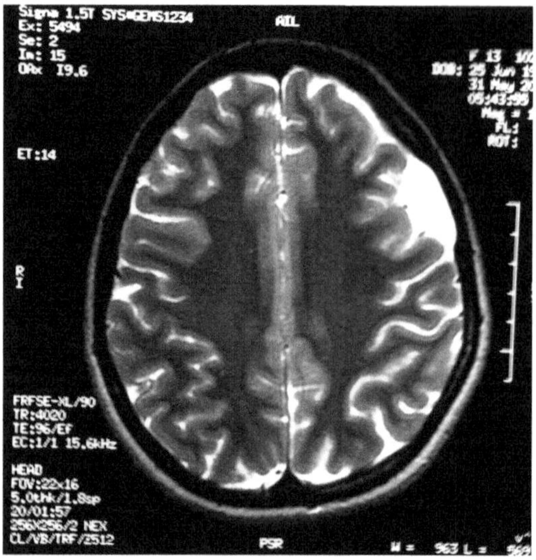

Fig. 4.8 Hemispheric convexity arachnoid cyst. T2-weighted axial MR image of a 13-year-old girl that was complaining of headaches. There is an arachnoid cyst in the left posterior frontal region that has caused indentation on the inner table of the overlying skull. It was considered that the cyst was not the cause of her symptoms and that surgery would not offer any improvement. Hence no surgery was performed. Her symptoms settled

ple arachnoid cysts [22]. Bilateral Sylvian cysts are encountered more often in children suffering from glutaric aciduria type 1 (GAT1).

Etiology and Pathogenesis

The formation of arachnoid cysts is hypothesized to result from abnormal embryologic development of the arachnoid membrane. Early in normal embryonic development, a loose layer of connective tissue called the meninx primitiva, or perimedullary mesh, a precursor to the pia and arachnoid mater, lines the surface of the dura and surrounds the neural tube. At about 15 weeks of gestation, the rhombic roof ruptures, CSF pulses through this mesh and the pia mater and arachnoid mater separate incompletely, resulting in the cobweb-like appearance of the arachnoid. The prevailing hypothesis for arachnoid cyst formation supports the aberrant separation of the arachnoid and pia, which are enclosed forming loculated chambers developing into a cystic mass. Another theory supports that the meninx primitiva formation is aberrant and leads to cyst formation.

Recent studies indicate that fluid secretion may be the main mechanism of filling of arachnoid cysts as increased expression of NKCC1 has been demonstrated in the plasma membranes of the cyst lining cells and that gene is implicated in fluid transport mechanisms [20]. It has been suggested that selective NKCC1 inhibitors could prevent the expansion of temporal arachnoid cysts, although this has not been demonstrated so far.

Natural History

Most arachnoid cysts have a benign natural history and remain stable in size. In a large study of incidentally discovered cerebral arachnoid cysts, in up to 80% of subjects, the arachnoid cysts do not enlarge with time and patients who were discovered over the age of 4 years did not develop any subsequent enlargement of the cyst [1, 22].

A small proportion of cysts increase in size in the first few years of life. This is believed to be due to a slit-valve mechanism that allows CSF to enter the cyst but not return to the subarachnoid space [18, 42]. This is often seen during endoscopic surgery, commonly in middle fossa arachnoid cysts where the valve mechanism is in the region of the carotid cistern and in suprasellar cysts in the vicinity of the basilar artery (Fig. 4.3d). The increase in size can cause symptoms due to mass effect or from secondary hydrocephalus from obstruction of CSF pathways.

Arachnoid cysts can be diagnosed antenatally (Figs. 4.5 and 4.7). Even in large cysts, no antenatal surgical treatment is performed currently, and the situation is reassessed after birth. Often, they increase in size after birth, as the intracranial cavity is exposed to the atmospheric pressure through the open fontanelle (Fig. 4.5). Some babies develop symptoms in association with that increase in size.

It is considered that if a child has not developed symptoms in the first few years of life, commonly he/she will not develop symptoms later.

However, that may not be true for middle fossa arachnoid cysts, which are known to cause symptoms in older children and adolescents, after minor head injury which can result in haemorrhage within the cyst, or rupture of the cyst and formation of subdural hygroma or haematoma.

Clinical Presentation

Many patients with arachnoid cysts are asymptomatic and are diagnosed incidentally when computerized tomography (CT) or magnetic resonance (MR) imaging is performed for an indication likely to be unrelated to the cyst. Some patients have only mild symptoms, even if the cyst is large, and cognition and neurological functions appear normal. This reflects the brain's ability to compensate slow changes of volume and pressure. As treatment for arachnoid cysts is only surgical, the presence of mild or vague symptoms often presents management dilemma, to operate or not.

In symptomatic patients, clinical presentation varies with age and location. Clinical symptoms and signs are related to either generalized increased ICP or to focal symptoms related to anatomical location of the cyst [46].

Infants may present with progressive macrocephaly, enlarged tense fontanelle, suture diastasis, irritability, failure to thrive and developmental delay. Developmental delay in the absence of symptoms of intracranial hypertension is not considered to be due to the cyst; hence it is not regarded an indication for surgery. Commonly infants are investigated first with ultrasound (US) scan, and if an arachnoid cyst is diagnosed, further imaging with MR scan is performed.

In older children and adults, the most frequent symptoms are those of raised intracranial pressure such as headache and dizziness [49] which can progress to nausea and vomiting, lethargy, sixth nerve palsy and papilledema especially in children. Patients with such symptoms are investigated with CT or MR scan depending on local availability, and the presence of arachnoid cyst is demonstrated.

The association between size of the cyst and raised intracranial pressure (ICP) as well as raised ICP and symptoms has not been clarified yet. Increased ICP has been documented in some studies only in patients with large cysts, whereas children with smaller cysts have a normal ICP [7, 14, 44]. Correlation between intracystic pressure and preoperative symptoms has been demonstrated in some studies [21]. Large middle fossa arachnoid cysts can cause shift of midline structures and signal change in the underlying white matter of the hemisphere, all indications of raised ICP, but the association of these findings with symptoms is unclear.

Several reports exist of patients with psychiatric manifestations, who were found to have arachnoid cysts and whose symptoms settled after successful surgical treatment of the arachnoid cyst [3, 51]. There is no obvious explanation of the cause of such psychiatric manifestations.

Arachnoid cysts of the middle cranial fossa may be associated with haemorrhage or rupture, following minor blunt head trauma. This is seen infrequently, mostly in children and adolescents who had previously undiagnosed arachnoid cyst and suffered minor trauma at school or during sports. They present with acute headaches and vomiting, and MR scan shows middle fossa arachnoid cyst with elements of haemorrhage within it or in association with it or subdural haematoma or hygroma due to rupture of the cyst (Fig. 4.1d). In a series reported by Parsch and colleagues, 2.43% of the subdural haematomas and hygromas observed were related to the rupture of a Sylvian fissure arachnoid cyst [36]. In a series of 168 temporal arachnoid cysts, 6.5% were found to have intracystic or subdural haematomas. The exact risk of haemorrhage or rupture of arachnoid cyst is unknown though as so far there has been no longitudinal study monitoring patients with asymptomatic arachnoid cysts to see how many will suffer haemorrhage or rupture.

Middle fossa arachnoid cysts can cause facial asymmetry due to focal bowing of the overlying temporal bone and distortion of the adjacent orbit in extreme cases.

Suprasellar arachnoid cysts can produce endocrinological symptoms (e.g. diabetes insipidus) or short stature (due to growth hormone deficiency) related to deformity of the pituitary stalk and visual disturbance from the displacement of the optic apparatus.

Quadrigeminal cistern arachnoid cysts can cause Parinaud syndrome from local pressure of the tectum.

Cerebello-pontine angle cysts have been associated with nystagmus, facial weakness, hearing loss and tinnitus from the seventh and eighth nerve compression [25, 35].

Posterior fossa arachnoid cysts can cause 6th and 12th cranial nerve compression [41, 48].

Suprasellar and posterior fossa cysts may cause symptomatic hydrocephalus (Figs. 4.2 and 4.3).

All these symptoms are reversible after surgical decompression of the cyst, except for endocrine disturbances in patients with suprasellar cysts, which have been shown not to reverse after treatment; hence they do not constitute indication for surgery anymore.

Epilepsy has been reported in association with arachnoid cysts, but it remains controversial if it is caused directly from the cyst; hence it is not regarded an indication for surgical treatment, and often epilepsy does not improve after successful surgical decompression of the cyst.

Radiological Features

Both on CT and MR scans, arachnoid cysts are well-demarcated, circumscribed, rounded lesions with smooth non-contrast-enhancing margins and content with homogeneous density similar to CSF. Similar features are seen on cranial US in babies. Before MR scanning, arachnoid cysts were investigated with CT scan and metrizamide CT cisternography, which could demonstrate the communication of the cyst cavity with the subarachnoid space. This is not practised anymore as it has been superseded by MR imaging. The three-dimensional relationship of arachnoid cysts to the basal cisterns, vessels and nerves is best visualized with the multiplanar MR scan, which is commonly performed even if the diagnosis is made with a CT or US scan. T2-weighted imaging and other similar sequences such as CISS or FIESTA can demonstrate the walls of the arachnoid cyst and the relationship with neighbouring cranial nerves, arteries and veins and cortical sulci in detail [5]. These anatomic relationships are of surgical importance. In middle fossa arachnoid cyst, the position of the ipsilateral carotid artery and optic nerve is important. In suprasellar cyst the position of the basilar artery should be ascertained. In quadrigeminal cistern cyst, the position of the internal cerebral veins is important. In all cases the relationship to the overlying cortex is important in designing the trajectory of surgical approach.

Some cysts can cause mass effect evidenced by midline shift or compression of nearby cerebral tissue or cerebrospinal fluid (CSF) compartments (Fig. 4.1c).

Intracranial arachnoid cysts can be diagnosed in utero by ultrasound as early as 13 weeks of gestation, but most are diagnosed during the second trimester. Nowadays with the advent of antenatal MR scanning, once a cyst is diagnosed in ultrasound, it is a common practice to obtain an MR scan of the foetus after the 21st week of gestation, to examine the lesion in more detail. Arachnoid cysts are shown well in antenatal MR scans (Figs. 4.5 and 4.7). If the cyst increases in size postnatally, the neurosurgeon will have to decide if early intervention is indicated if there are signs of intracranial hypertension (Fig. 4.5).

Middle fossa/Sylvian fissure cysts were classified by Galassi and associates in 1982 based on their appearance and apparent communication with adjacent normal CSF spaces [12].

Type I cysts are small, spindle shaped, limited to the anterior aspect of the middle cranial fossa and not associated with calvarial deformities, and they do not require treatment (Fig. 4.1a).

Type II cysts are larger triangular or quadrangular, extend along the Sylvian fissure, may cause temporal bone distortion and may require treatment (Fig. 4.1b).

Type III cysts are large, fill the entire middle cranial fossa, cause thinning and lateral expansion of the temporal bone and typically present with marked mass effect and midline shift (Fig. 4.1c). About 30% of arachnoid cysts fall within this category, and they often require surgical treatment.

Posterior fossa cysts can be in the midline or laterally. In the midline are either overlying the vermis (Fig. 4.2a) or intraventricular within the fourth ventricle. Laterally they are in the cerebello-pontine angle (Fig. 4.2b, c) or retrocerebellar over the cerebellar hemisphere (Fig. 4.2d). Midline lesions may need to be differentiated from Dandy-Walker syndrome. Posterior fossa cysts can cause hydrocephalus from compression of the aqueduct or distortion of the fourth ventricle.

Suprasellar cysts occupy most of the region of the third ventricle as they push upwards the floor of the third ventricle. They displace the basilar artery and the anterior aspect of the brain stem posteriorly, and they cause hydrocephalus by obstructing the foramen of Monro.

Occasionally, differential diagnosis from other cystic lesions may have to be made. Differentiation from other cystic lesions is usually easy. Proton density-weighted sequences, diffusion-weighted imaging (DWI) and measurement of apparent diffusion coefficient (ADC) values can be valuable in such circumstances and are part of standard imaging protocols in most units.

In the suprasellar region, craniopharyngioma and Rathke's cleft cyst are encountered. Rathke's cyst which has content with signal density that of CSF anatomically is in relation to the pituitary stalk, much lower from the location where a suprasellar cyst is located, does not extend up to the third ventricle and does not cause hydrocephalus. A small intrasellar arachnoid cyst can be confused with a Rathke's cyst, but on most occasions, surgical treatment is not required.

The presence of calcification on CT scan is diagnostic of craniopharyngioma. Arachnoid cysts do not contain calcium flecks in their walls. In MR images the walls of a cystic craniopharyngioma enhance with contrast in contrast to arachnoid cysts that their walls never enhance. In addition, the cholesterol crystal containing fluid of a craniopharyngioma returns high signal on proton density sequences.

In the posterior fossa, especially the cerebellopontine angle, epidermoid cyst can be found which contains proteinaceous fluid, which commonly returns high signal on proton density sequences. Some epidermoid cysts have dense walls which enhance with contrast.

In DWI sequences epidermoid cysts (and other cystic lesions with proteinaceous and lipid content such as abscesses) have hyperintense signal, whereas arachnoid cysts have hypointense signal [4, 28]. Arachnoid cysts have higher ADC values, whereas epidermoid cysts have restricted diffusion and appear dark on apparent diffusion coefficient (ADC) maps [17].

Ependymal and choroid plexus cysts are intraventricular lesions and commonly are smaller than arachnoid cysts. Ependymal cysts are always attached to one ventricular wall. Choroid plexus cysts are always attached to the choroid plexus. Both these lesions do not merit surgical treatment. In contrast, intraventricular arachnoid cysts fill the trigone or the frontal horn of the lateral ventricle or the cavity of the third ventricle and are considerably larger than the other two pathologies.

Benign intraparenchymal cysts can be found in the lobes of the cerebrum or cerebellum, and they have thick walls of neuroglial tissue and commonly do not merit surgical treatment as they do not cause intracranial hypertension.

Effect of Arachnoid Cysts on Cerebral Perfusion and Metabolism

Cerebral single-photon emission computerized tomography (SPECT) scans that investigate rCBF (regional cerebral blood flow) have demonstrated that arachnoid cysts reduce perfusion and metabolism in surrounding cortical regions, and this is restored to normal after successful surgical treatment of the cyst even though the size of the cysts was moderately reduced [31, 44, 45]. It is uncertain if the hypoperfusion is due to local compression of cerebral blood vessels by the cyst or due to a global effect of intracranial hypertension because it has been observed even in vascular territories away from the cyst. The improvement of hypoperfusion is correlated to the improvement of the patient in neuropsychological testing and cognition [15, 40, 47].

In patients with middle fossa arachnoid cysts and language impairment and cognitive deficits, the study of cerebral metabolism with ^{18}F-fludeoxyglucose positron emission tomography (PET) scan has demonstrated defects in cerebral metabolism, which improved after successful surgical cyst decompression, and this was correlated with clinical improvement of the cognitive defects [30].

Effect of Arachnoid Cysts on Language Organization

A study performed in five asymptomatic patients with left temporal arachnoid cyst investigated the influence of the cyst on the cortical organization of language [23]. Four of these patients had a clear left hemisphere language mapping, despite the presence of the cyst. The other patient had bilateral representation. While in the left side there was decreased cortical thickness in association with the cyst, the surface area of the inferior frontal gyrus, which is regarded as the substrate for language, namely, the pars triangularis and pars opercularis, was larger on the left side with the cyst, in comparison to the normal other right side. In other words, the presence of the cyst did not disturb the normal asymmetry of hemisphere language organization. This corresponds to clinical observations that children with temporal arachnoid cysts do not have speech problems and their school performance is normal.

Surgical Management of Intracranial Cysts

The primary goal of surgical treatment is improvement of clinical symptoms or at least prevention of further deterioration, without additional morbidity. Radiological reduction of the cyst, although not the primary aim of any surgery, is desirable and considered a form of treatment success. Any coexisting hydrocephalus will need treatment in its own merits. The threshold for surgical intervention usually is lower in children, compared to adults [1].

Indications for surgical management of arachnoid cysts remain an issue of controversy and debate.

Absolute Indications

- Presence of neurological symptoms and signs which can be clearly attributed to the anatomic location of the cyst
- Increased intracranial pressure (ICP) as evidenced by:
  - Symptoms and clinical signs of intracranial hypertension (headaches, vomiting, papilledema in older children, macrocrania, bulging fontanelle and Parinaud syndrome in smaller children)
  - Invasive recording with ICP bolt
- Coexisting symptomatic hydrocephalus (ventriculomegaly with increased intracranial pressure)

Relative Indications

- Increases in size of the cyst, seen in serial imaging, in the absence of new or progressive symptoms (this is uncommon after the first few years of age)
- Evidence of previous bleeding into or in proximity with the cyst or rupture of the cyst (more often seen in older children who have been asymptomatic for a long time, and they develop symptoms after minor head injury). Decision for surgery will depend on the presence of associated symptoms.

Controversial Indications

- Non-specific headaches in older children and adults
- Epilepsy
- Developmental delay in young children

In cases with such controversial symptoms, surgical treatment commonly does not offer any improvement. For this reason, most neurosurgeons avoid operation in such circumstances.

Surgical Techniques

Once a decision is made to proceed with treatment, three main surgical options are available:

- Endoscopic fenestration
- Insertion of a cyst-peritoneal shunt
- Microsurgical cyst fenestration/marsupialization

With proliferation of endoscopic techniques during the last decade, endoscopic fenestration has become the treatment of choice for most cranial arachnoid cysts with improved success rate. Even multiple neuroendoscopic attempts are a reasonable option for recurrent cases. Only if endoscopic fenestration has failed, shunt or microsurgical removal is employed.

Endoscopic Fenestration

The biggest advantage of neuroendoscopic surgery is minimal invasiveness, associated with a good chance of permanent cyst reduction and avoidance of shunt. The goal is a wide communication of the cyst with the basal cisterns (cysto-cisternostomy (CC)) and/or the ventricles (ventriculo-cystostomy (VC)). Effective management of any associated hydrocephalus can be performed as well (third ventriculostomy (ETV) in posterior fossa cysts and ventriculo-cysto-cisternostomy (VCC) in suprasellar cysts, which in effect becomes the third ventriculostomy).

In preparation for endoscopy, special MR sequences that reveal thin walls or septations (e.g. CISS, FIESTA) are very useful as they offer better imaging of the anatomic relations of the cyst walls to the surrounding structures [5].

Neuronavigation is used increasingly to plan entry and trajectory, but also while the endoscope is inside the cyst, especially in some deep-seated lesions such as intraventricular cysts where intraoperatively the anatomy can be confusing and it is helpful to have radiological guidance or quadrigeminal cysts where commonly the cyst wall is in contact with the deep veins and often due to the thickness of the cyst wall intraoperatively is not easy to appreciate the anatomic relationship; hence radiological guidance is important to avoid injury to the veins during fenestration. Increasingly, neuronavigation is used in all types of cysts by colleagues worldwide.

Planning of the burr hole is performed in such location so that if needed it can be easily converted to mini-craniotomy although in practice it is rare to have to abandon endoscopy and revert to mini-craniotomy.

During the procedure, it is important to keep CSF loss to minimum. For this reason, a small incision is performed on the cortical surface, and the endoscopic sheath is carefully introduced. If much CSF is lost, the danger for subdural collections increases, the cyst walls interfere with the endoscopic view and the accuracy of the neuronavigation further decreases. In large posterior fossa cysts with significant mass effect over the brain stem, excess CSF loss during the procedure can cause rapid brain stem shift which will manifest with episodes of bradycardia and can lead even to cardiac arrest.

The fenestration on the cyst walls and the basal cisterns should be done with great care to avoid vascular or nerve damage. In middle fossa cysts, the wall can be in contact with the carotid artery, the optic and the third nerve (Fig. 4.1b). In suprasellar cysts the inferior aspect of the cyst wall can be in contact with the basilar artery, the third nerves and the hypothalami (Fig. 4.3d). In quadrigeminal cysts the cyst wall can be in contact with the internal cerebral veins. Care should be exercised in all these circumstances. The optimal instruments for more "atraumatic" opening are, in order of smoothness: the balloon catheter, a blunt probe, the scissors, the laser (if available) and lastly the monopolar diathermy. The blunt monopolar diathermy electrode can be used also without electricity as a blunt probe. The diathermy use should be kept at minimum in general. The laser has the advantage over the monopolar coagulation that it does not shrink the cyst wall when performing the fenestration, thus ensuring bigger diameter of fenestration. In addition, it does not cause thermal damage to vessels and nerves. It is not universally available though. After fenestration, balloon dilatation and division of arachnoid strands with endoscopic scissors are often required to enlarge the stoma. In all cases, fenestrations should be performed down to free subarachnoid space, the opening should be as wide as possible to avoid closure with time and CSF flow should be verified by the free pulsations of the stoma edges.

In cases of posterior fossa cyst and hydrocephalus, an ETV may have to be performed at the same time with the cyst fenestration [26].

In suprasellar cysts causing obstructive hydrocephalus, an ETV is performed at the same time with the cyst fenestration, by opening the inferior part of the cyst wall which is commonly in contact to the floor of the third ventricle (Fig. 4.3d). A septostomy should be considered as well if it is felt that communication of the two lateral ventricles is not free.

If there is a previous ventriculo-peritoneal (VP) or cyst-peritoneal (CP) shunt, and endoscopy is attempted during shunt malfunction, removal of the shunt can be considered after successful endoscopic treatment.

During endoscopy, if the cyst wall is thick, tough or adherent to the surrounding neurovascular structures or if the anatomical landmarks are not visible and the surgeon doesn't feel confident to proceed, the endoscopic procedure should be abandoned, and consideration should be given to switch to microsurgical fenestration or a shunt.

Postoperative CSF leakage can be avoided with careful closure. The cortical incision can be plugged with Gelfoam. In children the dural opening is sutured. More important is the tight closure of the galea over the burr hole. If persistent leakage or subgaleal collections occur, this may imply insufficient performance of the fenestration. The options are redo endoscopy or shunting with wound resuturing.

An insertion of a ventriculo-peritoneal shunt for hydrocephalus due to an arachnoid cyst can increase the cyst size if left untreated.

Immediate complications of endoscopy are haemorrhage and nerve damage. Most oculomotor nerve palsies are transient, in the absence of obvious surgical nerve damage. Later complications are CSF leaks with meningitis (5–7%) and subdural haematomas/hygromas (9–15%). The incidence of complications was found to be higher in ventriculo-cysto-cisternostomies (VCC) than ventriculo-cystostomies (VC) [8].

MRI scans with CSF flow studies are performed soon after operation. A scan performed within 6 weeks from surgery should show some decrease in cyst size. After that, it is the author's practice to perform yearly MR scans for a few years to monitor recurrent increase in size. Other surgeons prefer to leave the MR scan only for recurrence of symptoms.

Outcome of Endoscopic Treatment

The reported success rate of neuroendoscopy for suprasellar, quadrigeminal and posterior fossa cysts is more than 83%. Sylvian and interhemispheric cysts are around 75% [13].

In successful cases the identification on MR images of a flow void at the site of fenestration confirms communication between the arachnoid cyst and the adjacent subarachnoid space. ECG-gated cine-mode MRI sequence can demonstrate that communication further.

Children aged <2 years are more likely to end up with a shunt (Fig. 4.1c). CSF absorption can be deficient, and the endoscopic fenestration may not function, in a manner analogous to the failure of ETV in the first 2 years of life.

Following successful endoscopic fenestration, it has been reported in various studies that arachnoid cysts usually reduce in size, they sometimes remain stable and they very rarely disappear [6, 9, 10, 13, 16, 26, 27, 30, 32, 37, 38, 43]. In children the reduction is more evident than in adults. Studies with volumetric measurement of cyst have shown that following endoscopic fenestration of arachnoid cysts and successful symptom control, the cyst does not disappear but reduces in volume significantly in a period of up 3–6 months after treatment, and it reaches a plateau with no significant changes further on [37].

For the last two decades, the senior author's first choice for all intracranial arachnoid cysts is endoscopic fenestration, with an overall success rate of 70%. Since 2002 he has not performed a microsurgical fenestration, which was the first procedure of choice before that year. Shunting is reserved only in case of failure of endoscopic fenestration, which practically is seen only in young children in the first 2 years of life.

Alternate Procedures

Microsurgery for Cyst Fenestration: Marsupialization

Prior to the widespread utilization of endoscopy, it was a front-line option [11], and it remains a reliable option in experienced hands. Through a mini-craniotomy, using the microscope, a significant part of the cyst wall that is separating the cyst from the subarachnoid space is removed. Some surgeons prefer a small "cortical" fenestration to minimize the risk for subdural collections. The previously practised complete excision of cyst wall is not employed any more.

Cyst-Peritoneal Shunt

For many neurosurgeons shunting is the last option for recurrences after craniotomy or neuroendoscopy. It is a good first-line option for very large middle fossa arachnoid cysts that extend over the convexity of the hemisphere. Many neurosurgeons use an adjustable valve in these cases to avoid rapid cyst decompression and possible later problems of overdrainage [19]. A cyst-peritoneal shunt should be avoided in the posterior fossa, as the catheter may end up lying in proximity to the lower cranial nerves or the brain stem or even penetrate it, with consequent neurological defects. Cyst shunts have similar complications and problems with ventricular shunts for hydrocephalus (infection, obstruction, overdrainage).

Prior to the advent of endoscopy, treatment of suprasellar cysts was performed with insertion of a ventricular catheter longer than usual, to penetrate the dome of the cyst through the foramen of Monro and with holes in the third ventricle and extra holes in the lateral ventricle, to drain the cyst and the ventricles simultaneously. This is rarely practised these days.

Overall Outcome Following Treatment

Overall improvements of quality of life, as well as cognitive functions, have been observed in most patients following successful treatment of intracranial arachnoid cysts [24, 29, 33]. Most children with arachnoid cysts that were treated successfully have normal development. Any problems may be related to complications of the treatment and not to the cyst itself. These results are independent of surgical technique employed [11, 32].

Spinal Arachnoid Cysts

Spinal arachnoid cysts are rare in general and constitute an uncommon cause of spinal cord or nerve root compression in children. They rarely cause symptoms in adulthood.

Secondary spinal arachnoid cysts seem to occur more frequently following surgery, trauma and arachnoiditis and can be confused with true congenital ones.

Spinal arachnoid cysts are subdivided by their location into intra- or extradural cysts according to their relation to the dura and into anterior, posterior or lateral cysts in relation to the spinal cord. In most series, intradural arachnoid cysts are more common, both in children and adults. Intradural cysts could be extramedullary or intramedullary [57, 63]. Extradural location is infrequent [52, 62, 64, 68, 70, 73]. Most cysts are located at the thoracic spine followed by cervical and lumbar regions. Sacral and cervicomedullary sites are rare. Most of the thoracic (Fig. 4.9), lumbar and sacral cysts are located dorsally, whereas the cervical arachnoid cysts are much more seen anteriorly to the spinal cord (Fig. 4.10). Extradural arachnoid cysts are located posteriorly to the thecal sac usually (Fig. 4.11). Multiple cysts are very rare. A single case has been described of a 9-year-old girl whose spinal cord compression was caused by multiple extradural arachnoid cysts extending from the midthoracic region to the sacrum [65]. All cysts were located dorsally to the cord and thecal sac.

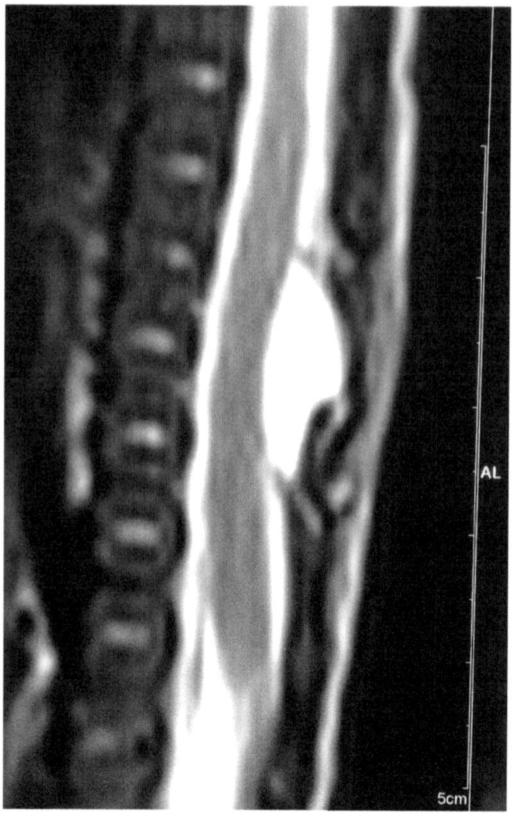

Fig. 4.9 Dorsal intradural thoracic arachnoid cyst. T2-weighted sagittal MR scan of an 8-month-old girl who presented in 2011 with reduced leg movement. There is an intradural cystic lesion with thick walls and contents with signal density similar to CSF, dorsally to the spinal cord at the level of T8 vertebra, causing compression. A microsurgical excision was performed through a laminotomy-laminoplasty. The girl developed normally with no spinal deformity. She is now a member of a swimming team

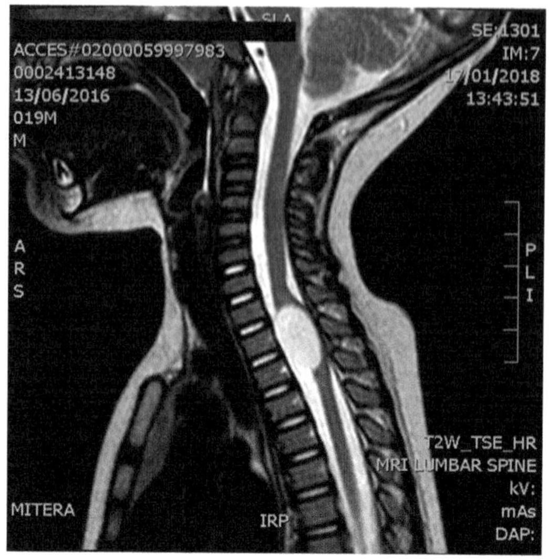

Fig. 4.10 Anterior intradural upper thoracic arachnoid cyst. T2-weighted sagittal MR scan of a 19-month-old boy who presented in 2018 with a 24-h history of paraplegia. On examination he was flexing his legs to pain. An anterior upper thoracic intradural arachnoid cyst is seen at the level of T2–T3, causing significant anterior cord compression. Through a laminotomy-laminoplasty, the cyst was approached dorsolaterally and was excised. Subtotal excision of the cyst wall was achieved. The child improved clinically initially. Later the cyst reformed, and this was associated with clinical deterioration. The second operation was performed 9 months later. He showed some clinical improvement after the second operation. Currently he can stand with support, and he is attempting a few steps

Familial occurrence [53, 61, 64], association with lymphedema and hereditary distichiasis [69] and neurocutaneous melanosis [59] have been reported as well as association with Marfan syndrome [67, 71, 72] and neural tube defects [66, 68] such as myelomeningocele [55], diastematomyelia [54, 66] or spina bifida occulta. The neural tube defect may be at a different spinal level to the arachnoid cyst. Foot deformities can be present in association with these congenital deformities. Association between extradural spinal arachnoid cysts and minor neural tube defects such as spina bifida occulta in the same region has been reported as well [52].

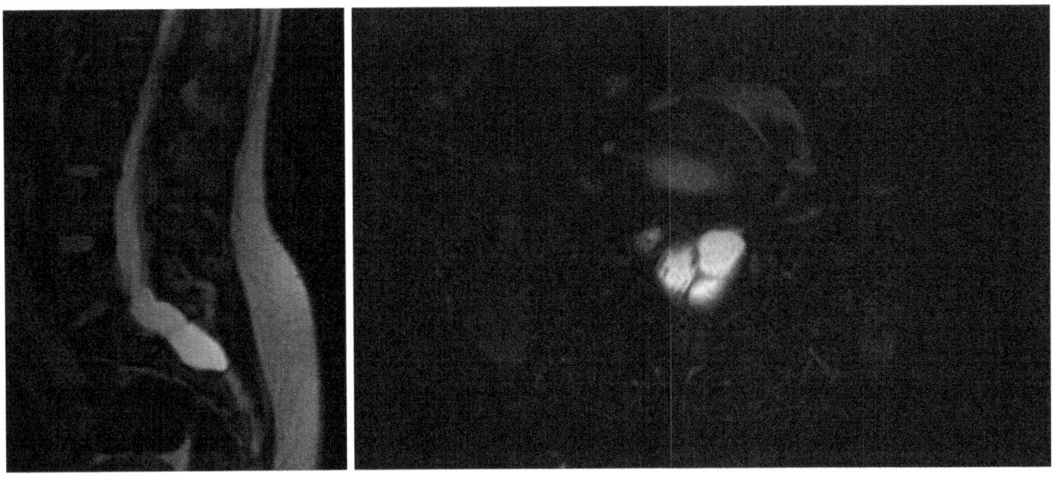

Fig. 4.11 Sacral extradural arachnoid cyst. T2-weighted sagittal and axial MR scans of a 12-year-old girl who presented in 2003 with an 18-month history of pain in the legs, predominantly on the left. She was an athlete, and as the symptoms deteriorated, she became unable to walk following intense sporting activity. There is an epidural arachnoid cyst in the sacral region, with septations, causing compression on the underlying roots on the left. During operation, a sizeable cyst was compressing the left S1 root, and there was a smaller cyst adjacent to the big one, so the septations seen in preoperative images were separate cysts in fact. After removal of the cysts, it became obvious that there was a defect in the axilla of the root, which was the site of origin of the cysts and which was sutured and sealed

Etiology and Pathogenesis

Etiology remains unclear. Intradural cysts have a pathogenesis similar to the intracranial arachnoid cysts [61]. Extradural cysts are outpouchings of the arachnoid membrane herniating to the extradural space through small defects within the dura mater [62, 70], so they have a narrow neck as a communication to the subarachnoid space [58]. This narrow neck is thought to function as a valve mechanism allowing the extradural cyst to enlarge due to pressure pulses within the cerebrospinal fluid. This fact could explain that many patients get asymptomatic by changing posture presuming the cyst empties itself [54, 56]. Once the cyst is too large and emptying is impossible, different postures of the patient do not produce relief of pain, and the patient remains symptomatic. However, many patients with large cysts do not present any symptoms, and the cyst is only an incidental finding. It is widely accepted that disturbances in the pattern of CSF flow contribute to the development of arachnoid cysts [68, 70].

Clinical Presentation

Most spinal arachnoid cysts are asymptomatic, and their cysts are diagnosed with the opportunity of an MR scan for some unrelated reason. A minority cause symptoms from cord or nerve root compression. A variety of symptoms can be present such as back pain, radicular and non-radicular pain, irritation or loss of sensation, weakness with muscle atrophy, paraparesis, quadriplegia and spasticity, gait disturbance and urinary and faecal dysfunction or perianal anaesthesia. Children can develop foot deformity secondary to neurological dysfunction. History can vary from acute sudden onset of pain or neurological deficit to long-standing or gradual deterioration of symptoms.

Radiological Features

Plain radiographs show non-specific findings which constitute indirect indications of the existence of an arachnoid cyst. Increased distances of pedicles [52, 56], absence of spinous process [52], widening of the spinal canal particularly in the sacrum or neural foramina, scalloped vertebral arches [65] or even scoliosis which is often seen in combination with neural tube defects all raise suspicions of intraspinal pathology and prompt the acquisition of MR scan.

Prior to MR scanning, CT scan and CT myelography at different postures allowing the contrast medium to fill the cyst revealed the cyst and the communication site in extradural cysts [60]. This is not practised anymore as all necessary information is seen on MR scan.

On MR images spinal arachnoid cysts have an equal or slightly more hyperintense signal than CSF in T1- and T2-weighted imaging due to their equal or slightly higher amount of protein [58, 60, 61]. Location, relation to the cord and thecal sac, size and extent are demonstrated very well. Intradural cysts can be large enough to cause cord compression and distortion of the spinal cord (Fig. 4.10) and can cause syringomyelia due to disturbance of cranio-caudal flow of CSF. In extradural cysts, often a narrow communicating neck to the subarachnoid space can be identified which seemed to be critical for satisfactory surgical treatment [65].

Surgical Management

Once it has been decided that the spinal arachnoid cyst is responsible for the symptoms and clinical signs of the patient, surgical treatment should be pursued. There are several surgical options including microsurgical excision of the cyst, microsurgical fenestration to the subarachnoid space or shunting the cyst fluid to the pleura cavity, peritoneum or atrium [61].

Microsurgical excision of intradural arachnoid cysts should be performed with care to avoid injury of the cord. Neuromonitoring should be employed to avoid operative nerve or cord damage. Laminotomy and laminoplasty are performed in children to avoid late spinal deformities. In case of difficulty of excision (e.g. adherence to anterior spinal artery), fenestration by partial wall excision is a satisfactory option, although it carries high risk or relapse [57] (Fig. 4.10). In case of failure of microsurgical excision, a cyst-peritoneal shunt can be placed.

Anterior cervical or thoracic arachnoid cysts can be difficult to excise completely or place a shunt tube, and even fenestration can be impossible to be performed in the presence of extensive scarring or hydrosyringomyelia. Cyst shunting carries the usual problems of shunt infection and malfunction as in hydrocephalus.

In extradural cyst it is important to identify the dural defect and the neck of the cyst and repair it during surgery following complete excision of the cyst [52].

Prognosis

Symptomatic patients improve after surgery [52, 63]. Duration and gravity of symptoms and neurological defects are important. If myelopathy or spasticity has been established before treatment, these may not recover in full. The longer the neurological deficits last, the higher the risk of the absence of recovery [61, 70]. Incomplete excision carries a high degree of relapse by reformation of the cyst wall, which may necessitate repeat surgery [57].

Questions

1. What percentage of arachnoid cysts enlarge over time
   (a) 10%
   (b) 20%
   (c) 40%
   (d) 60%
2. What is the most common location for arachnoid cysts?
   (a) Cerebello-pontine angle
   (b) Sylvian fissure/Middle fossa
   (c) Posterior fossa
   (d) Suprasellar

3. Indications for surgical management of arachnoid cysts include all of the following, but
   (a) Increased intracranial pressure
   (b) Neurological deficit attributed to the cyst location
   (c) Headaches
   (d) Increase in cyst size
   (e) Developmental delay

Answers

1. (a)
2. (b)
3. (e)

References

Intracranial Arachnoid Cysts

1. Al-Holou WN, Yew AY, Boomsaad ZE, Garton HJ, Muraszko KM, Maher CO. Prevalence and natural history of arachnoid cysts in children. J Neurosurg Pediatr. 2010;5(6):578–85.
2. Al-Holou WN, Terman S, Kilburg C, Garton HJ, Muraszko KM, Maher CO. Prevalence and natural history of arachnoid cysts in adults. J Neurosurg. 2013;118:222–31.
3. Baquero GA, Molero P, Pla J, Ortuno F. A schizophrenia-like psychotic disorder secondary to an arachnoid cyst remitted with neurosurgical treatment of the cyst. Open Neuroimaging J. 2014;8:1–4.
4. Bergui M, Zhong J, Bradac GB, Sales S. Diffusion-weighted images of intracranial cyst-like lesions. Neuroradiology. 2001;43(10):824–9.
5. Cinalli G, Peretta P, Spennato P, Savarese L, Varone A, Vedova P, Grimaldi G, Ragazzi P, Ruggiero C, Cianciulli E, Maggi G. Neuroendoscopic management of interhemispheric cysts in children. J Neurosurg Pediatr. 2006;105(3 Suppl):194–202.
6. Ciricillo SF, Cogen PH, Harsh GR, Edwards MS. Intracranial arachnoid cysts in children. A comparison of the effects of fenestration and shunting. J Neurosurg. 1991;74:230–5.
7. Di Rocco C, Tamburrini G, Caldarelli M, Velardi F, Santini P. Prolonged ICP monitoring in Sylvian arachnoid cysts. Surg Neurol. 2003;60(3):211–8.
8. El-Ghandour NM. Endoscopic treatment of middle cranial fossa arachnoid cysts in children. J Neurosurg Pediatr. 2012;9(3):231–8.
9. El-Ghandour NM. Endoscopic treatment of intraparenchymal arachnoid cysts in children. J Neurosurg Pediatr. 2014;14:501–7.
10. Fernández Molina G. Neuroendoscopic management of middle fossa arachnoid cysts. World Neurosurg. 2013;79(2 Suppl):S19.e19–23.
11. Galarza M, Pomata HB, Pueyrredón F, Bartuluchi M, Zuccaro GN, Monges JA. Symptomatic supratentorial arachnoid cysts in children. Pediatr Neurol. 2002;27:180–5.
12. Galassi E, Tognetti F, Gaist G, Fagioli L, Frank F, Frank G. CT scan and metrizamide CT cisternography in arachnoid cysts of the middle cranial fossa: classification and pathophysiological aspects. Surg Neurol. 1982;17(5):363–9.
13. Gangemi M, Seneca V, Colella G, Cioffi V, Imperato A, Maiuri F. Endoscopy versus microsurgical cyst excision and shunting for treating intracranial arachnoid cysts. J Neurosurg Pediatr. 2011;8(2):158–64.
14. Germanò A, Caruso G, Caffo M, Baldari S, Calisto A, Meli F, Tomasello F. The treatment of large supratentorial arachnoid cysts in infants with cyst-peritoneal shunting and Hakim programmable valve. Childs Nerv Syst. 2003;19(3):166–73.
15. Gjerde PB, Schmid M, Hammar Å, Wester K. Intracranial arachnoid cysts: impairment of higher cognitive functions and postoperative improvement. J Neurodev Disord. 2013;5:21.
16. Greenfield J, Souweidane MM. Endoscopic management of intracranial cysts. Neurosurg Focus. 2005;19:1–9.
17. Hakyemez B, Yildiz H, Ergin N, Uysal S, Parlak M. [Flair and diffusion weighted MR imaging in differentiating epidermoid cysts from arachnoid cysts]. Tani Girisim Radyol. 2003;9(4):418–26. (Article in Turkish, abstract in English).
18. Halani SH, Safain MG, Heilman CB. Arachnoid cyst slit valves: the mechanism for arachnoid cyst enlargement. J Neurosurg Pediatr. 2013;12:62–6.
19. Hamid NA, Sgouros S. The use of an adjustable valve to treat over-drainage of a cyst-peritoneal shunt in a child with a large sylvian fissure arachnoid cyst. Childs Nerv Syst. 2005;21:991–4.
20. Helland CA, Aarhus M, Knappskog P, Olsson L, Lund-Johansen M, Amiry-Moghaddam M, Wester K. Increased NKCC1 expression in arachnoid cysts supports secretory basis for cyst formation. Exp Neurol. 2010;224:424–8.
21. Helland CA, Wester K. Intracystic pressure in patients with temporal arachnoid cysts: a prospective study of preoperative complaints and postoperative outcome. J Neurol Neurosurg Psychiatry. 2007;78(6):620–3.
22. Huang JH, Mei WZ, Chen Y, Chen JW, Lin ZX. Analysis on clinical characteristics of intracranial arachnoid cysts in 488 pediatric cases. Int J Clin Exp Med. 2015;8:18343–50.
23. Hund-Georgiadis M, Yves Von Cramon D, Kruggel F, Preul C. Do quiescent arachnoid cysts alter CNS functional organization?: a fMRI and morphometric study. Neurology. 2002;59(12):1935–9.
24. Isaksen E, Leet TH, Helland CA, Wester K. Maze learning in patients with intracranial arachnoid cysts. Acta Neurochir (Wien). 2013;155(5):841–8.
25. Jallo GI, Woo HH, Meshki C, Epstein FJ, Wisoff JH. Arachnoid cysts of the cerebellopon-

tine angle: diagnosis and surgery. Neurosurgery. 1997;40(1):31–7.
26. Karabatsou K, Hayhurst C, Buxton N, O'Brien DF, Mallucci CL. Endoscopic management of arachnoid cysts: an advancing technique. J Neurosurg Pediatr. 2007;106(6 Suppl):455–62.
27. Kim MH, Jho HD. Endoscopic management of cranial arachnoid cysts using extra-channel method. J Korean Neurosurg Soc. 2010;47:433–6.
28. Lai PH, Hsu SS, Ding SW, Ko CW, Ko CW, Fu JH, Weng MJ, Yeh LR, Wu MT, Liang HL, Chen CK, Pan HB. Proton magnetic resonance spectroscopy and diffusion-weighted imaging in intracranial cystic mass lesions. Surg Neurol. 2007;68(Suppl 1):S25–36.
29. Laporte N, De Volder A, Bonnier C, Raftopoulos C, Sebire G. Language impairment associated with arachnoid cysts: recovery after surgical treatment. Pediatr Neurol. 2012;46:44–7.
30. Li Y, Chen X, Xu B. The efficacy of neuroendoscopic treatment for middle cranial fossa arachnoid cysts assessed by MRI 3D segmentation and modeling. Childs Nerv Syst. 2014;30:1037–44.
31. Martínez-Lage JF, Valentí JA, Piqueras C, Ruiz-Espejo AM, Román F, Nuño de la Rosa JA. Functional assessment of intracranial arachnoid cysts with Tc99 m-HMPAO SPECT: a preliminary report. Childs Nerv Syst. 2006;22(9):1091–7.
32. Mohsin A, Bennardo M, Almenawer SA, Zagzoog N, Smith AA, Dao D, Ajani O, Farrokhyar F, Singh SK. Exploring predictors of surgery and comparing operative treatment approaches for pediatric intracranial arachnoid cysts: a case series of 83 patients. J Neurosurg Pediatr. 2015;16:275–82.
33. Mørkve SH, Helland CA, Amus J, Lund-Johansen M, Wester KG. Surgical decompression of arachnoid cysts leads to improved quality of life: a prospective study. Neurosurgery. 2016;78(5):613–25.
34. Morris Z, Whiteley WN, Longstreth WT Jr, Weber F, Lee YC, Tsushima Y, Alphs H, Ladd SC, Warlow C, Wardlaw JM, Al-Shahi SR. Incidental findings on brain magnetic resonance imaging: systematic review and metaanalysis. BMJ. 2009;339:b3016.
35. Olaya JE, Ghostine M, Rowe M, Zouros A. Endoscopic fenestration of a cerebellopontine angle arachnoid cyst resulting in complete recovery from sensorineural hearing loss and facial nerve palsy. J Neurosurg Pediatr. 2011;7(2):157–60.
36. Parsch CS, Krauss J, Hofmann E, Meixensberger J, Roosen K. Arachnoid cysts associated with subdural hematomas and hygromas: analysis of 16 cases, long-term follow-up, and review of the literature. Neurosurgery. 1997;40(3):483–90.
37. Pitsika M, Sgouros S. Volume change of cranial arachnoid cysts after successful endoscopic fenestration in symptomatic children. Childs Nerv Syst. 2019;35:2313–8.
38. Pradilla G, Jallo G. Arachnoid cysts: case series and review of the literature. Neurosurg Focus. 2007;22:E7.
39. Rabiei K, Jaraj D, Marlow T, Jensen C, Skoog I, Wikkelsø C. Prevalence and symptoms of intracranial arachnoid cysts; a population-based study. J Neurol. 2016;263(4):689–94.
40. Raeder MB, Helland CA, Hugdahl K, Wester K. Arachnoid cysts cause cognitive deficits that improve after surgery. Neurology. 2005;64:160–2.
41. Raveenthiran V, Reshma KB. Sixth cranial nerve palsy due to arachnoid cyst. J Pediatr Ophthalmol Strabismus. 2014;51 Online:e58–61.
42. Schroeder HW, Gaab MR. Endoscopic observation of a slit-valve mechanism in a suprasellar prepontine arachnoid cyst: case report. Neurosurgery. 1997;40:198–200.
43. Schroeder HW, Gaab MR, Niendorf WR. Neuroendoscopic approach to arachnoid cysts. J Neurosurg. 1996;85:293–8.
44. Sgouros S, Chamilos C. Pathophysiology of intracranial arachnoid cysts: hypoperfusion of adjacent cortex. In: Wester K, editor. Arachnoid cysts. Epidemiology, biology and neuroimaging. London: Academic; 2018. p. 67–74.
45. Sgouros S, Chapman S. Congenital middle fossa arachnoid cysts may cause global brain ischaemia: a study with 99Tc-hexamethylpropyleneamineoxime single photon emission computerised tomography scans. Pediatr Neurosurg. 2001;35(4):188–94.
46. Sgouros S, Tsitouras V. Congenital intracranial cysts. In: Cohen AR, editor. Pediatric neurosurgery. Tricks of the trade. New York: Thieme; 2016. p. 325–9.
47. Soukup VM, Patterson J, Trier TT, Chen JW. Cognitive improvement despite minimal arachnoid cyst decompression. Brain Dev. 1998;20:589–93.
48. Tarantino R, Marruzzo D, Colista D, Mancarella C, Delfini R. Twelfth nerve paresis induced by an unusual posterior fossa arachnoid cyst: case report and literature review. Br J Neurosurg. 2014;28(4):528–30.
49. Tunes C, Flønes I, Helland C, Wilhemsen K, Goplen F, Wester KG. Pre- and post-operative dizziness and postural instability in temporal arachnoid cyst patients. Acta Neurol Scand. 2014;129(5):335–42.
50. Vernooij MW, Ikram MA, Tanghe HL, Vincent AJ, Hofman A, Krestin GP, Niessen WJ, Breteler MM, van der Lugt A. Incidental findings on brain MRI in the general population. N Engl J Med. 2007;357:1821–8.
51. Vidrih B, Karlovic D, Pasic MB. Arachnoid cyst as the cause of bipolar affective disorder: case report. Acta Clin Croat. 2012;51(4):655–9.

Spinal Arachnoid Cysts

52. Apel K, Sgouros S. Extradural spinal arachnoid cysts associated with spina bifida occulta. Acta Neurochir. 2006;148:221–6.
53. Bergland RM. Congenital intraspinal extradural cyst. Report of three cases in one family. J Neurosurg. 1968;28:495–9.
54. Cilluffo JM, Gomez MR, Reese DF, et al. Idiopathic ("congenital") spinal arachnoid diverticula: clinical diagnosis and surgical results. Mayo Clin Proc. 1981;56:93–101.

55. Duncan AW, Hoare RD. Spinal arachnoid cysts in children. Radiology. 1978;126:423–9.
56. Fortuna A, Mercuri S. Intradural spinal cysts. Acta Neurochir (Wien). 1983;68(3–4):289–314.
57. Ichinose T, Miyashita K, Tanaka S, Oikawa N, Oishi M, Nambu I, Kinoshita M, Nakada M. Recurrent spinal intramedullary arachnoid cyst: case report and literature review. World Neurosurg. 2020;138:68–72.
58. Jena A, Gupta RK, Sharma A, Prakesh VE, Khushu S. Magnetic resonance diagnosis of spinal arachnoid cyst—a report of two cases. Childs Nerv Syst. 1990;6(2):107–9.
59. Kasantijul V, Shuangshoti B, Pattanaruengial A, Kaoropthan S. Intraspinal melanotic arachnoid cyst and lipoma in neurocutaneous melanosis. Surg Neurol. 1989;31:138–41.
60. Khosla A, Wippold FJ 2nd. CT myelography and MR imaging of extramedullary cysts of the spinal canal in adult and pediatric patients. AJR Am J Roentgenol. 2002;178(1):201–7.
61. Lee HJ, Cho DY. Symptomatic spinal intradural arachnoid cysts in the pediatric age group: description of three new cases and review of the literature. Pediatr Neurosurg. 2001;35(4):181–7.
62. Lee MG, Cancina JE. Extradural spinal arachnoid cyst. West Indian Med J. 1980;29(1):67–72.
63. Lmejjati M, Aniba K, Haddi M, Hakkou M, Ghannane H, Ben Ali SA. Spinal intramedullary arachnoid cyst in children. Pediatr Neurosurg. 2008;44(3):243–6.
64. Menezes AH, Hitchon PW, Dlouhy BJ. Symptomatic spinal extradural arachnoid cyst with cord compression in a family: case report. J Neurosurg Spine. 2017;27(3):341–5.
65. Myles LM, Gupta N, Armstrong D, Rutka JT. Multiple extradural arachnoid cysts as a cause of spinal cord compression in a child. J Neurosurg. 1991;91(1 Suppl):116–20.
66. Perret G, Green D, Keller J. Diagnosis and treatment of intradural arachnoid cysts of the thoracic spine. Radiology. 1962;79:425–9.
67. Pyeritz RE, Fishman EK, Bernhardt BA, et al. Dural ectasia is a common feature of the Marfan syndrome. Am J Hum Genet. 1998;43:726–32.
68. Rabb CH, McComb JG, Raffel C, Kennedy JG. Spinal arachnoid cysts in the pediatric age group: an association with neural tube defects. J Neurosurg. 1992;77(3):369–72.
69. Schwartz JF, O'Brien MS, Hoffman JC Jr. Hereditary spinal arachnoid cysts, distichiasis and lymphedema. Ann Neurol. 1980;7:340–3.
70. Shih DY, Chen HJ, Lee TC, Chen L. Congenital spinal arachnoid cysts: a report of 2 cases with review of the literature. J Formos Med Assoc. 1990;89(7):588–92.
71. Smith MD. Large sacral dural defect in Marfan's syndrome—a case report. J Bone Joint Surg Am. 1993;75:1067–70.
72. Stern WE. Dural ectasia and the Marfan syndrome. J Neurosurg. 1988;69:221–7.
73. Ziv T, Watemberg N, Constantini S, Lerman-Sagie T. Cauda equina syndrome due to lumbosacral arachnoid cysts in children. Eur J Paediatr Neurol. 1999;3(6):281–4.

5 Management of Congenital Malformations (Cranial and Spinal)

Cameron Brimley and Samer Elbabaa

Introduction

Central nervous system development is complex with more than 100 billion neurons formed during in utero development. Over half the genome is devoted to the development of the CNS. There are multiple key developmental steps that, when a malfunction occurs, results in specific malformations. These include primary neurulation with formation of the neural tube during the third and fourth weeks of gestation and secondary neurulation with longitudinal cell condensations forming in the sacral and coccygeal regions in the sixth week of gestation. Neural tube defects (NTDs) result in *anencephaly*, *encephaloceles*, *dermal sinus tracts*, *meningoceles*, and *myelomeningoceles*.

Prosencephalic cleavage occurs at 6 weeks and results in *holoprosencephaly* if the cleavage does not occur properly. Midline prosencephalic development continues from 6 to 12 weeks with resultant *septo-optic dysplasia* if errors occur. The corpus callosum develops over 7–20 weeks of gestation with defects possibly causing *dysgenesis of the corpus callosum.*

Neuronal expansion and differentiation continue over 2–4 months of gestation with problems of development during this phase potentially resulting in *microcephaly*, *hemimegalencephaly*, *megalencephaly*, as well as *some cortical dysplasias*. Neuronal migration occurs between 3 and 5 months. Migrational disorders include various *neuronal heterotopias* and *lissencephaly*.

Cranial

Anencephaly results from rostral neural tube closure failure leading to the absence of major brain and skull portions. Neurulation occurs between the third and fourth weeks of gestation, beginning at the hindbrain-cervical junction, and proceeds both rostral and caudally. The anterior neuropore apices are designed to fuse at approximately gestational day 24. Failure of this fusion will result in anencephaly where amniotic fluid exposure causes significant injury and halted development. The residual tissue is poorly developed and disorganized, consisting of neuroblasts and vascular and glial tissues, surrounded by meninges. Anencephaly occurs in approximately 3/10,000 live births in the USA, with the fetus typically surviving only hours. The true incidence is difficult to estimate in the setting of spontaneous and planned abortions. Diagnosis is

C. Brimley (✉)
Geisinger Neuroscience Institute, Danville, PA, USA
e-mail: cjbrimley@geisinger.edu

S. Elbabaa
Pediatric Neurosurgery, Leon Pediatric Neuroscience Center of Excellence, Arnold Palmer Hospital for Children, Orlando, FL, USA
e-mail: samer.elbabaa@orlandohealth.com

N. Shimony, G. Jallo (eds.), *Pediatric Neurosurgery Board Review*,
https://doi.org/10.1007/978-3-031-23687-7_5

made with ultrasound as well as alpha fetoprotein. Folic acid supplementation has decreased the frequency of neural tube defects, including the incidence of anencephaly. There have not been any identifiable genetic mutations that account for NTDs and are more likely secondary to a combination of multiple genetic and environmental factors. Aside from folate supplementation as a preventative measure, there are no treatment options for anencephaly [1].

Encephalocele is another type of neural tube defect resulting from failure of the neuroectoderm to separate from the surface ectoderm during neural tube closure [2]. This leads to a mesodermal defect that prevents proper ossification of the skull, allowing cranial contents to protrude outside the cranium [3]. These defects typically occur along the midline and are usually covered by normal or dysplastic dermis. Different types include meningocele with herniation of the meninges, encephalomeningocele with herniation of the brain and meninges, and encephalomeningocystocele with herniation of the brain, ventricle, and meninges. Occipital location is more common in North America, while an anterior location most often occurs in Southeast Asia, India, and Africa. Anterior encephaloceles are given specific classifications based on location including naso-orbital, naso-frontal, naso-ethmoid, spheno-orbital, spheno-maxillary, and spheno-pharyngeal [4]. Occipital encephaloceles are associated with Chiari III malformations including displacement of the lower brainstem inferiorly into the foramen magnum (Fig. 5.1). If tested, maternal AFP is frequently within normal limits as the defect is covered by the dermis and not exposed to the amniotic fluid but can be diagnosed via ultrasound. Encephaloceles occur in approximately 1/10,000 births and account for 10–20% of all cranio-spinal dysraphisms with a female predominance and can be associated with monosomy x, trisomics 13, 18, and 21 as well as other mosaicisms. They are also associated with multiple syndromes including Meckel syndrome, Fraser syndrome, Roberts syndrome, and Walker-Warburg syndrome [5]. Up to 60% of patients with encephaloceles develop hydrocephalus.

Treatment consists of removing the herniated tissue, dysplastic dermal covering with subsequent dural repair, possible cranioplasty, and skin closure. If the skin layer is intact providing protection for the herniated elements, surgery may be undertaken after the baby had grown and increased in weight, waiting up to 4 months old. If the dermis covering is ruptured, the surgery should be completed as soon as possible. Other important aspects to consider are the amount of brain tissue that is herniated, the location and relationship of the venous sinuses, the size of the dural, and bone defect. Although the herniated tissue is frequently non-functional, this should be evaluated to determine if it is removable or not. Opinions vary regarding a cranioplasty at the time of resection vs waiting to see if the defect heals with new bone growth if the defect is small enough [6].

Holoprosencephaly (HPE) is the most common developmental defect of forebrain resulting from incomplete midline cleavage of the prosencephalon into two distinct hemispheres. The pathogenesis is thought to be secondary to disruption of the prechordal plate during early gastrulation and neural plate during neurulation. Disruption of the prechordal mesoderm disrupts neural induction and regional patterning which can lead to failure of midline cleavage [7, 8]. HPE is classified into three different subgroups (DeMyer classification) based on severity. These include alobar, semilobar, and lobar holoprosencephaly. Individuals with alobar HPE have a single midline forebrain with a small cerebral ventricle lacking interhemispheric division, absence of the corpus callosum, and olfactory bulbs. The basal ganglia, hypothalamus, and thalamus are typically fused at the midline. This thalamic fusion often results in formation of a large dorsal cyst. Patients with hydranencephaly and severe hydrocephalus may have imaging that appears similar to alobar HPE but have normal thalamic cleavage and partial falx present that help distinguish between these two entities. Semilobar HPE is characterized by failure of separation of the fronto-parietal lobes and absence or hypoplasia of the corpus callosum and

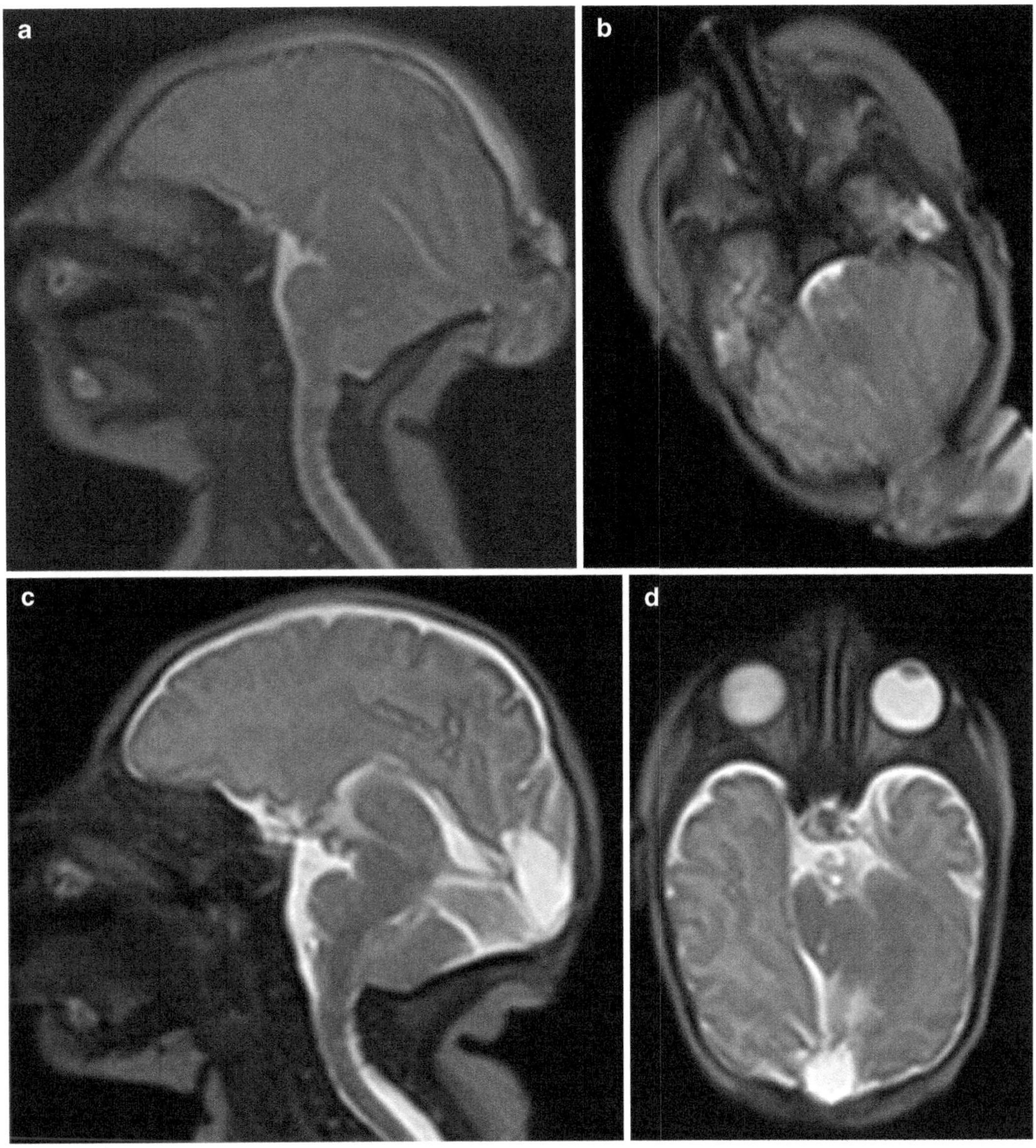

Fig. 5.1 Encephalocele. Pre-operative sagittal (**a**) and axial (**b**) T2 MRI showing an occipital encephalocele. Post-operative sagittal (**c**) and axial (**d**) T2 MRI after encephalocele repair

olfactory bulbs but with an interhemispheric fissure posteriorly (Fig. 5.2). Lobar HPE consists of more mild cleavage failure, frequently with persistence of continuity of the cingulate gyrus but with a distinct interhemispheric fissure and cleavage of the thalami. The fourth type is the middle interhemispheric variant (MIH), also called syntelencephaly, which involves midline interhemispheric fusion predominately of the posterior frontal and parietal lobes, while the focus of cleavage failure in alobar, semilobar, and lobar HPE is typically anteriorly located [9] (Fig. 5.3).

HPE is associated with facial abnormalities in approximately 80% of instances. The extent of midface hypoplasia abnormality is somewhat predictive of the severity of the holoprosencephaly. Severe midface abnormalities, such as cyclopia and ethmocephaly, are indicative of alobar

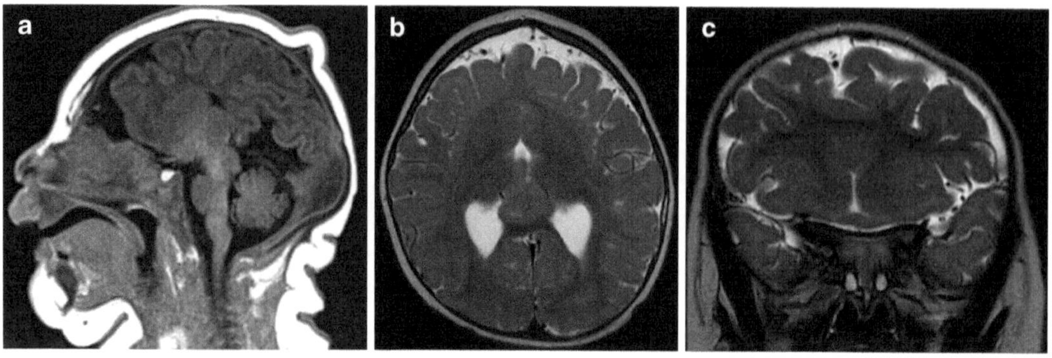

Fig. 5.2 Semilobar holoprosencephaly. Sagittal T1 (**a**), axial and coronal T2 (**b**, **c**) images showing fusion of bilateral anterior cerebral hemispheres, lack of anterior interhemispheric fissure and falx, partial fusion of the posterior aspect of the cerebral hemispheres, fusion of bilateral basal ganglia, and absent corpus callosum

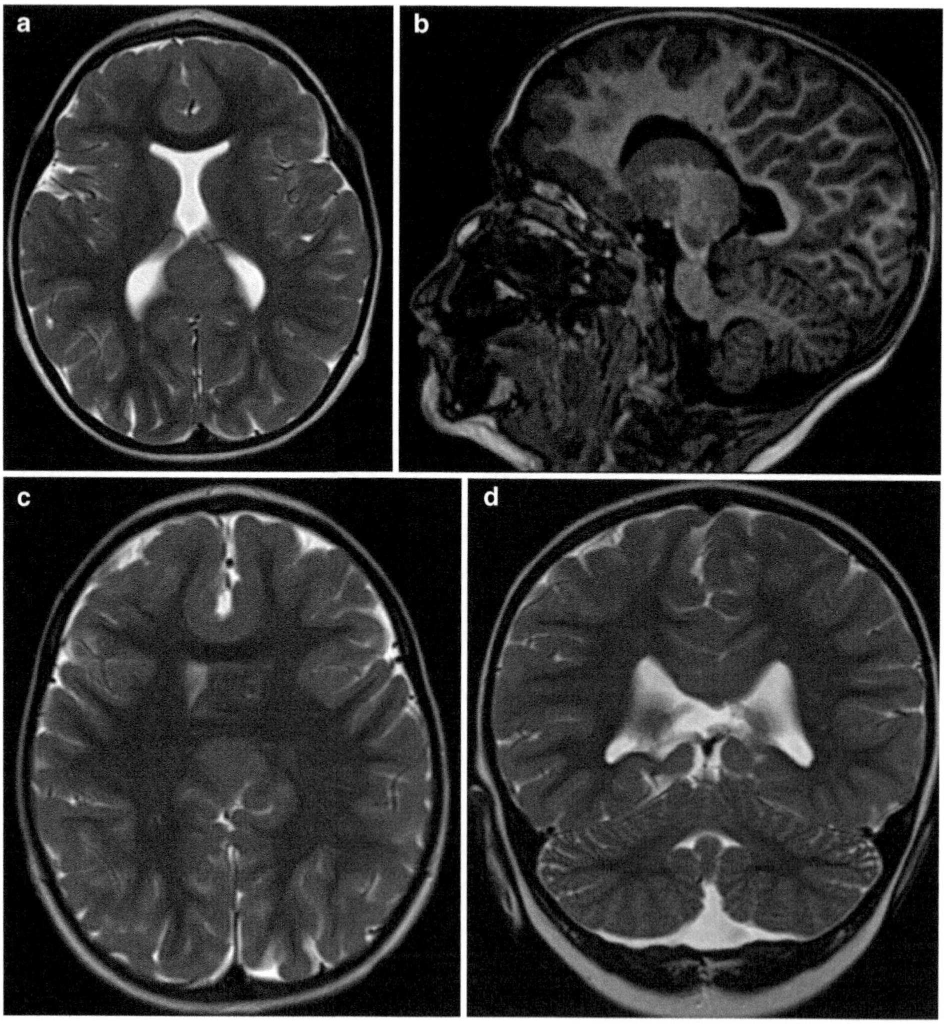

Fig. 5.3 Syntelencephaly. Axial T2 (**a**, **c**), Sagittal T1 (**b**), and Coronal T2 (**d**) images showing abnormal fusion of the frontal lobes across midline, dysgenesis of the corpus callosum with periventricular and subcortical nodular gray matter heterotopia, bifrontal polymicrogyria, absent septum pellucidum

HPE, while slightly milder midface abnormalities like cebocephaly, cleft lip, and single incisor can correlate with semilobar or lobar types including agenesis of the corpus callosum, mild pituitary abnormalities, and hypotelorism. These patients frequently have endocrinopathies (particularly diabetes insipidus), macrocephaly, hydrocephalus, seizures, spasticity, and developmental delay.

HPE occurs in approximately 1/250 conceptions, although most of these pregnancies do not proceed to birth. Only 1/10,000 live births are diagnosed with HPE and are more common in female, nonwhite, and multi-gestation pregnancies. Patients with HPE are genotypically and phenotypically heterogeneous. Similar to many other pathologies, a multiple-hit hypothesis accounts for development of holoprosencephaly through a combination of mutations in different genes with multiple environmental factors. Four major genes are thought to be the leading cause (ZIC2 (13q32), SIX3 (2p21), SHH (7q36), and TGIF (18p11.3) and are particularly more frequent in patients with chromosomal abnormalities such as trisomies 13 and 18 [10]. Environmental factors include maternal alcoholism, diabetes, and exposure to certain drugs like retinoic acid and cholesterol biosynthesis inhibitors [7].

Ultrasound is the primary modality for identifying HPE. When there is a concern for HPE on an ultrasound, obtaining a fetal MRI and doing karyotypic and mutation analysis can establish the diagnosis.

Prognosis is generally poor, particularly with alobar HPE. Some studies report up to 50% survival at 1 year in patients with semilobar or lobar HPE. These patients experience a high rate of hydrocephalus with around 20% needing CSF diversion surgeries [9].

Septo-optic dysplasia (SOD) is a congenital malformation consisting of a triad of optic nerve hypoplasia (ONH), endocrine dysfunction secondary to involvement of the pituitary and hypothalamus, and midline brain defects, particularly the absence of septum pellucidum and agenesis of the corpus callosum (Figs. 5.4 and 5.5). Patients experience a significant variation in phenotype with around 60% having hypothalamic or pituitary dysplasia with endocrinopathies, while almost 100% have optic nerve involvement. Only about 30% have all three aspects of the malformation, but at least two of the three aspects need to be present for the diagnosis. The main clinical manifestations are hypopituitarism (62–80%) with growth hormone being the most common hormone deficiency, while vision deficit and

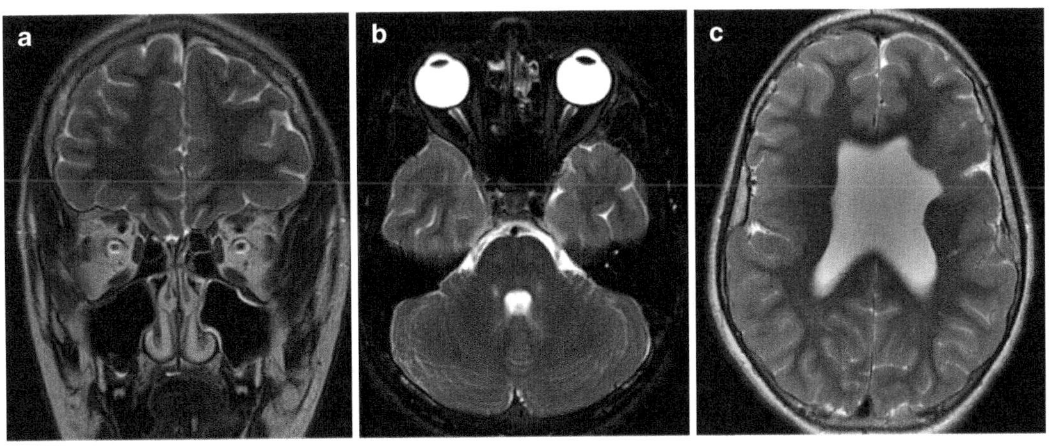

Fig. 5.4 Septo-optic dysplasia. Coronal T2 (**a**) and Axial T2 (**b**, **c**) images demonstrating absence of the septum pellucidum, bilateral schizencephaly of the frontal lobes with heterotopic gray matter, hypoplastic right optic nerve compared to the left

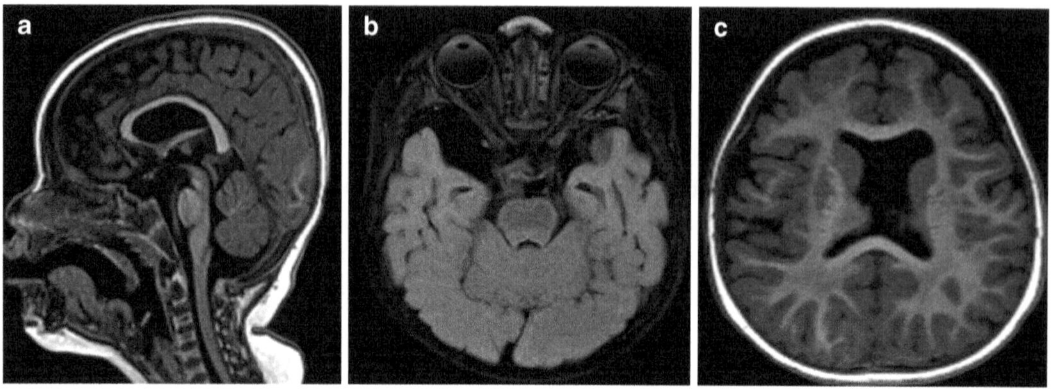

Fig. 5.5 Septo-optic dysplasia. Sagittal T1 (**a**), Axial T2 flair (**b**), and Axial T1 (**c**) images showing absence of the septum pellucidum, marked hypoplasia of the optic apparatus, and associated pituitary abnormalities with small pituitary gland, severe hypoplasia or absence of the pituitary infundibulum, and ectopia or absence of the normal posterior pituitary bright spot

developmental delay are also frequently present (20–50% of cases) [11]. Visual disturbances in SOD consist of nystagmus (bilateral ONH), strabismus (unilateral ONH), decreased visual acuity, amblyopia, and astigmatism and are the most frequent causes of congenital vision loss in developed countries [12]. SOD+ is a classification of patients who also have developmental delay and potentially additional malformations such as schizencephaly or cortical dysplasia. Diagnosis can be made with a brain MRI and endocrine labs [13].

The development of SOD is multifactorial and potentially related to young maternal age (<22), maternal DM, CMV, and exposure to other toxins in combination with mutations in HESX1, SOX2, SOX3, and OTX2 genes, although a genetic diagnosis is made in <1% of cases. SOD occurs in approximately 1/10,000 live births.

Treatment primarily focuses on management of endocrinopathies and providing vision aids.

Hydranencephaly is the resorption of a hemisphere or both hemispheres from destruction of previously normally developing brain in utero secondary to vascular occlusion, hemorrhage, infection, or maternal exposure to radiation or drugs. Although the hemisphere is resorbed and replaced with CSF, the thalamus, brainstem, cerebellum, and meninges are typically spared. Depending on the etiology of damage, a small amount of residual cortex may persist. On imaging, hydranencephaly may look similar to holoprosencephaly (HPE), but the presence of the falx and separate non-fused thalami, as well as the absence of midline facial anomalies, differentiates from HPE and indicates hydranencephaly [14] (Fig. 5.6).

The destruction event typically occurs during the second trimester with an incidence of approximately 1/5000 of pregnancies and around 1/50,000 live births. Although most cases are thought to occur from a spontaneous vascular occlusion or infection, genetic mutations in the COL4A1 gene, LAMB1 gene, and the PI3K-Akt3-mTOR pathway have been linked to some cases [15].

Most fetuses with hydranencephaly die before birth. Infants who survive are frequently born with macrocephaly but may otherwise appear normal with appropriate spontaneous reflexes. After a few weeks, infants will likely develop hyperirritability, abnormal muscle tone, and expanding head circumference. These babies are typically diagnosed via ultrasound with MRI completed after birth.

Management of these patients consists of treating seizures with antiepileptic medications and managing the likely development of hydrocephalus. Shunts are the most common approach to treating the hydrocephalus, but studies also show some efficacy of endoscopic choroid plexus coagulation [16, 17].

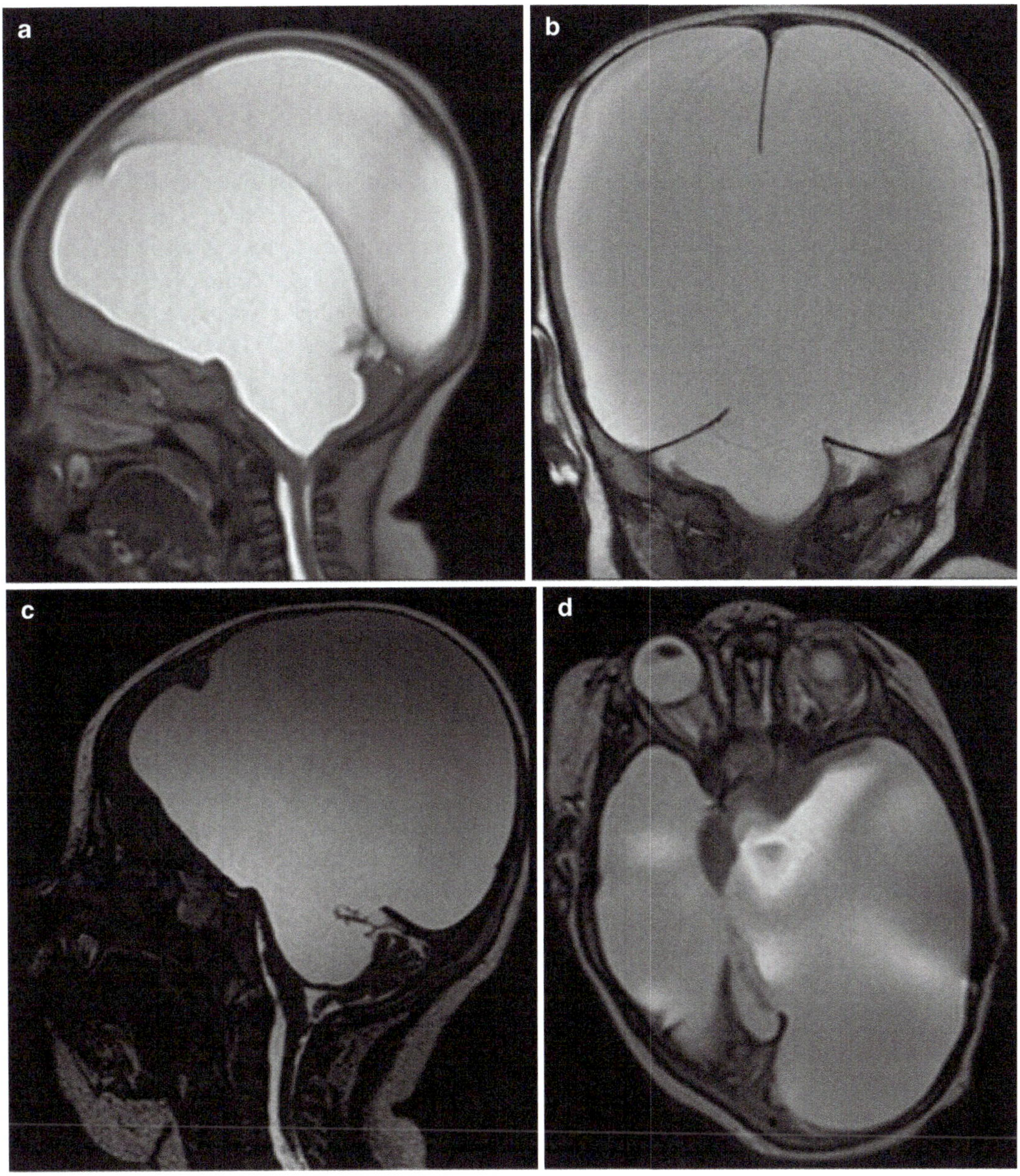

Fig. 5.6 Hydranencephaly. Sagittal T2 (**a**, **c**), Coronal T2 (**b**), and Axial T2 (**d**) images showing thin anterior cortical mantel, non-fused thalami, and presence of a falx

Spinal

Spinal dysraphism is a broad term that entails a fusion failure of dorsal spinal elements. These congenital malformations include closed neural tube defects such as spina bifida occulta as well as open defects including myelomeningoceles and multiple other malformations described below.

The pathogenesis centers around primary and secondary neurulation. Primary neurulation begins approximately on post-fertilization day 22 where the neural plate folds and starts to fuse into a neural tube, starting at the top of what will be the cervical cord and spreads cranially with closure of the tube at 24 days and caudally with closure of the neural tube at 26 days. Failure to close the caudal neuropore results in open spinal dysraphisms. Secondary neurulation occurs after the neural tube has closed and involves formation of the neural tube in the sacral and coccygeal regions with longitudinal cell condensations forming from mesenchymal cells. This process is completed in the sixth week after fertilization. Defects in organization of this mesenchyme from neuro-mesodermal cells can result in failed formation of posterior spinal element but with the successful development of a dermal/skin layer. These patients have closed dysraphisms such as spina bifida occulta. In addition to defective bone development, aberrant adipose tissue may develop becoming a lipoma.

In open spinal dysraphism patients, motor and sensory neuronal development and differentiation typically continue below the abnormal level. The amniotic fluid is relatively benign around the time the neural tube fails to close but becomes toxic as the pregnancy progresses and causes death of exposed neuronal tissue over the following weeks prior to delivery.

Neural tube defects (NTDs) as a whole present in 1/1000 live births in the USA and Europe, while spina bifida cases are reported in 0.5/1000 live births. There is a significant variance around the globe with reports noting the incidence in some regions to be up to 20 times higher.

Consistent with many congenital malformations, neural tube defects result from the interaction of multiple genetic and environmental factors. Some element of heritability exists, particularly in first-degree relatives, as there is a 2–5% risk for siblings born after a child with an NTD, representing a 20–50-fold increased risk compared to the general population. The risk increases to 10% for a subsequent pregnancy if two previous children are affected. Successful neural tube closure requires more than 200 genes, and multiple mutation pathways have resulted in neural tube defects making a specific gene target or heritability pattern very difficult to identify. The most significant environmental risk factors are insufficient folate and maternal obesity and diabetes. Valproic acid is the medication that has a high risk associated with development of NTDs if taken during the first trimester.

Certain spinal dysraphisms, especially closed malformations, may have minimal clinical significance and low impact on a patient's function, essentially amounting to an incidental finding. A large proportion of patients, however, have significant neurologic dysfunction including lower extremity weakness, sensory loss, bowel and bladder dysfunction, and unrelenting pain as a result of their NTD. Additionally, these patients often have multiple secondary developmental defects including Chiari II malformations, hydrocephalus, hypogenesis of the corpus callosum, and cognitive and developmental delay. They frequently exhibit hip dysplasia and dislocation, as well as lower extremity malformations, club feet, and spine malformations such as scoliosis.

The spectrum of spinal dysraphism is broad. Closed defects include spina bifida occulta, which results from failure of secondary neurulation with defective neuro-mesodermal and mesenchyme cell organization. Fusion of posterior vertebrae elements does not proceed, but the dermal layer still develops successfully. These do not require surgical repair but are important to take into consideration if the patient undergoes other spine surgeries.

Tethered cord is a broad term that includes many pathologies including any connection of the spinal cord to the spinal canal that results in spinal cord tension. This can occur after a MMC repair secondary to scarring, adhesion from spinal lipomas, and multiple other complex sources which will be discussed in more detail in their respective sections. Regarding closed spinal defects specifically, tethered cord most frequently refers to a thickened or fatty filum terminale attached to the caudal aspect of the conus medullaris extending down to its sacral terminating point [18] (Fig. 5.7). The thickened or fatty filum does not extend or have enough laxity such that when a patient grows, the filum exerts tension forces on the conus and caudal aspect of the spinal cord with the potential of causing neuronal injury [19]. This results in lower extremity weakness, sensory loss, problems with coordination, back pain, and bladder dysfunction. A filum typically needs to be thicker than 2 mm or contains lipomatous material to be considered patho-

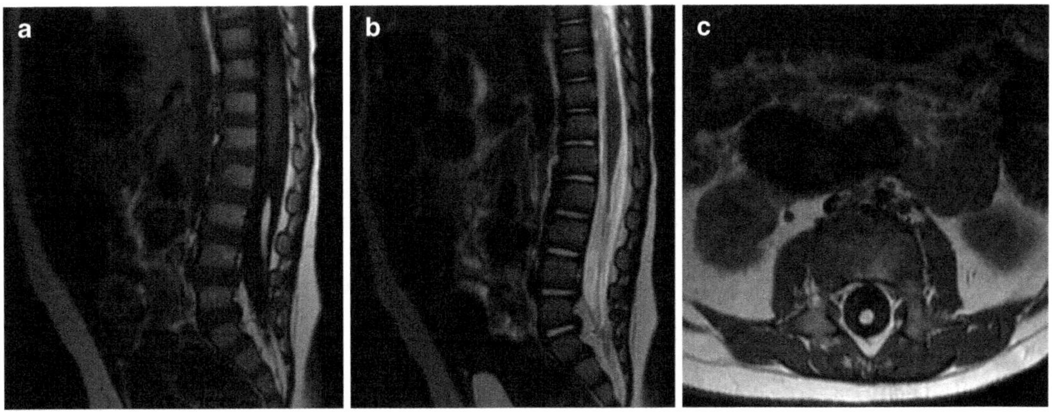

Fig. 5.7 Fatty filum. Sagittal T1 (**a**), Sagittal T2 (**b**), and Axial T1 (**c**) MRI demonstrating a thickened and fatty filum terminale with a low-lying conus indicating a tethered cord

logic. These filum features, combined with a low-lying conus at L2 or below, indicate a tethered cord. Some reports in the literature indicate that patients with a thickened filum may still incur tethering symptoms without a low-lying conus and may still benefit from surgery [20]. The incidence of tethered cord is difficult to ascertain as there are frequently no external signs and the diagnosis is made when the symptoms are appropriately identified and imaging subsequently obtained. One case series with more than 3000 patients with radiological tethered cord determined that only 15% of these patients underwent surgical release [21]. If a patient has a syrinx associated with the tethered cord, they are more likely to undergo surgery. No specific genes or mutations have been associated with tethered cord, although siblings of patients with other types of spinal dysraphisms have a slightly higher rate of occurrence. Surgery typically consists of one- or two-level laminectomy below the conus, linear durotomy, and visual identification of the filum terminale confirmed by intra-operative neuromonitoring, with subsequent coagulation and cutting of the filum.

Split cord malformations are closed spinal dysraphisms, sometimes referred to as diastematomyelia. These are divided into two subgroups. Type 1 includes two hemicords separated by an osteocartilaginous median septum, housed in a separate dural sheath (Fig. 5.8). Type 2 consists of two hemicords contained within the same dural envelope separated by a fibrous septum. Patients with type 1 have a slightly higher propensity of developing symptoms of tethered cord. Patients presenting with tethered cord symptoms can sometimes be distinguished by findings that lateralized to the left or right depending upon which aspect of the cord is tethered [22]. Embryologically, hemicords are formed because of persistent adhesions between the ectoderm and endoderm, leading to an accessory neurenteric canal around which condenses an endomesenchymal tract that bisects the developing notochord and causes formation of two hemineural plates [23]. Symptomatic patients are taken for surgery for removal of the osteocartilaginous septum and repair of the dura [24].

Dermal sinus tracts are defects that extend from the skin, lined by keratinized squamous epithelium (Fig. 5.9). They may occur anywhere between columella of the nose and coccyx with variable intracranial or intraspinal extension. These tracts develop from adhesion and incomplete dissolution of the continuity between the neural and cutaneous ectoderms during neurulation, around the fourth week of gestation. Nearly all reported cranial cases occur in the midline and commonly involve the external occipital protuberance. If a dermal sinus tract penetrates deeply, it can attach to the spinal cord or midline brain structures and serve as a source of cord tethering. In these instances, surgical resection may be necessary for cord detethering. Occasionally, dermal

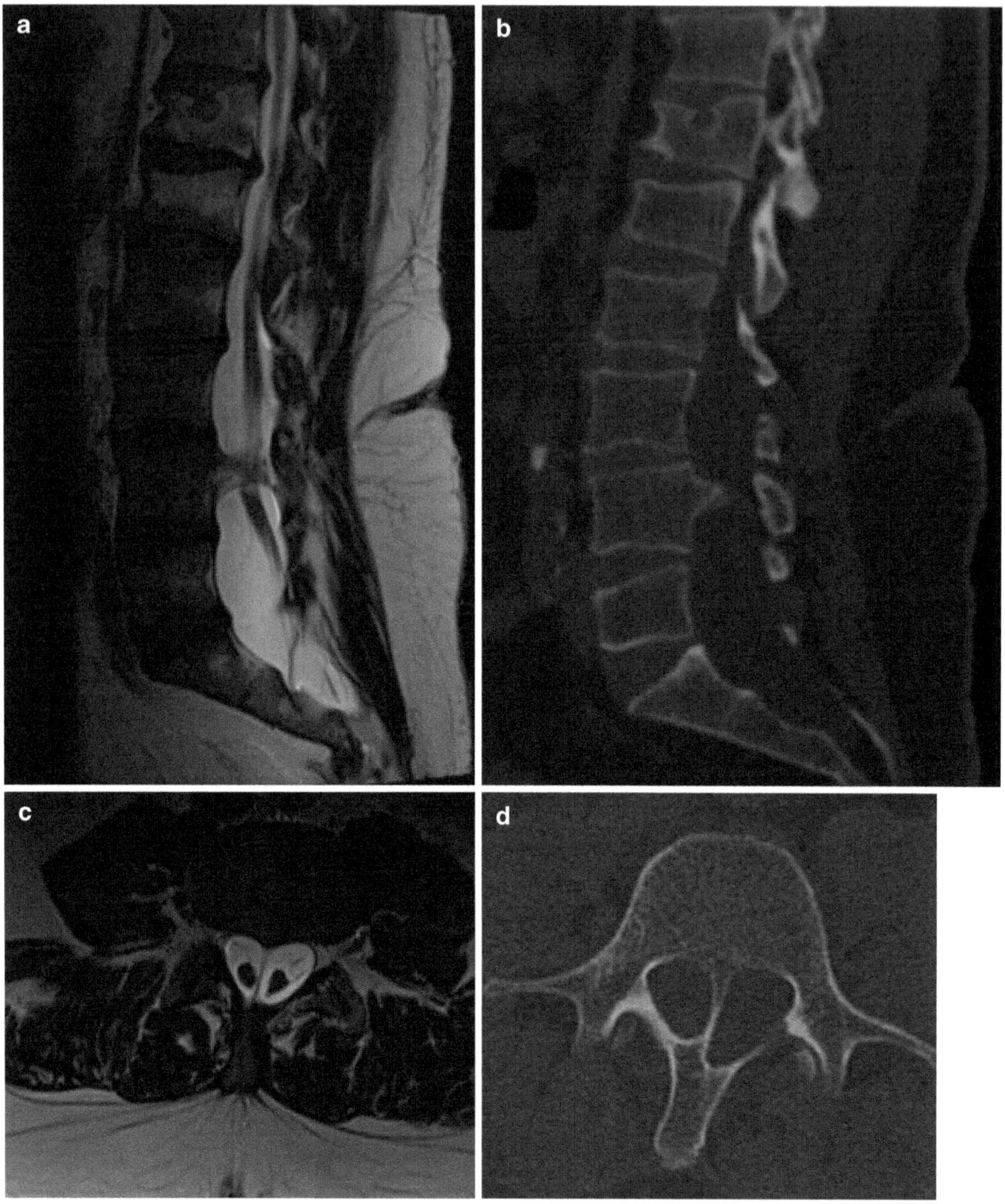

Fig. 5.8 Diastematomyelia. Sagittal T2 MRI (**a**), Sagittal CT (**b**), Axial T2 MRI (**c**), and Axial CT (**d**) of the lumbar spine showing a Type 1 diastematomyelia at L4 with an osteocartilagenous median septum extending from the dorsal vertebral body to the lamina with a two hemicords encased in their own dural envelopes. The patient also had a dermal sinus tract with cord tethering at L3

sinus tracts may create an open pathway to the spinal canal, and patients may have an additional risk of developing meningitis, necessitating early operative intervention [25]. Inclusion cysts can also occur in many cases of patients with dermal sinus tracts. These tracts are estimated to occur in 1 in 2500 live births and associated with other dysraphisms in approximately 11% of cases [26]. Sacral dimples are seen frequently prompting neurosurgical evaluation to determine if these

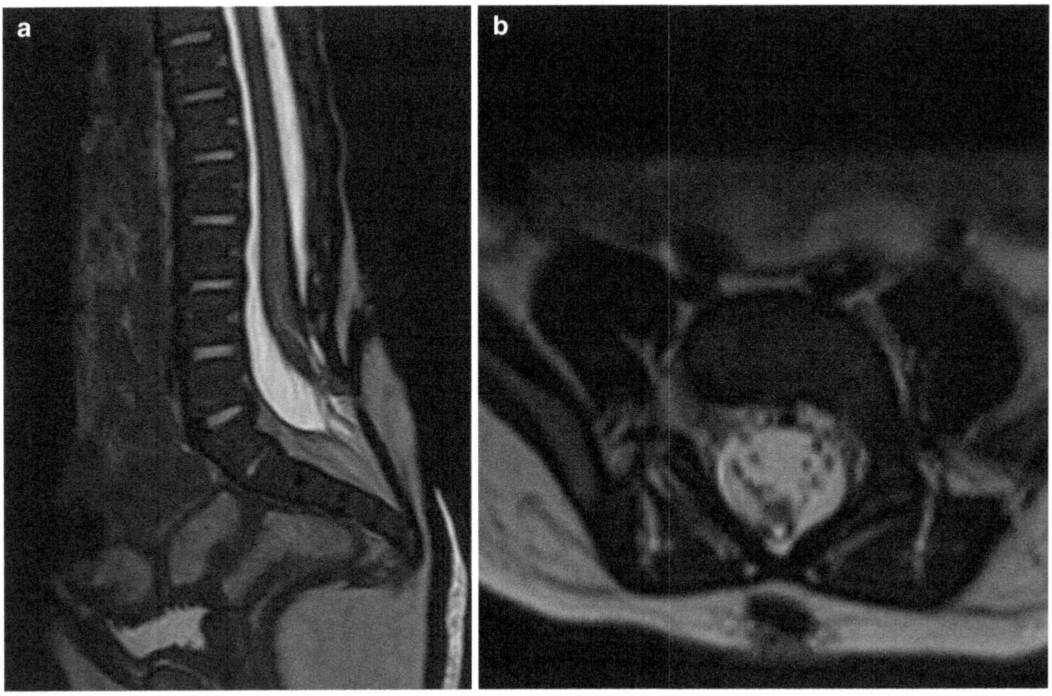

Fig. 5.9 Dermal sinus tract. Sagittal T2 (**a**) and Axial T2 (**b**) MRI showing a dermal sinus tract with spinal cord tethering

represent dermal sinus tracts. One multicenter study evaluated all patients who underwent ultrasound for sacral dimples and found that only 0.1% of these patients had significant findings, including dermal sinus tracts that prompted surgical exploration and detethering [27].

Spinal lipomas and lipomyelomeningocele are types of closed neural tube defects consisting of lipoma formation in the posterior cord. These occur secondary to premature dysjunction of epithelial ectoderm from neural ectoderm prior to neurulation/neural tube formation. This allows mesenchyme cells to contact the inner portion of developing neural tube, which induces fat development in the posterior aspect of the spinal cord, impeding neural tube closure. The fat typically extends through the spine and into the subcutaneous space. This fatty attachment tethers the spinal cord to that level where it leaves the canal. These are rare with a rate estimated to be between 0.3 and 0.6/10,000 live births and are associated with split cord malformations, dermal sinus tracts, diastematomyelia, and terminal hydromyelia [28]. The patients commonly have a lipomatous mass located at the lumbar sacral region, often with a harry nevus or dimple. Because of these signs, the diagnosis is often made prior to symptom onset.

Spinal lipomas are divided into subtypes including dorsal, transitional, caudal/terminal, and chaotic. Dorsal type includes lipomas that attach to the dorsal aspect of the spinal cord at the area of the myeloschisis and extend posteriorly through the dura, boney defect, and fascia to be in continuity with the subcutaneous tissue (Fig. 5.10). Transitional lipomas are similar with extension through the dura, bone, and fascia into the subcutaneous space but also have a component that extends intradural to the conus. Caudal or terminal lipomas attach at the base of the conus and may extend through the dura or potentially be encased in the dura [28]. Terminal lipomas do not involve the dorsal parts of the spinal cord or nerve roots. The extension of the fatty connection from the cord to the subcutaneous fat results in a tethered cord with associated symp-

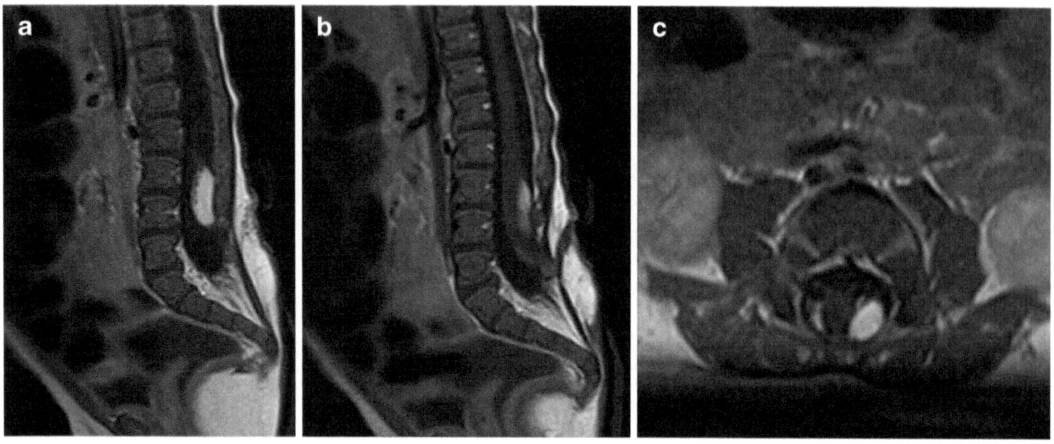

Fig. 5.10 Spinal Lipoma. Sagittal T1 (**a**, **b**) and Axial T1 (**c**) MRI demonstrating a dorsal spinal lipoma

toms if not corrected. Chaotic lipomas are similar to dorsal or transitional lipomas but have a portion that penetrates through the placode to the ventral aspect of the cord. The final category is lipomyelomeningocele which involves a spinal lipoma connected to a neural placode that protrudes posteriorly through the bone and fascia to connect to the subcutaneous fat. In these circumstances, the neural placode resides outside the spinal canal until it is repaired.

Surgery involves the removal of the dorsal subcutaneous mass of adipose tissue, followed by identification of the fascial, bony, and dural defects. The lipoma-spinal or cord/neural placode interface is identified and as much of the lipomatous tissue is removed while avoiding damaging the neural tissue. After the lipoma is removed, the neural placode should be folded with the placode edges touching and the pia sewn together to form a tube. The dura is repaired either primarily or with duraplasty if additional space is needed to help reduce retethering. It is important to note that total or near-total resection of a lipoma tends to reduce the incidence of retethering, which tends to occur at a high rate in patients with only partial resections [29].

The best surgical timing has yet to be determined in patients with lipomyelomeningoceles or spinal lipomas who do not exhibit signs or symptoms of cord tethering. Spinal lipomas are a progressive disease with 33–40% of asymptomatic patients deteriorating over the following 9 years. When these patients develop neurologic dysfunction, recovery may take many months with many patients never returning to their baseline. Some groups advocate for early preventative surgery prior to symptom onset with the expectation that these patients would inevitably develop symptoms over time. The data in the literature is mixed regarding this but trending toward performing earlier surgery with improved long-term stability of neurological function [30].

The literature also indicates that earlier surgery for patients exhibiting tethered cord symptoms results in better long-term lower extremity function and sensation, although also noting that patients with pre-operative bowel and bladder dysfunction often do not fully recover these functions. Patients with lipomyelomeningoceles who undergo surgery have approximately 20–30% retethering rate over 3–8 years [28].

Open spinal dysraphism consists of meningocele (herniation of meninges through a defect in the bony elements without herniation of the neural elements) or myelomeningocele (consists of herniation of neural elements). These can occur throughout the spinal canal from cervical to sacral regions and may be either ventral, lateral, or dorsal. The pathophysiology is likely different based on the location of formation. Posterior lumbar and sacral meningoceles likely develop from a secondary neurulation problem, while ventral and lateral defects are from generalized mesenchymal abnormalities such as NF1 and Marfan's disease.

Myelomeningocele (MMC) results from the failure of primary neurulation of the caudal aspect of the neural plate into a neural tube around 26 days of gestation. This leads to an exposed neural placode that remains open to the environment as the mesoderm and ectoderm do not receive the appropriate signals to form the bone, muscle, fascia, and skin over the open neural tissue. The neuroepithelium initially continues to undergo normal neuronal differentiation, but as the amniotic fluid become more toxic over the pregnancy, neurons start becoming hemorrhagic and undergo cell death. The incidence of MMC is approximately 3.4/10,000 live births with an early death rate of approximately 10%. Diagnosis is typically made with fetal ultrasound with subsequent follow-up with fetal MRI (Fig. 5.11). Maternal serum AFP screening can be done at 16–18 weeks with a sensitivity of 75% with false positives occurring secondary to other fetal disorders or an underestimated gestational age. After the MMC is identified, closure is either performed in utero or within 24–48 h after birth [31].

Fetal closure of MMC was demonstrated in the MOMs study in 2011 to have significant advantages by decreasing the need of cerebrospinal fluid shunting with lower rates of hindbrain herniation and better lower extremity motor function. Specifically, patients with prenatal closure had a shunt placement rate of 40% while postnatal

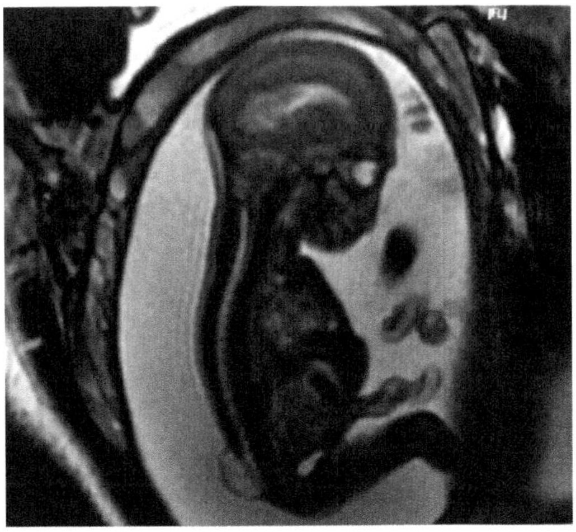

Fig. 5.11 Myelomeningocele. Sagittal T2 fetal MRI showing a lower lumbar myelomeningocele

patients underwent shunts in 82% of cases. The subsequent need for a shunt revision was also less frequent in the prenatal repair group (15.4% vs 40.2%). Although the fetal surgery group had a more severe affected level of the MMC, they were found to have function at two or more levels beyond what was expected and had likelihood of being able to walk without orthotics or devices in 42% of cases compared to 21% of patients who were repaired postnatally. Fetuses who underwent surgery prenatally had a higher rate of preterm birth with an average gestational age of 34.1 weeks compared to 37.3 weeks for the postnatal repair group. Approximately one fifth of the prenatal repair group experienced respiratory distress syndrome initially, but no other significant differences existed between groups secondary to prematurity. The prenatal closure patients were also noted to have a higher rate of surgery for delayed spinal cord tethering. Inclusion criteria for the study were a singleton pregnancy, the myelomeningocele upper boundary located between T1 and S1, evidence of hindbrain herniation, a gestational age between 19 and 25.9 weeks, a normal karyotype, and maternal age of at least 18. Patients were excluded if they had a fetal anomaly unrelated to the MMC, sever kyphosis, risk of preterm birth, placental abruption, a BMI of 35 or more, and a prior hysterotomy [32–35]. Subsequent evaluation of patients in the study noted that fetuses with ventricle size of >15 mm had a shunt rate of 79.4% in spite of fetal closure indicating these patients may not receive benefit from an in utero repair. Many more centers around the country are developing the ability to perform fetal surgery and prenatal MMC closure. Of those women referred for fetal MMC repair, 17.7% were deemed appropriate candidates and elected to undergo this surgery.

Surgical closure, either in utero or postnatal, involves separating and isolating the neural placode and then folding and suturing the edges to simulate the creation of a neural tube. The dural remnants are then identified, and the spinal canal is reconstructed (Fig. 5.12). The muscle, fascia, and dermal layers are then identified and undermined to allow the edges to be opposed to each other and closed in sequential order (Fig. 5.13).

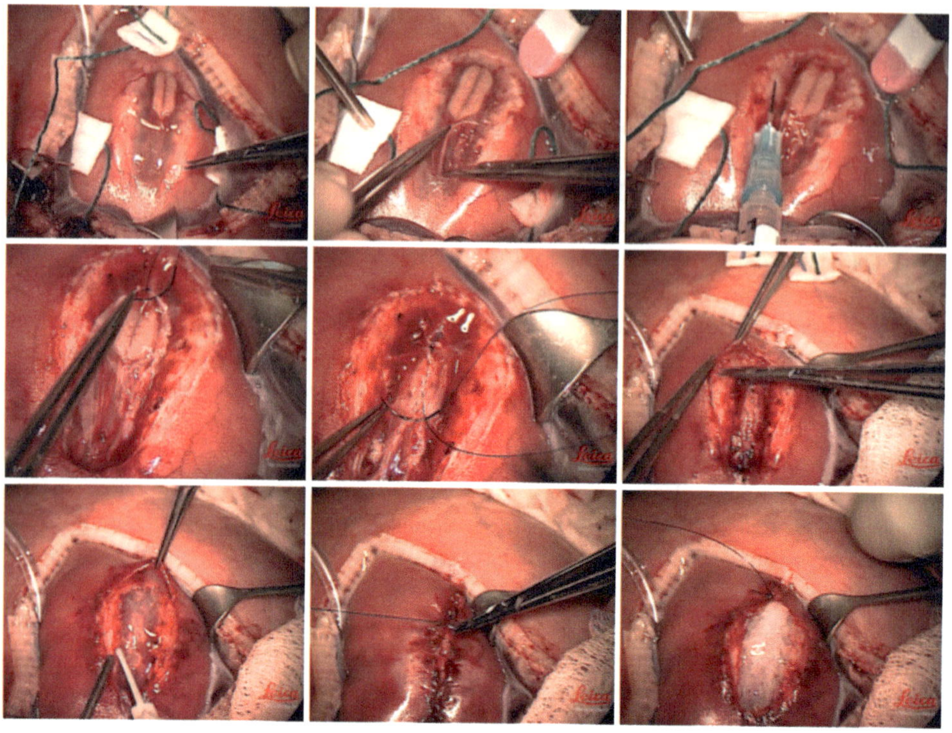

Fig. 5.12 Myelomeningocele fetal closure 1. Images from a fetal MMC closure illustrating placode isolation, construction of a neural tube, separation of dura, muscle, and fascia

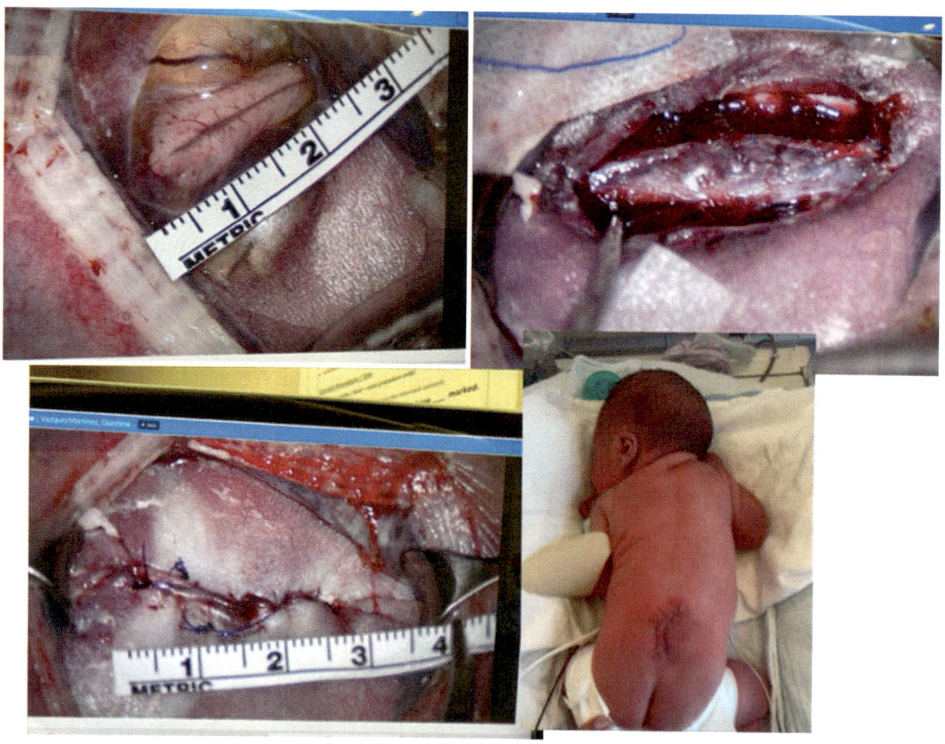

Fig. 5.13 Myelomeningocele fetal closure 2. Images showing the MMC prior to closure, the neural placode reconstructed into the neural tube. Fascia, muscle, and skin closed

Patients with MMC experience significant long-term disabilities including lower extremity dysfunction and paralysis, bowel and bladder dysfunction, and a high rate of scoliosis and hip dysplasia. Associated brain anomalies include Chiari II malformations with hindbrain herniation, small posterior fossa, tectal beaking, and hydrocephalus (Fig. 5.14) requiring shunting in approximately 75% of cases.

Essentially all MMC patients also develop spinal cord tethering radiographically with approximately 30% becoming symptomatic during periods of high growth rates with a slightly higher rate in patients who underwent fetal MMC closure (Fig. 5.15). Symptoms include bladder/urinary dysfunction, motor dysfunction with worsening of gait, sensory dysfunction with increased pain, numbness, paresthesia, and scoliosis [36]. These patients undergo detethering operations with subsequent improvement of symptoms occurring in 10–25%, symptoms stabilizing in 60–80%, and worsening in approximately 10%. Symptomatic retethering occurs in 15–30% of patients and requires additional detethering surgeries. Operations involve exploration of the prior MMC repair including additional laminectomies and intradural exploration to identify areas of spinal cord tethering. The goal is to release the placode and spinal cord in all directions, particularly in areas that are causing tension, without causing nerve damage while attempting to reduce the risk of retethering. This surgery is difficult with distorted anatomy, scar tissue, and aberrant nerve pathways with a high likelihood of not achieving a

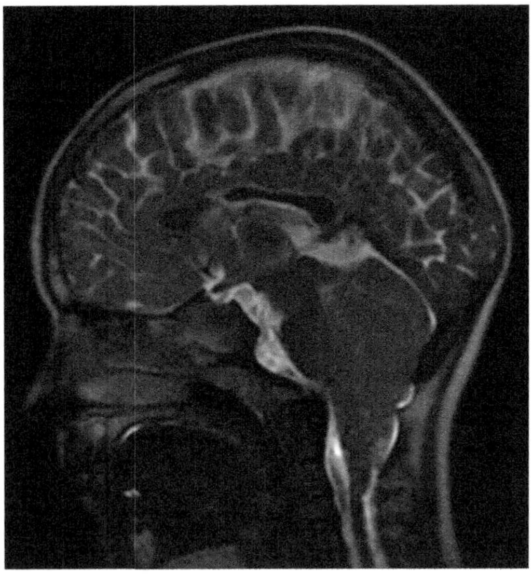

Fig. 5.14 MMC Chiari II. Sagittal T2 MRI illustrating the hindbrain herniation and medullary kinking, small posterior fossa, tectal beaking, and moderate hydrocephalus

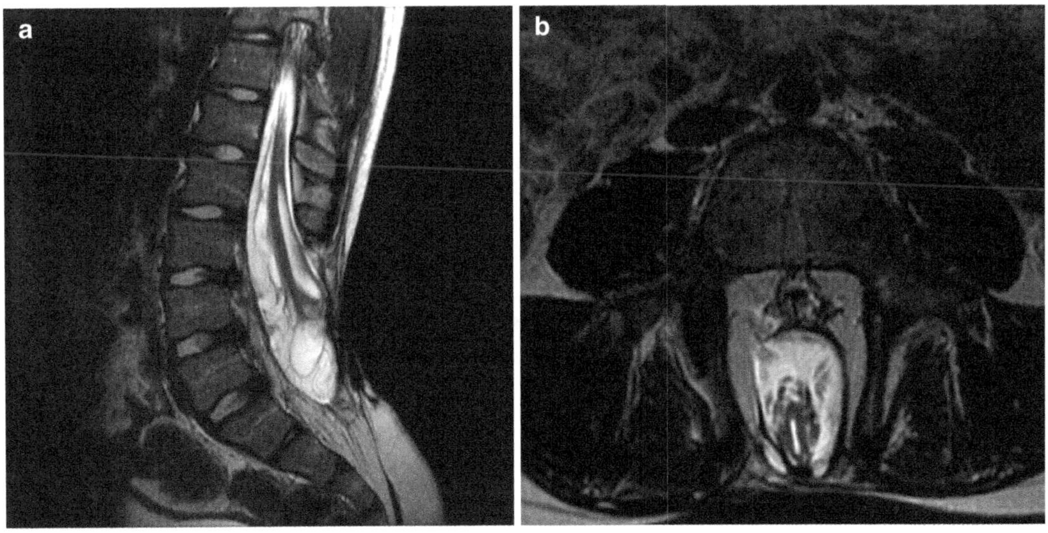

Fig. 5.15 MMC rethetering. Sagittal T2 (**a**) and Axial T2 (**b**) images that show a prior MMC repair with subsequent spinal cord adhesion and tethering to the dorsal aspect of the spinal canal

complete detethering. Detethering operations have a post-op wound breakdown, CSF leak, and infection rate of 10–35% [37].

An additional management strategy for tethered cord syndrome has been proposed with the aim to reduce the tension on the spinal cord through spinal column shortening [38]. Patients undergo two- to three-level laminectomies at the thoraco-lumbar junction followed by either pedicle subtraction osteotomies or vertebral column resection [39]. With screws and rods placed above and below this level, compression is applied to the screws with the aim of decreasing the interval by 1.5–2.5 cm [40]. This procedure is typically performed at the thoraco-lumbar junction which allows the surgeon to avoid operating at the prior tethered cord location, removing the need to dissect through layers of scar tissue, enter the dura, or manipulate nerves. Thus, these patients have a significantly lower rate of CSF leaks and wound infections. Approximately 70–80% of patients experience improvement of pre-operative symptoms, while 10–30% experience stability or worsening of their symptoms [41] (Figs. 5.16 and 5.17).

Scoliosis is the most common and severe skeletal complication related to MMC, resulting in respiratory compromise, decreased mobility, and worsening of neurologic symptoms. The prevalence is reported in the literature at 52.8% but varies significantly by study with the larger studies noting a prevalence closer to 25%. The level of the MMC correlates with the risk of developing scoliosis with a higher likelihood in patients with thoracic lesions (93%) compared to upper lumbar (72%), lower lumbar (43%), or sacral (8%) lesions. Treatment includes tethered cord release with resultant improvement of the scoliosis in approximately 15% of cases, stability of the curvature in 60% of patients, and worsening of the curve in 25%. Retethering often occurs earlier in patients with scoliosis. Posterior, anterior, or combination instrumentation techniques are frequently applied in conjunction with detethering operations. Scoliosis correction surgery improves the Cobb angle from 70–90° to 35–45° but has a significant complication rate around 50% [42].

Hydrocephalus in patients with myelomeningoceles is typically treated with cerebrospinal fluid shunting. Endoscopic third ventriculostomies and choroid plexus cautery have been attempted but without significant success [43].

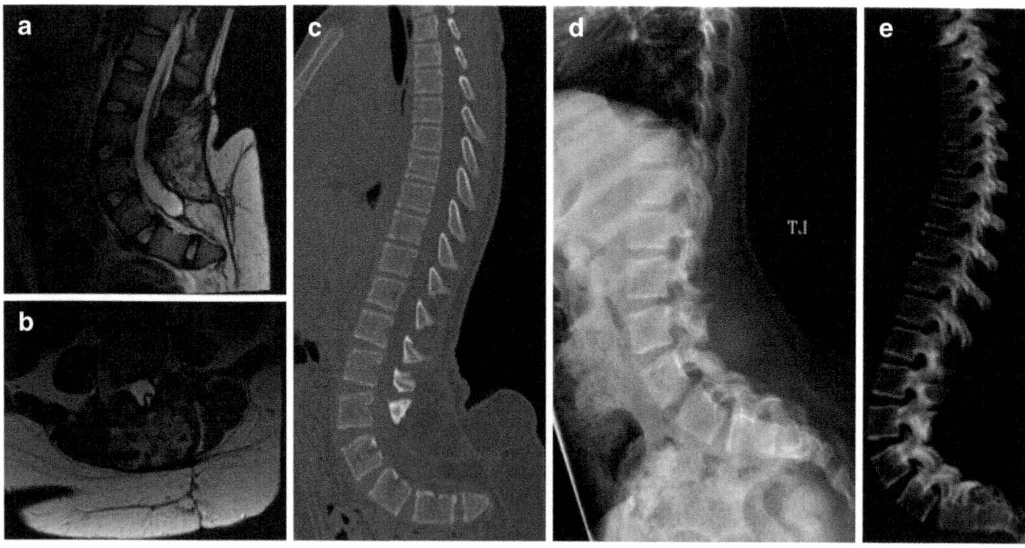

Fig. 5.16 MMC spinal shortening 1. Sagitta T2 (**a**), Axial T2 (**b**), Sagittal T/L spine CT (**c**), Sagittal 3-D CT reconstruction (**d**), and Lateral x-ray (**e**) demonstrating prior lumbar laminectomies with persistent complex tethered cord. Pre-operative images prior to a spinal shortening surgery

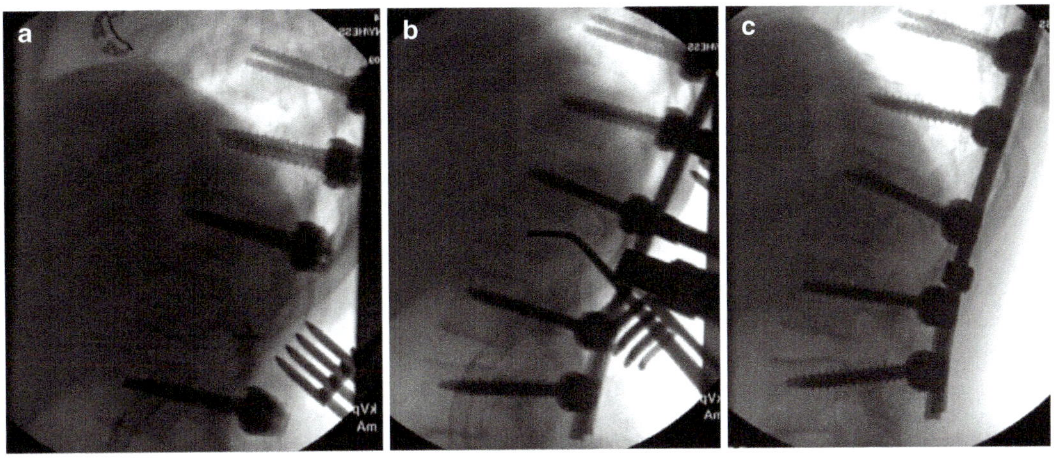

Fig. 5.17 MMC spinal shortening 2. Lateral intraoperative fluoroscopic images showing pedicle screw placement from T9 to L2 (**a**), T12 superior 2/3 corpectomy with partial compression of the instrument construct (**b**), and completed compression of the instrument construct with resultant 2.2 cm of shortening (**c**)

Review Questions

1. An infant is born at gestational age of 37 weeks with a head circumference in the 82nd percentile and has a full but soft fontanelle. He has decreased tone and reflexes. An MRI shows a very thin anterior cortical mantel and thalami connected by the thalamic adhesion, with preservation of the falx cerebri. This patient has:
   (a) Semilobar holoprosencephaly
   (b) Alobar holoprosencephaly
   (c) Hydranencephaly
   (d) Septo-optic dysplasia
2. Hydranencephaly results from:
   (a) An event that causes resorption of one or both hemispheres during the second trimester
   (b) Failure of closure of the anterior neuropore at 24 days of gestation
   (c) Failure of midline cleavage that arrests development of the hemispheres around the sixth week of gestation
   (d) Acute development of aqueductal stenosis at the end of the first trimester causing extreme hydrocephalus and neuronal regression
3. A 32-year-old pregnant female with estimated gestational age of 25 weeks is referred after an ultrasound notes a myelomeningocele. Which feature was an exclusion criterion to be involved in the MOMs study for fetal repair?
   (a) Gestational age of 25 weeks
   (b) Placenta previa
   (c) Prior cesarean section
   (d) Placenta located on the ventral aspect of the uterus
4. What is the primary outcome of the MOMs study that will help with counseling the patient?
   (a) A higher rate of patients regaining their lower extremity motor function and the ability to ambulate with minimal assistance
   (b) Fewer CNS infections during the newborn period
   (c) Decreased rate of PEG tube placement
   (d) Lower rate of ventriculoperitoneal shunt placement without a significant difference in infant mortality
5. Data has shown that fetal ventricular size may correlate with the rate of hydrocephalus development in patients with myelomeningoceles. What ventricular size correlates with a

higher rate of hydrocephalus and subsequent shunt placement that may make the utility of fetal repair less favorable?
   (a) >10 mm
   (b) >13 mm
   (c) >15 mm
   (d) >18 mm
6. After discussion, this mother decides to proceed with a fetal repair of her baby's myelomeningocele. What are some of the risks of proceeding?
   (a) Preterm birth with higher rate of short-term respiratory failure requiring respiratory support
   (b) A higher rate of CNS infections requiring longer-term suppressive antibiotics
   (c) Increased risk of damage to the fetal spinal cord causing spinal cord damage
   (d) Decreased fertility and ability to have subsequent children

Answers
1. (c)
2. (a)
3. (c)
4. (d)
5. (c)
6. (a)

References

1. Munteanu O, Cîrstoiu MM, Filipoiu FM, Neamţu MN, Stavarache I, Georgescu TA, Bratu OG, Iorgulescu G, Bohîlţea RE. The etiopathogenic and morphological spectrum of anencephaly: a comprehensive review of literature. Rom J Morphol Embryol. 2020;61(2):335–43. https://doi.org/10.47162/RJME.61.2.03. PMID: 33544785; PMCID: PMC7864317.
2. Avagliano L, Massa V, George TM, Qureshy S, Bulfamante GP, Finnell RH. Overview on neural tube defects: from development to physical characteristics. Birth Defects Res. 2019;111(19):1455–67. https://doi.org/10.1002/bdr2.1380. Epub 2018 Nov 12. PMID: 30421543; PMCID: PMC6511489.
3. Lo BW, Kulkarni AV, Rutka JT, Jea A, Drake JM, Lamberti-Pasculli M, Dirks PB, Thabane L. Clinical predictors of developmental outcome in patients with cephaloceles. J Neurosurg Pediatr. 2008;2(4):254–7. https://doi.org/10.3171/PED.2008.2.10.254. PMID: 18831658.
4. Mahapatra AK. Anterior encephalocele—AIIMS experience a series of 133 patients. J Pediatr Neurosci. 2011;6(Suppl 1):S27–30. https://doi.org/10.4103/1817-1745.85706. PMID: 22069427; PMCID: PMC3208910.
5. Markovic I, Bosnjakovic P, Milenkovic Z. Occipital encephalocele: cause, incidence, neuroimaging and surgical management. Curr Pediatr Rev. 2020;16(3):200–5. https://doi.org/10.2174/1573396315666191018161535. PMID: 31656152; PMCID: PMC8193807.
6. Rehman L, Farooq G, Bukhari I. Neurosurgical interventions for occipital encephalocele. Asian J Neurosurg. 2018;13(2):233–7. https://doi.org/10.4103/1793-5482.228549. PMID: 29682014; PMCID: PMC5898085.
7. Geng X, Oliver G. Pathogenesis of holoprosencephaly. J Clin Invest. 2009;119(6):1403–13. https://doi.org/10.1172/JCI38937. Epub 2009 Jun 1. PMID: 19487816; PMCID: PMC2689134.
8. Grinblat Y, Lipinski RJ. A forebrain undivided: unleashing model organisms to solve the mysteries of holoprosencephaly. Dev Dyn. 2019;248(8):626–33. https://doi.org/10.1002/dvdy.41. Epub 2019 May 1. PMID: 30993762.
9. Winter TC, Kennedy AM, Woodward PJ. Holoprosencephaly: a survey of the entity, with embryology and fetal imaging. Radiographics. 2015;35(1):275–90. https://doi.org/10.1148/rg.351140040. PMID: 25590404.
10. Dubourg C, Kim A, Watrin E, de Tayrac M, Odent S, David V, Dupé V. Recent advances in understanding inheritance of holoprosencephaly. Am J Med Genet C Semin Med Genet. 2018;178(2):258–69. https://doi.org/10.1002/ajmg.c.31619. Epub 2018 May 22. PMID: 29785796.
11. Webb EA, Dattani MT. Septo-optic dysplasia. Eur J Hum Genet. 2010;18(4):393–7. https://doi.org/10.1038/ejhg.2009.125. Epub 2009 Jul 22. PMID: 19623216; PMCID: PMC2987262.
12. Ganau M, Huet S, Syrmos N, Meloni M, Jayamohan J. Neuro-ophthalmological manifestations of septo-optic dysplasia: current perspectives. Eye Brain. 2019;11:37–47. https://doi.org/10.2147/EB.S186307. PMID: 31695544; PMCID: PMC6805786.
13. Gutierrez-Castillo A, Jimenez-Ruiz A, Chavez-Castillo M, Ruiz-Sandoval JL. Septo-optic dysplasia plus syndrome. Cureus. 2018;10(12):e3727. https://doi.org/10.7759/cureus.3727. PMID: 30800538; PMCID: PMC6384050.
14. Gezmu AM, Shifa JZ, Kgwarae C, Siamisang A. Hydranencephaly in a neonate: a literature review. Neurol India. 2020;68(1):199–201. https://doi.org/10.4103/0028-3886.279698. PMID: 32129279.
15. Omar AT 2nd, Manalo MKA, Zuniega RRA, Reyes JCB, Brillante EMB, Khu KJO. Hydranencephaly: clinical features and survivorship in a retrospective cohort. World Neurosurg. 2020;144:e589–96. https://doi.org/10.1016/j.wneu.2020.09.029. Epub 2020 Sep 8. PMID: 32916366.

16. Sandoval JI, De Jesus O. Hydranencephaly. 2021 Aug 30. In: StatPearls [Internet]. Treasure Island (FL): StatPearls Publishing; 2021. PMID: 32644417.
17. Sandberg DI, Chamiraju P, Zoeller G, Bhatia S, Ragheb J. Endoscopic choroid plexus coagulation in infants with hydranencephaly or hydrocephalus with a minimal cortical mantle. Pediatr Neurosurg. 2012;48(1):6–12. https://doi.org/10.1159/000339850. Epub 2012 Jul 21. PMID: 22832209.
18. Bui CJ, Tubbs RS, Oakes WJ. Tethered cord syndrome in children: a review. Neurosurg Focus. 2007;23(2):E2. https://doi.org/10.3171/foc.2007.23.2.2. PMID: 17961017.
19. Hertzler DA 2nd, DePowell JJ, Stevenson CB, Mangano FT. Tethered cord syndrome: a review of the literature from embryology to adult presentation. Neurosurg Focus. 2010;29(1):E1. https://doi.org/10.3171/2010.3.FOCUS1079. PMID: 20593997.
20. Michael MM, Garton ALA, Kuzan-Fischer CM, Uribe-Cardenas R, Greenfield JP. A critical analysis of surgery for occult tethered cord syndrome. Childs Nerv Syst. 2021;37(10):3003–11. https://doi.org/10.1007/s00381-021-05287-5. Epub 2021 Jul 15. PMID: 34268593.
21. Kashlan ON, Wilkinson DA, Morgenstern H, Khalsa SS, Maher CO. Predictors of surgical treatment in children with tethered fibrofatty filum terminale. J Neurosurg Pediatr. 2019:1–8. https://doi.org/10.3171/2019.8.PEDS19292. Epub ahead of print. PMID: 31675690.
22. Pang D, Dias MS, Ahab-Barmada M. Split cord malformation: part I: a unified theory of embryogenesis for double spinal cord malformations. Neurosurgery. 1992;31(3):451–80. https://doi.org/10.1227/00006123-199209000-00010. PMID: 1407428.
23. Pang D. Split cord malformation: part II: clinical syndrome. Neurosurgery. 1992;31(3):481–500. https://doi.org/10.1227/00006123-199209000-00011. PMID: 1407429.
24. Mahapatra AK, Gupta DK. Split cord malformations: a clinical study of 254 patients and a proposal for a new clinical-imaging classification. J Neurosurg. 2005;103(6 Suppl):531–6. https://doi.org/10.3171/ped.2005.103.6.0531. PMID: 16383252.
25. Tisdall MM, Hayward RD, Thompson DN. Congenital spinal dermal tract: how accurate is clinical and radiological evaluation? J Neurosurg Pediatr. 2015;15(6):651–6. https://doi.org/10.3171/2014.11.PEDS14341. Epub 2015 Mar 13. PMID: 26030333.
26. Muñoz Montoya JE, Jara MA, Vargas Osorio MP, Franco FR. Dermal sinus tract associated with type I and type II split cord malformation. Asian J Neurosurg. 2020;15(1):172–5. https://doi.org/10.4103/ajns.AJNS_287_19. PMID: 32181196; PMCID: PMC7057908.
27. Kucera JN, Coley I, O'Hara S, Kosnik EJ, Coley BD. The simple sacral dimple: diagnostic yield of ultrasound in neonates. Pediatr Radiol. 2015;45(2):211–6. https://doi.org/10.1007/s00247-014-3110-1. Epub 2014 Jul 5. PMID: 24996813.
28. Sarris CE, Tomei KL, Carmel PW, Gandhi CD. Lipomyelomeningocele: pathology, treatment, and outcomes. Neurosurg Focus. 2012;33(4):E3. https://doi.org/10.3171/2012.7.FOCUS12224. PMID: 23025444.
29. Pang D. Surgical management of complex spinal cord lipomas: how, why, and when to operate. A review. J Neurosurg Pediatr. 2019;23(5):537–56. https://doi.org/10.3171/2019.2.PEDS18390. PMID: 31042665.
30. Talamonti G, D'Aliberti G, Nichelatti M, Debernardi A, Picano M, Redaelli T. Asymptomatic lipomas of the medullary conus: surgical treatment versus conservative management. J Neurosurg Pediatr. 2014;14(3):245–54. https://doi.org/10.3171/2014.5.PEDS13399. Epub 2014 Jun 27. PMID: 24971607.
31. Copp AJ, Adzick NS, Chitty LS, Fletcher JM, Holmbeck GN, Shaw GM. Spina bifida. Nat Rev Dis Primers. 2015;1:15007. https://doi.org/10.1038/nrdp.2015.7. PMID: 27189655; PMCID: PMC4898641.
32. Adzick NS, Thom EA, Spong CY, Brock JW 3rd, Burrows PK, Johnson MP, Howell LJ, Farrell JA, Dabrowiak ME, Sutton LN, Gupta N, Tulipan NB, D'Alton ME, Farmer DL, MOMS Investigators. A randomized trial of prenatal versus postnatal repair of myelomeningocele. N Engl J Med. 2011;364(11):993–1004. https://doi.org/10.1056/NEJMoa1014379. Epub 2011 Feb 9. PMID: 21306277; PMCID: PMC3770179.
33. Farmer DL, Thom EA, Brock JW 3rd, Burrows PK, Johnson MP, Howell LJ, Farrell JA, Gupta N, Adzick NS, Management of Myelomeningocele Study Investigators. The Management of Myelomeningocele Study: full cohort 30-month pediatric outcomes. Am J Obstet Gynecol. 2018;218(2):256.e1–256.e13. https://doi.org/10.1016/j.ajog.2017.12.001. Epub 2017 Dec 12. PMID: 29246577; PMCID: PMC7737375.
34. Moldenhauer JS, Adzick NS. Fetal surgery for myelomeningocele: after the Management of Myelomeningocele Study (MOMS). Semin Fetal Neonatal Med. 2017;22(6):360–6. https://doi.org/10.1016/j.siny.2017.08.004. Epub 2017 Oct 12. PMID: 29031539.
35. Houtrow AJ, Thom EA, Fletcher JM, Burrows PK, Adzick NS, Thomas NH, Brock JW 3rd, Cooper T, Lee H, Bilaniuk L, Glenn OA, Pruthi S, MacPherson C, Farmer DL, Johnson MP, Howell LJ, Gupta N, Walker WO. Prenatal repair of myelomeningocele and school-age functional outcomes. Pediatrics. 2020;145(2):e20191544. https://doi.org/10.1542/peds.2019-1544. PMID: 31980545; PMCID: PMC6993457.
36. Mehta VA, Bettegowda C, Ahmadi SA, Berenberg P, Thomale UW, Haberl EJ, Jallo GI, Ahn ES. Spinal cord tethering following myelomeningocele repair. J Neurosurg Pediatr. 2010;6(5):498–505. https://doi.org/10.3171/2010.8.PEDS09491. PMID: 21039176.
37. Ferreira Furtado LM, Da Costa Val Filho JA, Dantas F, Moura de Sousa C. Tethered cord syndrome

after myelomeningocele repair: a literature update. Cureus. 2020;12(10):e10949. https://doi.org/10.7759/cureus.10949. PMID: 33072445; PMCID: PMC7560491.
38. Aldave G, Hansen D, Hwang SW, Moreno A, Briceño V, Jea A. Spinal column shortening for tethered cord syndrome associated with myelomeningocele, lumbosacral lipoma, and lipomyelomeningocele in children and young adults. J Neurosurg Pediatr. 2017;19(6):703–10. https://doi.org/10.3171/2017.1.PEDS16533. Epub 2017 Mar 31. PMID: 28362188.
39. Zhang C, Chang CC, Mummaneni PV, Yuan C, Dhall S, Jian F, Gupta N, Chou D. Spinal column shortening versus revision detethering for recurrent adult tethered cord syndrome: a preliminary comparison of perioperative and clinical outcomes. J Neurosurg Spine. 2020:1–7. https://doi.org/10.3171/2019.12.SPINE19659. Epub ahead of print. PMID: 32032960.
40. Archer J, Jea A. Spinal column shortening for secondary tethered cord syndrome in children: 2-dimensional operative video. Oper Neurosurg (Hagerstown). 2019;16(6):E168. https://doi.org/10.1093/ons/opy247. PMID: 30169877.
41. Theodore N, Cottrill E, Kalb S, Zygourakis C, Jiang B, Pennington Z, Lubelski D, Westbroek EM, Ahmed AK, Ehresman J, Sciubba DM, Witham TF, Turner JD, Groves M, Kakarla UK. Posterior vertebral column subtraction osteotomy for recurrent tethered cord syndrome: a multicenter, retrospective analysis. Neurosurgery. 2021;88(3):637–47. https://doi.org/10.1093/neuros/nyaa491. PMID: 33372221; PMCID: PMC7884146.
42. Mummareddy N, Dewan MC, Mercier MR, Naftel RP, Wellons JC 3rd, Bonfield CM. Scoliosis in myelomeningocele: epidemiology, management, and functional outcome. J Neurosurg Pediatr. 2017;20(1):99–108. https://doi.org/10.3171/2017.2.PEDS16641. Epub 2017 Apr 28. PMID: 28452655.
43. Kulkarni AV, Drake JM, Kestle JR, Mallucci CL, Sgouros S, Constantini S, Canadian Pediatric Neurosurgery Study Group. Predicting who will benefit from endoscopic third ventriculostomy compared with shunt insertion in childhood hydrocephalus using the ETV Success Score. J Neurosurg Pediatr. 2010;6(4):310–5. https://doi.org/10.3171/2010.8.PEDS103. Erratum in: J Neurosurg Pediatr. 2011;7(2):221. PMID: 20887100.

6 Management of Chiari Malformation

Andrew M. Hersh, George Jallo, and Nir Shimony

Abbreviations

CSF Cerebrospinal fluid
ETV Endoscopic third ventriculostomy
MRI Magnetic resonance imaging

A. M. Hersh (✉)
Department of Neurosurgery, Johns Hopkins University School of Medicine, Baltimore, MD, USA
e-mail: ahersh2@jhmi.edu

G. Jallo
Department of Neurosurgery, Johns Hopkins University School of Medicine, Baltimore, MD, USA

Department of Neurosurgery, Johns Hopkins Medicine, Institute for Brain Protection Sciences, Johns Hopkins All Children's Hospital, St. Petersburg, FL, USA

David Goldenberg Family Endowed Chair, Institute for Brain Protection Sciences, Johns Hopkins All Children's Hospital, St, Petersburg, FL, USA
e-mail: gjallo1@jhmi.edu

N. Shimony
Department of Neurosurgery, University of Tennessee - Health Science Center, Memphis, TN, USA

Department of Surgery, St. Jude Children's Research Hospital, Memphis, TN, USA

Le Bonheur Neuroscience Institute, Le Bonheur Children's Hospital, Memphis, TN, USA

Department of Neurosurgery, The Johns Hopkins University - School of Medicine, Baltimore, MD, USA

Semmes-Murphey Clinic, Memphis, TN, USA
e-mail: nshimony@semmes-murphy.com

Introduction

Hans Chiari reported over 100 years ago three types of anatomical alterations in the hindbrain that he noticed in association with hydrocephalus. The first type, known presently as a Chiari 1, was described in 1891 as featuring "elongation of the tonsils and medial divisions of the inferior lobules of the cerebellum into cone-shaped projections" which herniate into the spinal canal. He argued that these cerebellar changes could cause bulbar symptoms. The second type, or Chiari 2, was characterized by "displacement of portions of the cerebellum within the elongated fourth ventricle into the widened spinal canal." Substantial hydrocephalus was noted, along with a lumbar myelomeningocele with diastematomyelia. In the same article, Chiari described a third type featuring substantial hydrocephalus with a cervical encephalocele. Later, he would describe a fourth type featuring marked cerebellar hypoplasia [1, 2].

These findings set the stage for a century of scientific and surgical advancements in treatment of the so-called Chiari malformations. Chiari believed that hydrocephalus resulted in the cerebellar changes he witnessed. This view increasingly fell out of favor, as cases featuring the cerebellar malformations but lacking hydrocephalus were reported. Additionally, the malformations were noted to occur in association with a wide range of pathologies, including syringomyelia, craniosynostosis, scoliosis, genetic syn-

N. Shimony, G. Jallo (eds.), *Pediatric Neurosurgery Board Review*,
https://doi.org/10.1007/978-3-031-23687-7_6

dromes, and anomalies of the craniocervical junction. Posterior fossa decompression emerged as the mainstay of treatment for symptomatic patients. Nonetheless, debate over the primary contributors to Chiari malformations has led to controversy over the appropriate treatment paradigm. Over 100 years since Chiari described his eponymic malformations, consensus is still lacking on the pathophysiology of Chiari malformations. Moreover, some argue that the malformations are more properly represented as deformations, alterations, or formations, given the progressive natural history observed in many patients, whereas a malformation denotes a static congenital anomaly [3]. These different terminologies reflect the ongoing debate in the field and highlight how much more remains to be discovered. In this chapter, we discuss the subtypes of Chiari malformations and theories of pathogenesis, highlight associated conditions and appropriate workup for pediatric neurosurgeons, and describe surgical treatments and principles for patients with Chiari malformations.

Chiari Subtypes

Chiari 1

The majority of Chiari malformations are Chiari 1, although several other subtypes exist. The Type 1 malformation represents the simplest subtype and features extension of the cerebellar tonsils into the upper cervical spinal canal [4]. The exact definition of pathological tonsillar herniation is of debate. Radiographic descent ≥5 mm is usually considered the cutoff for Chiari 1 malformations. However, it should be recognized that variations exist, and some argue that patients with lesser degrees of herniation can develop symptoms that would benefit from surgery [5]. Herniation below 2 mm is unlikely to be of significance. Moreover, variability exists across examiners in measurement of tonsillar herniation, and the diagnosis is ideally supported by independent measurements from at least two clinicians [6].

Syringomyelia accompanies approximately 70–80% of Type I malformations. Chiari 1 is often found incidentally, with a reported incidence of nearly 3% of children displaying radiographic evidence of Chiari 1, even though not all are symptomatic [7]. Therefore, thorough workup in symptomatic patients is important to diagnosing a Chiari 1 malformation as responsible for the onset of symptoms.

Chiari 2, 3, and 4

The Chiari 2 malformation is less common than Chiari 1 but is more life-threatening. This subtype is present in almost all infants born with a myelomeningocele and involves downward displacement of the cerebellar vermis and brainstem through the foramen magnum ("peg"-like appearance) [8]. There can also be cerebellar hypoplasia, elongation of the medulla and lower pons, displacement of the fourth ventricle into the spinal canal, and beaking or hypoplasia of the tectum [9, 10]. Diastematomyelia occurs in around 15–20% of patients with Chiari 2 [11]. Folate supplementation during pregnancy has contributed to a decline in the appearance of myelomeningoceles and consequently a decline in the incidence of Chiari 2 malformations in developed countries [12].

The next two subtypes are considerably rare. An occipital or high cervical encephalocele with posterior fossa herniation is characteristic of Chiari 3 malformations, along with a small posterior fossa. Prognosis is poor and respiratory failure is common [13, 14]. Chiari 4 malformations were described by Chiari in 1895 in a second paper after publication of his original three classifications, although the terminology has now fallen out favor [15] and features severe cerebellar hypoplasia with posterior fossa herniation [16].

New Classification Schemes

Since Chiari's publication of the traditional four classifications, new entities have been proposed with some controversy. Chiari 0 malformations represent syringomyelia in the absence of cerebellar tonsil ectopia, yet they improve with posterior fossa decompression. The pathophysiology and treatment response may reflect crowding of the posterior fossa and arachnoid adhesions at the foramen of Magendie resulting in altered flow of cerebrospinal fluid (CSF) without tissue herniation. Careful workup should be undertaken to ensure the absence of tonsillar herniation and other potential etiologies of syringomyelia, including tumors, vascular malformations, and cysts [17].

Chiari 1.5 malformations feature the tonsillar herniation seen in Chiari 1 in addition to brainstem herniation through the foramen magnum, which can result in an elongated brainstem and fourth ventricle. Patients may progress over time from a diagnosis of Chiari 1 to imaging findings characteristic of a Chiari 1.5, and surgeons should be vigilant about this diagnosis [18]. Overall clinical and imaging features are similar, and it is disputed whether it truly warrants a separate classification [19]. Some authors do suggest differences in treatment outcomes compared to the Chiari 1 phenotype, including a higher likelihood of repeat reoperations for persistent syringomyelia after posterior decompressive surgery. A more aggressive surgical intervention at the outset may be warranted in these patients [20, 21].

A Chiari 5 has also been recently proposed, representing occipital lobe herniation through the foramen magnum [22]. Most recently, a Chiari 0.5 has been described involving ventral herniation of the tonsils which can cause similar symptoms as Chiari and respond to decompressive therapy [23].

The types of Chiari malformations are summarized in Table 6.1. Controversies abound regarding newer classification schema, and most Chiari cases encountered by pediatric neurosurgeons are Chiari 1 and 1.5 malformations. These represent the focus of the present chapter.

Table 6.1 Summary of the classification schemes for Chiari malformations

Type	Key features
Traditional categories	
Chiari 1	• Cerebellar tonsillar herniation into the foramen magnum • Variable definition of herniation—usually ≥5 • Often presents in adulthood • Often asymptomatic • Headache and pain are common initial symptoms • High frequency of syringomyelia • Most common
Chiari 2 (Arnold-Chiari)	• Nearly always presents with myelomeningocele • Herniation of the cerebellum and brainstem through the foramen magnum • Tectal beaking/hypoplasia • Displacement of the fourth ventricle into spinal canal • Diastematomyelia (15–20% of patients)
Chiari 3	• Severe herniation with occipital or high cervical encephalocele • Life-threatening complications
Chiari 4	• Cerebellar hypoplasia/aplasia
Proposed new categories	
Chiari 0	• Syringomyelia without tonsillar herniation • May benefit from posterior decompression
Chiari 0.5	• Ventral tonsillar herniation • May benefit from posterior decompression
Chiari 1.5	• Chiari 1 (tonsillar herniation) + brainstem herniation through the foramen magnum • Similar clinical and imaging features as Chiari 1 • Higher risk of repeat reoperation for persistent syringomyelia
Chiari 5	• Herniation of the occipital lobe through the foramen magnum

Pathogenesis and Pathophysiology

The array of Chiari subtypes and intermediary classifications reflects our limited understanding of the pathogenesis of the disease. Several theories have been proposed and are actively debated; however, no single theory can account for all features and associations of Chiari malformations. Moreover, theories of pathogenesis often struggle to explain the large number of asymptomatic patients with radiographic evidence of Chiari 1 malformations. Chiari attributed the malformations he discovered to hydrocephalus, believing that the CSF pressure differential between the brain and spine caused by hydrocephalus results in herniation of the cerebellum. The rise in intracranial pressure results in tonsillar herniation, blocking CSF flow through the foramen magnum, which can cause syringomyelia and worsen the hydrocephalus in a vicious cycle [24]. Hydrocephalus can occur in association with Chiari malformations; however, it is not universally present, and herniation often precedes radiographic evidence of hydrocephalus. On the other hand, hydrocephalus has also been argued to result from, rather than cause, Chiari malformations, due to the blockage of CSF flow from the herniated cerebellum [25, 26].

A popular theory attributes Chiari 1 malformations to underdevelopment of the posterior fossa and para-axial mesoderm. The small space cannot accommodate the brainstem and cerebellar components, resulting in herniation of the cerebellar tonsils. Indeed, the mean posterior fossa volume in children with Chiari 1 malformations is smaller than control patients [27]. Nonetheless, the findings of incidental Chiari malformations in asymptomatic adults suggest that tonsillar herniation alone may not be responsible for the clinical symptoms. Traditionally, Chiari 1 malformations have been defined as featuring ≥5 mm of tonsillar descent on radiographic imaging. However, this definition excludes patients with fewer millimeters of herniation yet nonetheless presenting symptomatically and cannot account for those patients with radiographic evidence that are asymptomatic [28]. Moreover, this explanation does not account for the association of Chiari malformations with genetic syndromes and other anomalies of the central nervous system [24].

Other theories have been purported to explain the development of Chiari malformations. One such theory argues that tethered cord can result in downward traction on the brainstem, producing cerebellar herniation. Another maintains that events that lower intrathecal pressure, such as lumbar-to-peritoneal shunts, can promote herniation, a mechanism that is analogously reverse to the intracranial hydrocephalus theory [25]. Still an alternative theory maintains that craniocervical abnormalities produce tonsillar herniation and chronic cervical instability that can present asymptomatically for long periods [29]. Similarly, a new theory maintains that instability of the atlantoaxial spine initiates a cascade of events that can cause Chiari malformations. This theory posits that stabilization of the upper cervical spine is the true treatment for Chiari malformations and is discussed further below [30].

Comorbidities and Associations

Regardless of etiology, the symptoms arising from Chiari malformations are often attributable to direct compression of the cervical spinal cord and neurological tissue surrounding the foramen magnum by the herniated tonsils. Obstruction of CSF flow can result in syringomyelia or syringobulbia causing associated symptoms [31]. Chiari malformations are also associated with scoliosis, spinal instability, and craniosynostosis and can manifest as a component of several genetic syndromes that warrant multidisciplinary treatment.

Syringomyelia

Syringomyelia, defined as fluid-filled cysts that form within the spinal cord, is commonly seen in Chiari malformations (Fig. 6.1), with a lower estimated incidence in children (40%) compared to adults (69%) [32]. Syrinx formation in the brainstem, or syringobulbia, can also occur but is infrequently seen in the absence of syringomy-

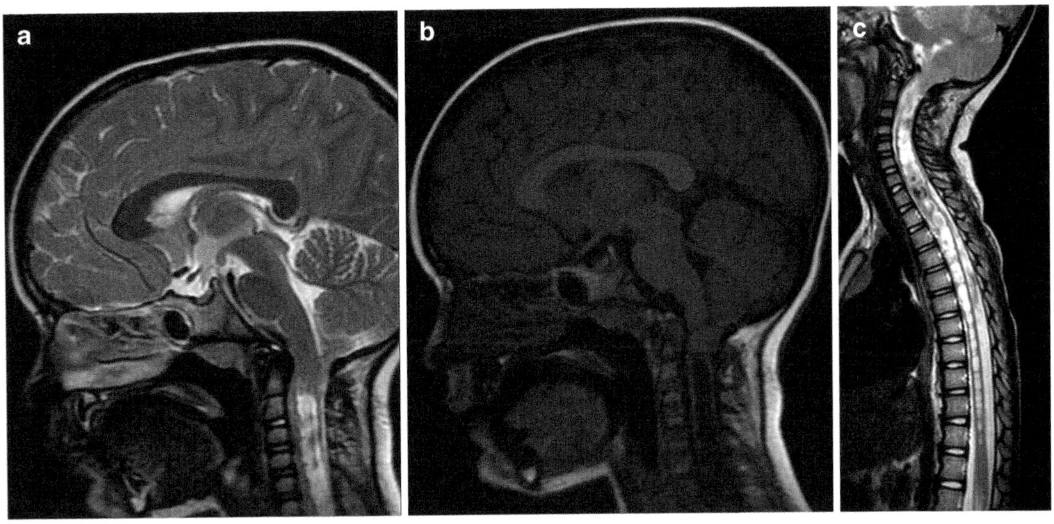

Fig. 6.1 MRI of a patient with a Chiari malformation and syringomyelia. (**a**) Sagittal T2-weighted MRI and (**b**) sagittal T1-weighted MRI illustrating tonsillar herniation and a cervical syrinx. (**c**) MRI of the cervical and thoracic spine illustrating extensive syringomyelia. Decompression of the posterior fossa often suffices to improve or resolve the syrinx; however, at times, a repeat decompression, fourth ventricular stent, or syringosubarachnoid shunt may be needed

elia [33]. Other risk factors for syrinx formation besides age include female sex, extent of tonsillar descent, and basilar invagination [34]. Communication of the syrinx with the fourth ventricle was once presumed, but autopsy specimens and magnetic resonance imaging (MRI) have shown that the syrinx is usually noncommunicating. More recent theories postulate that the pulsatility of the cerebellar tonsils or arteries pushes fluid into the spinal cord [32]. Syringomyelia in the setting of Chiari malformations generally occurs in the cervical or cervicothoracic cord, given its location adjacent to the cervicomedullary abnormality, although caudal syrinxes are seen in the thoracic and lumbar cord in around 20% of cases [35]. Holocord syringomyelia is also frequently encountered [35]. Syringomyelia can cause pain, upper extremity weakness, and loss of temperature sensation, while syringobulbia confers a worse prognosis and can cause sudden-onset symptoms including irregular breathing, vocal cord paralysis, and difficulty swallowing [33, 36]. Surgery is an effective means of improving symptoms and reducing the size of syrinxes [37].

Notably, syrinx formation is encountered in a wide range of central nervous system pathologies, including tumors, trauma, infection, spinal stenosis, and other craniocervical abnormalities. Given that tonsillar herniation is often an incidental finding, a thorough workup should be completed in patients with tonsillar herniation and syringomyelia to ensure that no other attributable causes are detected [33].

Scoliosis

Patients with a Chiari malformation and syringomyelia frequently have underlying scoliosis, with estimates ranging from 14 to 65% of patients with Chiari 1 malformations and a higher incidence in Chiari 2 malformations [38]. Conversely, around 10% of patients with a presumed diagnosis of idiopathic scoliosis are discovered to harbor a Chiari malformation and/or syringomyelia on MRI [39]. The precise etiology for scoliosis in the setting of a Chiari malformation is unclear, and both tonsillar herniation and syringomyelia have been proposed as inciting factors. Tonsillar herniation may compress the posterior column pathways and produce abnormal intramedullary pressure which can impair proper maintenance of posture and contribute to scoliosis [40]. Alternatively, some argue that asymmetric expansion of the syrinx can cause asymmetric dysfunction of the anterior horn cells resulting in uneven denervation of the paraspinal and deep back musculatures, ultimately resulting in scoliosis [39, 41].

Infantile and juvenile cases may present with symptoms related to obstructive or restrictive lung diseases, depending on the Cobb angle. In the setting of Chiari malformations, scoliosis can present with atypical features, including early onset, kyphotic curvature, and neurological deficits. Scoliosis may be the only initial complaint in patients with Chiari malformations, and a thorough workup should therefore be performed in patients with scoliosis to evaluate for craniocervical abnormalities and syringomyelia [39]. Similarly, patients with Chiari malformations should be assessed for scoliosis given their propensity to co-occur.

Assessment of the scoliotic deformity should include X-rays of the spine to measure the clavicle angle, Cobb angle, and sagittal balance. Although disagreement arises concerning the value of MRI for scoliosis, patients with a suspected Chiari malformation would anyway receive MRI to evaluate for tonsillar herniation and craniocervical anomalies [39]. Patients with mild scoliosis should be closely monitored with follow-up exams, while high-risk patients at risk of worsening progression or complications should be referred to specialists and can be treated conservatively with bracing or operatively with spinal fusion. Younger patients less than 10 years old are generally at lower risk for curve progression [39]. Furthermore, early treatment of syringomyelia and the Chiari malformation can be effective in halting progression of the scoliosis [38].

Craniosynostosis

Chiari malformations are also frequently encountered alongside craniosynostosis, with a greater incidence in syndromic and multisuture craniosynostosis compared to isolated nonsyndromic or single-suture cases. Chiari malformations can be encountered with premature closure of any of the sutures, although the greatest frequency is seen with lambdoid craniosynostosis. Therefore, workup for Chiari malformations is suggested in all patients with syndromic and/or multisuture craniosynostosis, and some advocate in patients with isolated lambdoid craniosynostosis as well [42]. It is hypothesized that the Chiari malformation develops in these patients because of the abnormally small posterior fossa that results from premature suture fusion, resulting in crowding of the hindbrain and tonsillar herniation. A strong genetic association with Chiari malformations has also been observed in certain syndromic forms of craniosynostosis, such as Crouzon, Apert, or Pfeiffer syndrome [43, 44]. In particular, a specific mutation has been found within a subset of patients with Crouzon syndrome linked to development of the Chiari malformation in these patients, although the pathogenesis has not been entirely elucidated [43].

Consensus is lacking on the management of patients with both Chiari malformations and craniosynostosis. Patients with symptomatic Chiaris generally are treated for both the craniosynostosis and Chiari malformation. In asymptomatic patients, some suggest that resolution of the synostosis is sufficient and may even improve the Chiari malformation, while others recommend simultaneous correction of both the synostosis and Chiari [42].

Hydrocephalus

Hydrocephalus is noted in an estimated 10% of patients with Chiari malformations [45]. This association was recognized early by Hans Chiari, who suggested that hydrocephalus is responsible for the malformations he observed. Indeed, hydrocephalus can increase intracranial pressure and cause reversible displacement of the cerebellar tonsils; however, this is distinct from the anatomical abnormality of Chiari malformations. Hydrocephalus in the setting of Chiari malformations may result from obstruction of the fourth ventricular outflow tract or aqueductal stenosis stemming from tonsillar herniation [46]. Cases with only partial obstruction would not develop hydrocephalus, explaining the occurrence of hydrocephalus in only a minority of Chiari patients [47]. Additionally, surgical treatment of Chiari malformations can result in post-operative hydrocephalus in a subset of patients that may warrant management with extraventricular drainage [45]. Similarly, repair of craniosynostosis may cause hydrocephalus which can contribute to tonsillar displacement [42].

Optimal management of the hydrocephalus seen in Chiari malformations is debated. Often, the hydrocephalus is treated first to reduce intracranial pressure and decrease the syringomyelia. Children with syndromic craniosynostosis with concomitant Chiari malformation and hydrocephalus may have worsening skull growth and crowding of the posterior fossa after treatment of the hydrocephalus using a ventriculoperitoneal shunt, and therefore the craniosynostosis should be treated first. However, this concern may not hold for treatment with endoscopic third ventriculostomies or treatment of single-suture craniosynostosis [47].

Spinal Instability

Craniovertebral junction instability is reported in around 10–14% of patients presenting with Chiari 1 malformations, some of whom warrant stabilization [48]. Instability of the craniovertebral junction can result in cervical and occipital pain, which can be difficult to distinguish from symptoms caused by the Chiari malformation or syringomyelia, as well as myelopathy, hyperreflexia, and downbeat nystagmus [49]. Several genetic syndromes have a propensity for craniovertebral instability in occurrence with Chiari malformations, particularly hereditary connective tissue disorders such as Ehlers-Danlos syndrome. However, controversy has arisen regarding the term "instability" in the setting of Ehlers-Danlos syndrome, where patients can have inherent hypermobility with increased range of joint movement that should not be mistakenly classified as pathological instability warranting surgical intervention [50].

Complicating the matter is a lack of agreement on the precise workup for craniocervical instability in the setting of Chiari malformations. Corroboration of clinical and radiographic findings, including dynamic imaging, can help determine the appropriate treatment, particularly in those patients with hereditary connective tissue disorders [49]. Basilar invagination is commonly reported in patients requiring stabilization of the craniovertebral junction, and several unique radiographic parameters have been proposed for assessment of instability, such as the clivoaxial angle and the basion-axial interval [51].

A new theory explaining the pathophysiology of Chiari malformation has been proposed with atlantoaxial dislocation as the central driver of tonsillar herniation. The theory posits that craniovertebral junction can adapt to subtle cases of dislocation to minimize damage to critical neural structures from compression by the odontoid process and upper cervical spine. Herniation of the tonsils serves to protect the spinal cord, functioning analogously to an "airbag" [30]. Proponents of the theory maintain that stabilization of the atlantoaxial spine is required for definitive treatment of the Chiari malformation and to prevent re-occurrence without a need for a posterior fossa decompression. Other surgeons who consider the two entities distinct may perform a posterior fossa decompression with posterior stabilization either during the initial surgery or at a later time when clinical symptoms warrant intervention [48].

Associated Syndromes

Chiari malformations, although generally appearing in isolation, can occur in association with several syndromes and diseases, including hereditary genetic syndromes, hydrocephalus, skeletal anomalies, neurofibromatosis type 1, brain tumors, tethered cord, and endocrinopathies (Table 6.2). The association of Chiari malformations with syndromic craniosynostosis, hydro-

Table 6.2 Genetic conditions commonly associated with Chiari malformations

Genetic disease	Gene	Locus	Description
Achondroplasia	*FGFR3*	4p16.3	Short-limb skeletal dysplasia
Beckwith-Wiedemann	*ICR1, KCNQ1OT1, CDKN1C*	11p15.5	Macrosomia, macroglossia, renal anomalies, increased risk of childhood cancer
Crouzon syndrome	*FGFR2*	10q26.13	Syndromic craniosynostosis, facial alterations (e.g., hypertelorism)
Ehlers-Danlos	Numerous, often collagen genes	Numerous	Hereditary connective tissue disorder, joint hypermobility, stretchy skin, impairment of wound healing, easy bruising. Be wary of pathologic craniocervical instability vs benign hypermobility
Klippel-Feil anomaly	*GDF6*	8q22.1	Congenital fusion of cervical vertebrae
Neurofibromatosis type 1	*NF1*	17q11.2	Café-au-lait spots, Lisch nodules, scoliosis, neurofibromas, optic gliomas, pheochromocytomas, scoliosis
Noonan's syndrome	*PTPN11*	12q24.13	Short stature, facial dysmorphism, congenital heart defects
Paget disease of the bone	Numerous	Numerous	Dysregulated bone remodeling, excessive bone breakdown
Scoliosis	Numerous	Numerous	Sideways curvature of thespine
Williams syndrome	Deletion of multiple genes	7q11.23	Intellectual disability, supravalvular aortic stenosis, facial features (e.g., broad forehead)

cephalus, and hereditary connective tissue disorders has been discussed. Skeletal anomalies associated with Chiari malformations include scoliosis and craniocervical instability, as described previously, as well as Klippel-Feil anomaly, which is noted in 3% of cases of Chiari 1 malformations [45]. This anomaly involves congenital fusion of the cervical spine and can be associated with a short neck, low posterior hairline, and reduced neck movements [52]. Approximately 8% of cases of the autosomal dominant disease neurofibromatosis type 1 also feature a Chiari malformation, while a slightly smaller number of patients treated for Chiari malformations were also found to have neurofibromatosis type 1 [53]. Other genetic syndromes include Beckwith-Wiedemann, Noonan, Williams, and Crouzon syndromes [54]. Rare cases of Chiari malformations following Paget's disease have also been reported [55]. Careful consideration should be afforded to patients presenting with syndromes or associated anomalies to determine the influence of the Chiari malformation on symptoms and assess priorities for surgical intervention.

Diagnosis and Workup

Symptoms

Not all Chiari malformations diagnosed radiographically will present symptomatically. Studies of large imaging databases have shown that anywhere from 14% to nearly 68% of patients with radiographic findings of tonsillar herniation more than 5 mm below the foramen magnum will be clinically asymptomatic [42, 56]. Asymptomatic patients generally remain asymptomatic over time, although most studies have only analyzed follow-up over a few years, and long-term changes are less clear [57]. In the remaining patients, symptoms are attributed to the compression of neural structures by the herniated tonsils and, in certain cases, the associated syringomyelia. Female gender, syringomyelia, older age in pediatric cohorts, and extent of tonsillar herniation are associated with a greater likelihood of symptomatic presentation [42].

Most commonly, patients report occipital or cervical dull, persistent pain and headaches, which may stem from dural irritation in the posterior fossa. Infants may present with irritability and crying. Valsalva maneuvers worsen the pain [35]. Other symptoms include sensory deficits, hyperreflexia, weakness, and a positive Babinski sign. Compression of cranial nerves in the posterior fossa can cause dysarthria, vocal cord paralysis, tongue atrophy, hiccups, sensorineural hearing loss, bradycardia, and syncope. Cerebellar symptoms include downbeating nystagmus and, less frequently, ataxia. Syringomyelia can result in "cape-like" loss of sensation, radicular pain, and weakness, although these symptoms may not present when the Chiari malformation is diagnosed early [39, 58]. Other symptoms result from associated conditions, including scoliosis, hydrocephalus, and craniocervical abnormalities.

Imaging

MRI of the brain and cervical spine illustrates the position of the cerebellar tonsils and is routinely used in workup of Chiari malformations [59]. MRIs are increasingly being performed at younger ages, enabling early diagnoses of Chiari 1 malformations prior to the onset of significant neurological symptoms [58]. Chiari 1 malformations are generally diagnosed when tonsillar herniation exceeds 5 mm in adults or 6 mm in children, typically measured on sagittal slices from the lowest level of the foramen magnum to the lowest position of the tonsils, although coronal cuts are also helpful. However, lesser degrees of herniation can still cause symptoms in some patients and may benefit from surgical intervention [6]. The location of the foramen magnum is identified by the line of McRae from the basion to opisthion [60]. Of note, some patients will be symptomatic with only 3–5 mm of displacement, while others with greater amounts of displacement will be diagnosed with anatomical Chiari malformations but will remain asymptomatic [59].

In addition to the degree of displacement, the morphology of the tonsils should be assessed, including the degree of crowding and whether they develop a peg-like, or pointed, appearance, suggestive of a tendency to restrict CSF flow and compress the medulla and cervical cord, resulting in neurological symptoms [60]. A small posterior fossa with peg-like tonsils suggests the diagnosis of a Chiari malformation rather than tonsillar ectopia or development of the tonsils in an abnormal location [59]. Additionally, MRIs can detect the presence of syringomyelia, hydrocephalus, abnormalities of the craniocervical junction, cord compression, and scoliosis [59, 60].

Other imaging modalities can be performed for adjunctive workup. Computed tomography scans of the head can assess tonsillar crowding, while cine-MRIs can capture the flow of CSF. Standard radiographs can also be acquired to investigate scoliosis, cervical fusion, and other vertebral abnormalities. Furthermore, workup should examine potential etiologies of secondary tonsillar herniation, such as tumors, hydrocephalus, and intracranial hypertension [61].

Complex Chiari Malformations

In recent years, the classification of some Chiaris as "complex Chiari malformations" has arisen, referring to patients with concomitant craniovertebral anomalies that would benefit from occipitocervical fusion. These patients may also have brainstem herniation and are often considered a Chiari 1.5 malformation. Ventral brainstem compression can be illustrated on MRI in these patients. Several radiographic parameters have been proposed to assess for instability at the craniocervical junction and determine the need for fusion, including the clivoaxial angle and pB-C2 line. The clivoaxial angle refers to the angle between the clivus and the spine, with smaller angles reflecting ventral compression. Clivoaxial angles less than 125° have been proposed as markers of complex Chiari malformations [62]. The pB-C2 line is a perpendicular line to the line from the basion to the posteroinferior C2 vertebral body and extends from the ventral dural edge. This measurement reflects the presence of a retroflexed odontoid and ventral brainstem compression. Various authors have suggested lengths above 5 or 9 mm as suggestive of a complex Chiari malformation [63, 64].

Sleep Studies

Sleep studies are important to assess for sleep-disordered breathing, which presents in as many as 70% of patients with Chiari malformations, a far greater rate than the general population. Medullary compression by the herniated tonsils can affect the central respiratory drive, while compression of cranial nerves IX and X can weaken the pharyngeal muscles and reduce vocal cord function. Polysomnography and respiratory polygraphy can assist with screening for sleep-disordered breathing. Sleep-disordered breathing phenomena in these patients include central and obstructive sleep apnea, with obstructive sleep apnea from cranial nerve compression constituting the more common finding. Indeed, some argue that obstructive sleep apnea causes a transient increase in intracranial pressure which can worsen the positioning of the cerebellar tonsils and contribute to progression of the Chiari malformation and development of syringomyelia [65]. Sleep-disordered breathing often improves after surgery; however, the level of impairment warranting surgery has not been definitively established [66]. Additionally, evidence suggests that surgical decompression of Chiari malformations can contribute to an increased incidence of post-operative respiratory failure in patients with sleep-disordered breathing, highlighting the importance of screening for sleep-disordered breathing preoperatively to plan appropriately for respiratory disturbances [67].

Ophthalmological Evaluation

Evaluation by an ophthalmologist is not strictly warranted but can be helpful in some cases. Ocular disturbances are common among patients and include retro-orbital pain, floaters and flashing lights, diplopia, blurry vision, and reduced visual fields [28]. Papilledema is rarely detected but can signal a severe malformation [68]. Chiari malformations can also present with nystagmus, particularly a gaze-evoked nystagmus, downbeat nystagmus, or periodic alternating nystagmus, as well as strabismus. Treatment options are limited for strabismus and include specialized strabismus surgery following posterior decompression of the Chiari malformation. Pharmacological treatment and posterior decompression can improve nystagmus associated with Chiari malformations [69].

Treatment

The decision-making process for treatment of Chiari malformations (Fig. 6.2) should consider (1) the patient's symptoms and neurological deficits, (2) associated conditions and comorbidities, and (3) choice of surgical technique. The goals of surgery are to decompress the brainstem and cervical spine, restore adequate flow of CSF, stabilize or reduce the syrinx if present, and restore the normal morphology of the craniovertebral junction [62, 70]. Additionally, treatment of concomitant anomalies, such as scoliosis, should be considered. Given the frequency of incidental Chiari malformations, asymptomatic patients without syringomyelia do not undergo surgery. Routine long-term follow-up should be offered, as around 5% of asymptomatic patients will eventually develop symptoms [71]. The timing of follow-up differs by surgeons but generally should be performed annually for several years, followed by longer intervals between visits. In adulthood, follow-up may be limited to symptomatic presentation.

Surgical intervention is warranted for patients with neurological deficits regardless of the presence of syringomyelia. However, treatment of patients with only pain or headaches but lacking syringomyelia is controversial [62]. Surgery may be avoided in tolerable headaches, whereas unrelenting headaches may benefit from intervention [72]. Still, some surgeons are more aggressive and favor intervention in patients with suboccipital headaches [71].

Consensus is lacking on surgical treatment for asymptomatic patients with syringomyelia. The

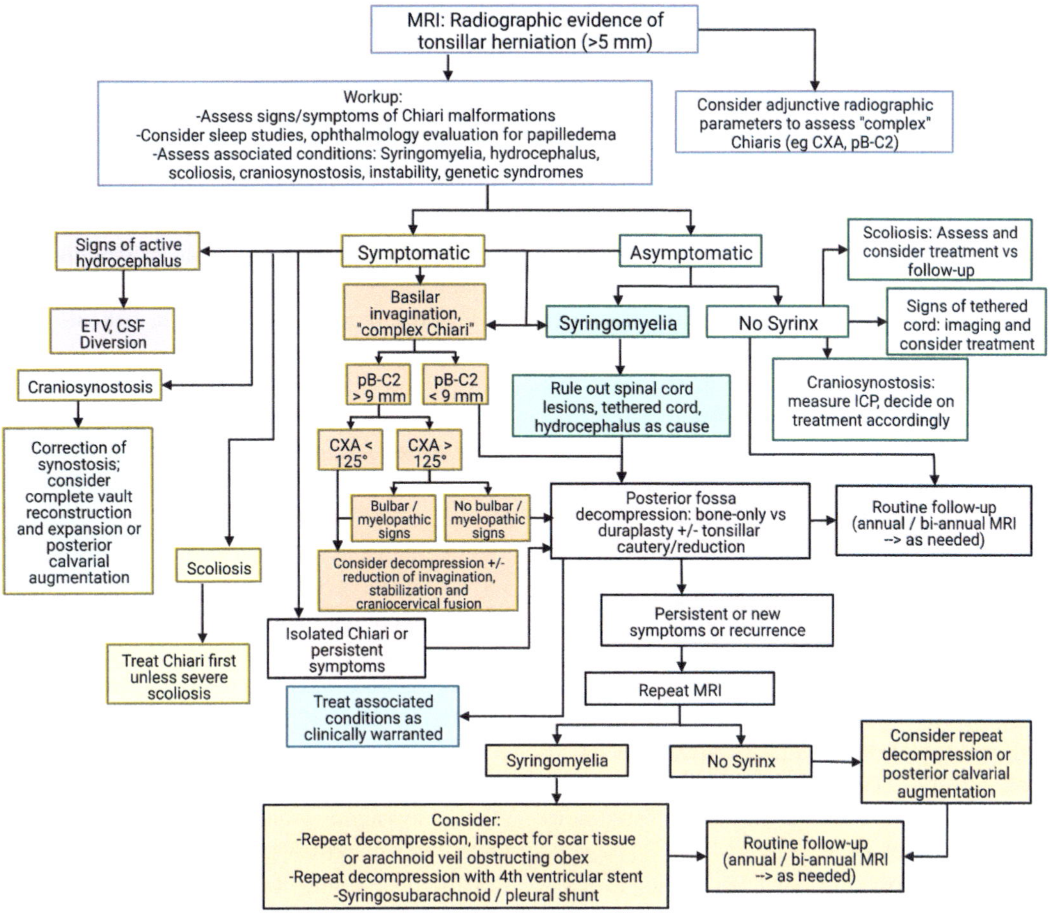

Fig. 6.2 Flowchart illustrating the decision-making process for patients with Chiari malformations

size of the syrinx impacts some surgeons' choice, with more surgeons favoring operating on larger syrinxes compared to smaller ones in asymptomatic patients [62]. Syringomyelia is often felt to progress in the absence of intervention, favoring treatment in asymptomatic patients [72]. Treatment for isolated symptomatic Chiari malformations, with or without syringomyelia, generally consists of a posterior fossa decompression. Patients with a designated complex Chiari malformation as reflected by the clivoaxial line, pB-C2 line, or other radiographic parameters may benefit from concomitant occipitocervical fusion, as these patients have a high risk of developing craniocervical kyphosis [62, 63].

Posterior Fossa Decompression

The mainstay of treatment and most commonly accepted form of surgical intervention for symptomatic Chiari malformations consists of posterior fossa decompression. A suboccipital craniectomy with a C1 laminectomy can effectively decompress the cervicomedullary junction and restore adequate CSF flow [72]. Coagulation or resection of the cerebellar tonsils can be performed for cases with significantly low-lying tonsils to reduce their size [73]. Tonsillar resection is believed to improve CSF flow but can result in increased morbidity; therefore, some surgeons avoid manipulation of the tonsils and instead prefer duraplasty. Microsurgical and minimally invasive techniques can help minimize morbidity associated with tonsillar resection [74].

Bone-Only vs Decompression with Duraplasty

Decompression can be achieved either with removal of the bony contents alone or can include a duraplasty. Advocates of duraplasty argue that it affords greater decompression and restores the flow of CSF into the subarachnoid spaces, particularly when the tonsils extend below the lamina of C1. Opening the dura also allows the surgeon to address the potential presence of arachnoid veils and webs contributing to the fourth ventricular outlet obstruction [70, 75]. Arachnoid webs obstructing the flow of CSF should be divided [73]. Of note, duraplasty is more invasive compared to bony decompression only and is associated with a greater risk of a CSF leak, infection, cerebellar slump, and arachnoid adhesions [76]. A watertight dural closure mitigates the risk of a CSF leak.

Intraoperative ultrasound can be used to determine if the tip of the tonsils are visible and whether sufficient decompression has been performed to assess the need for a duraplasty [77]. Evidence of a sufficient decompression includes the presence of a CSF space anterior to the brainstem and dorsal to the tonsils—that is, CSF pulsatility around the tonsils. Thereby, ultrasound can be used to ensure that duraplasty is only performed in patients without adequate decompression. Following duraplasty, intraoperative ultrasound can be used again to determine the adequacy of the decompression [78].

Decompression of the posterior fossa (Fig. 6.3) can improve symptoms in around 80% of cases, with a reoperation rate varying from 3 to 7% for persistent symptoms or syringomyelia [49, 73]. Some studies have suggested greater rates of clinical and syringomyelia improvement in patients receiving posterior fossa decompression with duraplasty compared to those receiving bony decompression only, along with lower rates of reoperation. Data from the Park-Reeves Syringomyelia Research Consortium registry suggests that decompression with duraplasty is an independent predictor of syrinx improvement. Overall, decompression with duraplasty resulted in syrinx resolution in 86% of patients, while bony decompression alone resulted in resolution in 77% of patients. Additionally, although most patients in both cohorts had resolution of their syrinx, resolution was quicker in patients with duraplasty [79].

Outcomes After Decompression

Radiological resolution of the syrinx is achieved in most patients. Studies have not consistently shown a difference in clinical outcomes between patients with and without a preoperative syrinx, although patients with shorter syrinxes tend to have better outcomes than those with more extensive syringomyelia [37, 80]. Occipital and cervical pain, sleep apnea, and mild scoliosis also benefit from decompressive surgery, whereas ataxia, nystagmus, and muscle atrophy have lower rates of post-operative improvement [73]. In particular, young children under 10 years old and patients with Cobb angles under 40° tend to have lower rates of curve progression requiring spinal fusion compared to older children and patients with Cobb angles greater than 40°. Therefore, patients in these latter two categories should particularly be monitored closely post-operatively for progression of scoliosis. Additionally, early decompression is recommended to reduce the risk of a subsequent spinal fusion operation. Posterior fossa decompression may be particularly beneficial toward halting the natural history of scoliosis in patients with associated syringomyelia [39].

Following surgery, patients should be closely monitored with regular MRI scans and clinical visits for at least 10 years [33]. Patients with recurrence of symptoms or progression of syringomyelia may benefit from a repeat decompression. Placement of a stent from the fourth ventricle to the subarachnoid space of the cervical spine during a reoperation has been shown to

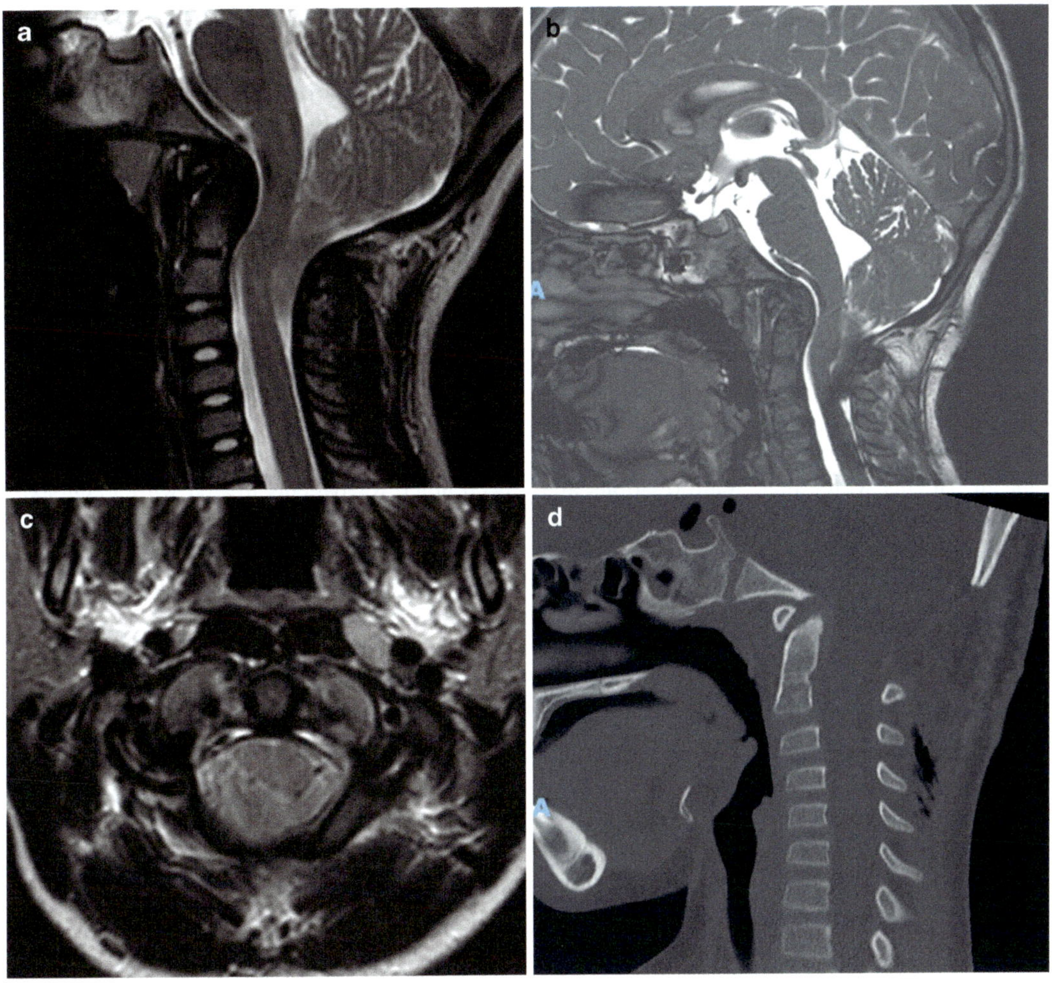

Fig. 6.3 Images before and after decompression of an 8-year-old girl initially presenting with Valsalva headaches. (**a**, **b**) Sagittal T2-weighted MRI showing significant tonsillar herniation extending to the C2 vertebral level with significant lower brainstem compression, basilar invagination, and a steep clivoaxial angle. (**c**) Axial T2-weighted MRI showing crowding of the foramen magnum with compression of the brainstem. (**d**) Post-operative sagittal CT scan illustrating wide decompression of the foramen magnum following a suboccipital craniectomy and C1 laminectomy. The patient's headaches resolved after surgery. The clivoaxial angle remains steep, and the patient may eventually benefit from craniocervical instrumentation and fusion

effectively treat persistent syringomyelia by altering the flow of CSF away from the central canal. Occasionally, patients will require stent replacement for recurrent syrinxes [81]. Alternatively, placement of a syringosubarachnoid shunt is performed by some surgeons when decompression fails to improve syringomyelia and imaging confirms obliteration of the subarachnoid space at the syrinx level [73].

Endoscopic Third Ventriculostomies

Endoscopic third ventriculostomies (ETV) can help manage obstructive hydrocephalus associated with Chiari 1 malformations with a 90% success rate. Success rates are lower in the presence of a myelomeningocele [82]. Ventriculoperitoneal shunts can also be used; however, ETVs are less invasive and consequently preferred. Although the causal direction between hydrocephalus and Chiari malformations is unclear, ETVs can not only treat hydrocephalus but also reduce tonsillar herniation and improve Chiari symptoms and syringomyelia [47].

Posterior Calvarial Distraction

The complex craniosynostosis encountered in some patients with Chiari malformations may require remodeling of the calvarium to reduce the synostosis. Posterior calvarial distraction has been described to improve posterior fossa volume in patients with Chiari malformations and craniosynostosis. The osteotomy can be extended to the foramen magnum to directly increase the size of the posterior fossa. In turn, the expanded volume reduces the tonsillar herniation and improves the syringomyelia, with complete improvement in tonsillar herniation observed in some patients [83]. Posterior cranial vault releases can improve the symptoms of Chiari malformations and restore CSF flow without requiring a suboccipital decompression, allowing for simultaneous treatment of the complex craniosynostosis and Chiari malformation [84]. Therefore, posterior calvarial distraction has been recommended by some authors as a potential first-line therapy in patients with Chiari malformations and complex craniosynostosis [85].

Craniocervical Fusion

Patients with a "complex" Chiari malformation display abnormalities of the craniocervical junction, most commonly basilar invagination, brainstem herniation, and a retroflexed odontoid. Patients who are initially treated for complex Chiari malformations with suboccipital decompressions can eventually progress to develop symptomatic craniocervical instability warranting occipitocervical fusion. Consequently, some surgeons recommend considering combining the standard suboccipital decompression with craniocervical fusion in this patient cohort [64]. A C1–C2 or occiput-C2 fusion can be performed.

Recently, a recommendation for occipitocervical fusion as the main treatment modality for all cases of Chiari malformations has been proposed, based on the underlying proposition that atlantoaxial instability drives the morphological changes that result in Chiari malformations. This recommendation is maintained even in the absence of overt radiographic signs of basilar invagination. Studies of atlantoaxial fixation as the primary treatment for Chiari malformations have shown post-operative improvement in the vast majority of cases, including in both the pediatric and adult literature [30, 86]. Significant improvements in neurological function have also been noted for patients treated with atlantoaxial fixation after failing initial surgery with foramen magnum decompression [87].

Although reported outcomes are positive, the Pediatric Craniocervical Society recommends against this approach, noting that the patient population reported in the aforementioned studies are fundamentally distinct from the general population of patients with Chiari malformations [88]. Morbidity is substantially greater with atlantoaxial fixation compared to suboccipital decompression, and the risk of mortality is increased, particularly due to potential injuries to the vertebral artery [30]. The topic remains an area of active discussion, and continued investigations are ongoing to determine the optimal treatment paradigm.

Conclusion

Chiari malformations can be divided into an ever-increasing array of subtypes, with Chiari 1 malformations most commonly encountered in clinical practice. Although first described in the late 1800s, the pathophysiology remains incompletely understood, with various competing theories offered to explain the disease mechanism. Moreover, Chiari malformations can be associated with a large number of other conditions, including hydrocephalus, craniosynostosis, scoliosis, craniocervical instability, and hereditary connective tissue disorders. MRIs are used to confirm the diagnosis; however, many patients will be diagnosed incidentally without developing symptoms. The mainstay of treatment consists of a posterior fossa decompression to restore CSF flow and reduce neural compression. The operation can be performed with or without a duraplasty. Decompressive surgery can improve neurological symptoms, as well as syringomyelia and scoliosis. New treatment paradigms have recently been proposed and are a subject of active discussion and investigation, highlighting the ongoing controversies and developments in the field.

Review Questions

1. A Chiari 2 malformation is characterized by which of the following?
   (a) Occipital encephalocele
   (b) Syrinx formation without tonsillar herniation
   (c) Tonsillar herniation alone
   (d) Tonsillar and brainstem herniation
   (e) Severe cerebellar hypoplasia
2. Single-suture synostosis of which of the following sutures is most frequently associated with Chiari malformations?
   (a) Lambdoid
   (b) Sagittal
   (c) Metopic
   (d) Coronal
3. A patient presents with radiographic findings of a Chiari 1 malformation and syringomyelia but is otherwise asymptomatic. What is the next best step?
   (a) Observation with follow-up MRI
   (b) Posterior fossa decompression, bone-only
   (c) Posterior fossa decompression with duraplasty
   (d) MRI spinal cord to rule out spinal cord lesions
   (e) Occipitocervical fusion
4. A 6-year-old girl was discovered to have moderate scoliosis on a screening test. A follow-up MRI reveals extensive syringomyelia with an associated Chiari 1 malformation. The patient is otherwise asymptomatic. No spinal cord lesions or other etiologies responsible for syringomyelia are identified. What is the appropriate next step?
   (a) Observation with repeat MRI in 1 year
   (b) Posterior fossa decompression
   (c) Treatment of scoliosis followed by decompression
   (d) Decompression with craniocervical fusion
   (e) Posterior calvarial reconstruction
5. Which of the following interventions can be considered in patients with recurrent or progressive syringomyelia following posterior fossa decompression for a Chiari malformation?
   (a) Endoscopic third ventriculostomy
   (b) Stenting from the fourth ventricle to cervical subarachnoid space
   (c) Ventriculoperitoneal shunt
   (d) Repeat decompression with syrinx drainage

Answer Keys

1. d
2. a
3. d
4. b
5. b

References

1. Arnett B. Arnold-Chiari malformation. Arch Neurol. 2003;60:898–900. https://doi.org/10.1001/ARCHNEUR.60.6.898.
2. Chiari H. Concerning alterations in the cerebellum resulting from cerebral hydrocephalus. Pediatr Neurosci. 1891;17:1172–5. https://doi.org/10.1159/000120293.
3. Goel A. Is Chiari a "formation" or a "malformation?". J Craniovertebr Junction Spine. 2017;8:1. https://doi.org/10.4103/0974-8237.199881.
4. Zhao JL, Li MH, Wang CL, Meng W. A systematic review of Chiari I malformation: techniques and outcomes. World Neurosurg. 2016;88:7–14. https://doi.org/10.1016/J.WNEU.2015.11.087.
5. Aitken LA, Lindan CE, Sidney S, et al. Chiari type I malformation in a pediatric population. Pediatr Neurol. 2009;40:449. https://doi.org/10.1016/J.PEDIATRNEUROL.2009.01.003.

6. Lawrence BJ, Urbizu A, Allen PA, et al. Cerebellar tonsil ectopia measurement in type i Chiari malformation patients show poor inter-operator reliability. Fluids Barriers CNS. 2018;15:1–10. https://doi.org/10.1186/S12987-018-0118-1/FIGURES/5.
7. Leonard JR, Limbrick DD. Chiari I malformation: adult and pediatric considerations. Neurosurg Clin N Am. 2015;26:xiii–xiv. https://doi.org/10.1016/J.NEC.2015.07.002.
8. Stevenson KL. Chiari Type II malformation: past, present, and future. Neurosurg Focus. 2004;16:E5. https://doi.org/10.3171/FOC.2004.16.2.6.
9. Geerdink N, van der Vliet T, Rotteveel JJ, et al. Essential features of Chiari II malformation in MR imaging: an interobserver reliability study—part 1. Childs Nerv Syst. 2012;28:977–85. https://doi.org/10.1007/S00381-012-1761-5.
10. Kuhn J, Emmady PD. Chiari II malformation. StatPearls; 2022.
11. Zaleska-Dorobisz U, Bladowska J, Biel A, et al. MRI diagnosis of diastematomyelia in a 78-year-old woman: case report and literature review. Pol J Radiol. 2010;75:82.
12. Hidalgo JA, Tork CA, Varacallo M. Arnold Chiari malformation. StatPearls; 2022.
13. Andica C, Soetikno RD. Chiari malformation type III: case report and review of the literature. Radiol Case Rep. 2013;8:831. https://doi.org/10.2484/RCR.V8I3.831.
14. Jeong DH, Kim CH, Kim MO, et al. Arnold-Chiari malformation type III with meningoencephalocele: a case report. Ann Rehabil Med. 2014;38:401. https://doi.org/10.5535/ARM.2014.38.3.401.
15. Arora R. Imaging spectrum of cerebellar pathologies: a pictorial essay. Pol J Radiol. 2015;80:142. https://doi.org/10.12659/PJR.892878.
16. Tubbs RS, Demerdash A, Vahedi P, et al. Chiari IV malformation: correcting an over one century long historical error. Childs Nerv Syst. 2016;32:1175–9. https://doi.org/10.1007/S00381-015-2765-8/FIGURES/4.
17. Chern JJ, Gordon AJ, Mortazavi MM, et al. Pediatric Chiari malformation Type 0: a 12-year institutional experience: clinical article. J Neurosurg Pediatr. 2011;8:1–5. https://doi.org/10.3171/2011.4.PEDS10528.
18. Kim IK, Wang KC, Kim IO, Cho BK. Chiari 1.5 malformation: an advanced form of Chiari I malformation. J Korean Neurosurg Soc. 2010;48:375. https://doi.org/10.3340/JKNS.2010.48.4.375.
19. Liu W, Wu H, Aikebaier Y, et al. No significant difference between Chiari malformation Type 1.5 and Type I. Clin Neurol Neurosurg. 2017;157:34–9. https://doi.org/10.1016/J.CLINEURO.2017.03.024.
20. Bordes S, Jenkins S, Tubbs RS. Defining, diagnosing, clarifying, and classifying the Chiari I malformations. Childs Nerv Syst. 2019;35:1785–92. https://doi.org/10.1007/S00381-019-04172-6/FIGURES/11.
21. Tubbs RS, Iskandar BJ, Bartolucci AA, Oakes WJ. A critical analysis of the Chiari 1.5 malformation. J Neurosurg Pediatr. 2004a;101:179–83. https://doi.org/10.3171/PED.2004.101.2.0179.
22. Tubbs RS, Muhleman M, Loukas M, Oakes WJ. A new form of herniation: the Chiari V malformation. Childs Nerv Syst. 2012;28:305–7. https://doi.org/10.1007/S00381-011-1616-5/FIGURES/1.
23. Morgenstern PF, Tosi U, Uribe-Cardenas R, Greenfield JP. Ventrolateral tonsillar position defines novel Chiari 0.5 classification. World Neurosurg. 2020;136:444–53. https://doi.org/10.1016/J.WNEU.2020.01.147.
24. Shoja MM, Tubbs RS, Oakes WJ. Embryology and pathophysiology of the Chiari I and II malformations. The Chiari Malformations. 2013;9781461463696:55–72. https://doi.org/10.1007/978-1-4614-6369-6_4/FIGURES/00046.
25. Buell TJ, Heiss JD, Oldfield EH. Pathogenesis and cerebrospinal fluid hydrodynamics of the Chiari I malformation. Neurosurg Clin N Am. 2015;26:495. https://doi.org/10.1016/J.NEC.2015.06.003.
26. Mancarella C, Delfini R, Landi A. Chiari malformations. Acta Neurochir Suppl. 2019;125:89–95. https://doi.org/10.1007/978-3-319-62515-7_13.
27. Trigylidas T, Baronia B, Vassilyadi M, Ventureyra ECG. Posterior fossa dimension and volume estimates in pediatric patients with Chiari I malformations. Childs Nerv Syst. 2008;24:329–36. https://doi.org/10.1007/S00381-007-0432-4/TABLES/7.
28. Milhorat TH, Chou MW, Trinidad EM, et al. Chiari I malformation redefined: clinical and radiographic findings for 364 symptomatic patients. Neurosurgery. 1999;44:1005–17. https://doi.org/10.1097/00006123-199905000-00042.
29. Labuda R, Nwotchouang BST, Ibrahimy A, et al. A new hypothesis for the pathophysiology of symptomatic adult Chiari malformation Type I. Med Hypotheses. 2022;158:110740. https://doi.org/10.1016/J.MEHY.2021.110740.
30. Goel A. Is atlantoaxial instability the cause of Chiari malformation? Outcome analysis of 65 patients treated by atlantoaxial fixation. J Neurosurg Spine. 2015;22:116–27. https://doi.org/10.3171/2014.10.SPINE14176.
31. Ciaramitaro P, Ferraris M, Massaro F, Garbossa D. Clinical diagnosis—part I: what is really caused by Chiari I. Childs Nerv Syst. 2019;35:1673–9. https://doi.org/10.1007/S00381-019-04206-Z/FIGURES/3.
32. Holly LT, Batzdorf U. Chiari malformation and syringomyelia: JNSPG 75th Anniversary Invited Review Article. J Neurosurg Spine. 2019;31:619–28. https://doi.org/10.3171/2019.7.SPINE181139.
33. Ciaramitaro P, Massimi L, Bertuccio A, et al. Diagnosis and treatment of Chiari malformation and syringomyelia in adults: international consensus document. Neurol Sci. 2022;43:1327–42. https://doi.org/10.1007/S10072-021-05347-3/FIGURES/2.
34. Kahn EN, Muraszko KM, Maher CO. Prevalence of Chiari I malformation and Syringomyelia. Neurosurg Clin N Am. 2015;26:501–7. https://doi.org/10.1016/J.NEC.2015.06.006.

35. Pindrik J, Johnston JM. Clinical presentation of Chiari I malformation and Syringomyelia in children. Neurosurg Clin N Am. 2015;26:509–14. https://doi.org/10.1016/J.NEC.2015.06.004.
36. George TM, Higginbotham NH. Defining the signs and symptoms of Chiari malformation type I with and without syringomyelia. Neurol Res. 2011;33:240–6. https://doi.org/10.1179/016164111X12962202723760.
37. Lara-Reyna J, Chae J, Tosi U, et al. Syringomyelia resolution following Chiari surgery: a novel scale for communication and research. Neurosurgery. 2021;88:E60–6. https://doi.org/10.1093/NEUROS/NYAA326.
38. Hankinson TC, Klimo P, Feldstein NA, et al. Chiari malformations, syringohydromyelia and scoliosis. Neurosurg Clin N Am. 2007;18:549–68. https://doi.org/10.1016/J.NEC.2007.04.002.
39. Noureldine MHA, Shimony N, Jallo GI, Groves ML. Scoliosis in patients with Chiari malformation Type I. Childs Nerv Syst. 2019;35:1853–62. https://doi.org/10.1007/S00381-019-04309-7.
40. Eule JM, Erickson MA, O'Brien MF, Handler M. Chiari I malformation associated with syringomyelia and scoliosis: a twenty-year review of surgical and nonsurgical treatment in a pediatric population. Spine (Phila Pa 1976). 2002;27:1451–5. https://doi.org/10.1097/00007632-200207010-00015.
41. Brockmeyer DL. Editorial: Chiari malformation Type I and scoliosis: the complexity of curves. J Neurosurg Pediatr. 2011a;7:22–3. https://doi.org/10.3171/2010.9.PEDS10383.
42. Strahle J, Muraszko KM, Buchman SR, et al. Chiari malformation associated with craniosynostosis. Neurosurg Focus. 2011a;31:E2. https://doi.org/10.3171/2011.6.FOCUS11107.
43. Cinalli G, Spennato P, Sainte-Rose C, et al. Chiari malformation in craniosynostosis. Childs Nerv Syst. 2005;21:889–901. https://doi.org/10.1007/S00381-004-1115-Z/FIGURES/12.
44. Engel M, Castrillón-Oberndorfer G, Hoffmann J, et al. Chiari malformation in nonsyndromal single craniosynostosis-Much Ado about Nothing? Acta Neurochir. 2012;154:1803–7. https://doi.org/10.1007/S00701-012-1439-5/FIGURES/3.
45. Tubbs RS, Beckman J, Naftel RP, et al. Institutional experience with 500 cases of surgically treated pediatric Chiari malformation Type I: clinical article. J Neurosurg Pediatr. 2011;7:248–56. https://doi.org/10.3171/2010.12.PEDS10379.
46. Loukas M, Shayota BJ, Oelhafen K, et al. Associated disorders of Chiari Type I malformations: a review. Neurosurg Focus. 2011;31:E3. https://doi.org/10.3171/2011.6.FOCUS11112.
47. Massimi L, Pennisi G, Frassanito P, et al. Chiari Type I and hydrocephalus. Childs Nerv Syst. 2019b;35:1701–9. https://doi.org/10.1007/S00381-019-04245-6/TABLES/1.
48. Klekamp J. Chiari I malformation with and without basilar invagination: a comparative study. Neurosurg Focus. 2015;38:E12. https://doi.org/10.3171/2015.1.FOCUS14783.
49. Goldstein HE, Anderson RCE. Craniovertebral junction instability in the setting of Chiari I malformation. Neurosurg Clin N Am. 2015;26:561–9. https://doi.org/10.1016/J.NEC.2015.06.001.
50. Brodbelt AR, Flint G. Ehlers Danlos, complex Chiari and cranio-cervical fixation: how best should we treat patients with hypermobility? vol. 31. Taylor & Francis; 2017. p. 397.
51. Henderson FC Sr, Austin C, Benzel E, et al. Neurological and spinal manifestations of the Ehlers–Danlos syndromes. Am J Med Genet C Semin Med Genet. 2017;175(1):195–211. Wiley Online Library.
52. Frikha R. Klippel-Feil syndrome: a review of the literature. Clin Dysmorphol. 2020;29:35–7. https://doi.org/10.1097/MCD.0000000000000301.
53. Tubbs RS, Rutledge SL, Kosentka A, et al. Chiari I malformation and neurofibromatosis Type 1. Pediatr Neurol. 2004b;30:278–80. https://doi.org/10.1016/J.PEDIATRNEUROL.2003.09.013.
54. Saletti V, Viganò I, Melloni G, et al. Chiari I malformation in defined genetic syndromes in children: are there common pathways? Childs Nerv Syst. 2019;35:1727–39. https://doi.org/10.1007/S00381-019-04319-5/FIGURES/6.
55. Richards PS, Bargiota A, Corrall RJM. Paget's disease causing an Arnold-Chiari Type 1 malformation: radiographic findings. AJR Am J Roentgenol. 2001;176:816–7. https://doi.org/10.2214/AJR.176.3.1760816.
56. Meadows J, Kraut M, Guarnieri M, et al. Asymptomatic Chiari type I malformations identified on magnetic resonance imaging. J Neurosurg. 2000;92:920–6. https://doi.org/10.3171/JNS.2000.92.6.0920.
57. Strahle J, Muraszko KM, Kapurch J, et al. Natural history of Chiari malformation Type I following decision for conservative treatment. J Neurosurg Pediatr. 2011b;8:214–21. https://doi.org/10.3171/2011.5.PEDS1122.
58. Steinbok P, Steinbok P. Clinical features of Chiari I malformations. Childs Nerv Syst. 2004;20(5):329–31. https://doi.org/10.1007/S00381-003-0879-X.
59. Fakhri A, Shah MN, Goyal MS. Advanced imaging of Chiari 1 malformations. Neurosurg Clin N Am. 2015;26:519–26. https://doi.org/10.1016/J.NEC.2015.06.012.
60. Raybaud C, Jallo GI. Chiari 1 deformity in children: etiopathogenesis and radiologic diagnosis. Handb Clin Neurol. 2018;155:25–48. https://doi.org/10.1016/B978-0-444-64189-2.00002-0.
61. McVige JW, Leonardo J. Imaging of Chiari Type I malformation and syringohydromyelia. Neurol Clin. 2014;32:95–126. https://doi.org/10.1016/J.NCL.2013.07.002.
62. Hersh DS, Groves ML, Boop FA. Management of Chiari malformations: opinions from different centers—a review. Childs Nerv Syst. 2019;35:1869–73. https://doi.org/10.1007/S00381-019-04176-2.

63. Bollo RJ, Riva-Cambrin J, Brockmeyer MM, Brockmeyer DL. Complex Chiari malformations in children: an analysis of preoperative risk factors for occipitocervical fusion: clinical article. J Neurosurg Pediatr. 2012;10:134–41. https://doi.org/10.3171/2012.3.PEDS11340.
64. Brockmeyer DL. The complex Chiari: issues and management strategies. Neurol Sci. 2011b; 32:345–7. https://doi.org/10.1007/S10072-011-0690-5/FIGURES/2.
65. Abel F, Tahir MZ. Role of sleep study in children with Chiari malformation and sleep disordered breathing. Childs Nerv Syst. 2019;35(10):1763–8. https://doi.org/10.1007/S00381-019-04302-0.
66. Khatwa U, Ramgopal S, Mylavarapu A, et al. MRI findings and sleep apnea in children with Chiari I malformation. Pediatr Neurol. 2013;48:299–307. https://doi.org/10.1016/J.PEDIATRNEUROL.2012.12.009.
67. Dauvilliers Y, Stal V, Abril B, et al. Chiari malformation and sleep related breathing disorders. J Neurol Neurosurg Psychiatry. 2007;78:1344. https://doi.org/10.1136/JNNP.2006.108779.
68. Zhang JC, Bakir B, Lee A, Yalamanchili SS. Unusual association of diseases/symptoms: papilloedema due to Chiari I malformation. BMJ Case Rep. 2011;2011:bcr0820114721. https://doi.org/10.1136/BCR.08.2011.4721.
69. Shaikh AG, Ghasia FF. Neuro-ophthalmology of type 1 Chiari malformation. Expert Rev Ophthalmol. 2015;10:351. https://doi.org/10.1586/17469899.2015.1057505.
70. Yilmaz A, Kanat A, Musluman AM, et al. When is duraplasty required in the surgical treatment of Chiari malformation Type I based on tonsillar descending grading scale? World Neurosurg. 2011;75:307–13. https://doi.org/10.1016/J.WNEU.2010.09.005.
71. Saletti V, Farinotti M, Peretta P, et al. The management of Chiari malformation Type 1 and syringomyelia in children: a review of the literature. Neurol Sci. 2021;42:4965–95. https://doi.org/10.1007/S10072-021-05565-9.
72. Albert GW. Chiari malformation in children. Pediatr Clin North Am. 2021;68:783–92. https://doi.org/10.1016/J.PCL.2021.04.015.
73. Poretti A, Ashmawy R, Garzon-Muvdi T, et al. Chiari Type 1 deformity in children: pathogenetic, clinical, neuroimaging, and management aspects. Neuropediatrics. 2016;47:293–307. https://doi.org/10.1055/S-0036-1584563.
74. Galarza M, Gazzeri R, Alfieri A, Martínez-Lage JF. "Triple R" tonsillar technique for the management of adult Chiari I malformation: surgical note. Acta Neurochir. 2013;155:1195–201. https://doi.org/10.1007/S00701-013-1749-2/FIGURES/4.
75. Massimi L, Frassanito P, Bianchi F, et al. Bony decompression vs duraplasty for Chiari I malformation: does the eternal dilemma matter? Childs Nerv Syst. 2019a;35:1827–38. https://doi.org/10.1007/S00381-019-04218-9/TABLES/1.
76. Lu VM, Phan K, Crowley SP, Daniels DJ. The addition of duraplasty to posterior fossa decompression in the surgical treatment of pediatric Chiari malformation Type I: a systematic review and meta-analysis of surgical and performance outcomes. J Neurosurg Pediatr. 2017;20:439–49. https://doi.org/10.3171/2017.6.PEDS16367.
77. McGirt MJ, Attenello FJ, Datoo G, et al. Intraoperative ultrasonography as a guide to patient selection for duraplasty after suboccipital decompression in children with Chiari malformation Type I. J Neurosurg Pediatr. 2008;2:52–7. https://doi.org/10.3171/PED/2008/2/7/052.
78. Yeh DD, Koch B, Crone KR. Intraoperative ultrasonography used to determine the extent of surgery necessary during posterior fossa decompression in children with Chiari malformation Type I. J Neurosurg Pediatr. 2006;105:26–32. https://doi.org/10.3171/PED.2006.105.1.26.
79. Hale AT, David Adelson P, Albert GW, et al. Factors associated with syrinx size in pediatric patients treated for Chiari malformation Type I and syringomyelia: a study from the Park-Reeves Syringomyelia Research Consortium. J Neurosurg Pediatr. 2020;25:629–39. https://doi.org/10.3171/2020.1.PEDS19493.
80. Atchley TJ, Alford EN, Rocque BG. Systematic review and meta-analysis of imaging characteristics in Chiari I malformation: does anything really matter? Childs Nerv Syst. 2020;36:525–34. https://doi.org/10.1007/S00381-019-04398-4.
81. Riordan CP, Michael Scott R. Fourth ventricle stent placement for treatment of recurrent syringomyelia in patients with Type I Chiari malformations. J Neurosurg Pediatr. 2018;23:164–70. https://doi.org/10.3171/2018.7.PEDS18312.
82. Rei J, Pereira J, Reis C, et al. Endoscopic third ventriculostomy for the treatment of hydrocephalus in a pediatric population with myelomeningocele. World Neurosurg. 2017;105:163–9. https://doi.org/10.1016/J.WNEU.2017.05.107.
83. Park H, Oh S, Woo Choi J, Shin Ra Y. Complete posterior cranial vault distraction osteogenesis to correct Chiari malformation Type I associated with craniosynostosis. J Neurosurg Pediatr. 2021;29:298–304. https://doi.org/10.3171/2021.10.PEDS21443.
84. Levitt MR, Niazi TN, Hopper RA, et al. Resolution of syndromic craniosynostosis-associated Chiari malformation Type I without suboccipital decompression after posterior cranial vault release. J Neurosurg Pediatr. 2012;9:111–5. https://doi.org/10.3171/2011.11.PEDS11268.
85. Lo WB, Thant KZ, Kaderbhai J, et al. Posterior calvarial distraction for complex craniosynostosis and cerebellar tonsillar herniation. J Neurosurg Pediatr. 2020;26:421–30. https://doi.org/10.3171/2020.4.PEDS19742.
86. Goel A, Gore S, Shah A, et al. Atlantoaxial fixation for Chiari 1 formation in pediatric age-group patients: report of treatment in 33 patients. World Neurosurg.

2018;111:e668–77. https://doi.org/10.1016/J.WNEU.2017.12.137.
87. Goel A, Vutha R, Shah A, et al. Atlantoaxial fixation for failed foramen magnum decompression in patients with Chiari formation. J Craniovertebr Junction Spine. 2020;11:186–92. https://doi.org/10.4103/JCVJS.JCVJS_113_20.
88. Brockmeyer DL, Oakes WJ, Rozzelle C, et al. Letter to the Editor: Chiari malformation Type 1 and atlantoaxial instability: a letter from the Pediatric Craniocervical Society. J Neurosurg Spine. 2015;23:820–3. https://doi.org/10.3171/2015.3.SPINE15233.

7 Management of Head Shape Deformity and Craniosynostosis

Edward S. Ahn and Archis R. Bhandarkar

Introduction

The principles behind managing children who present with developmental abnormalities of the cranial vault such as deformational plagiocephaly and craniosynostosis are important topics for neurosurgeons to master. In this chapter, we will review several concepts such as (1) key definitions and diagnostic criteria for deformational plagiocephaly and craniosynostosis; (2) approaches to non-operative management such as repositioning, physical therapy, and helmet therapy; and (3) surgical techniques for craniosynostosis repair including both open and endoscopic techniques.

Readers should be able to answer the following questions by the end of this chapter:

Self-Learning Questions

1. What are the diagnostic criteria and techniques to diagnose deformational plagiocephaly and craniosynostosis?
2. When is surgical management appropriate for children with craniofacial anomalies, and what is the role of non-operative techniques?
3. What are the different surgical techniques and osteotomy designs for craniosynostosis repair?
4. What clinical factors would make an open approach to craniosynostosis repair preferred over endoscopic techniques and vice versa?

Deformational Plagiocephaly

Introduction

Epidemiology and Definitions Deformational plagiocephaly ("oblique head" in Greek) is a condition diagnosed in newborns who present with asymmetry of the face and/or cranial vault due to prolonged exposure to external mechanical pressure. For example, posterior deformational plagiocephaly is characterized by flattening of the occiput and can be associated with chronic exposure to pressure on the back of the head from laying in the supine position [1]. The incidence of posterior deformational plagiocephaly has been estimated at roughly 8.2 in every 100 children. Some have theorized that there has been a rise in cases since the American Academy of Pediatrics (AAP)'s "Back to Sleep" campaign in 1992 which encouraged newborns to sleep in the supine position to prevent sudden infant death syndrome [2].

E. S. Ahn (✉) · A. R. Bhandarkar
Mayo Clinic Department of Neurologic Surgery, Rochester, MN, USA
e-mail: ahn.edward@mayo.edu; bhandarkar.Archis@mayo.edu

N. Shimony, G. Jallo (eds.), *Pediatric Neurosurgery Board Review*,
https://doi.org/10.1007/978-3-031-23687-7_7

Diagnosis

The diagnosis of posterior deformational plagiocephaly can largely be made from appropriate physical exam technique. Of note, it is critical to distinguish posterior deformational plagiocephaly from craniosynostosis especially of the lambdoid suture as the two conditions have different natural histories and require different approaches to management. A thorough physical exam of the newborn with suspected posterior deformational plagiocephaly should include an assessment of facial and cranial vault symmetry, palpation of the sutures, and cranial measurements [1].

Physical exam findings that support a diagnosis of posterior deformational plagiocephaly include (1) a classic "parallelogram"-shaped head on an aerial view, (2) protruding of the forehead on the flattened side, (3) ear on the flattened side being anterior to the ear on the contralateral side, and (4) flattening of the occiput with a unilateral bald spot. Findings that would support a diagnosis of lambdoid craniosynostosis include (1) a classic "trapezoid"-shaped head on aerial view, (2) a palpable ridge on palpation of the lambdoid suture, (3) ear on the flattened side being posterior to the ear on the contralateral side, and (4) the presence of an occipitomastoid bulge [3].

Imaging has a nuanced role in the diagnosis of posterior deformational plagiocephaly, and a recent guideline has been issued and endorsed in 2016 on the topic by the Congress of Neurological Surgeons (CNS) and American Association of Neurological Surgeons (AANS). In the guideline, the authors argue that there is class III evidence that "clinical examination is most often sufficient to diagnose plagiocephaly." In cases where clinical examination cannot appropriately resolve between posterior deformational plagiocephaly and craniosynostosis, ordering skull x-rays or ultrasound is appropriate to assess whether the suture is fused. CT imaging should be reserved for skull x-rays and ultrasound prove non-diagnostic [4].

Therapy

Therapy for positional deformational plagiocephaly includes physical and helmet therapy. Physical therapy is the initial mode of treatment and consists of exercises and behavioral modifications designed to strengthen the ipsilateral sternocleidomastoid which can shorten on the flattened side of a newborn with positional deformational plagiocephaly. These exercises include encouraging prone playing ("tummy time") and offering food in a way that discourages a particular side preference [1].

Some experts recommend that if improvements are not noted in a child's plagiocephaly after attempting physical therapy for 4–8 weeks, then imaging may be ordered to confirm that the sutures are in fact not fused. In the case that sutures are indeed not fused, then providers should pursue helmet therapy [1]. Helmet therapy consists of using a custom-fit head orthosis to apply mechanical pressures that encourage appropriate growth of the cranial vault. Additionally, a 2016 guideline written and endorsed by the CNS and AANS recommends that helmet therapy also be offered to children who present with moderate to severe plagiocephaly at an advanced age [5].

Summary: Clinical Pearls for the Treatment of Deformational Plagiocephaly

- Posterior deformational plagiocephaly is a condition in newborns characterized by flattening of the occiput and can be associated with chronic exposure to pressure on the back of the head from laying in the supine position.
- Current guidelines support that clinical examination is sufficient to diagnose positional deformational plagiocephaly. Imaging is only recommended when the clinical exam is equivocal.
- Physical exam findings that support a diagnosis of posterior deformational plagiocephaly

compared to craniosynostosis include a classic "parallelogram"-shaped head with protruding of the forehead on the flattened side, as well as the ear on the flattened side being anterior to the ear on the contralateral side.

- Treatment for posterior deformational plagiocephaly consists of repositioning and physical therapy. Helmet therapy may be warranted for moderate to severe cases, as well as those that are not responsive to physical therapy.

Craniosynostosis

Introduction

Craniosynostosis is a condition characterized by a defect in the growth of the newborn skull wherein there is early fusion of one or more of the cranial sutures. The calvarial vault uniquely develops via the process of membranous ossification with the cranial sutures serving as growth centers for new bone. Skull growth is driven by increase in volume of the underlying brain with new bone generated at the sutures ideally matching the growth of the brain. Craniosynostosis occurs when there is early fusion of the cranial sutures at any point during this process [6].

Epidemiology and Definitions Craniosynostosis occurs on average in 1 out of every 2500 live child births [6]. Craniosynostosis most commonly involves fusion of the sagittal suture ("scaphocephaly," 40–60% of cases) but also can involve the coronal ("anterior plagiocephaly," 20–30% of cases), metopic ("trigonocephaly," 10% of cases), and rarely the lambdoid suture [7]. Craniosynostosis can be subdivided by single-suture craniosynostosis and multiple-suture craniosynostosis based upon the number of sutures involved. Craniosynostosis can occur as part of a larger syndrome such as Apert's syndrome, Crouzon's syndrome, and Pfeiffer's syndrome in which case the condition is appropriately called syndromic craniosynostosis but more often presents as an isolated defect and is designated as non-syndromic craniosynostosis [7].

Diagnosis

Diagnosis of craniosynostosis involves a combination of both a thorough clinical exam and radiologic studies. In the sections below, we will describe several considerations and principles for appropriately diagnosing craniosynostosis.

Clinical Exam in Craniosynostosis

A three-step conceptual framework for diagnosing craniosynostosis has been previously described in the literature including assessing "(1) whether a craniosynostosis is present, (2) whether there are additional features suggesting an associated syndrome, and (3) whether urgent or elective management is required" [8].

Assessing Head Shape and Presence of Fused Suture The presence of a fused suture can be assessed via palpation of a ridge along the suture, as well as careful examination of the child's head shape that may support a diagnosis of craniosynostosis. For example, as described in section "Diagnosis", unilambdoid synostosis is characterized by ipsilateral occipitoparietal flattening, contralateral frontal and parietal bossing, and ipsilateral displacement of the ear posteriorly. Additionally, the changes in head shape noted in sagittal craniosynostosis include bitemporal narrowing as well as frontal and occipital bossing. Metopic synostosis results in a trigone-shaped skull and associated parieto-occipital bossing. Bilateral coronal synostosis can result in a prominent frontal bone, displacement of the vertex anteriorly, and flattening of the occiput [7]. Knowledge of these common changes in head shape can support the clinical diagnosis of craniosynostosis.

Assessing for Syndromic Features An assessment of syndromic features is important as syndromic craniosynostosis has a different natural history compared to non-syndromic craniosynostosis. *Crouzon's* and *Apert's syndromes* are the most common craniosynostosis syndromes. Crouzon's phenotype is characterized by "brachycephalic craniosynostosis, significant hypertelorism, proptosis, maxillary hypoplasia, beaked nose and, possibly, cleft palate… as well as intracranial anomalies including hydrocephalus, Chiari 1 malformation, and hind-brain herniation" [7]. Hallmarks of Apert's syndrome include craniosynostosis alongside syndactyly of the extremities. Physical exam findings that may be present include "coronal suture synostosis, wide-set eyes, mid-face hypoplasia, choanal stenosis, and shallow orbits" [7]. The presence of syndromic features like these may warrant genetic testing for genes known to be associated with craniosynostosis such as the FGF receptor genes (FGFR3 and FGFR2).

Assessing for Findings That May Prompt Emergent Management A thorough clinical exam of the patient with suspected craniosynostosis also involves assessing for features that may prompt emergent management. The scalp should be assessed for any prominent blood vessels, and the fontanelles should have their shape, size, and tension characterized. Additionally, it is important to assess for signs of increased intracranial pressure through an appropriate ophthalmologic exam [8].

Radiologic Studies in Craniosynostosis

Imaging studies may be used in the clinical workup of a patient with suspected craniosynostosis to assess for the patency of the sutures, as well as assist with surgical planning. Many centers forego imaging if the physical examination reveals enough characteristics of the disorder. Several imaging modalities such as *computerized tomography (CT) with three-dimensional reconstruction, ultrasound, and plain film x-rays* may be used to work up a possible diagnosis of craniosynostosis. Of these modalities, CT allows providers to assess all cranial sutures for patency but can be more expensive than x-rays, as well as carry more radiation risk compared to ultrasound [8]. One study at a tertiary medical center found that non-syndromic craniosynostosis patients on average undergo two CT scans, which is "equivalent to 1.5 years of the average annual background radiation dose a person living in the USA will encounter from environmental radiation, medical exposures, and consumer products" [9]. Additionally, the authors recommend delaying imaging to the point of pre-surgical planning instead of initial presentation given that there are higher effective radiologic doses associated with CTs obtained before 6 months of age.

Ultrasound is an emerging technology for the diagnosis of craniosynostosis that is promising because it is fast, inexpensive, and non-radiating. One study in a small cohort of 26 infants demonstrated that ultrasound imaging with a Siemens Elegra, 7.5 MHz linear scanner, could appropriately detect partial or total fusion of cranial sutures with good correspondence with CT imaging [10]. In a larger study of 126 patients of which 115 patients had normal sutures and 8 had craniosynostosis, the sensitivity of ultrasound imaging with a 12-MHz linear Philips HealthCare transducer was 100% and specificity 98% with good concordance with four-view skull radiography [11].

Management

Management options for craniosynostosis include a variety of operative approaches which together can achieve good correction of head shape. Operative approaches include both open and endoscopic approaches.

Operative Management: Open Approaches

In open approaches to craniosynostosis repair, large skin incisions are made to expose the skull so that the surgeon may remove and rearrange significant portions of the bone through osteotomies. The overall purpose of different osteotomy designs is to create bone windows that allow for normal development of the cranial vault and appropriate expansion of the underlying brain. In this section, we will describe several common osteotomy techniques used in open repair such as strip craniectomy, "pi" osteotomies, as well as the Melbourne technique.

Open Strip Craniectomy Open strip craniectomies and suturectomies are one of the earliest described open surgical approaches for treating craniosynostosis which involve either removal of the fused bone or release of the fused suture, respectively. Surgical texts describing this approach date as far back as 1890. Among open approaches, open strip craniectomy is not as common in modern practice as "pi" osteotomies and the Melbourne technique which we describe below. However, the principle behind the open strip craniectomy lives on in endoscopic approaches that use the technique [12].

"Pi" Osteotomies Pi osteotomies are commonly used in the treatment of single-suture sagittal craniosynostosis. The techniques get their name for the shape of the osteotomies which resemble the Greek symbol for "Pi" (π). In a pi osteotomy for the treatment of sagittal craniosynostosis, two paramedian osteotomies are made on either side of the fused sagittal suture from the coronal suture to the lambdoid suture. The osteotomies are then extended laterally and bitemporally to form the classic "pi" shape. Then, "barrel stave" osteotomies (which are given that name as they are thin sequential osteotomies that resemble barrel staves) are performed in the parietal bone in order to allow for preferential expansion along the sides rather than in the anterior-posterior direction [3].

The Melbourne Technique The Melbourne technique is a technique described by the Melbourne Craniofacial Unit that is a form of radical cranial vault remodeling which may be preferred in patients who present with serious deformity or advanced age. The goal of the technique is to correct several deformities that may accompany the fused suture such as occipital and frontal deformities in one procedure [13]. Core aspects of the procedure involve (1) removal of a large precoronal frontal segment to treat frontal bossing and (2) removal of bone immediately posterior to the coronal suture which is used in the recontouring of a new occiput [3].

Operative Management: Endoscopic Approaches

Endoscopic approaches for craniosynostosis repair use minimally invasive approaches to release or remove fused sutures at an early age followed by months of helmet therapy. Endoscopic suture repair works to correct cranial vault deformities by (1) surgically releasing the fused suture impeding growth and (2) leveraging the rapid growth in newborn brain through serial helmeting [14].

Operative Approach Endoscopic strip craniectomy is the most commonly performed technique for endoscopic craniosynostosis repair. The general steps in a two-incision approach to endoscopically repair a sagittally fused suture include (1) creating small skin incisions at the coronal and lambdoid sutures so that the surgeon has proximal and distal visualization of the fused suture, (2) subgaleal dissection followed by burr hole creation is performed directly under the incisions, (3) enlargement of the burr holes with a rongeur so that an endoscope may be introduced, (4) introduction of the endoscopic which is used for visualization as well to separate bone from dura, and (5) osteotomies of the bone with a rongeur or scissors under visualization with the endoscope. A similar approach is followed for endoscopic repair of other cranial sutures [15].

Helmet Therapy Following Endoscopic Repair Serial helmeting is a key component of postoperative protocols following endoscopic craniosynostosis repair. Generally, helmeting will continue until at least 1 year of age, and serial laser scans are used to guide adjustments in the size and shape of the child's helmet. The duration and frequency of adjustments in helmet timing can vary between institutions. In one protocol published by staff at Boston Children's Hospital, the authors describe that children at their institution are fit with initial helmet between 1 and 5 days after discharge with return visits to the "orthotist every two to three weeks until the surgeon discontinues helmet therapy" [14].

Principles of Patient Selection While no formal clinical guideline has yet to be issued on the appropriateness of performing open versus endoscopic repair, data does exist in the literature that generally support endoscopic approaches as safe.

For example, a systematic review comparing endoscopic approaches to open repair found that endoscopic approaches were associated with "statistically significant reductions in blood loss (mean difference = 162.4 mL), operative time (mean difference = 112.38 min), length of stay (mean difference = 2.56 days), and rates of perioperative complications (odds ratio = 0.58), reoperation (odds ratio = 0.37) and transfusion (odds ratio = 0.09)" [16]. Guidelines can vary between institutions, but generally endoscopic repair is recommended to children who present with craniosynostosis at an early age (less than 3 months), whereas open cranial vault modeling is reserved for "children older than eight months whose brains have significantly matured in size" [14]. Of note, endoscopic approaches offer less visualization than open approaches, and factors like the number of sutures involved as well as the severity of the disease should be considered by the individual surgeon before selecting an approach.

Operative Management: Flexible Springs and Distractor Devices

For both endoscopic and open approaches to cranial vault repair, refusion of the repaired suture is critical to avoid. In the evolution of craniosynostosis repair, devices such as flexible springs and distractors were invented to mechanically push bones apart in order to avoid refusion [6]. In this subsection, we describe some principles for surgeons to know about the role of flexible springs and distractor devices in craniosynostosis repair. Of note, craniosynostosis repair involving springs and distractors are often multi-staged because both flexible springs and distractor devices need to be removed in a second planned surgery.

Flexible Springs The use of flexible springs has a good safety profile with low morbidity in patients who receive craniosynostosis repair. In one study that compared 20 patients who received spring-assisted cranioplasty versus 20 patients who received pi-plasty for isolated sagittal craniosynostosis, the authors concluded "the two groups of surgery resulted in a quite similar morphologic outcome… (and that) the spring group was superior with respect to blood loss, transfusion requirements, operative time, ICU time, recovery time, and total hospital stay" [17]. More recently, groups have reported using biomechanical computational modeling to predict the effect of spring forces on skull growth in order to optimize surgical planning [18].

Distractor Devices The role of distractor devices in craniosynostosis repair relies on the principle of distraction osteogenesis which uses "internal or external distractor plates to gradually expand the cranial vault over a series of weeks" [19]. Distractor devices can be combined with minimally invasive techniques for surgeons who seek to avoid the large incisions associated with open cranial vault repair. In one small case series, ten patients with coronal craniosynostosis were treated with endoscopic craniosynostosis repair as well as with a unidirectional bone distraction system. The external distractor system was placed where the incision was made, and parents were instructed on how to move the device at a rate of a distraction rate of 1 mm per day. Hence, distraction of the frontal bone was achieved gradually with an external fixation system rather than at the initial surgery. The authors concluded that "anthropometric results were satisfactory both for the families and the medical team" through this minimally invasive approach [20]. A systematic review comparing similar distraction osteogenesis techniques to open cranial vault modeling for unilateral coronal craniosynostosis concluded that the techniques had relatively similar outcomes overall with distraction osteogenesis achieving better Whitaker aesthetic outcomes [19].

Measuring Clinical Outcomes in Craniosynostosis

Surgeons should be aware of several standardized and commonly used measures to evaluate outcomes after craniosynostosis repairs. Measurements to assess clinical improvement include craniometric measurements as well as the Whitaker aesthetic classes.

Craniometric Outcomes Commonly collected craniometric measurements to track improvements in head shape in patients with craniosynostosis include the *cephalic index* and the *cranial vault asymmetry index*. The cephalic index is defined as the maximum anterior-posterior length divided by the maximum head breadth times 100. The cranial vault asymmetry index is defined by first calculating two frontozygomatic-to-contralateral occipital diagonal distances and represents the absolute difference in diagonal distance divided by the shorter diagonal distance times 100 [21, 22]. Mean cephalic index values in normal children are 85 in newborns aged 0–3 months, 84 in newborns aged 4–6 months, 83 in newborns aged 7–12 months, 82 in newborns aged 13–18 months, and 81 in newborns aged 19–24 months [23].

Whitaker Aesthetic Classes The Whitaker aesthetic classification is a subjective yet standardized reporting system for aesthetic outcomes after craniosynostosis where patients are assigned to four classes. Whitaker Class 1 patients are those "where no refinements or surgical revisions considered advisable or necessary by the surgeon or the patient." Whitaker Class 2 patients are those where "soft-tissue or lesser bone-contouring revisions desirable, whether performed or not." Whitaker Class 3 patients are those where "major alternative osteotomies or bone-grafting procedures needed or performed." Lastly, Whitaker Class 4 patients are those for whom "major procedure duplicating or exceeding in extent the original surgery necessary" [24, 25]. While the Whitaker classification of craniosynostosis outcomes is imperfect and has been shown to have low interrater reliability [24], it is still commonly used in the literature, and readers interested in engaging with the primary craniosynostosis literature should be knowledgeable of it.

Summary: Clinical Pearls for Craniosynostosis Repair

- Craniosynostosis is a condition characterized by a defect in the growth of the newborn skull wherein there is early fusion of one or more of the cranial sutures.
- Craniosynostosis most commonly involves fusion of the sagittal suture ("scaphocephaly," 40–60% of cases) but also can involve the coronal ("anterior plagiocephaly," 20–30% of cases), metopic ("trigonocephaly," 10% of cases), and rarely the lambdoid suture.
- The clinical exam of a child with suspected craniosynostosis should include assessing for (1) the presence of a fused suture through a palpable ridge, (2) other clinical signs that may suggest syndromic diseases, and (3) clinical signs such as raised intracranial pressure that would suggest the need for emergent intervention.
- Imaging studies such as computerized tomography (CT) with three-dimensional reconstruction, ultrasound, and plain film x-rays may be used to work up a possible diagnosis of craniosynostosis.
- Surgical management for craniosynostosis includes both open approaches (open strip craniectomy, pi osteotomies, and the Melbourne technique) and endoscopic approaches. Patients who receive endoscopic repair require postoperative helmet therapy.
- There are several factors a surgeon should consider while picking an open versus endoscopic approach for craniosynostosis repair including age, presence of multiple fused sutures, and others. Endoscopic techniques have generally been associated with reduced blood loss, operative time, and length of stay.
- Cranial measurements such as cephalic index and cranial vault asymmetry index are commonly used metrics to assess the efficacy of craniosynostosis repair.

Multiple-Choice Questions

Question 1: Which of the following is *not* a physical exam finding expected in a child with posterior deformational plagiocephaly?

a) "Parallelogram"-shaped head on aerial inspection
b) Ear on the flattened side anterior to the ear on the contralateral side

c) Palpable ridge at the lambdoid suture
d) Protruding of the forehead on the flattened side

Question 2: Which of the following genes have been found to have strong associations with syndromic craniosynostosis?
a) FGF3
b) VEGF
c) KRAS
d) MGMT

Question 3: The most commonly fused cranial suture in unilateral craniosynostosis is:
a) Coronal
b) Sagittal
c) Lambdoid
d) None of the above

Question 4: Systematic reviews have shown that endoscopic craniosynostosis repair generally has reduced what compared to open repair:
a) Hospital length of stay
b) Intraoperative blood loss
c) Operative time
d) All of the above

Answer keys: c, a, b, d

References

1. Biggs WS. Diagnosis and management of positional head deformity. Am Fam Physician. 2003;67(9):1953–6.
2. Kalra R, Walker ML. Posterior plagiocephaly. Childs Nerv Syst. 2012;28(9):1389–93.
3. Bertrand AA, Hu AC, Lee JC. Planning and osteotomy designs in the correction of single-suture craniosynostosis. Ann Plast Surg. 2021;86(2):226–32.
4. Mazzola C, Baird LC, Bauer DF, et al. Congress of neurological surgeons systematic review and evidence-based guideline for the diagnosis of patients with positional plagiocephaly: the role of imaging. Neurosurgery. 2016;79(5):E625–6.
5. Tamber MS, Nikas D, Beier A, et al. Congress of neurological surgeons systematic review and evidence-based guideline on the role of cranial molding orthosis (helmet) therapy for patients with positional plagiocephaly. Neurosurgery. 2016;79(5):E632–3.
6. Proctor MR, Meara JG. A review of the management of single-suture craniosynostosis, past, present, and future. J Neurosurg Pediatr. 2019;24(6):622–31.
7. Kabbani H, Raghuveer TS. Craniosynostosis. Am Fam Physician. 2004;69(12):2863–70.
8. Kajdic N, Spazzapan P, Velnar T. Craniosynostosis—recognition, clinical characteristics, and treatment. Bosn J Basic Med Sci. 2018;18(2):110–6.
9. Bruce MK, Mittal AM, Whitt DS, et al. Computed tomography associated radiation exposure in children with craniosynostosis. Childs Nerv Syst. 2021;37(8):2635–41.
10. Regelsberger J, Delling G, Helmke K, et al. Ultrasound in the diagnosis of craniosynostosis. J Craniofac Surg. 2006;17(4):623–5; discussion 626–8.
11. Rozovsky K, Udjus K, Wilson N, Barrowman NJ, Simanovsky N, Miller E. Cranial ultrasound as a first-line imaging examination for craniosynostosis. Pediatrics. 2016;137(2):e20152230.
12. Mehta VA, Bettegowda C, Jallo GI, Ahn ES. The evolution of surgical management for craniosynostosis. Neurosurg Focus. 2010;29(6):E5.
13. Greensmith AL, Holmes AD, Lo P, Maxiner W, Heggie AA, Meara JG. Complete correction of severe scaphocephaly: the Melbourne method of total vault remodeling. Plast Reconstr Surg. 2008;121(4):1300–10.
14. Brown L, Proctor MR. Endoscopically assisted correction of sagittal craniosynostosis. AORN J. 2011;93(5):566–79; quiz 580–1.
15. Jimenez DF, Barone CM. Endoscopic techniques for craniosynostosis. Atlas Oral Maxillofac Surg Clin North Am. 2010;18(2):93–107.
16. Goyal A, Lu VM, Yolcu YU, Elminawy M, Daniels DJ. Endoscopic versus open approach in craniosynostosis repair: a systematic review and meta-analysis of perioperative outcomes. Childs Nerv Syst. 2018;34(9):1627–37.
17. Windh P, Davis C, Sanger C, Sahlin P, Lauritzen C. Spring-assisted cranioplasty vs pi-plasty for sagittal synostosis—a long term follow-up study. J Craniofac Surg. 2008;19(1):59–64. https://doi.org/10.1097/scs.0b013e31815c94c8.
18. Bozkurt S, Borghi A, van de Lande LS, Jeelani NUO, Dunaway DJ, Schievano S. Computational modelling of patient specific spring assisted lambdoid craniosynostosis correction. Sci Rep. 2020;10(1):18693.
19. Corkum JP, Burke E, Samargandi O, Retrouvey H, Bezuhly M. Comparison of distraction osteogenesis and single-stage remodeling for correction of unilateral coronal craniosynostosis. J Craniofac Surg. 2019;30(2):370–6.

20. Tellado MG, Lema A. Coronal suturectomy through minimal incisions and distraction osteogenesis are enough without other craniotomies for the treatment of plagiocephaly due to coronal synostosis. J Craniofac Surg. 2009;20(6):1975–7.
21. Kim MJ, Kang MK, Deslivia MF, Kim YO, Choi JW. Applicative factors of helmet molding therapy in late-diagnosed positional plagiocephaly. J Korean Med Sci. 2020;35(36):e295.
22. Bookland MJ, Ahn ES, Stoltz P, Martin JE. Image processing and machine learning for telehealth craniosynostosis screening in newborns. J Neurosurg Pediatr. 2021;27(5):581–8. Published online March 19.
23. Pindrik J, Molenda J, Uribe-Cardenas R, Dorafshar AH, Ahn ES. Normative ranges of anthropometric cranial indices and metopic suture closure during infancy. J Neurosurg Pediatr. 2016;25(6):667–73.
24. Wes AM, Naran S, Sun J, et al. The Whitaker classification of craniosynostosis outcomes: an assessment of interrater reliability. Plast Reconstr Surg. 2017;140(4):579e–86e.
25. Whitaker LA, Bartlett SP, Schut L, Bruce D. Craniosynostosis: an analysis of the timing, treatment, and complications in 164 consecutive patients. Plast Reconstr Surg. 1987;80(2):195–212.

Pediatric Brain and Brainstem Tumors

8

Nir Shimony, Cameron Brimley, George Jallo, and Paul Klimo Jr.

Introduction

Pediatric brain tumors are now the leading cancer-related pathology to lead to pediatric mortality [1]. In recent years, there has been a significant progress in pediatric central nervous system (CNS) tumors and more specifically brain tumors, leading to better understanding and in some cases to promising treatment options, such as targeted treatment. The recent update for the WHO CNS tumor classification incorporated many changes for pediatric brain tumors and in particular for medulloblastomas, low-grade gliomas, and ependymomas [2]. Yet, other tumors are

N. Shimony
Department of Neurosurgery, University of Tennessee - Health Science Center, Memphis, TN, USA

Department of Surgery, St. Jude Children's Research Hospital, Memphis, TN, USA

Le Bonheur Neuroscience Institute, Le Bonheur Children's Hospital, Memphis, TN, USA

Department of Neurosurgery, The Johns Hopkins University - School of Medicine, Baltimore, MD, USA

Semmes-Murphey Clinic, Memphis, TN, USA
e-mail: nshimony@semmes-murphey.com

C. Brimley
Department of Neurosurgery, Geisinger Commonwealth School of Medicine, Scranton, PA, USA

G. Jallo
Department of Neurosurgery, The Johns Hopkins University School of Medicine, Baltimore, MD, USA

David M Goldenberg Family Endowed Chair, Institute for Brain Protection Sciences, Johns Hopkins All Children's Hospital, St. Petersburg, FL, USA

David Goldenberg Family Endowed Chair, Institute for Brain Protection Sciences, Johns Hopkins All Children's Hospital, St., Petersburg, FL, USA
e-mail: gjallo1@jhmi.edu

P. Klimo Jr. (✉)
Division of Pediatric Neurosurgery, Department of Surgery, St. Jude Children's Research Hospital, Memphis, TN, USA

Department of Neurosurgery, The University of Tennessee Health Science Center, Memphis, TN, USA

Department of Neurosurgery, Le Bonheur Children's Hospital, Memphis, TN, USA

Semmes Murphey, Memphis, TN, USA
e-mail: pklimo@semmes-murphey.com

N. Shimony, G. Jallo (eds.), *Pediatric Neurosurgery Board Review*,
https://doi.org/10.1007/978-3-031-23687-7_8

still lack of meaningful understanding and hence new treatment modalities.

Recent years brought significant progress in our understanding and knowledge regarding the biological behavior of different tumors. We now know much more about some of the transcriptional activation and suppression through chromatin modifications and the role of epigenetic regulation in the development of these tumors, their behavior, and response to treatment [1]. Research in recent years showed great progress in our knowledge of the alterations in epigenetic modifiers or heritable changes in the epigenome, including changes in DNA methylation, chromatin remodeling, microRNAs, and long non-coding RNAs [3]. We have a better understanding of the role of surgery, extent of resection, need for second-look surgery, adjuvant chemotherapy or radiation therapy, as well as the timing of utilizing targeted treatment. Yet, in many cases the main treatment modality is still surgery which is indicative of the lack of better treatment modalities to match the biological behavior of the different tumors. It is well established that pediatric brain tumors lack the same abounded tumor mutations [3]. The distinction among the different age groups is now much better established due to our better understanding of the epigenetic regulation. Embryonal tumors are known to be completely distinct from adult brain parenchymal tumors and are rarely seen in the adult subgroup. Even for tumors that have similar histological features and sometimes names (e.g., high-grade gliomas or pilocytic astrocytomas), the significant progress we have made regarding the different histone mutations as well as BRAF-related changes has led to the understanding that those are completely different tumors across the different age groups, with different behaviors, and hence in many cases different types of treatment modalities are needed [4].

The evolution of targeted treatment can take many years, and even today with the significant knowledge expansion, relevant treatment for the different tumor subtyping is missing in many of the cases. One of the known examples for this long process is with atypical teratoid/rhabdoid tumors (ATRT). The recurrent mutations in SMARCB1 that were identified in a majority of ATRT tumors as well as other rhabdoid tumors were first found and published almost two decades ago [5]. Yet, the understanding of the importance of loss of SMARCB1/INI1 in the evolution of these tumors came only in recent years. Our understanding regarding loss of INI1, H3K27 trimethylation, as well as the involvement of EZH2 in the evolution of these tumors led to the opening of several trials using tazemetostat as a potential targeted treatment for these tumors (NCT02601937, NCT03213665). These findings further support that pediatric brain tumors are different entities from adult brain tumors.

Main Players: Methylation, Histone Mutation, MEK/BRAF, FGFR, and Other Alterations

The new classification WHO update in 2021 introduced many changes in the way that we classify pediatric brain tumors. In the update that was published in 2016, molecular subtyping became part of the diagnostic criteria for some tumors. The introduction of H3K27M mutant with the new definition of midline glioma changed the way we define midline structures involved with aggressive tumors, such as the previously known DIPG. In the new classification, this is defined as a distinct diagnosis which resembles the aggressive behavior these tumors tend to have. Alterations in histone genes are recognized as the most common mutation in children with diffuse midline gliomas [2]. Further understanding of the importance of histone mutations as well as ATRX and DAXX in pediatric brain tumors led to nowadays definition of pediatric glioma as biologically unique entities that differed from adult tumors [6]. We better understand the importance of defects in chromatin architecture as possible mechanism in the creation of pediatric gliomas [7]. The methylation changes we see in these tumors are thought to be the major cause for the treatment-related resistance we see in these tumors. One of the promising agents to face this problem is the panobinostat that is currently being evaluated in a phase I trial in children with diffuse pontine gliomas [8]. Very similar methylation changes (H3K27M trimethylation paucity very similar to the finding in H3K27M positive gliomas) among others were seen in posterior fossa ependymoma subtype group A that in a way act biologically very similar to midline

H3K27M tumors with similar resistance to current adjuvant therapy, frequent recurrence tumor, and overall poor prognosis. Hence, potential utilization of targeted therapy in these tumors is now considered, and future studies are intended to target these potential treatment modalities that are considered in midline gliomas [9].

One of the other major changes was in the way we define medulloblastomas with the introduction of the four main groups (WNT, SHH, group 3, and group 4), now further delineated by subgroups according to their molecular subtype and epigenetic behavior.

The field of neuro-oncology and in particular pediatric neuro-oncology is thriving and constantly changing in light of the new data and research emerging in recent years. In the following sections of this chapter, we will focus on summarizing the major changes and the possible treatments that are considered nowadays.

Medulloblastoma

What Is the Current Knowledge?

The historic differentiation of medulloblastomas (MB) to five histological subtypes (classic, desmoplastic, nodular, large cell, anaplastic) has gradually been replaced by the four molecular subtypes (WNT, SHH, non-SHH/non-WNT group 3, and non-SHH/non-WNT group 4) starting from a consensus paper back in 2012 [10, 11]. The appearance in MRI is different as well across the different subtypes (Figs. 8.1 and 8.2). Today, with much more information about the different subgroups in relation to epidemiological factors, it was shown that each subgroup can be further be divided according to demographic and genetic alterations (WNT α, β; SHH α, β, γ, δ; group 3 α, β, γ; group 4 α, β, γ) [10, 12, 13]. Group 4 and SHH are the most common diagnoses among patients with MB. WNT tend to have the best prognosis with more than 95% overall survival at 5 years, with SHH and group 4 following with around 75%, and group 3 having the worse prognosis with around 50% OS in 5 years. Yet, within each subgroup there are subtypes that show good prognosis (e.g., group 3 type α, mostly in infants) and such that show bad prognosis (e.g., SHH type β, mostly in infants). Currently, it is important to describe a patient with MB using the subgroup, demographic, metastatic, and genetic alteration. One example is from the HIT-SIOP PET 4 European trial that shows that when further delineating the WNT group by the age of 16 years old the event-free survival of the patients less than 16 years was close to 100% in 5 years vs. the 88% for the whole group [14]. Another example that has significant ramifications for prognosis is having a patient with SHH MB with or without TP53 mutation. The presence of the mutation changes the overall

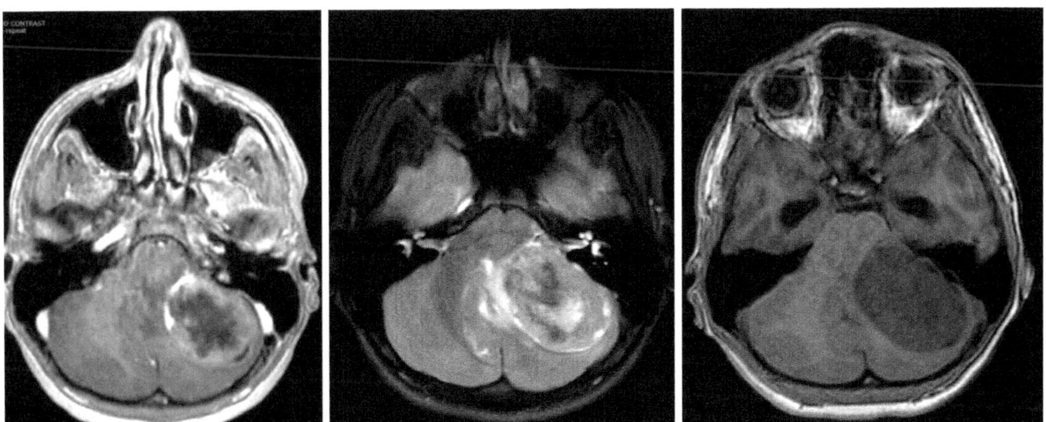

Fig. 8.1 Medulloblastoma in the posterior fossa. Axial slides from the left: T1 with gadolinium shows heterogenic enhancement, T2 relatively hyperintense and contains areas suspicious for intratumoral bleeding, and T1 usually hypointense to the brain

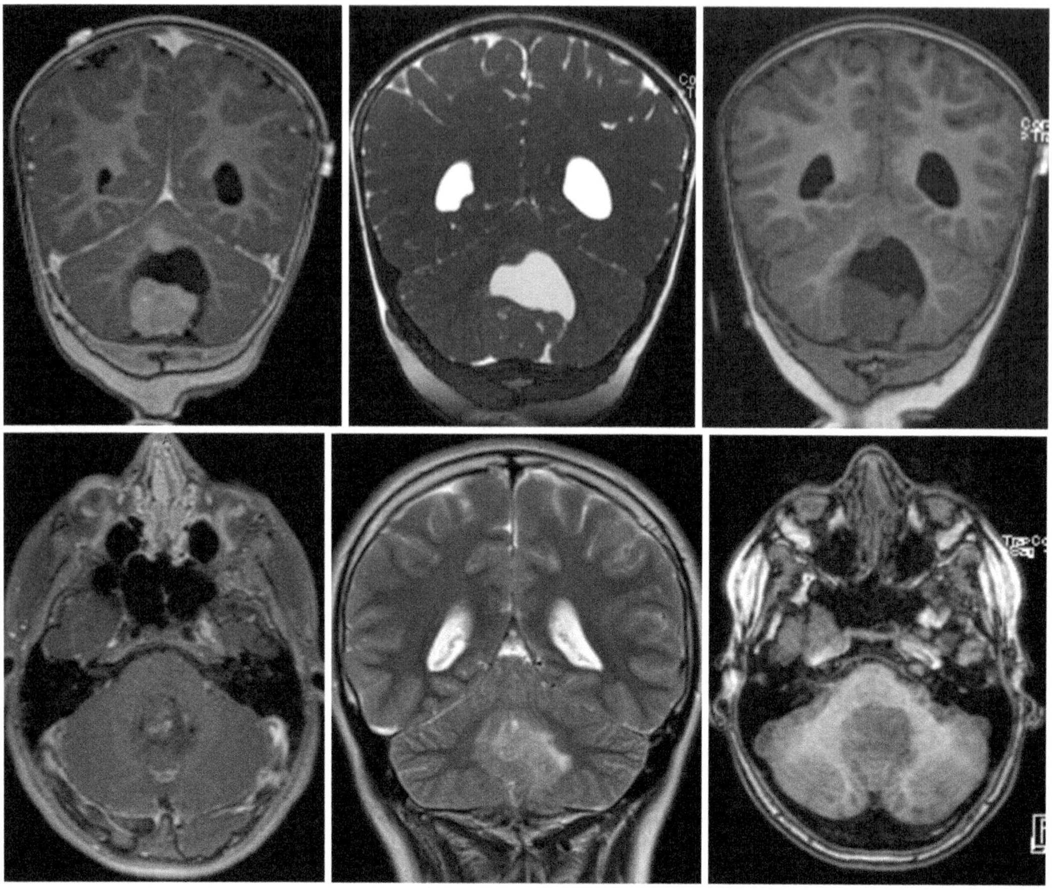

Fig. 8.2 Different medulloblastoma subtypes will have a different appearance on MRI. The upper row shows SHH TP53-negative tumor, whereas the bottom row non-SHH, non-WNT, group 4 subtype

survival almost in twofold (81% OS without the mutation vs. 41% with it). In 2019, Sharma et al. further discussed the differentiation of groups 3 and 4 to eight subgroups, showing that the presence of MYC amplification creates significantly poor prognosis within these groups (around 50% OS in 5 years). On the other hand, good prognostic factors will include chromosome 7 gain, chromosome 8 loss, and chromosome 11 loss.

As the information is still evolving, we believe the discussion for each case should include thorough details about these features and not just the definition of MB initial subgroup.

Role of Surgical Intervention

Surgery for medulloblastoma is still one of the foundations for optimal treatment. It is crucial for good diagnosis, having enough tissue for molecular testing as well as genetic alteration, relieving hydrocephalus that is quite common in these cases, and lowering the overall tumor burden allowing for better response for the adjuvant therapy. The main benefit today of the broad knowledge we have about the tumor molecular and genetic thumb print is in the discussion what to do next after the initial surgery—chemotherapy, radiation therapy, targeted therapy, and even second- and even third-look surgery when it is known that the current adjuvant therapy is not beneficial.

Neurological morbidity for pediatric patient going for MB resection is 24% overall and is described as high as 44% when achieving GTR [15]. Hence, understanding the role of extent of resection for the OS and PFS is crucial.

In the past the risk stratification of MB was much in accordance with the residual tumor left (more or less than 1.5 cm^2 residual disease) and the presence of metastases as well as the age of the patient. The cutoff for the residual tumor came from a well-described publication back in 1996. Yet, over the years and especially now with the new understanding of the different subgroups, many critiques suggest this cutoff is obsolete although still being used at the present time. In 2016, a large cohort study by Thompson et al. (787 patients—86 with WNT tumors, 242 with SHH tumors, 163 with group 3 tumors, and 296 with group 4 tumors) concluded that when taking into consideration the different subgroups in MB, there is not much benefit of aggressive surgical approach when dealing with MB [16]. Their findings showed that GTR had benefit only in PFS and not OS when compared to STR (using the <1.5 cm^2 residual cutoff to define NTR and above to STR), with no benefit at all when compared to NTR. The benefit for GTR over STR according to their findings was shown only for group 4. Yet, many arguments against their findings are still being held today. In 2018, Patel et al. published their experience going for second-look surgery for MB regardless of the initial subgroup [17]. They found tumor remnant in almost all the patients that were taken for second look even in those where the preoperative imaging was questionable (only 1 patient out of 14 patients had negative exploration). Their findings question our true ability to define the extent of resection especially with the extensive use of coagulative materials that is widely practiced nowadays. Another recent large literature review found association between EOR and PFS in specific subgroups but no benefit in OS [15]. Yet, the major problem that stays in concluding information from these studies remained the lack of stratification regarding measurement techniques for residual tumors.

Taking into consideration of everything that is currently known, we conclude that maximal safe resection should be the aim of surgery, including possible transfer of patients to a more experienced center if the surgeon does not feel comfortable in achieving the best possible resection for the patient. Until the current armamentarium of adjuvant therapy will show better results in achieving good OS, surgery will stay one of the mainstays of treatment.

Management of Adjuvant Therapy

One of the main discussions in the decision about adjuvant treatment after the surgical resection for MB is the role of radiation therapy. In the past, radiation-sparing protocols were utilized mainly for patients less than 3 years old, with some protocols utilizing chemotherapy only and others adding the use of intrathecal chemotherapy [18]. Nowadays the improved knowledge regarding the different subgroups allow us to use radiation-sparing protocols in more favorable MB subtypes like WNT and specific SHH especially in young children [19].

Targeted therapy emerged in recent years as possible promising avenue in LGG. Unfortunately, in MB the current knowledge does not support the use of targeted therapy, except in a very specific subset of tumors (e.g., vismodegib for SHH in adults only) [20].

Low-Grade Gliomas

This group of tumors is the most common brain tumor in the pediatric age group. The knowledge base for these tumors expanded quite significantly in the recent decade, especially with the incorporation of the mitogen-activated protein kinase (MAPK) pathway in the diagnosis and recently in the treatment algorithm [4]. For the low-grade gliomas excluding glioneuronal tumors, the tumors can be found as part of two groups of tumors—"circumscribed astrocytic gliomas" (e.g., pilocytic astrocytoma) and "pediatric-type diffuse low-grade gliomas" (Fig. 8.3). The recent WHO classification system that was published in 2021 introduced 14 newly recognized tumor types. Almost half of these newly recognized tumors can be related as low-grade tumors either low-grade gliomas or glioneuronal tumors. Among the newly recognized low-grade tumors, there is a subset of tumors falling under the "pediatric-type diffuse low-grade gliomas"—"diffuse astrocytoma, MYB, or MYBL1-altered"; "polymorphous low-grade neuroepithelial tumor of the young (PLNTY)"; and "diffuse low-grade glioma MAPK-altered" [2]. This change was necessary

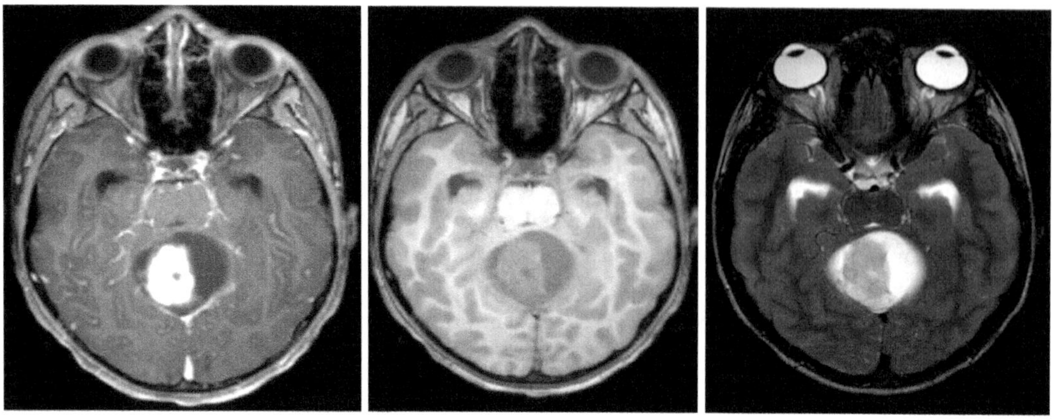

Fig. 8.3 Pilocytic astrocytoma. From the left: axial—T1 with gadolinium, usually significantly enhanced. T1 usually iso- to hypointense, and T2 usually hyperintense

in order to distinguish the relatively indolent and almost benign course the diffuse low-grade gliomas have in the "pediatric type" when compared to the "adult type" that is IDH wild-type diffuse glioma [21]. These new subsets of tumors have features that before this new classification led to different diagnoses. For example, some of the now-known PLNTY tumors were diagnosed in the past as oligodendrogliomas. PLNTY indeed harbors prominent oligodendrocyte-like changes, among other features, that resemble fibrillary, spindled, and pleomorphic astrocytic tumors [22]. These groups of tumors, as the rest of the LGG, have high activation of the MAPK pathway, and more distinctively FGFR-related fusion changes, and mainly will affect children and young adults presenting with tumors located mainly in the temporal lobe, related to the new onset of seizures and situated in the subcortex [2].

For the pediatric patient diagnosed with low-grade glioma, just until recently the treatment paradigm was surgery (aimed for maximal safe resection when feasible vs. just biopsy for other cases), cytotoxic chemotherapy, and rarely radiotherapy. Unfortunately, although most of these tumors don't have aggressive biological behavior, in many cases when meaningful surgery is not feasible, the results of the adjuvant therapy for progression-free survival and overall survival are not very encouraging. The recent progress in our understanding of the MAPK pathway and the possible utilization of different agents (MEK or BRAF inhibitors) modifying its activity allow us to stop or slow cell proliferation for these tumors. So far, the main targets are point mutation at BRAF V600E, somatic driver mutations such as BRAF:KIAA1549, as well as other mutations related to FGFR1 and MYB [23]. Maybe the most studied and known MEK inhibitor is selumetinib which was first studied and used for refractory or inoperable plexiform neurofibromas and recently has been used, mainly as part of open trials, in the treatment of LGG. The results we have so far are a bit more promising for the NF1-related tumors. In 2019, a phase 2 multi-center study tested the use of selumetinib in non-de novo pilocytic astrocytomas harboring either the fusion-related protein (KIAA1549) or the point mutation at BRAF V600E [24]. It found that about a third of the patients (36%) that had non-NF1 LGG had sustainable response while on treatment vs. 40% in the NF group. Other agents from the MEK inhibitors or BRAF inhibitors (e.g., dabrafenib) are currently being tested both for recurrent/inoperable tumors and the first line of defense. It is important to mention that as of now there is no significant shift in the way we treat patients with newly diagnosed LGG in the pediatric age group, but the combination and utilization of targeted therapy need to happen early in the discussion about adjuvant therapy.

High-Grade Gliomas

Pediatric HGG include a group of tumors that comprise aggressive biological activity and usually dismal prognosis (Fig. 8.4). The previous histological diagnoses such as glioblastoma and anaplastic astrocytoma are now being diverted into discussion regarding genetic and molecular subtypes. In the recent decade, a groundbreaking finding sculptured the way that we understand these tumors with the new knowledge coming about the mutations in the chromatin remodeling pathway and more specifically in the Histone 3 variant H3.3 [1]. The mutation of H3K27M, which was previously mainly related to midline gliomas, now is well known to be a driving force in many aggressive tumors. The new WHO classification describes pediatric HGG as four different subgroups [2]:

1. Diffuse midline glioma, H3 K27-altered
2. Diffuse hemispheric glioma, H3 G34-mutant
3. Diffuse pediatric-type high-grade glioma, H3 wild type and IDH wild type
4. Infant-type hemispheric glioma

It is clear that the driving force is the differentiation of which tumor harbors histone mutations and IDH mutations. Yet, the new classifications still show that we need to incorporate both histopathological and molecular data. This is especially true for the third subtype with both H3 and IDH wild-type tumors. In the last classification, a new term by age group became official, infant-type hemispheric glioma, compromised from ALK, ROS1, NTRK1/2/3, MET, and other changes [25, 26].

Historically, the main treatment modalities for most pHGG were surgical resection and radiation therapy. Yet, in recent years there have been a number of chemotherapy protocols as part of clinical trials or consortiums, usually with the combination of radiation therapy. The historic Children's Oncology Group (CCG-943) study protocol that included radiation therapy combined with lomustine (CCNU), vincristine, and prednisone showed efficacy in both OS and EFS for pHGG [27]. Successive trials aimed in different agents including temozolomide (TMZ) showed promising results in adult methylated MGMT HGG in the combination of resection and radiation therapy (STUPP protocol) [28], which lack the previous promising results of CCG-943. TMZ was found not to be effective in pHGG, although its combination with CCNU showed relative efficacy. This finding led to the fact that surgical resection still remains the mainstay of the current treatment.

When taking into consideration the recent findings and classifications, different agents are now being tested where surgical resection (unless DIPG or extensively diffuse) and radiation (for patients above 3 years of age) therapy still makes the mainstay of treatment. The H3K27M mutation is so common (~80%) in patients with diffuse intrinsic pontine glioma (DIPG) that the nomen-

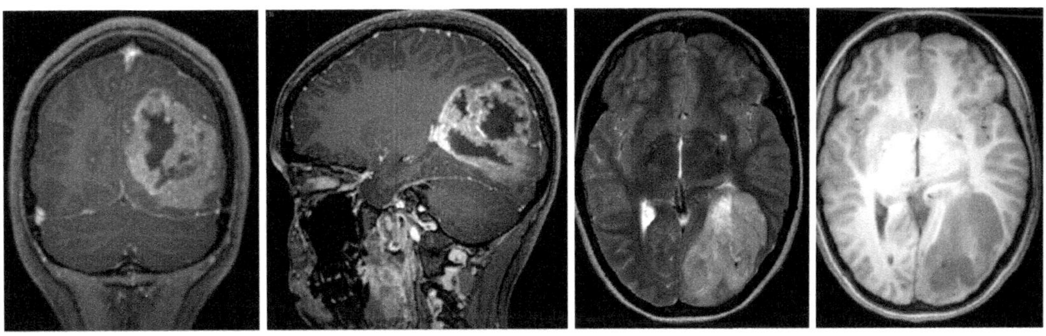

Fig. 8.4 Left occipital high-grade glioma. Histologic diagnosis—glioblastoma. From left to right: coronal T1 with gadolinium, sagittal T1 with gadolinium, axial T2, and axial T1. Tumor is enhanced with mixed signal secondary to areas of necrosis. The tumor is hyperintense on T2 and usually hypo- to isointense on T1

clature is for diffuse midline glioma and H3K27M mutant/alteration. The mortality rate for these tumors is close to 100%, secondary to the fact that surgical resection is not feasible for most of these tumors and the response to chemotherapy is quite poor. Within the H3K27M mutants, the specific histone mutation (H3.1, H3.2, or H3.3) is important. For example, H3.1K27M is more common in young children and tends to have better prognosis secondary to better response for radiation therapy and chemotherapy [29, 30]. Another example is mutation at H3.3 but at glycine 34 resulting in tumors with a valine or arginine substitution (H3G34R/V). These tumors tend to present in adolescence and to be located in the cerebral hemispheres. Different promotors were found to be involved such as MYCN, ATRX, P53, and PDGFRA. These tumors tend to have much better overall survival (OS) than H3K27M, but as for the latest type of tumors, we lack good chemotherapeutic agents to get significant response [31, 32]. Our current understanding of the histone mutation triggers is the idea behind using panobinostat (histone deacetylase (HDAC) inhibitor) that showed promising results in vitro to normalize K27M gene expression, reduce cell proliferation and viability, and also crossing the notorious blood-brain barrier (BBB). Unfortunately, so far in humans, this agent doesn't show good efficacy in crossing the BBB [33]. At the present time, no other HDAC inhibitor has been found to have a promising response for diffuse midline gliomas. Many studies are now being conducted to find better solution to diffuse midline gliomas, so far without significant results. One study in recent years is ONC201 (use of DRD2 antagonist) showed encouraging results in different adult high-grade tumors, and now initial results are showing promising results for pediatric midline gliomas. Yet, further follow-up and trials are needed [26–28].

For the *IDH mutant pHGG*, the overall prognosis is much better than the H3K27M subtype. Compared to adult HGG where the IDH1/2 mutation is fairly common and usually present in secondary tumors, in pediatric HGG the IDH mutation is fairly rare [29, 34]. In pHGG when the IDH mutation is present, it is usually present in the adolescent age group, and these tumors tend to have MGMT methylation, hence showing good response to TMZ [35]. Across the years many studies are aimed at targeting the IDH complex (e.g., vorasidenib, enasidenib), yet none of these agents was yet to show significant efficacy over time. Recent years revealed other possible targeted treatments with ongoing trials such as PARP (poly-adenosine 50-diphosphate-ribose) inhibitors, such as olaparib, with or without radiation (NCT03155620 and NCT03233204) [32, 36].

For the *non-H3 and non-IDH mutations*, it is very important to get a full panel of their molecular parameters. Some advocate for further delineating this group into three subtypes. The first group has some similar features like pediatric LGG with either BRAF V600E mutation, NF1, MET, FGFR2, or NTRK2/3. This potentially allows for the use of targeted treatment, such as BRAF or MEK inhibitors. This as well as the fact that those are usually hemispheric gives overall much better prognosis [37].

The second group and the third group have poor prognosis. The second is composed of amplifications of EGFR, CDK6, and MYCN. Several studies are now aiming at the use of EGFR inhibitors, some with few promising results, but further investigation and follow-up are needed. The third group has chromosome 1p and 20q loss and 17q gain, resulting in PDGFRA and MET amplifications [37]. The prognosis is poor. There are some trials aiming at PDGFRA inhibitors, but results are still too preliminary.

To summarize, the overall prognosis of pHGG is pretty poor. There are many trials for the different subgroups and surgery still plays a major role. Hence, as of now the best treatment paradigm is to have maximal safe resection when amenable and start adjuvant treatment while enrolling the patients for clinical trials. As for DIPG, there is an ongoing debate about the use of biopsy as part of the treatment. The authors' recommendation is to enroll these patients to trials and then act accordingly if biopsy is needed.

Ependymomas

The most recent changes in CNS tumor classification now define ependymomas both by molecular parameters and by anatomical location. As such this group of tumors is subcategorized into supratentorial, infratentorial, and spinal (Fig. 8.5). In this chapter we will cover only the brain-related ependymomas [2]. Ependymomas are 2.5 times more common in the pediatric age group, and within this group, most of the ependymomas are intracranial (~90%) and usually in the posterior fossa, with distinct difference in OS across age groups, most likely secondary to the different molecular subtypes (in children below the age of 3, the 5-year OS rate is 42–55%, whereas around 70% 10-year OS in older age and around 80% in adults) [38–40].

Supratentorial ependymomas were subclassified into RELA fusion and Yap1 in the past. Now it is defined as ZFTA and Yap1. ZFTA, now being the substitute for RELA fusion, is the new designation for C11orf95 and considered more representative since there are other fusion possibilities rather than RELA [2]. Yap1 has the same designation as in the previous 2016 WHO classification. The ZFTA tumors are more common and have overall lower survival when compared to Yap1 that has excellent prognosis [1, 41, 42].

Posterior fossa or infratentorial ependymomas, after many years, are differentiated into group A (PFA) and group B (PFB). Another subgroup is PF-SE that includes mainly subependymomas [43, 44]. PFA is characterized by lack of H3K27 trimethylation (aberrant expression of EZHIP or in rare cases by H3K27M mutations) and is known to be with overall balanced genome, less responsive for adjuvant treatment with poorer prognosis and high recurrence rate (56% 10-year overall survival) [38]. This draws some similarities to midline gliomas, although there are obvious differences as well. PFA is also more common in infants and young children, whereas PFB is more common in older children and has much better outcome (10-year OS ~88%) [38]. Two markers that have been diagnosed as poor prognostic factors are gain of chromosome 1q (which defines bad prognosis within PFA group where it is quite common but not in PFB) as well as loss of chromosome 6q [45–47]. In recent years, there are findings that further subclassify PFA and PFB, giving us better understanding regarding the poor and better outcome markers in each group [41].

The current treatment paradigm for ependymomas is pretty similar to what was recommended a decade ago, which means maximal safe surgery and then treatment as needed, with the main adjuvant treatment is postoperative radiation therapy. Yet, the current understanding we have about the biology of these tumors helps us shape the treatment in a more tailored way.

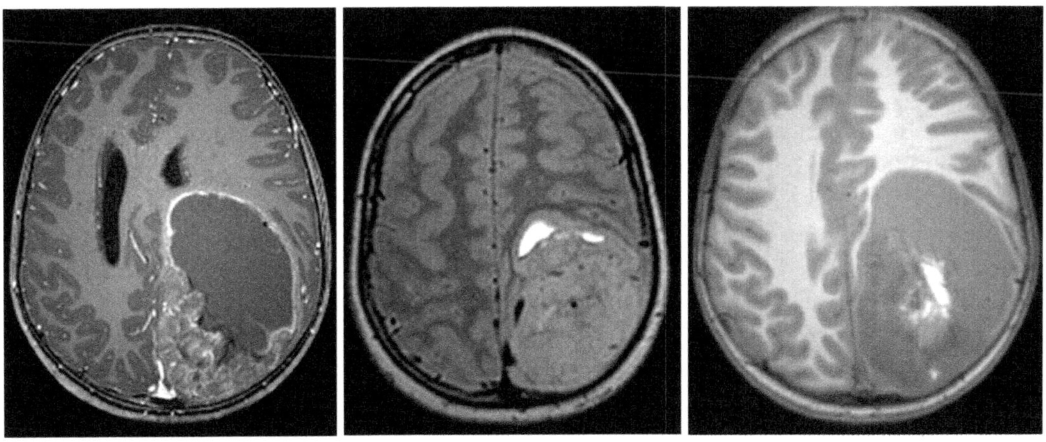

Fig. 8.5 Supratentorial ependymoma. From the left: axial—T1 with gadolinium, usually with heterogenic enhancement. T2 usually hyperintense, and T1 usually iso- to hypointense

The main tool is still surgery regardless of the actual subtype. Once the pathology diagnosis is determined, there are several post-surgical treatment options.

For *supratentorial ependymomas*, when the diagnosis is ZFTA aggressive, post-surgical treatment is warranted including consideration for pre-treatment second-look surgery when there is large residual. The treatment will include radiation therapy (proton or photon beam), follow-up, and then surgical intervention or chemotherapy in case of recurrent tumor. For Yap1, because of the excellent prognosis after gross total surgical resection, follow-up only is warranted with consideration for another surgery or radiation when there is a recurrence.

For *posterior fossa ependymomas*, PFA has poor prognosis and relatively poor response for adjuvant treatment. Hence, the best tool is to perform second-look surgery when needed and feasible and start radiation therapy with or without chemotherapy after maximizing surgical results. For PFB, if the results of the surgical resection are gross total removal, there is no need for adjuvant therapy, just serial imaging follow-up. In other cases, radiation should be considered since the tumors respond very well to this adjuvant therapy.

Glioneuronal and Neuronal Tumors

Low-grade tumors and glioneuronal tumors represent more than a third of pediatric CNS tumors. The glioneuronal group of tumors usually presents with seizures. This group of tumors is often considered as LEAT, which stands for long-term epilepsy-associated tumors. The common presentation will be in young patients, indolent behavior usually without overt symptoms or signs, a tendency to occur in the neocortex with a predilection for the temporal lobes, and relatively high association with cortical disorganization such as dysplasia [48]. Similar to low-grade tumors, the latest changes of the WHO classification are primarily based on underlying genetic alteration (FGFR1, MYB/MYBL1, BRAF, or IDH1/2) [23]. Most of these tumors have low MIB or Ki-67 (usually less than 3%) and are defined as low-grade tumors classified as WHO I. Glioneuronal and neuronal tumors are still grouped together, with three new subtypes that are now defined in the new classification: "diffuse glioneuronal tumor with oligodendroglioma-like features and nuclear clusters (DGONC)," "myxoid glioneuronal tumor (MGT)," and "multinodular and vacuolating tumor (MVNT)." The other tumors that fall under the group of glioneuronal and neuronal tumors are ganglioglioma, desmoplastic infantile ganglioglioma, dysembryoplastic neuroepithelial tumor, papillary glioneuronal tumor, rosette-forming glioneuronal tumor, diffuse leptomeningeal glioneuronal tumor, gangliocytoma, dysplastic cerebellar gangliocytoma, central neurocytoma, extraventricular neurocytoma, and cerebellar liponeurocytoma.

The glioneuronal tumors usually will harbor the BRAFV600E mutation or alteration in the FGFR1 [49]. Diffuse leptomeningeal glioneuronal tumors, on the other hand, are rare glioneuronal tumors that mostly will have the KIAA1549-BRAF fusion and loss of chromosome 1p [50]. The treatment paradigm is very much dependent of the presenting symptoms. For those that presented with seizures, the usual course of action is for gross total resection when it is amenable in a safe manner. In cases of intractable epilepsy, consideration should be given not just for the resection of the tumor but also for potential disconnection of other cortical or parenchymal areas that might be already involved as part of the epileptogenic zone. The indolent nature of these tumors in many cases leads to "wait and see" approach whenever the tumor is asymptomatic or there is no progression over sequential follow-ups. Hence, the use of adjuvant therapy or targeted therapy is usually avoided unless surgical resection is not feasible but needed [2]. When adjuvant treatment is being considered, care should be taken to consider the use the targeted therapy such as dabrafenib (BRAF inhibitor) or trametinib (MEK inhibitor) when suited rather conventional chemotherapy or radiation therapy [51].

Craniopharyngiomas

This group of tumors is one of the most challenging brain tumors among children. The tumors are thought to rise from embryological remnants of Rathke's pouch [52]. There are two distinctive types of craniopharyngiomas—adamantinomatous and papillary. They were considered two subtypes of the same tumor in the previous WHO classifications. In the recent 2021 update, they are now classified as distinct tumor types. This change was driven out of their different clinical demographics, radiologic features, histopathologic findings, genetic alterations, and methylation profiles [53, 54]. The adamantinomatous craniopharyngioma is more common in the pediatric age group with genetic and molecular alteration in CTNNB1, whereas the papillary craniopharyngioma is much more common in the adult age group and is positive for BRAF V600E mutation. The later finding potentially allows for targeted treatment to be part of the armamentarium treating these tumors.

Craniopharyngiomas are counted as benign tumors from histology perspective, yet taking into consideration their biological tendency to harbor the sellar and parasellar region, in close proximity to critical neurovascular structures, invading the hypothalamus, optic pathways, and ventricular system, making craniopharyngiomas a high-risk aggressive tumor with significant morbidities [52, 55–57]. It was advocated for years that the best treatment is gross total resection. Recent years raised debates and arguments against this aggressive approach mainly because the high recurrence (recurrence after GTR was reported to be 17–34%) and progression of pediatric craniopharyngiomas even with extensive resection [58, 59]. The overall survival has been reported to be between 88 and 94% at 5 years and between 70 and 92% at 10 years [52]. The relatively high overall survival was part of the argument against aggressive surgical treatment that leads to significant morbidity including hypothalamic-hypophyseal axis dysfunction, visual impairment, and cerebrovascular pathologies.

The current treatment paradigm for pediatric craniopharyngiomas advocates for maximal safe resection utilizing the endonasal approach when it is feasible and the surgeon feels good sealing of the sella, and prevention of CSF leak will be possible. After surgery in most of the cases, it is advisable to consider radiation therapy. Radiotherapy (XRT) as an adjuvant treatment is reported to have favorable results in terms of tumor control but also to have possible high long-term morbidities, such as neurocognitive and radiation-induced vasculopathies (Moyamoya-like picture) [60]. This is especially significant in small children and should be taken into consideration when choosing the right treatment methodology [61, 62]. In recent years there is a growing use of proton beam as a possible solution for the post-radiation morbidities. The local control for both photon and proton beam radiation is reported to be 77–100% [62]. The toxicity profile with proton beam is pretty much similar to the conventional radiation therapy but was found to have benefits in reducing injury to the neurocognitive function of the patients. Since the recurrence rate is quite high as mentioned before, treating recurrence tumor is not unusual. In a recent study, a treatment paradigm was suggested stating that in case of recurrence or progression of a tumor in a symptomatic patient, immediate intervention is warranted (usually surgery or radiation therapy). In case of asymptomatic patient, if the progression is significant (at least 30% increase in size), treatment should be initiated immediately; if less significant (25–30%), close MRI should be done, and the parents should be instructed to look for any new symptom; and if the following MRI (3 months) shows significant progression, then treatment is needed. In case the tumor mildly progresses (less than 25%), close follow-up should be initiated [52].

Choroid Plexus Carcinoma/ Papilloma

This subset of tumors is pretty much the same when compared to previous classifications by the WHO. The majority of choroid plexus tumors are sporadic, yet it is important to remember that CPC has strong association with Li-Fraumeni syndrome, which is a well-known syndrome to be associated with different kinds of cancer driven by mutations of the TP53 tumor suppressor gene [63]. Another important genetic syndrome that is related to higher association with CPPs is Aicardi syndrome. It is not part of the neuroepithelial tumors anymore. These tumors represent 10–20% of the brain tumors arising in infancy [40]. This group of tumors is more common in the pediatric age group. Choroid plexus papilloma (CPP) is five times more common from the aggressive form of these tumors, the choroid plexus carcinomas (CPCs) [64, 65]. Majority of the patients will be less than 5 years of age, where the more aggressive form of these groups of tumors tends to happen much earlier around infancy. The classic anatomical location in pediatric CPP is around the atrium of the lateral ventricle (Fig. 8.6), while in adult it tends to be in the posterior fossa along the fourth ventricle and its outlets [66]. CPC on the other end is usually located in the lateral ventricles. Although there is some progress in our understanding of the epigenomic of these tumors including frequent chromosome-wide copy-number alterations and *TP53* mutations, much is still unknown [67]. Currently, for pediatric CPP/CPC, it is well established that alteration for TP53 is more likely to be found but not much beyond that. On recent studies, like in other tumor types, it was found that there is most likely a different type of mutations in adults (e.g., *TERT* promotor mutations) that are almost not seen in the pediatric choroid plexus tumors [67]. Several research studies

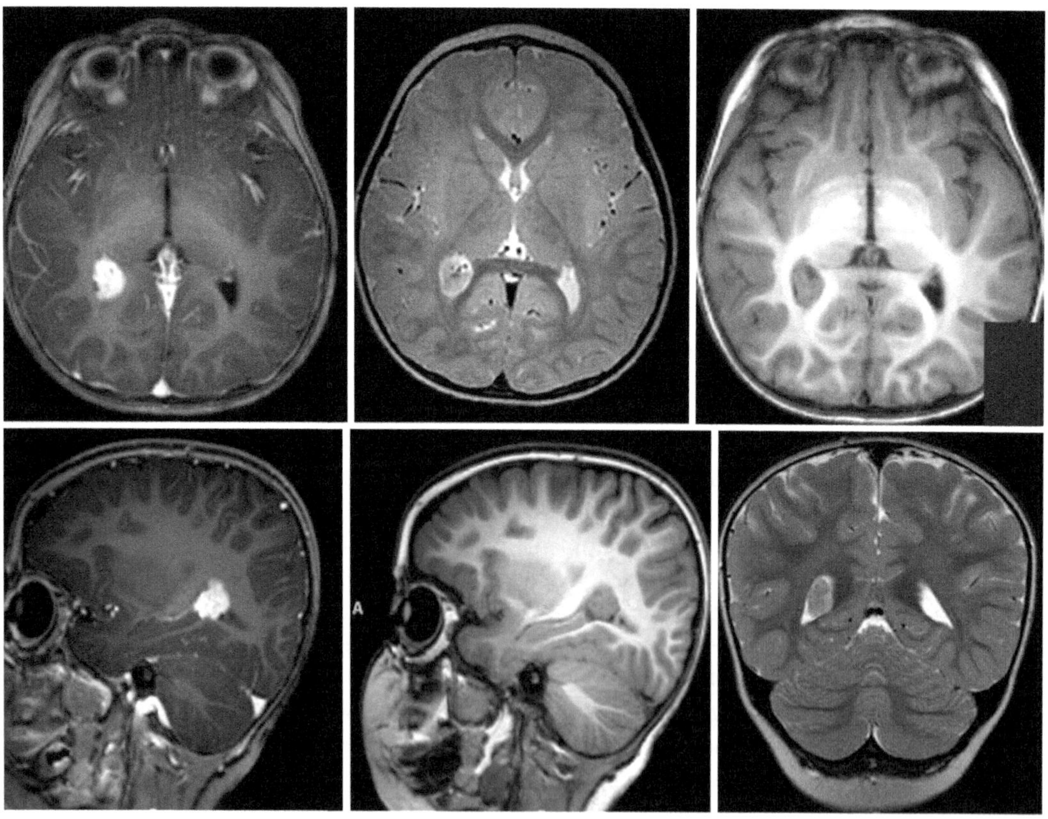

Fig. 8.6 Choroid plexus papilloma. Upper row: axial—T1 with gadolinium, T2, T1. The tumor is vividly enhanced, iso- to hyperintense on T2, and isointense on T1. Second row: sagittal T1 with gadolinium, sagittal T1, and coronal T2

found different genetic alterations, including longer survival in CPC cases when there is gain of chromosome 9p and loss of chromosome 10q [68]. On the other end, loss of chromosome 12q was associated with significant shorter survival among patients with CPC according to a different study [69].

With the lack of new information that will allow us to better diagnose and treat these tumors, the old classification system is still valid—CPP which is WHO I, atypical CPP which is WHO II, and the aggressive CPC which is grade III—and has poor prognosis (5-year survival is 56%). There are some suggestions nowadays, that consider the age as well as the location for distinction between three subgroups. The use of DNA methylation profiling helps further segregate these three groups in a more distinctive way—supratentorial pediatric low-risk choroid plexus tumors (CPP, aCPP; "pediatric A"), supratentorial high-risk choroid plexus tumors (CPP, aCPP, and CPC; "pediatric B"), and infratentorial low-risk choroid plexus tumors in adults (CPP and aCPP, "adult") [69].

The treatment paradigm includes surgery for resection aiming for complete removal when feasible. For both CPP and aCPP when gross total resection is achieved, no more treatment is needed. For aCPP that had partial resection, there is a debate regarding the need for adjuvant therapy especially for those that are older than 3 years old. With CPC, chemotherapy as adjuvant therapy was found to be beneficial in several papers. There are different types of treatment protocols by either the Children's Oncology Group (CCG99703) that include high-dose chemotherapy and autologous hematopoietic stem cell rescue as a way to avoid radiation therapy at young age. Still, because of the rarity of this disease, more data is needed to better understand the best treatment methodology. For CPP, complete removal usually leads to very good prognosis (5-year overall survival of 90–100%), with very rare recurrence rate and extremely rare malignancy transformation (6% and <1%, respectively) [70]. For aCPP, the recurrence rate is very high especially in kids 3 years of age and older [71]. The main different between CPP and aCPP is the mitotic index. Yet, the value of the mitotic index as prognostic factor was found to be just for the patients that are older than 3 years old [72]. As mentioned, the prognosis for CPC is much less favorable with a 5-year survival of 56–64%, with many of the survivors suffering from long-term deficits [73]. In an attempt to better understand the behavior of CPC, a study done by Tabori and colleagues stratifying the patients by the existence of TP53 mutation found that patients with TP53 wild-type CPCs survived significantly better over 5 years than those that had TP53 mutation (>80% vs. 0%) [73]. One of the major problems in the treatment of CPC is the tendency (>20%) to have metastatic disease at time of diagnosis [74].

Review Questions

1. According to the latest WHO classification, which combination is correct?
   (a) Medulloblastoma—WNT, SHH, group 3, group 4, group 5
   (b) Ependymoma—RELA, posterior fossa group A, anaplastic
   (c) Pediatric HGG—diffuse midline glioma H3K27M altered, diffuse hemispheric glioma, H3G34 mutant
   (d) Pediatric LGG—IDH mutant, IDH wild type, PLTNY
2. A 2-year-old previously known to meet all his milestones is now being admitted for lethargy and repeated vomiting episodes. His MRI shows large intraventricular tumor located in the atrium of the lateral ventricle with associated hydrocephalus. The tumor is vividly enhanced on T1 with gadolinium, isointense on T1, and mildly hyperintense on T2. What is true about the possible diagnosis?
   (a) CPC is much more common in adults and then in the pediatric age group.
   (b) CPP is twice as common as CPC.
   (c) Classic treatment paradigm will be—biopsy and once established radiation therapy and chemotherapy.
   (d) If GTR was achieved for CPP at the age group of infancy, the overall survival is excellence.

3. A 15-year-old is being admitted for recent lethargy and headaches. He is rushed to the CT scan and a large suprasellar and third ventricle tumor with associated hydrocephalus. The tumor has several areas with calcifications. MRI shows a large tumor extending from the sellar region with mixed intensity on T2 and vivid enhancement on T1 with gadolinium. What is true about the possible diagnosis?
   (a) CSF diversion should be done instantly, and the overall survival from these tumors is poor. Hence, a biopsy, shunt, and chemotherapy should be started immediately.
   (b) There are two distinct types: adamantinomatous and papillary. The adamantinomatous is with high alteration of BRAF V600E mutation.
   (c) The current WHO classification defines three subtypes—adamantinomatous, papillary, and anaplastic.
   (d) The most common type in the pediatric age group is adamantinomatous which is defined with high alteration rate of CTNNB1.

Answer keys: (1) c, (2) d, (3) d

References

1. Kilburn LB, Packer RJ. JNO special issue: an update on pediatric neuro-oncology. J Neurooncol. 2020;150(1):1–4.
2. Louis DN, Perry A, Wesseling P, Brat DJ, Cree IA, Figarella-Branger D, et al. The 2021 WHO classification of tumors of the central nervous system: a summary. Neuro Oncol. 2021;23(8):1231–51.
3. La Madrid AM, Kieran MW. Epigenetics in clinical management of children and adolescents with brain tumors. Curr Cancer Drug Targets. 2018;18(1):57–64.
4. Jones DTW, Kieran MW, Bouffet E, Alexandrescu S, Bandopadhayay P, Bornhorst M, et al. Pediatric low-grade gliomas: next biologically driven steps. Neuro Oncol. 2018;20(2):160–73.
5. Biegel JA, Kalpana G, Knudsen ES, Packer RJ, Roberts CW, Thiele CJ, et al. The role of INI1 and the SWI/SNF complex in the development of rhabdoid tumors: meeting summary from the workshop on childhood atypical teratoid/rhabdoid tumors. Cancer Res. 2002;62(1):323–8.
6. Schwartzentruber J, Korshunov A, Liu XY, Jones DT, Pfaff E, Jacob K, et al. Driver mutations in histone H3.3 and chromatin remodelling genes in paediatric glioblastoma. Nature. 2012;482(7384):226–31.
7. Khuong-Quang DA, Buczkowicz P, Rakopoulos P, Liu XY, Fontebasso AM, Bouffet E, et al. K27M mutation in histone H3.3 defines clinically and biologically distinct subgroups of pediatric diffuse intrinsic pontine gliomas. Acta Neuropathol. 2012;124(3):439–47.
8. Grasso CS, Tang Y, Truffaux N, Berlow NE, Liu L, Debily MA, et al. Functionally defined therapeutic targets in diffuse intrinsic pontine glioma. Nat Med. 2015;21(6):555–9.
9. Jain SU, Do TJ, Lund PJ, Rashoff AQ, Diehl KL, Cieslik M, et al. PFA ependymoma-associated protein EZHIP inhibits PRC2 activity through a H3 K27M-like mechanism. Nat Commun. 2019;10(1):2146.
10. Taylor MD, Northcott PA, Korshunov A, Remke M, Cho YJ, Clifford SC, et al. Molecular subgroups of medulloblastoma: the current consensus. Acta Neuropathol. 2012;123(4):465–72.
11. Kool M, Korshunov A, Remke M, Jones DT, Schlanstein M, Northcott PA, et al. Molecular subgroups of medulloblastoma: an international meta-analysis of transcriptome, genetic aberrations, and clinical data of WNT, SHH, Group 3, and Group 4 medulloblastomas. Acta Neuropathol. 2012;123(4):473–84.
12. Duke ES, Packer RJ. Update on pediatric brain tumors: the molecular era and neuro-immunologic beginnings. Curr Neurol Neurosci Rep. 2020;20(8):30.
13. Cavalli FMG, Remke M, Rampasek L, Peacock J, Shih DJH, Luu B, et al. Intertumoral heterogeneity within medulloblastoma subgroups. Cancer Cell. 2017;31(6):737–54.e6.
14. Goschzik T, Schwalbe EC, Hicks D, Smith A, Zur Muehlen A, Figarella-Branger D, et al. Prognostic effect of whole chromosomal aberration signatures in standard-risk, non-WNT/non-SHH medulloblastoma: a retrospective, molecular analysis of the HIT-SIOP PNET 4 trial. Lancet Oncol. 2018;19(12):1602–16.
15. Thompson EM, Bramall A, Herndon JE 2nd, Taylor MD, Ramaswamy V. The clinical importance of medulloblastoma extent of resection: a systematic review. J Neurooncol. 2018;139(3):523–39.
16. Thompson EM, Hielscher T, Bouffet E, Remke M, Luu B, Gururangan S, et al. Prognostic value of medulloblastoma extent of resection after accounting for molecular subgroup: a retrospective integrated clinical and molecular analysis. Lancet Oncol. 2016;17(4):484–95.
17. Patel P, Wallace D, Boop FA, Vaughn B, Robinson GW, Gajjar A, et al. Reoperation for medulloblastoma prior to adjuvant therapy. Neurosurgery. 2019;84(5):1050–8.
18. Naung H, Cohen KJ. An intrathecal limited postoperative chemotherapy regimen for the treatment of young children with nodular/desmoplastic medulloblastoma and medulloblastoma with extensive nodularity. J Neurooncol. 2021;152(3):567–72.

19. Lafay-Cousin L, Smith A, Chi SN, Wells E, Madden J, Margol A, et al. Clinical, pathological, and molecular characterization of infant medulloblastomas treated with sequential high-dose chemotherapy. Pediatr Blood Cancer. 2016;63(9):1527–34.
20. Robinson GW, Orr BA, Wu G, Gururangan S, Lin T, Qaddoumi I, et al. Vismodegib exerts targeted efficacy against recurrent sonic hedgehog-subgroup medulloblastoma: results from phase II pediatric brain tumor consortium studies PBTC-025B and PBTC-032. J Clin Oncol. 2015;33(24):2646–54.
21. Ellison DW, Hawkins C, Jones DTW, Onar-Thomas A, Pfister SM, Reifenberger G, et al. cIMPACT-NOW update 4: diffuse gliomas characterized by MYB, MYBL1, or FGFR1 alterations or BRAF(V600E) mutation. Acta Neuropathol. 2019;137(4):683–7.
22. Johnson DR, Giannini C, Jenkins RB, Kim DK, Kaufmann TJ. Plenty of calcification: imaging characterization of polymorphous low-grade neuroepithelial tumor of the young. Neuroradiology. 2019;61(11):1327–32.
23. Qaddoumi I, Orisme W, Wen J, Santiago T, Gupta K, Dalton JD, et al. Genetic alterations in uncommon low-grade neuroepithelial tumors: BRAF, FGFR1, and MYB mutations occur at high frequency and align with morphology. Acta Neuropathol. 2016;131(6):833–45.
24. Fangusaro J, Onar-Thomas A, Young Poussaint T, Wu S, Ligon AH, Lindeman N, et al. Selumetinib in paediatric patients with BRAF-aberrant or neurofibromatosis type 1-associated recurrent, refractory, or progressive low-grade glioma: a multicentre, phase 2 trial. Lancet Oncol. 2019;20(7):1011–22.
25. Clarke M, Mackay A, Ismer B, Pickles JC, Tatevossian RG, Newman S, et al. Infant high-grade gliomas comprise multiple subgroups characterized by novel targetable gene fusions and favorable outcomes. Cancer Discov. 2020;10(7):942–63.
26. Guerreiro Stucklin AS, Ryall S, Fukuoka K, Zapotocky M, Lassaletta A, Li C, et al. Alterations in ALK/ROS1/NTRK/MET drive a group of infantile hemispheric gliomas. Nat Commun. 2019;10(1):4343.
27. Sposto R, Ertel IJ, Jenkin RD, Boesel CP, Venes JL, Ortega JA, et al. The effectiveness of chemotherapy for treatment of high grade astrocytoma in children: results of a randomized trial. A report from the Childrens Cancer Study Group. J Neurooncol. 1989;7(2):165–77.
28. Stupp R, Mason WP, van den Bent MJ, Weller M, Fisher B, Taphoorn MJ, et al. Radiotherapy plus concomitant and adjuvant temozolomide for glioblastoma. N Engl J Med. 2005;352(10):987–96.
29. Mackay A, Burford A, Carvalho D, Izquierdo E, Fazal-Salom J, Taylor KR, et al. Integrated molecular meta-analysis of 1,000 pediatric high-grade and diffuse intrinsic pontine glioma. Cancer Cell. 2017;32(4):520–37 e5.
30. Castel D, Philippe C, Calmon R, Le Dret L, Truffaux N, Boddaert N, et al. Histone H3F3A and HIST1H3B K27M mutations define two subgroups of diffuse intrinsic pontine gliomas with different prognosis and phenotypes. Acta Neuropathol. 2015;130(6):815–27.
31. Bjerke L, Mackay A, Nandhabalan M, Burford A, Jury A, Popov S, et al. Histone H3.3. mutations drive pediatric glioblastoma through upregulation of MYCN. Cancer Discov. 2013;3(5):512–9.
32. Chen CCL, Deshmukh S, Jessa S, Hadjadj D, Lisi V, Andrade AF, et al. Histone H3.3G34-mutant interneuron progenitors co-opt PDGFRA for gliomagenesis. Cell. 2020;183(6):1617–33.e22.
33. Chatwin HV, Cruz Cruz J, Green AL. Pediatric high-grade glioma: moving toward subtype-specific multimodal therapy. FEBS J. 2021;288(21):6127–41.
34. Paugh BS, Qu C, Jones C, Liu Z, Adamowicz-Brice M, Zhang J, et al. Integrated molecular genetic profiling of pediatric high-grade gliomas reveals key differences with the adult disease. J Clin Oncol. 2010;28(18):3061–8.
35. Korshunov A, Ryzhova M, Hovestadt V, Bender S, Sturm D, Capper D, et al. Integrated analysis of pediatric glioblastoma reveals a subset of biologically favorable tumors with associated molecular prognostic markers. Acta Neuropathol. 2015;129(5):669–78.
36. Wang Y, Wild AT, Turcan S, Wu WH, Sigel C, Klimstra DS, et al. Targeting therapeutic vulnerabilities with PARP inhibition and radiation in IDH-mutant gliomas and cholangiocarcinomas. Sci Adv. 2020;6(17):eaaz3221.
37. Korshunov A, Schrimpf D, Ryzhova M, Sturm D, Chavez L, Hovestadt V, et al. H3-/IDH-wild type pediatric glioblastoma is comprised of molecularly and prognostically distinct subtypes with associated oncogenic drivers. Acta Neuropathol. 2017;134(3):507–16.
38. Jenseit A, Camgoz A, Pfister SM, Kool M. EZHIP: a new piece of the puzzle towards understanding pediatric posterior fossa ependymoma. Acta Neuropathol. 2022;143(1):1–13.
39. Gatta G, Botta L, Rossi S, Aareleid T, Bielska-Lasota M, Clavel J, et al. Childhood cancer survival in Europe 1999-2007: results of EUROCARE-5—a population-based study. Lancet Oncol. 2014;15(1):35–47.
40. Ostrom QT, Gittleman H, Liao P, Rouse C, Chen Y, Dowling J, et al. CBTRUS statistical report: primary brain and central nervous system tumors diagnosed in the United States in 2007-2011. Neuro Oncol. 2014;16(Suppl 4):iv1–63.
41. Pajtler KW, Wen J, Sill M, Lin T, Orisme W, Tang B, et al. Molecular heterogeneity and CXorf67 alterations in posterior fossa group A (PFA) ependymomas. Acta Neuropathol. 2018;136(2):211–26.
42. Zheng T, Ghasemi DR, Okonechnikov K, Korshunov A, Sill M, Maass KK, et al. Cross-species genomics reveals oncogenic dependencies in ZFTA/C11orf95 fusion-positive supratentorial ependymomas. Cancer Discov. 2021;11(9):2230–47.
43. Cavalli FMG, Hubner JM, Sharma T, Luu B, Sill M, Zapotocky M, et al. Heterogeneity within the PF-EPN-B ependymoma subgroup. Acta Neuropathol. 2018;136(2):227–37.
44. Witt H, Mack SC, Ryzhova M, Bender S, Sill M, Isserlin R, et al. Delineation of two clinically and molecularly distinct subgroups of posterior fossa ependymoma. Cancer Cell. 2011;20(2):143–57.

45. Pajtler KW, Witt H, Sill M, Jones DT, Hovestadt V, Kratochwil F, et al. Molecular classification of ependymal tumors across all CNS compartments, histopathological grades, and age groups. Cancer Cell. 2015;27(5):728–43.
46. Rajeshwari M, Sharma MC, Kakkar A, Nambirajan A, Suri V, Sarkar C, et al. Evaluation of chromosome 1q gain in intracranial ependymomas. J Neurooncol. 2016;127(2):271–8.
47. Baroni LV, Sundaresan L, Heled A, Coltin H, Pajtler KW, Lin T, et al. Ultra high-risk PFA ependymoma is characterized by loss of chromosome 6q. Neuro Oncol. 2021;23(8):1360–70.
48. Thom M, Blumcke I, Aronica E. Long-term epilepsy-associated tumors. Brain Pathol. 2012;22(3):350–79.
49. Rivera B, Gayden T, Carrot-Zhang J, Nadaf J, Boshari T, Faury D, et al. Germline and somatic FGFR1 abnormalities in dysembryoplastic neuroepithelial tumors. Acta Neuropathol. 2016;131(6):847–63.
50. Deng MY, Sill M, Chiang J, Schittenhelm J, Ebinger M, Schuhmann MU, et al. Molecularly defined diffuse leptomeningeal glioneuronal tumor (DLGNT) comprises two subgroups with distinct clinical and genetic features. Acta Neuropathol. 2018;136(2):239–53.
51. Mamdouhi T, Vagrecha A, Johnson AA, Levy CF, Atlas M, Krystal JI. Successful use of crushed formulation of dabrafenib and trametinib in a pediatric glioneural tumor. Pediatr Blood Cancer. 2021;68(10):e29187.
52. Fouda MA, Karsten M, Staffa SJ, Scott RM, Marcus KJ, Baird LC. Management strategies for recurrent pediatric craniopharyngioma: new recommendations. J Neurosurg Pediatr. 2021;27(5):548–55.
53. Muller HL, Merchant TE, Warmuth-Metz M, Martinez-Barbera JP, Puget S. Craniopharyngioma. Nat Rev Dis Primers. 2019;5(1):75.
54. Holsken A, Sill M, Merkle J, Schweizer L, Buchfelder M, Flitsch J, et al. Adamantinomatous and papillary craniopharyngiomas are characterized by distinct epigenomic as well as mutational and transcriptomic profiles. Acta Neuropathol Commun. 2016;4:20.
55. Ali ZS, Lang SS, Kamat AR, Adappa ND, Palmer JN, Storm PB, et al. Suprasellar pediatric craniopharyngioma resection via endonasal endoscopic approach. Childs Nerv Syst. 2013;29(11):2065–70.
56. Fouda MA, Riordan CP, Zurakowski D, Goumnerova LC. Analysis of 2141 pediatric craniopharyngioma admissions in the USA utilizing the Kids' Inpatient Database (KID): predictors of discharge disposition. Childs Nerv Syst. 2020;36(12):3007–12.
57. Gonc EN, Yordam N, Ozon A, Alikasifoglu A, Kandemir N. Endocrinological outcome of different treatment options in children with craniopharyngioma: a retrospective analysis of 66 cases. Pediatr Neurosurg. 2004;40(3):112–9.
58. Caldarelli M, Massimi L, Tamburrini G, Cappa M, Di Rocco C. Long-term results of the surgical treatment of craniopharyngioma: the experience at the Policlinico Gemelli, Catholic University, Rome. Childs Nerv Syst. 2005;21(8–9):747–57.
59. Cohen M, Guger S, Hamilton J. Long term sequelae of pediatric craniopharyngioma—literature review and 20 years of experience. Front Endocrinol (Lausanne). 2011;2:81.
60. Cohen M, Bartels U, Branson H, Kulkarni AV, Hamilton J. Trends in treatment and outcomes of pediatric craniopharyngioma, 1975-2011. Neuro Oncol. 2013;15(6):767–74.
61. Kiehna EN, Merchant TE. Radiation therapy for pediatric craniopharyngioma. Neurosurg Focus. 2010;28(4):E10.
62. Jimenez RB, Ahmed S, Johnson A, Thomas H, Depauw N, Horick N, et al. Proton radiation therapy for pediatric craniopharyngioma. Int J Radiat Oncol Biol Phys. 2021;110(5):1480–7.
63. Malkin D. Li-fraumeni syndrome. Genes Cancer. 2011;2(4):475–84.
64. Rickert CH, Paulus W. Tumors of the choroid plexus. Microsc Res Tech. 2001;52(1):104–11.
65. Thomas C, Metrock K, Kordes U, Hasselblatt M, Dhall G. Epigenetics impacts upon prognosis and clinical management of choroid plexus tumors. J Neurooncol. 2020;148(1):39–45.
66. Nagib MG, O'Fallon MT. Lateral ventricle choroid plexus papilloma in childhood: management and complications. Surg Neurol. 2000;54(5):366–72.
67. Thomas C, Soschinski P, Zwaig M, Oikonomopoulos S, Okonechnikov K, Pajtler KW, et al. The genetic landscape of choroid plexus tumors in children and adults. Neuro Oncol. 2021;23(4):650–60.
68. Rickert CH, Wiestler OD, Paulus W. Chromosomal imbalances in choroid plexus tumors. Am J Pathol. 2002;160(3):1105–13.
69. Ruland V, Hartung S, Kordes U, Wolff JE, Paulus W, Hasselblatt M. Choroid plexus carcinomas are characterized by complex chromosomal alterations related to patient age and prognosis. Genes Chromosomes Cancer. 2014;53(5):373–80.
70. Jeibmann A, Wrede B, Peters O, Wolff JE, Paulus W, Hasselblatt M. Malignant progression in choroid plexus papillomas. J Neurosurg. 2007;107(3 Suppl):199–202.
71. Siegfried A, Morin S, Munzer C, Delisle MB, Gambart M, Puget S, et al. A French retrospective study on clinical outcome in 102 choroid plexus tumors in children. J Neurooncol. 2017;135(1):151–60.
72. Thomas C, Ruland V, Kordes U, Hartung S, Capper D, Pietsch T, et al. Pediatric atypical choroid plexus papilloma reconsidered: increased mitotic activity is prognostic only in older children. Acta Neuropathol. 2015;129(6):925–7.
73. Tabori U, Shlien A, Baskin B, Levitt S, Ray P, Alon N, et al. TP53 alterations determine clinical subgroups and survival of patients with choroid plexus tumors. J Clin Oncol. 2010;28(12):1995–2001.
74. Wrede B, Hasselblatt M, Peters O, Thall PF, Kutluk T, Moghrabi A, et al. Atypical choroid plexus papilloma: clinical experience in the CPT-SIOP-2000 study. J Neurooncol. 2009;95(3):383–92.

Pediatric Spine, Spinal Cord, and Peripheral Nervous System Tumors

9

Nir Shimony and George Jallo

Introduction

Intradural spinal tumors are rare entities in the pediatric population, which typically have been diagnosed after many months of symptoms. Pediatric spinal tumors can be classified in different ways based on the anatomic location in relation to the dura (extra- or intradural). Spinal tumors that are extradural can include sarcoma, lymphoma, metastasis, osteoblastoma, and more. In this chapter we will focus on the management and care of pediatric spinal intradural tumors. The intradural tumors are further subclassified as intradural-extramedullary lesions or intramedullary lesions. The former usually will manifest neurological deficit because of either cord compression or nerve involvement/compression, whereas the latter will ensue neurological deficit because of direct involvement of the spinal cord, since these lesions arise from cells within the spinal cord itself, which can lead to progressive neurological decline due to their expansile and infiltrative destructive nature.

Overall, in the adult population, the prominent tumor type that affects the spine is metastatic disease that usually affects the extradural compartment usually with significant bony involvement. In this age group, it is less likely to find intramedullary tumors affecting the cord itself. The opposite is true for the pediatric age group, and hence it is more common for a child with a newly diagnosed spinal tumor to have a true spinal cord tumor than extradural tumor. In the recent report by the CBTRUS discussing CNS and PNS tumors among age group of 0–19 years of age, it was found that tumors of the spinal cord and cauda equina accounted for 5.1% of all brain and other CNS tumors [1].

The focus of this chapter will be to give the reader updates and highlights for the manage-

N. Shimony (✉)
Department of Neurosurgery, University of Tennessee - Health Science Center, Memphis, TN, USA

Department of Surgery, St. Jude Children's Research Hospital, Memphis, TN, USA

Le Bonheur Neuroscience Institute, Le Bonheur Children's Hospital, Memphis, TN, USA

Department of Neurosurgery, The Johns Hopkins University - School of Medicine, Baltimore, MD, USA

Semmes-Murphey Clinic, Memphis, TN, USA
e-mail: nshimony@semmes-murphey.com; nshimony@uthsc.edu

G. Jallo
Department of Neurosurgery, University of Tennessee Health Science Center, Memphis, TN, USA

David Goldenberg Family Endowed Chair, Institute for Brain Protection Sciences, Johns Hopkins All Children's Hospital, St. Petersburg, FL, USA
e-mail: gjallo1@jhu.edu

N. Shimony, G. Jallo (eds.), *Pediatric Neurosurgery Board Review*,
https://doi.org/10.1007/978-3-031-23687-7_9

ment of pediatric spinal intradural tumors including pearls for surgical principles associated with resection of intradural spinal lesions.

Intramedullary Spinal Cord Tumors

Epidemiology

Intramedullary spinal cord tumors (IMSCTs) are quite rare in children. Spinal cord and cauda equina tumors responsible for 5.1% of all CNS tumors in the pediatric age group [1]. The distinction between spinal cord tumors and intramedullary spinal cord tumors is not clear in many previous publications. According to current data, intramedullary spinal cord tumors account for 5–10% of all central nervous system (CNS) lesions [1]. The most frequently encountered IMSCTs are gliomas, predominantly astrocytomas, and ependymomas. The predominant histology among the pediatric age group is of astrocytic tumors of the spinal cord, whereas ependymomas are relatively more common in the adult population. In a recent publication by CBTRUS evaluating the epidemiology and distribution of CNS tumors, there was almost no difference between astrocytomas (19.7%) and ependymal tumors (19.6%) among the pediatric age group of 0–19 years of age in the USA. When separating pilocytic astrocytomas from the rest of the astrocytomas, ependymal tumors are the most prominent histology for all age groups followed by meningeal tumors for the pediatric age group, while in adults the meningeal tumors and nerve sheath tumors are the most prominent histology followed by ependymal tumors [1]. Contrary to the pediatric population, in the adult population, it is relatively rare to find an astrocytic spinal cord tumor. The prevalence of different spinal cord tumors changes over the different age groups, where among infancy to age 10 years old most of the IMSCT will be astrocytomas, with higher rate of malignant and aggressive tumors among infants and toddlers [1, 2]. This trend shifts toward almost equal predominance with ependymomas among adolescent years, with ependymomas becoming the more dominant IMSCT among adults [3]. Other IMSCTs include gangliogliomas, lipomas, subependymomas, hemangioblastomas, dermoids, teratomas, and in extremely rare cases intramedullary metastases. There is no apparent gender predilection for such lesions, while some describe slight male predominance [4, 5].

Risk Factors

Different conditions are known to have higher propensity for the development of spinal cord tumors. Conditions such as neurofibromatosis are well related to the development of spinal tumors. In the spinal cord, NF1 is known to have predilection for the development of spinal cord astrocytomas and the development of neurofibromas or plexiform neurofibromas that are not usually intradural tumors but can involve the spinal column and the nerve roots. On the other hand, NF2 is known to be related to the development spinal schwannomas, meningiomas, as well as spinal cord ependymomas. The NF2 gene is well known to be related to the development of spinal cord ependymomas and in many of the cases will be found in sporadic non-syndromic spinal cord ependymomas [6].

von Hippel-Lindau (VHL) disease can also be related to spinal cord tumors, with isolated or multiple spinal hemangioblastomas, but on rare occasion, there exists some astrocytomas. Hence, it is recommended that an annual screening of brain and spinal MRI be done for all VHL patients. Other inherited syndromes like Li-Fraumeni have been described to be related to spinal cord tumors, as well as anecdotal cases that were described in other syndromes such as Turcot's syndrome [7].

Clinical Presentation

Pediatric patients with IMSCTs are diagnosed in a late fashion in many cases accounting for the indolent course in the majority of these tumors. The reported average duration of symptoms until diagnosis of spinal cord tumors is between 2 and 37 months [4, 8, 9]. The median time according to most publications is around 10 months. Typically, IMSCTs exhibit indolent growth, unless a higher-grade histology is present and then the presentation is relatively acute. Pediatric patients, especially at a young age, are known to have a good compensatory system allowing them to withstand progressing pain and even deficits for a long period of time before symptoms are reviled. Pain is the most frequent presenting symptom, often with axial back or neck pain and occasionally radicular pain due to nerve root impingement. Nocturnal pain can also be present, and its presence is an alarming sign at all age groups. The presenting signs and symptoms differ over different age groups. In toddlers and infants, it was shown that a head tilt or even a true newly diagnosed torticollis, delayed or regress of motor milestones, and early handedness can be hazardous signs for potential spinal-related pathology [4]. Hence, for a growing kid experiencing excessive clumsiness or repeated falls or having progressive spinal deformity, a thorough investigation for possible spinal cord pathology needs to be taken [10]. Even unexplainable abdominal pain or newly diagnosed hydrocephalus of unclear etiology can be the result of an IMSCT in the pediatric population [8, 11].

Investigation

The main diagnostic assessment if there is a clinical concern for possible spinal-related pathology is magnetic resonance imaging (MRI) of the relevant spinal anatomic location (cervical, thoracic, or lumbar) with consideration to include the full spinal column when there are no specific localizing sings and especially if the pediatric patient requires general anesthesia. In the pediatric population, IMSCTs most commonly arise in the cervical and thoracic spine, mainly because of the relative predominance of astrocytomas that in 50–60% of the cases will originate in the cervical cord or the cervico-thoracic junction. Ependymomas will usually be found in the cervical cord and the lumbar spine usually as myxopapillary ependymomas. Beside the anatomical location, the MRI can provide "clues" regarding possible diagnosis, yet the actual diagnosis still relied on tissue diagnosis. Table 9.1 summarizes the most common parameters for pediatric IMSCTs. Figure 9.1 demonstrates a simplified way to see the anatomical distribution of the different types of the more common pediatric spinal tumors.

In recent years there is a growing interest in the use of advanced imaging in order to better define spinal cord tumors. The use of techniques that are widely used for brain imaging recently was described in few publications for spinal cord pathologies including the use of MR diffusion tensor imaging (DTI), MR perfusion-weighted imaging (PWI), and sequences like apparent diffusion coefficient (ADC), fractional anisotropy (FA), axial diffusivity (AD), and radial diffusivity (RD). Tractography of the spinal cord can show, for example, that spinal cord astrocytoma will usually encase the spinal cord fibers, whereas ependymoma will displace them [12].

Learn to Know the "Tumor Fingerprint"

In recent years there is a significant progress in the way we understand spinal cord tumors, especially in regard to the genetic and molecular biology of spinal cord glial tumors. The current diagnosis and grading are more than ever relaying on specific genetic mutation rather than only the morphologic features of the tumor. Yet, this progress is, as mentioned, mainly for glial tumors (e.g., ependymomas, astrocytomas). For the rare tumors involving the pediatric spinal cord, such as epidermoid cysts, lipomas, or even lymphoma, the diagnosis in many cases is still mainly histological. Table 9.2 summarizes the main molecular and genetic parameters known for pediatric intramedullary tumors.

Astrocytoma

The knowledge regarding spinal cord astrocytomas still lags behind as compared to the brain

Table 9.1 Most common parameters for pediatric IMSCTs

Tumor	Anatomical location	Intramedullary distribution	T1 appearance	T2 appearance	Contrast enhancement	Unique imaging features
Astrocytoma (Fig. 9.2)	Cervical and thoracic cord	Eccentric, sometimes with exophytic portion	Isointense, *hypo*intense	Isointense, *hyper*intense	Heterogeneous enhancement, usually not with clear borders (up to 30% will not have enhancement)	Intralesional or tumor perimeter cysts can be found. Syrinx can be found Peritumoral edema common in 40–50% of the cases Hemorrhage is not common
Ependymoma [13, 14] (Fig. 9.2)	Cervical and thoracic cord	Centrally located	Isointense, *hypo*intense	Usually *hyper*intense	Symmetrical enhancement with sharp borders	"Cap sign"[a] in 20% of the cases Associated cysts in 50% of the cases[b]
Hemangioblastoma [15, 16]	Thoracic and then cervical cord	Eccentric usually partially exophytic on the dorsal aspect of the cord (up to 25% of the cases will be purely intramedullary)	Hypo- and isointense most common (75%)	Iso- to *hypo*intense (tumor nodule)	Both patterns of homogenous and patchy enhancement can be found. The nodule usually will enhance vividly	"Cap sign"[a] possible Cysts (very common) can be seen usually same density and intensity as the CSF Syrinx is very common In the majority of the cases, there is a solitary nodule; otherwise there is a significant concern for vHL disease
Ganglioglioma [14]	Cervico-thoracic	Eccentric	Mixed signal intensity	*Hyper*intense	Heterogeneous patchy enhancement, up to 15% will not have enhancement	The tumors tend to involve very long segments with sometimes greater than eight vertebral body segments. SWI or GRE might show calcifications, and 40–50% will have tumoral cysts
Rare tumors						
AT/RT [17, 18]	Cervical and then thoracolumbar	Varied, leptomeningeal spread is common	Mixed signal, iso-density/ slightly high signal	Mixed signals, slightly higher/ iso-density signals	Vary, some will have striking enhancement and others almost none Meningeal and nerve root enhancement are a common finding; CSF involvement is common as well	Almost all the cases will have some degree of intratumoral and peritumoral hemorrhage Cauda equina syndrome presentation is quite characteristic when there is lumbar or sacral involvement

Lipoma (not related to spinal dysraphism)[c]	Cervical cord and filum terminale	Dorsal cord exophytic or even dural based on cord involvement or significant compression	*Hyper*intense	*Hypo*intense	No enhancement	Fat suppression sequence will show significant hypointensity
Paraganglioma	Filum terminale and cauda equina	Encapsulated usually attached to the filum terminale	Hypo- to *iso*intense	Iso- to *hyper*intense	Relative homogeneous and vividly enhanced	Hemosiderin cap can be seen "Salt and pepper" appearance on T2, due to the hypervascularity and the flow void that can be seen as a result
Neuroenteric cysts	Usually thoracic and then cervical cord	The cyst is usually ventral to the cord or involves the ventral portion of it as eccentric lesion (can be misdiagnosed as astrocytoma)	*Hypo*intense (can be variable depending on the protein content)	*Hyper*intense (can be variable depending on the protein content)	Non-enhancing (rare reports of the cyst wall that is enhancing)	Usually intradural extramedullary, less than 5–10% of these tumors will be with true intramedullary involvement
Dermoid/epidermoid cysts	Thoracic cord and cauda equina	Well-defined lesion, usually without any edema For intramedullary dermoids intensity is variable because of possible fat contents and possible associated infection that can lead to enhancement, perilesional edema, and heterogeneous intensity on T1 and T2	Looks like CSF—*hypo*intense	Looks like CSF—*hyper*intense	No enhancement or very thin one along the cyst wall	Classic bright on DWI and dark (low intensity) on ADC map Classically will be associated with dermal sinus
Subependymomas [19]	Usually cervical and then thoracic cord	Eccentric subpial growth	*Iso*intense	*Hyper*intense	Variable	"Bamboo leaf sign"[d] may be present Syrinx can be found

[a] "Cap sign," hemosiderin deposition that looks dark (extreme hypointense signal) on T2-weighted imaging)

[b] Different types of cysts can be seen. Intratumoral cysts can be a combination of necrotic tumor cells and old hemorrhagic products, hence important to address in treatment. Peritumoral cysts (rostral or caudal) usually will not enhance as vividly as the tumor itself and will have xanthochromic fluid or even more recent hemorrhagic content but does not contain tumor cells [20, 21]

[c] Lipomas that are related to spinal dysraphism, such as lipomeningocele, are considered by many to be hamartomas rather than true spinal cord lipomas. Lumbo-sacral is the classic location for lipomas related to spinal dysraphism

[d] "Bamboo leaf sign," steep expansion of the affected cord as a result of the subpial growth

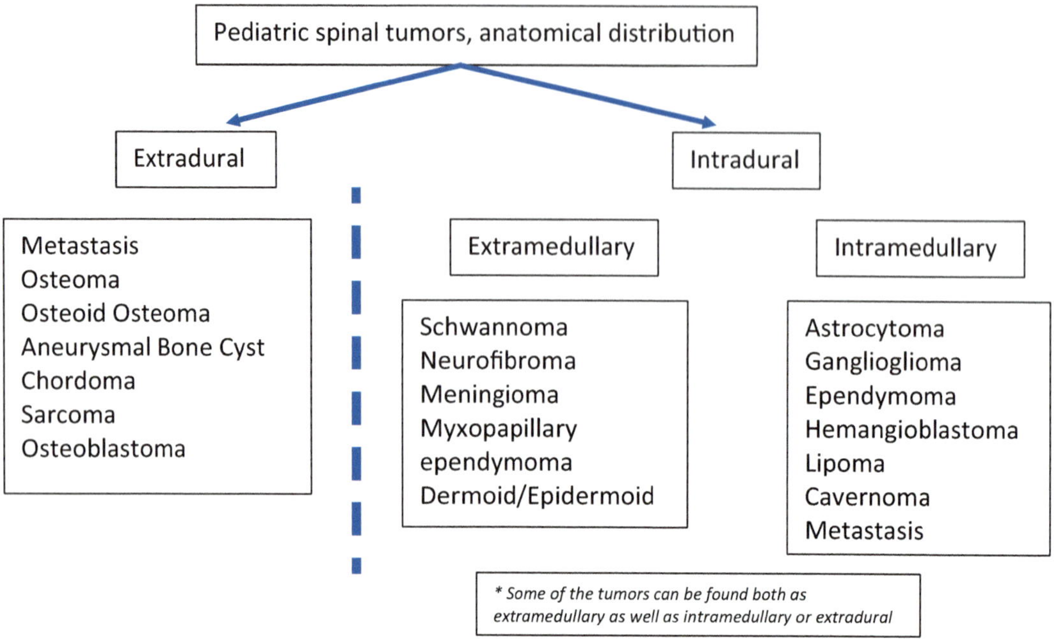

Fig. 9.1 Simplified view on the anatomical distribution of different pediatric spinal tumors. Some tumors (e.g., metastases) can be found in different compartments and not solely by the anatomical category that is described in the figure

astrocytic tumors. The involvement of one of the major mutations for intracranial astrocytomas, IDH1/2, is still not completely clear in regard to spinal cord astrocytomas. In several case series of spinal cord astrocytomas, IDH mutations were not found, which raise the question of spinal cord astrocytomas being a separate entity than the same histology lesions that are found in the brain [25]. Previous studies showed that supratentorial pilocytic astrocytomas are more likely to harbor the BRAF V600E mutation than same histology lesions that can be found in the posterior fossa or the spinal cord. As it appears that BRAF-KIAA1549 translocation is much more common in spinal cord tumors than the BRAF V600E, this understanding might help us better tailor future targeted treatment for these patients [26]. The H3F3A K27M is found mainly in high-grade spinal cord tumor histology astrocytomas, in which BRAF is almost never found and hence serves as another possible way to delineate this subgroup.

Ependymoma

In recent years there is a growing body of data and knowledge regarding the different subtypes of ependymomas. This has led to further classification of ependymomas into nine molecular subgroups according to age, CNS location, and biology, with important implications for prognostic stratification [27]. It is well established that the ST-EP can be mainly divided for expression of Yap or RELA mutations and that most of the ST-EP exhibits C11orf95-RELA fusion. For IT-EP it is now well established to designate them into group A and group B, with much more favorable outcome for group B. IT-EP-A tumors feature a generally balanced genome, with occasional gain of 1q, while IT-EP-B tumors typically display numerous chromosomal aberrations [28]. It was found in recent studies that the number of somatic mutation did not vary much across the different subtypes of spinal ependymomas and that these somatic mutations were different

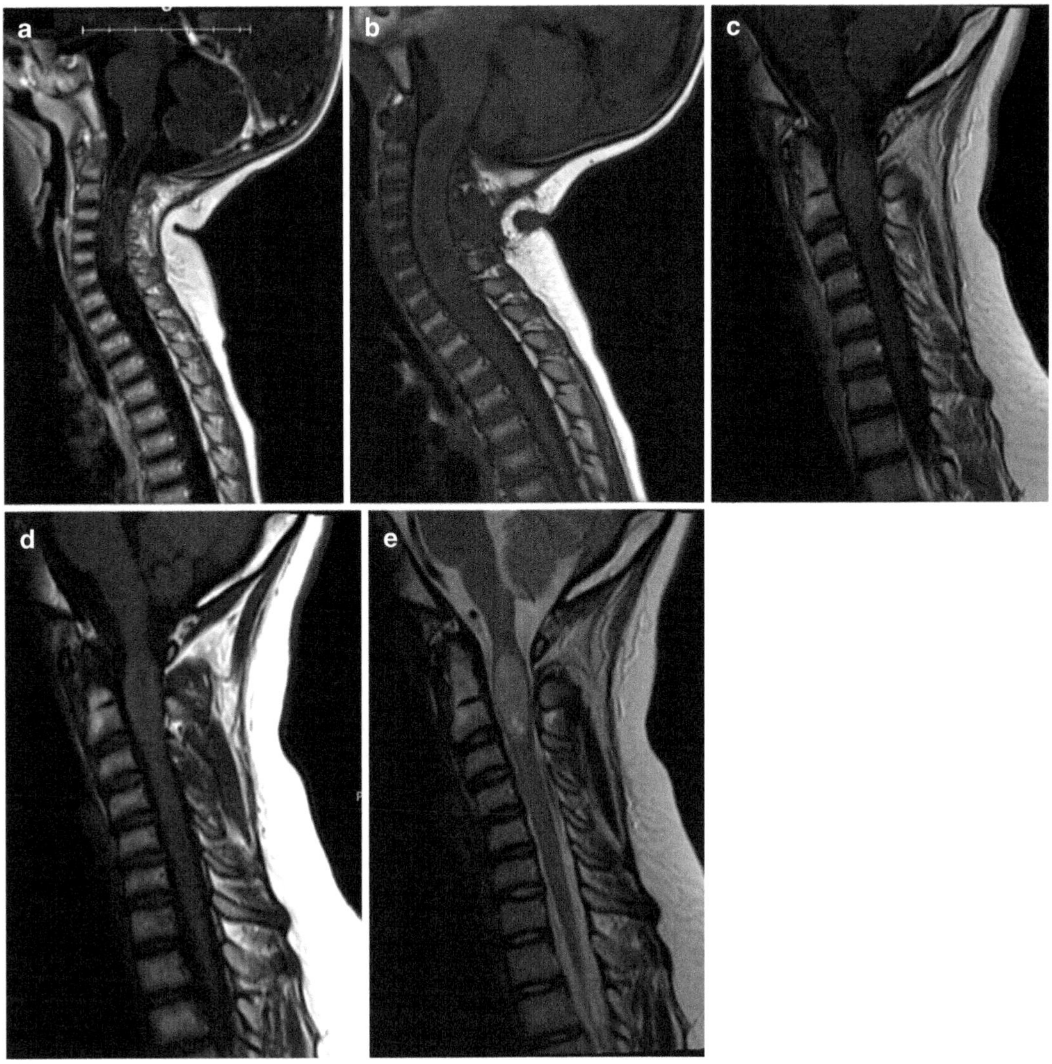

Fig. 9.2 Imaging example of the most common intramedullary tumors. (**a**, **b**) Cervical intramedullary pilocytic astrocytoma. T1-weighted post-contrast (**a**) and T1-weighted without gadolinium (**b**) sagittal magnetic resonance (MR) images demonstrating a well-defined heterogenic enhancing intramedullary spinal cord tumor with surrounding spinal cord edema. (**c**, **d**, **e**) Cervical intramedullary ependymoma. T1-weighted post-contrast (**c**), T1-weighted without gadolinium (**d**), and T2-weighted sagittal magnetic resonance (MR) images demonstrating a well-defined relatively homogenous enhancing intramed ullary spinal cord tumor with surrounding spinal cord edema

from those that were found for the intracranial ependymomas. The current knowledge regarding spinal cord ependymomas' molecular, biological, and genetic parameters is still lacking when compared to the intracranial ependymomas. In summary, it is known that SC-EP with MYCN amplification most likely should be distinct as a separate type of SC-EP with poor prognosis [29]. Spinal cord myxopapillary ependymomas and the very rare subependymomas should be still identified using morphological testing since so far there is not enough data to distinct them by molecular parameters. Spinal cord myxopapillary ependymomas should also be defined as WHO II, because clinical trial datasets do not support a WHO I clinical behavior [29].

Table 9.2 Most common molecular and genetic parameters for pediatric IMSCTs

Tumor type	WHO grade, histological subtype	Molecular and genetics features	Special considerations
Astrocytomas	*I—pilocytic* *II—diffuse, pilomyxoid* *III—anaplastic* *IV—glioblastoma*	*IDH1* *BRAF v600e* *BRAF-KIAA1549* *H3F3A K27M mutation* *CDKN2A*	• *IDH1 much more common in brain astrocytomas* • *BRAF-KIAA1549 translocation, BRAF copy number gain, but not BRAF V600E mutation* • *H3K27M is associated with midline brain gliomas and predicts bad outcome regardless of histological grade* • *CDKN2A more common in spinal cord and usually predict poor prognosis in case of homozygous deletion*
Ependymomas	*I—subependymoma* *II—myxopapillary ependymoma*[a] *III—Anaplastic*	*NF2,* *MYCN* *(several genetic mutations and molecular features are being discussed, but data is not strong enough for further distinct the different tumor by it)*	• *Partial or complete loss of chromosome 6 most common for subependymomas* • *NEFL gene more common for myxopapillary than brain ependymomas* • *Mutations in NF2 (22q) are specific for spinal ependymomas (loss to low expression of NF2)* • *There is a growing consensus for a novel molecular subgroup of spinal ependymoma designated as SP-EPN-MYCN with histological features of ependymoma and a characteristic MYCN amplification* [22]
Gangliogliomas	*I—ganglioglioma* *III—anaplastic*	*BRAF V600E, KIAA1549-BRAF fusion, H3K27M (will be found in some of the anaplastic cases)*	• *BRAF V600E mutation can be found in 15–60% of cranial GGs but only rarely in spinal cord GGs* • *The anaplastic features usually are detectable in the glial component* • *For anaplastic tumors there are features that resemble high-grade glioma like TP53 mutations, CDKN2A deletions, H3K27M, and BRAF V600E mutations*
Hemangioblastomas	*I*	*HIF-α, VEGF*	• *Usually in adults* • *Of the patients that are having VHL disease and hemangioblastoma, in 20% the tumor will be in the spinal cord (the rest is in the posterior fossa)* • *VHL disease has an autosomal dominant inheritance (90% penetrance) and is caused by a mutation or loss of the tumor suppressor gene at 3p25–26* [23]
ATRT [24]	*IV*	*SMARCB1, loss of INI-1 nuclear expression, alteration of BRG1, cytogenetic abnormality in chromosome 22*	• *Currently being delineated to three groups lately described as SHH, TYR, and MYC*

[a] *The distinction of myxopapillary as WHO II is not yet part of WHO official classification but rather a growing consensus among world's experts*

ATRT

Atypical teratoid/rhabdoid tumors are highly malignant and aggressive tumors of the CNS, regardless of their anatomical location. They have a peak incidence in children younger than 2 years of age and are the most common CNS tumor in this age subgroup [30]. As only anecdotal data exists and the relatively low survival rate, there is not enough to discuss the spinal entity. Recent studies have shown promising results for diagnosis and possible more targeted treatment. DNA methylation and gene expression profiles help distinguish three distinct epigenetic subgroups of ATRT (ATRT-MYC, ATRT-SHH, and ATRT-TYR). Currently, there is no conclusive literature to further differentiate spinal cord ATRT from intracranial ATRT [31].

Hemangioblastoma

Currently, the diagnosis of intracranial and spinal cord hemangioblastomas is similar. There is no data to suggest different subgroups like what is seen with ependymomas and possibly astrocytomas. The VHL gene mutation leads to loss of inhibition of HIF-α, which then leads to elevated levels of this protein as well as VEGF, with the consequence of pathological blood vessel proliferation [25].

Management Paradigm for IMSCT

The first question that needs to be answered in the case of a newly diagnosed pediatric IMSCT—to treat or not to treat. In some cases of clinically silent, incidentally found lesions, serial monitoring, and watchful waiting may be appropriate. Yet, most of the pediatric IMSCT will eventually grow and will need treatment. Hence, if the decision is made for follow-up, a strict plan needs to be established, and the family needs to be educated regarding the hazardous signs of progression. Although significant progress in the field of neuro-oncology has been made, not much has changed regarding spinal cord tumors. Today, for most pediatric spinal cord tumors, excluding high-grade invasive tumors, despite our better understanding of the molecular subtyping, the best results are still achieved when maximal safe resection is the mainstay of treatment. The goals of surgery are to obtain a diagnosis and to decompress the spinal cord by performing a safe maximal tumor cytoreduction. For certain tumors, malignant tumors, the extent of resection remains controversial. The use of adjuvant therapy is not well supported in the literature for spinal cord tumors when compared to brain-related tumors; hence individual discussion is mandatory following surgery.

Extent of Resection for Pediatric IMSCT

Gross total resection (GTR) or near total resection (NTR) can be achieved in a significant fraction of IMSCTs (since a large portion of the IMSCTs are ependymomas and low-grade astrocytomas). Spinal ependymomas typically demonstrate clear surrounding cleavage planes that facilitate tumor extirpation in their entirety. On the other hand, low-grade astrocytomas given their infiltrative nature make total removal more difficult as the margins are often blurred with normal neural structures. Yet, several groups have reported their experience with surgical resection of low-grade IMSCTs [20, 32–34]. The use of intraoperative monitoring is helpful in aiding the surgeon to perform a maximal safe resection, especially the utilization of D-wave monitoring when it is feasible (use of D-wave for lesions close to the conus is usually not feasible). The careful evaluation of the radiographic features of the tumor, the intraoperative results of the frozen section, as well as the microscopic evaluation of the tumor can assist with the decision-making regarding the extent of resection. High-grade tumors with infiltrative nature without clear delineation from the spinal cord make a gross total resection difficult. As a near total resection will not change the course of the disease, a biopsy or even partial debulking (if there is a component of mass effect on the healthy cord) is a better surgical choice. In certain cases where the tumor is amenable for significant resection in a safe fashion, the surgeon is encouraged to try and achieve a maximal safe resection [35]. For spinal cord ependymomas (especially grade II and myxopapillary), it has been shown that, like the intracranial ependymomas, the best prognostic results are achieved with radical resection, sometimes with more than one surgery (second-look surgery) [36]. Since the current adjuvant treatment for IMSCT does not show a significant benefit in many cases, our recommendation is to peruse maximal safe resection in any case if feasible, unless the preoperative imaging suggests highly infiltrative and aggressive high-grade tumor not amenable for safe resection [37]. Special consideration needs to be given for the need for spinal instrumentation and fusion in cases when regular laminoplasty does not seem to be suffice.

Treatment Paradigm

There has been no real breakthrough regarding the treatment of pediatric spinal cord tumors, and no significant benefit with adjuvant chemotherapy and radiation therapy in this subgroup of tumors, as the main treatment tool for most pediatric spinal cord tumors is surgical resection. For tumors that are completely incidental without clinical signs and without significant radiographic ramifications (e.g., extensive syringomyelia), watchful waiting with strict follow-up can be initiated. This last statement is especially important in cases of multisite spinal cord tumor secondary for genetic predisposition (e.g., neurofibromatosis). Recent SEER database review for pediatric spinal cord astrocytomas advocate again for maximal safe resection for this subset of tumors [38]. Yet, since it is almost impossible to achieve in a safe manner GTR for diffuse astrocytomas and especially those with high-grade features or proven diagnosis of high-grade astrocytomas, it is strongly advocated to consider tumor debulking only/biopsy for high-grade spinal cord astrocytomas, but consideration for maximal safe resection needs to be taken by a case-by-case manner because of the potential benefit of cytoreduction for these tumors. Currently, the use of adjuvant chemotherapy is still controversial in the treatment of spinal cord astrocytomas, although different agents such as temozolomide, cisplatin, carboplatin, bevacizumab, and irinotecan have been used with some benefits [39, 40]. For pediatric spinal cord low-grade astrocytomas, patients who received adjuvant radiation therapy and chemotherapy after subtotal resection had longer survival times when compared with those that had only subtotal resection but worse than those GTR [41]. Hence, some centers advocate for either second-look surgery or watchful waiting for cases of low-grade spinal cord astrocytomas with near total or partial resection, where others will start treatment. In recent years there is a trend of gradually abandoning the use of chemotherapy for pediatric spinal cord astrocytomas, with advocating for more aggressive resection when feasible with the use of adjuvant radiation therapy as needed [38]. For the future the better understanding we currently have in regard to the specific molecular and genetic features of pediatric spinal cord astrocytomas hopefully will allow the use of targeted therapy in order to better control those cases where GTR is not amenable.

For ependymomas, the main treatment tool is surgery as well with possible second look for remnant tumor or recurrent tumor. When GTR cannot be achieved, the use of chemotherapy, radiotherapy, or the combination of the two is reasonable and was shown to have some benefits. There is still a great controversy for the use of radiation therapy for spinal cord ependymomas, as well as for the use of classic chemotherapy. Several agents are currently under investigation for possible efficacy for spinal cord ependymoma such as mTOR inhibitors, imatinib, and bevacizumab. Bevacizumab has also been shown to be effective in decreasing the size of cystic spinal cord ependymomas especially in NF2 patients. Hence, it is currently investigated for the use as adjuvant therapy in the treatment of spinal cord ependymomas regardless of NF2 syndrome [42, 43].

For spinal cord hemangioblastomas, surgery is the main tool as well, with GTR as the goal which in many cases is achievable. The use of radiation therapy, especially SRS, was described but had rarely been used, unless resection is not feasible, and the diagnosis is already known. As for adjuvant chemotherapy, the main agent that showed promising results is bevacizumab, but the data is still too anecdotal [44, 45]. Other agents are currently under investigation, but the rarity of this lesion and the relatively high likelihood of achieving GTR make any study like this hard to complete (e.g., thalidomide, pazopanib).

Figure 9.3 summarizes the decision-making flow chart for the newly diagnosed spinal intradural tumor in a pediatric patient.

Surgical Pearls for Intramedullary Tumors

There are different techniques for achieving maximal safe resection for spinal cord tumors. We summarize here some of our recommendation for resection of spinal cord tumors, which we follow for maximal resection as well as for restricted biopsy:

- The use of neuromonitoring is crucial for achieving this goal. We believe that the use of D-wave alongside the traditional MEPs and SSEPs can maximize the resection. In contrast to MEP/SSEP, the D-wave measurement is not influenced by blood pressure, heart rate, temperature, and anesthetics. Whenever there is a decrease of 50% or more in the D-waves in comparison to baseline, this is a warning sign to stop the specific manipulation that has been done before motor deficit will ensue.
- *Safe entry zones into the spinal cord*:

  If the tumor comes to the surface and this area is accessible, it is better to pursue the entry through it.

  The classic dorsal median sulcus. It is possible to observe it by following the small veins diving into the cord on both sides of the median sulcus. Another option that is advocated by some is to perform phase reversal using a strip to locate the two dorsal columns. When the spinal cord is rotated, or in cases where the normal anatomy is disturbed by the tumor, it is useful to identify the bilateral dorsal root entry zones in order to possibly locate the midline.

  Other options are through the dorsal intermediate sulcus or dorsolateral sulcus (DLS or posterolateral sulcus). The DLS is adjacent to the dorsal root entry zone, and a safe entry can be made just through it taking into consideration the trajectory of the dorsal horn of the spinal cord grey matter that is very close to it.

  The dorsal root entry zone can serve also as a possible marker for lateral approach with careful dissection just below it with mapping for the lateral corticospinal tracts. Some also published their experience with what they define as "ADREZotomy" (anterior to dorsal root entry zone myelotomy). The spinal cord is entered between the dorsolateral tract and the dorsal spinocerebellar tracts, anterior to the lateral proper fasciculus of the spinal cord and posterior to the lateral corticospinal tract [46, 47].

  In order to expose the lateral aspects of the cord, severing of the dentate ligaments at the same level and sometime below and above and even opposite side can assist. In cases the surgery is in the conus area, the sensory roots can be used for gentle retraction.

  For some tumors there is a cleavage plane between the tumor and the spinal cord which allows dissection and coagulation of some of the vascular feeders for the tumor, hence minimizing intratumoral bleeding while performing the tumor resection.

We advocate for laminoplasty after dural closure whenever feasible.

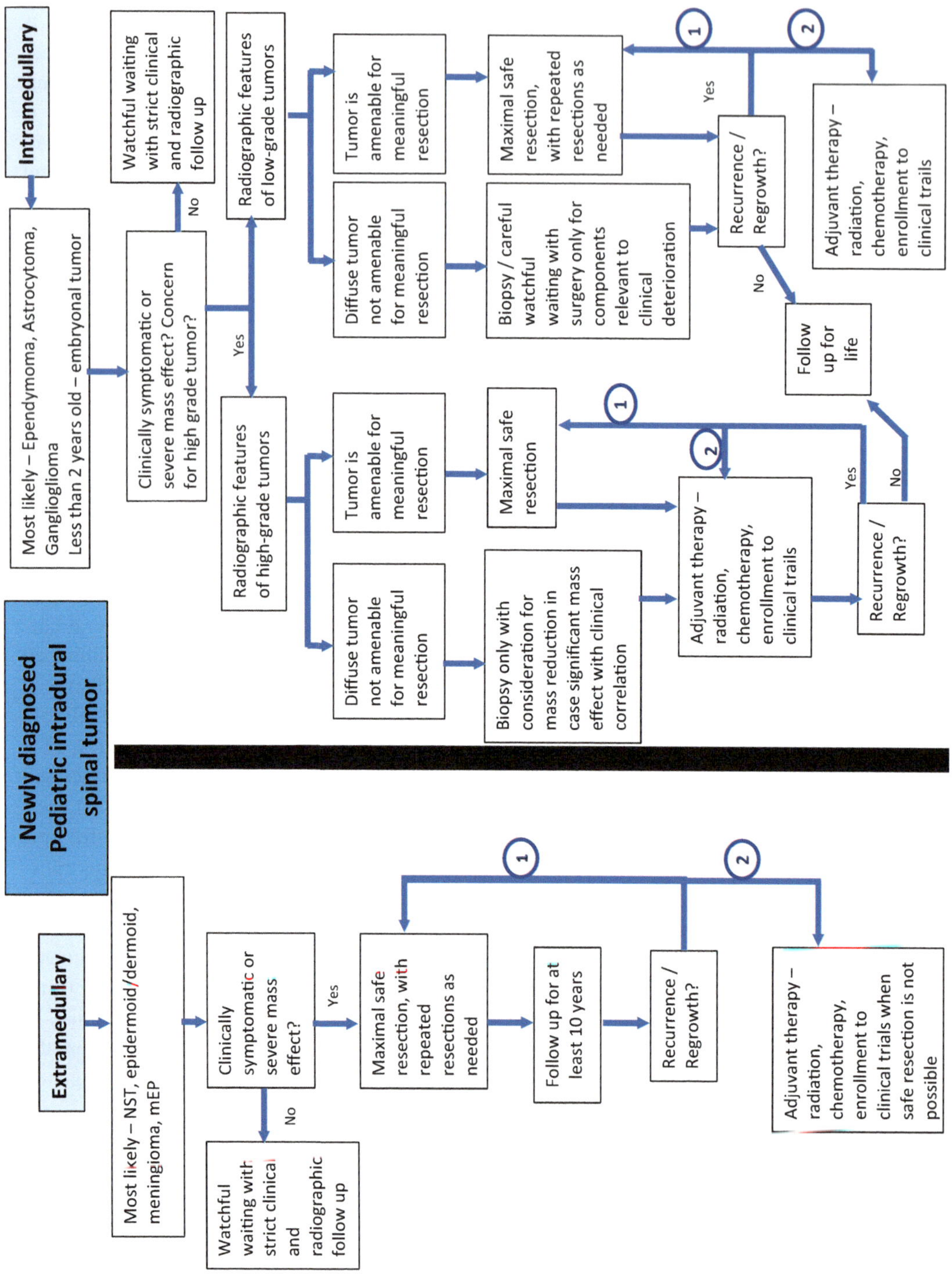

Fig. 9.3 Flow chart for decision-making in the treatment of spinal cord tumors

Intradural Extramedullary Tumors

In contrast to the adult population, most of the spinal tumors in children are intramedullary spinal cord tumors. Tumors of the spinal canal that reside within the thecal sac but not originating or involving the spinal cord are defined as intradural extramedullary tumors. These lesions are varied and include meningiomas, nerve sheath tumors (e.g., schwannoma, neurofibroma), dermoids/epidermoids (can also be intramedullary), teratomas, and myxopapillary ependymomas. The broad discussion about the management of nerve sheath tumors as part of neurofibromatosis is beyond the scope of this chapter and will be discussed as part of the chapter focusing on the management of NF. The classic symptoms related to the extramedullary tumors are a consequence of external compression on the spinal cord, the ventral or dorsal nerve roots, or the spinal nerve itself on its course throughout the vertebral foramen. Since the signs and symptoms are as a consequence of mechanical compression or stretch rather than actual parenchymal involvement, in many cases the presentation is relatively late in the course of the disease.

Meningiomas

Meningiomas of childhood are extremely rare, with less than 5% of all reported spinal meningiomas occurring in the pediatric population [48, 49]. Most of the publishable data regarding spinal meningiomas is anecdotal to small case series. Most of the data is in correlation to patients diagnosed with NF2, and only a fraction is related to truly sporadic spinal meningiomas of childhood. Hence, whenever a child is diagnosed with spinal meningioma, genetic consultation is advised to rule out NF2. A history of radiation therapy may also be a risk factor for development of these lesions. The most common presenting symptom is sensory deficit and associated pain. In a recently published case series, the mean duration between symptom onset and presentation was 9.7 months, which according to the authors is shorter than adult intraspinal meningioma lag time for diagnosis; hence they concluded that it might be related to the more aggressive nature pediatric spinal meningiomas have [50]. In contrast to the adult population, there is a male predilection for this disorder in children.

Like other spinal pathologies, the best tool for diagnosis is the MRI. On MRI, meningiomas are generally isointense to hypointense on T1WI and isointense on T2WI and with vivid enhancement on contrasted sequences. The main differential diagnosis by MRI for these features is for schwannomas and cavernous angiomas.

The most common variant of pediatric meningiomas is clear cell meningiomas [51]. This pathological variant has been reported to occur more in the lumbar region affecting the cauda equina, compared with other variants of meningiomas that occur in the cervical and thoracic regions [49, 51–54]. Clear cell meningiomas have a more aggressive nature and are pathologically considered as WHO grade II variants. In general, this is a rare subset of meningiomas, but within the small group of kids that will be affected with meningiomas, this is the usual pathological diagnosis [55, 56].

Complete surgical resection for all symptomatic or progressive pediatric meningiomas is the key for successful treatment result. The achievement of Simpson grade I is not feasible in many spinal meningiomas because of the difficulties of reconstructing well the dura in order to prevent CSF leak. Therefore, GTR may not be attainable in every patient, and serial post-operative monitoring with imaging is necessary. For recurrent disease, radiation, such as SRS, may be an appropriate alternate to repeat surgery, especially for lesions that are not amenable to repeat surgery. The use of routine post-operative radiotherapy needs to be carefully considered because of questionable therapeutic efficacy and possible radiation-induced toxicity especially for the pediatric population [50]. The use of chemotherapy for these lesions is not commonly advocated.

Nerve Sheath Tumors

The most common nerve sheath tumors in children are schwannomas and neurofibromas. Usually, these tumors are seen as part of either NF1 or NF2 pathologies. The more aggressive and relatively rare malignant peripheral nerve sheath tumor usually is seen more in adults. A thorough discussion about nerve sheath tumors as part of neurofibromatosis will be carried out in the chapter focusing on the management of neurofibromatosis.

Schwannomas and neurofibromas usually involve the dorsal sensory nerve root and affect the peripheral nerves as they exit the spinal cord and travel toward the neural foramina. The fact these tumors usually create motor deficit only late in the course of the disease leads commonly to lag in diagnosis and to the fact that by the time the patient is presented the tumor in many cases already gets to sizeable dimensions, which hinder achievement of GTR. MRI is the diagnostic tool most commonly used with the lesions usually isointense on T1- and hyperintense on T2-weighted imaging and has homogeneous enhancement. Sometimes it is hard to differentiate these tumors from spinal meningiomas.

The treatment of these tumors warrants complete surgical resection when feasible, with schwannomas sometimes being amenable for en bloc resection with or without sacrificing the sensory root. Yet, in many cases, the size of the tumor and the spinal cord compression don't allow for significant tumor manipulation (severing the dentate ligament can help) demanding surgical debulking rather than en bloc resection. Since in many cases there is a need to drill and expose the foramen, consideration for instrumentation and fusion needs to be taken for each case. Conversely, neurofibromas are often significantly involved within the nerve and hence cannot be fully resected without sacrificing the nerve. In cases where subtotal resection was performed, observation with serial MRI should be considered because of the slow-growing nature of these tumors. Adjuvant therapies such as chemotherapy and radiation therapy usually are reserved for the malignant peripheral nerve sheath tumors. For large plexiform neurofibromas that can be seen in NF1, recent years showed promising results with targeted treatment (*selumetinib*, MEK inhibitor) [57].

Myxopapillary Ependymomas

Myxopapillary ependymomas are considered WHO grade I lesions. Yet, recent advances in the understanding of ependymomas of the spinal cord are suggestive to change it for WHO I and II or add it as additional grade [58]. This is a rare pathology, representing only about 15% of pediatric spine tumors. Myxopapillary ependymomas usually reside at the conus medullaris, cauda equina, and filum terminale. Because of this anatomical location, the classic symptoms include back pain, radiculopathy, lower extremity paresis, and bowel or bladder dysfunction. Like with other intradural extramedullary tumors, there is commonly a long lag time for diagnosis secondary the slow grow and relative indolent course of this pathology [59]. Rarely the presentation can be as part of an acute event of subarachnoid hemorrhage. The treatment usually includes the attempt for GTR preferably as an en bloc resection to prevent seeding. Given the critical surrounding structures in the upper lumbar cistern, such as the conus, in some cases achieving GTR may not be feasible. Reports suggest a rate of GTR in approximately 35–60% of cases [60–62]. Adjunct therapy with radiation may be appropriate in cases of subtotal resection and especially in the pediatric population where the disease is more aggressive. A SEER database review and analysis from 2016 showed that pediatric patients affected by myxopapillary ependymoma had a significant increase in overall survival when a GTR was achieved in comparison to those that had STR and adjuvant radiation therapy [61]. The use of post-operative routine radiation therapy in order to prevent recurrence is still highly debatable.

Conclusions

Spinal tumors in the pediatric population are rare entities. Although we see significant advance in the knowledge base of the molecular and genetic features of these tumors, the treatment paradigm still relies on surgical intervention when symptomatic. In many cases the surgical goal is of maximal safe tumor resection. The low-grade nature of the majority of intradural spinal tumors in children can lead to delays in diagnosis due to their indolent growth. Hence, widespread education for the possibility for spinal tumor among pediatric patients is important. Improvements in diagnostic imaging, microsurgical techniques, and intraoperative monitoring have led to excellent outcomes in many cases, allowing for follow-up only with serial imaging after surgery without the need for adjuvant therapy in many cases. Yet, since surgery is not always enough for successful treatment, it is crucial to have a full knowledge of the genetic and molecular alterations of the tumor in order to tailor the best treatment for the patient.

Review Questions

1. The most common tumor in an 8-year-old child is:
   (a) Astrocytoma
   (b) Ependymoma
   (c) Hemangioblastoma
   (d) Myxopapillary ependymoma
2. The average time for the diagnosis of an intramedullary spinal cord tumor is:
   (a) 1 month
   (b) 2 months
   (c) 4 months
   (d) 10 months
3. Ependymomas of the spinal cord are known to:
   (a) To be subclassified as RELA and Yap1.
   (b) Usually not amenable for gross total removal.
   (c) When diagnosed with MYCN amplification, the prognosis is usually poor.
   (d) Will respond very well for adjuvant therapy, and hence a biopsy only paradigm with addition of adjuvant therapy usually leads to good prognosis.
4. A 5-month-old baby is presented to the emergency department with lethargy, severe torticollis, lack of spontaneous movement in his legs, and obvious decrease in arm movement. According to the parents, the signs started about 3 weeks ago and have been rapidly progressed. He is diagnosed with significant swelling of his cervical spinal cord over MRI with the following features for the scan—isointense on T1WI, slightly hyperintense on T2WI, and mixed enhancement on T1WI with gadolinium. There is a clear restriction on DWI imaging and signs for both patchy hemorrhage and possible leptomeningeal involvement. His brain MRI reveals signs for active hydrocephalus. Taking all the parameters into account, the most likely diagnosis is:
   (a) Myxopapillary ependymoma
   (b) ATRT
   (c) Low-grade astrocytoma
   (d) Ganglioglioma
5. A 16-year-old male is evaluated in the trauma bay after a car crash. He is GCS 15, without any neurological deficit. He is an athlete, currently playing basketball, and has no complaints regarding back pain or leg pain. The trauma team orders abdominal CT for possible intraperitoneal bleed. On the CT scan, there is a finding suggesting an intradural mass at the level of T9. He is sent to MRI which reveals the mass is intradural extramedullary with some cord compression but no surrounding edema. The mass is isointense on T1WI and T2WI, with clear enhancement on contrasted sequences. The family asks for your advice:
   (a) This is most likely a lipoma, and since he is asymptomatic, they can let it go.
   (b) He needs to go for surgery right now because of the radiographic cord compression.

(c) The main differential diagnoses are schwannoma and myxopapillary ependymoma.
(d) The possible diagnosis is meningioma, but since he is asymptomatic at this point, an organized follow-up to monitor symptoms and tumor growth is recommended.

Answer Keys

1. a
2. d
3. c
4. b
5. d

References

1. Ostrom QT, Patil N, Cioffi G, Waite K, Kruchko C, Barnholtz-Sloan JS. CBTRUS statistical report: primary brain and other central nervous system tumors diagnosed in the United States in 2013-2017. Neuro Oncol. 2020;22(12 Suppl 2):iv1–iv96. https://doi.org/10.1093/neuonc/noaa200.
2. Parsa AT, Lee J, Parney IF, Weinstein P, McCormick PC, Ames C. Spinal cord and intradural-extraparenchymal spinal tumors: current best care practices and strategies. J Neurooncol. 2004;69(1–3):291–318. https://doi.org/10.1023/b:neon.0000041889.71136.62.
3. Chang UK, Choe WJ, Chung SK, Chung CK, Kim HJ. Surgical outcome and prognostic factors of spinal intramedullary ependymomas in adults. J Neurooncol. 2002;57(2):133–9. https://doi.org/10.1023/a:1015789009058.
4. Crawford JR, Zaninovic A, Santi M, Rushing EJ, Olsen CH, Keating RF, et al. Primary spinal cord tumors of childhood: effects of clinical presentation, radiographic features, and pathology on survival. J Neurooncol. 2009;95(2):259–69. https://doi.org/10.1007/s11060-009-9925-1.
5. Auguste KI, Gupta N. Pediatric intramedullary spinal cord tumors. Neurosurg Clin N Am. 2006;17(1):51–61. https://doi.org/10.1016/j.nec.2005.10.004.
6. Lee CH, Chung CK, Kim CH. Genetic differences on intracranial versus spinal cord ependymal tumors: a meta-analysis of genetic researches. Eur Spine J. 2016;25(12):3942–51. https://doi.org/10.1007/s00586-016-4745-4.
7. Karsy M, Guan J, Sivakumar W, Neil JA, Schmidt MH, Mahan MA. The genetic basis of intradural spinal tumors and its impact on clinical treatment. Neurosurg Focus. 2015;39(2):E3. https://doi.org/10.3171/2015.5.FOCUS15143.
8. Segal D, Lidar Z, Corn A, Constantini S. Delay in diagnosis of primary intradural spinal cord tumors. Surg Neurol Int. 2012;3:52. https://doi.org/10.4103/2152-7806.96075.
9. Schick U, Marquardt G. Pediatric spinal tumors. Pediatr Neurosurg. 2001;35(3):120–7. https://doi.org/10.1159/000050404.
10. Yao KC, McGirt MJ, Chaichana KL, Constantini S, Jallo GI. Risk factors for progressive spinal deformity following resection of intramedullary spinal cord tumors in children: an analysis of 161 consecutive cases. J Neurosurg. 2007;107(6 Suppl):463–8. https://doi.org/10.3171/PED-07/12/463.
11. Wilne S, Walker D. Spine and spinal cord tumours in children: a diagnostic and therapeutic challenge to healthcare systems. Arch Dis Child Educ Pract Ed. 2010;95(2):47–54. https://doi.org/10.1136/adc.2008.143214.
12. Liu X, Tian W, Chen H, LoStracco TA, Zhang J, Li MY, et al. Advanced neuroimaging in the evaluation of spinal cord tumors and tumor mimics: diffusion tensor and perfusion-weighted imaging. Semin Ultrasound CT MR. 2017;38(2):163–75. https://doi.org/10.1053/j.sult.2016.07.006.
13. Kobayashi K, Imagama S, Kato F, Kanemura T, Sato K, Kamiya M, et al. MRI characteristics of spinal ependymoma in WHO grade II: a review of 59 cases. Spine (Phila Pa 1976). 2017;43:E525. https://doi.org/10.1097/BRS.0000000000002496.
14. Koeller KK, Rosenblum RS, Morrison AL. Neoplasms of the spinal cord and filum terminale: radiologic-pathologic correlation. Radiographics. 2000;20(6):1721–49. https://doi.org/10.1148/radiographics.20.6.g00nv151721.
15. Baker KB, Moran CJ, Wippold FJ, Smirniotopoulos JG, Rodriguez FJ, Meyers SP, et al. MR imaging of spinal hemangioblastoma. AJR Am J Roentgenol. 2000;174(2):377–82. https://doi.org/10.2214/ajr.174.2.1740377.
16. Do-Dai DD, Brooks MK, Goldkamp A, Erbay S, Bhadelia RA. Magnetic resonance imaging of intramedullary spinal cord lesions: a pictorial review. Curr Probl Diagn Radiol. 2010;39(4):160–85. https://doi.org/10.1067/j.cpradiol.2009.05.004.
17. Wu HY, Xu WB, Lu LW, Li HH, Tian JS, Li JM, et al. Imaging features of spinal atypical teratoid rhabdoid tumors in children. Medicine (Baltimore). 2018;97(52):e13808. https://doi.org/10.1097/MD.0000000000013808.
18. Babgi M, Samkari A, Al-Mehdar A, Abdullah S. Atypical teratoid/rhabdoid tumor of the spinal cord in a child: case report and comprehensive review of the literature. Pediatr Neurosurg. 2018;53(4):254–62. https://doi.org/10.1159/000488459.
19. Toi H, Ogawa Y, Kinoshita K, Hirai S, Takai H, Hara K, et al. Bamboo leaf sign as a sensitive magnetic resonance imaging finding in spinal subependymoma: case report and literature review. Case Rep Neurol Med. 2016;2016:9108641. https://doi.org/10.1155/2016/9108641.

20. McCormick PC, Torres R, Post KD, Stein BM. Intramedullary ependymoma of the spinal cord. J Neurosurg. 1990;72(4):523–32. https://doi.org/10.3171/jns.1990.72.4.0523.
21. Goy AM, Pinto RS, Raghavendra BN, Epstein FJ, Kricheff II. Intramedullary spinal cord tumors: MR imaging, with emphasis on associated cysts. Radiology. 1986;161(2):381–6. https://doi.org/10.1148/radiology.161.2.3763905.
22. Ghasemi DR, Sill M, Okonechnikov K, Korshunov A, Yip S, Schutz PW, et al. MYCN amplification drives an aggressive form of spinal ependymoma. Acta Neuropathol. 2019;138(6):1075–89. https://doi.org/10.1007/s00401-019-02056-2.
23. Westwick HJ, Giguère JF, Shamji MF. Incidence and prognosis of spinal hemangioblastoma: a surveillance epidemiology and end results study. Neuroepidemiology. 2016;46(1):14–23. https://doi.org/10.1159/000441147.
24. Louis DN, Perry A, Reifenberger G, von Deimling A, Figarella-Branger D, Cavenee WK, et al. The 2016 World Health Organization Classification of Tumors of the Central Nervous System: a summary. Acta Neuropathol. 2016;131(6):803–20. https://doi.org/10.1007/s00401-016-1545-1.
25. Abd-El-Barr MM, Huang KT, Moses ZB, Iorgulescu JB, Chi JH. Recent advances in intradural spinal tumors. Neuro Oncol. 2018;20(6):729–42. https://doi.org/10.1093/neuonc/nox230.
26. Shankar GM, Lelic N, Gill CM, Thorner AR, Van Hummelen P, Wisoff JH, et al. BRAF alteration status and the histone H3F3A gene K27M mutation segregate spinal cord astrocytoma histology. Acta Neuropathol. 2016;131(1):147–50. https://doi.org/10.1007/s00401-015-1492-2.
27. Pajtler KW, Witt H, Sill M, Jones DT, Hovestadt V, Kratochwil F, et al. Molecular classification of ependymal tumors across all CNS compartments, histopathological grades, and age groups. Cancer Cell. 2015;27(5):728–43. https://doi.org/10.1016/j.ccell.2015.04.002.
28. Zhang M, Iyer RR, Azad TD, Wang Q, Garzon-Muvdi T, Wang J, et al. Genomic landscape of intramedullary spinal cord gliomas. Sci Rep. 2019;9(1):18722. https://doi.org/10.1038/s41598-019-54286-9.
29. Ellison DW, Aldape KD, Capper D, Fouladi M, Gilbert MR, Gilbertson RJ, et al. cIMPACT-NOW update 7: advancing the molecular classification of ependymal tumors. Brain Pathol. 2020;30(5):863–6. https://doi.org/10.1111/bpa.12866.
30. Frühwald MC, Biegel JA, Bourdeaut F, Roberts CW, Chi SN. Atypical teratoid/rhabdoid tumors-current concepts, advances in biology, and potential future therapies. Neuro Oncol. 2016;18(6):764–78. https://doi.org/10.1093/neuonc/nov264.
31. Benesch M, Nemes K, Neumayer P, Hasselblatt M, Timmermann B, Bison B, et al. Spinal cord atypical teratoid/rhabdoid tumors in children: clinical, genetic, and outcome characteristics in a representative European cohort. Pediatr Blood Cancer. 2020;67(1):e28022. https://doi.org/10.1002/pbc.28022.
32. Kutluk T, Varan A, Kafali C, Hayran M, Soylemezoglu F, Zorlu F, et al. Pediatric intramedullary spinal cord tumors: a single center experience. Eur J Paediatr Neurol. 2015;19(1):41–7. https://doi.org/10.1016/j.ejpn.2014.09.007.
33. Constantini S, Miller DC, Allen JC, Rorke LB, Freed D, Epstein FJ. Radical excision of intramedullary spinal cord tumors: surgical morbidity and long-term follow-up evaluation in 164 children and young adults. J Neurosurg. 2000;93(2 Suppl):183–93.
34. McGirt MJ, Chaichana KL, Atiba A, Attenello F, Woodworth GF, Jallo GI. Neurological outcome after resection of intramedullary spinal cord tumors in children. Childs Nerv Syst. 2008;24(1):93–7. https://doi.org/10.1007/s00381-007-0446-y.
35. McGirt MJ, Goldstein IM, Chaichana KL, Tobias ME, Kothbauer KF, Jallo GI. Extent of surgical resection of malignant astrocytomas of the spinal cord: outcome analysis of 35 patients. Neurosurgery. 2008;63(1):55–60; discussion 60–1. https://doi.org/10.1227/01.NEU.0000335070.37943.09.
36. Safaee M, Oh MC, Mummaneni PV, Weinstein PR, Ames CP, Chou D, et al. Surgical outcomes in spinal cord ependymomas and the importance of extent of resection in children and young adults. J Neurosurg Pediatr. 2014;13(4):393–9. https://doi.org/10.3171/2013.12.PEDS13383.
37. Luksik AS, Garzon-Muvdi T, Yang W, Huang J, Jallo GI. Pediatric spinal cord astrocytomas: a retrospective study of 348 patients from the SEER database. J Neurosurg Pediatr. 2017;19(6):711–9. https://doi.org/10.3171/2017.1.PEDS16528.
38. Azad TD, Pendharkar AV, Pan J, Huang Y, Li A, Esparza R, et al. Surgical outcomes of pediatric spinal cord astrocytomas: systematic review and meta-analysis. J Neurosurg Pediatr. 2018;22(4):404–10. https://doi.org/10.3171/2018.4.PEDS17587.
39. Gwak SJ, An SS, Yang MS, Joe E, Kim DH, Yoon DH, et al. Effect of combined bevacizumab and temozolomide treatment on intramedullary spinal cord tumor. Spine (Phila Pa 1976). 2014;39(2):E65–73. https://doi.org/10.1097/BRS.0000000000000070.
40. Hassall TE, Mitchell AE, Ashley DM. Carboplatin chemotherapy for progressive intramedullary spinal cord low-grade gliomas in children: three case studies and a review of the literature. Neuro Oncol. 2001;3(4):251–7.
41. Ahmed R, Menezes AH, Torner JC. Role of resection and adjuvant therapy in long-term disease outcomes for low-grade pediatric intramedullary spinal cord tumors. J Neurosurg Pediatr. 2016;18(5):594–601. https://doi.org/10.3171/2016.5.PEDS15356.
42. The response of spinal cord ependymomas to bevacizumab in patients with neurofibromatosis Type 2. J Neurosurg Spine. 2017;26(4):474–82. https://doi.org/10.3171/2016.8.SPINE16589.

43. Farschtschi S, Merker VL, Wolf D, Schuhmann M, Blakeley J, Plotkin SR, et al. Bevacizumab treatment for symptomatic spinal ependymomas in neurofibromatosis type 2. Acta Neurol Scand. 2016;133(6):475–80. https://doi.org/10.1111/ane.12490.
44. Salim DK. Continuous angiogenesis inhibition in the treatment for von Hippel-Lindau-related hemangioblastomas of retina and spinal cord. J Oncol Pharm Pract. 2019;25(8):2049–51. https://doi.org/10.1177/1078155219827635.
45. Omar AI. Bevacizumab for the treatment of surgically unresectable cervical cord hemangioblastoma: a case report. J Med Case Rep. 2012;6:238. https://doi.org/10.1186/1752-1947-6-238.
46. Ren J, He C, Hong T, Li X, Ma Y, Yu J, et al. Anterior to Dorsal Root Entry Zone Myelotomy (ADREZotomy): a new surgical approach for the treatment of ventrolateral deep intramedullary spinal cord cavernous malformations. Spine (Phila Pa 1976). 2018;43(17):E1024–E32. https://doi.org/10.1097/BRS.0000000000002607.
47. Ren J, Hong T, He C, Li X, Ma Y, Yu J, et al. Surgical approaches and long-term outcomes of intramedullary spinal cord cavernous malformations: a single-center consecutive series of 219 patients. J Neurosurg Spine. 2019;31(1):123–32. https://doi.org/10.3171/2018.12.SPINE181263.
48. Ambekar S, Sharma M, Kukreja S, Nanda A. Complications and outcomes of surgery for spinal meningioma: a Nationwide Inpatient Sample analysis from 2003 to 2010. Clin Neurol Neurosurg. 2014;118:65–8. https://doi.org/10.1016/j.clineuro.2013.12.010.
49. Wang XQ, Zeng XW, Zhang BY, Dou YF, Wu JS, Jiang CC, et al. Spinal meningioma in childhood: clinical features and treatment. Childs Nerv Syst. 2012;28(1):129–36. https://doi.org/10.1007/s00381-011-1570-2.
50. Wu L, Yang C, Liu T, Fang J, Yang J, Xu Y. Clinical features and long-term outcomes of pediatric spinal meningiomas. J Neurooncol. 2017;133(2):347–55. https://doi.org/10.1007/s11060-017-2441-9.
51. Balogun JA, Halliday W, Bouffet E, Kulkarni AV. Spinal clear cell meningioma in a 3-year-old: a case report. Pediatr Neurosurg. 2013;49(5):311–5. https://doi.org/10.1159/000366452.
52. Colen CB, Rayes M, McClendon J Jr, Rabah R, Ham SD. Pediatric spinal clear cell meningioma. Case report. J Neurosurg Pediatr. 2009;3(1):57–60. https://doi.org/10.3171/2008.10.17668.
53. Park HC, Sohn MJ, Kim EY, Han HS, Park HS. Spinal clear cell meningioma presented with progressive paraparesis in infancy. Childs Nerv Syst. 2000;16(9):607–10. https://doi.org/10.1007/PL00007302.
54. Brusius CV, Pereira Filho AA, Barnewitz JP, Putten AC, Pitta Pinheiro C, Aesse FF. Intradural spinal meningioma in a 20-month-old female. Pediatr Neurosurg. 2008;44(3):247–52. https://doi.org/10.1159/000121385.
55. Kumar R, Das KK, Jaiswal AK, Mehrotra A, Sahu RN, Srivastava AK, et al. Clear cell meningioma in a child: a case report and review of literature. Asian J Neurosurg. 2015;10(1):53. https://doi.org/10.4103/1793-5482.151520.
56. Jallo GI, Kothbauer KF, Silvera VM, Epstein FJ. Intraspinal clear cell meningioma: diagnosis and management: report of two cases. Neurosurgery. 2001;48(1):218–21; discussion 21–2.
57. Walker JA, Upadhyaya M. Emerging therapeutic targets for neurofibromatosis type 1. Expert Opin Ther Targets. 2018;22(5):419–37. https://doi.org/10.1080/14728222.2018.1465931.
58. Neumann JE, Spohn M, Obrecht D, Mynarek M, Thomas C, Hasselblatt M, et al. Molecular characterization of histopathological ependymoma variants. Acta Neuropathol. 2020;139(2):305–18. https://doi.org/10.1007/s00401-019-02090-0.
59. Bagley CA, Wilson S, Kothbauer KF, Bookland MJ, Epstein F, Jallo GI. Long term outcomes following surgical resection of myxopapillary ependymomas. Neurosurg Rev. 2009;32(3):321–34; discussion 34. https://doi.org/10.1007/s10143-009-0190-8.
60. Lin Y, Smith ZA, Wong AP, Melkonian S, Harris DA, Lam S. Predictors of survival in patients with spinal ependymoma. Neurol Res. 2015;37(7):650–5. https://doi.org/10.1179/1743132815Y.0000000041.
61. Lucchesi KM, Grant R, Kahle KT, Marks AM, DiLuna ML. Primary spinal myxopapillary ependymoma in the pediatric population: a study from the Surveillance, Epidemiology, and End Results (SEER) database. J Neurooncol. 2016;130(1):133–40. https://doi.org/10.1007/s11060-016-2218-6.
62. Abdulaziz M, Mallory GW, Bydon M, De la Garza Ramos R, Ellis JA, Laack NN, et al. Outcomes following myxopapillary ependymoma resection: the importance of capsule integrity. Neurosurg Focus. 2015;39(2):E8. https://doi.org/10.3171/2015.5.FOCUS15164.

Pediatric Vascular Malformations

10

Ari D. Kappel, Alfred P. See, and Edward R. Smith

Arteriovenous Malformations (AVMs)

Background

AVMs are high-flow vascular lesions consisting of a nidus of tangled blood vessels with a direct arterial-to-venous connection. There are no intervening capillaries or functional parenchyma within the nidus, but the lesion may be surrounded by gliotic tissue or a hemosiderin ring. In the CNS they may occur in the cerebral hemispheres, brainstem, or spinal cord. Due to the lack of an intervening capillary bed, there is high-flow shunting of arterial blood and a lack of resistance that leads to increased pressure in the draining veins. Arteries and draining veins may become dilated with increased tortuosity, and veins may become arterialized over time with thick walls, smooth muscle proliferation, and collagen deposition [1].

A. D. Kappel
Department of Neurosurgery, Boston Children's Hospital, Boston, MA, USA

Harvard Medical School, Boston, MA, USA

Department of Neurosurgery, Brigham and Women's Hospital, Boston, MA, USA
e-mail: ari.kappel@childrens.harvard.edu

A. P. See · E. R. Smith (✉)
Department of Neurosurgery, Boston Children's Hospital, Boston, MA, USA

Harvard Medical School, Boston, MA, USA
e-mail: alfred.see@childrens.harvard.edu; edward.smith@childrens.harvard.edu

Epidemiology

The prevalence of brain AVMs is approximately 10–18 per 100,000 people and is the most common vascular lesion causing acute hemorrhagic stroke in pediatric patients [2, 3]. Patients with AVMs most often present intracranial hemorrhage (58%), seizures (34%), or other neurologic deficits (8%) [2].

Natural History

The risk of AVM rupture is approximately 2–4% per year [4–6], but rupture risk may vary widely based on risk factors and angioarchitectural features including deep or posterior fossa location, deep venous drainage, a single draining vein or venous outflow stenosis, history of previous hemorrhage, and associated aneurysms [7–9]. Aneurysms associated with AVMs are classified as intranidal aneurysms (type I), proximal or distal flow-related aneurysms (type II), and unrelated aneurysms (type III) [10] and may be associated with rupture later in life compared to AVMs with deep locations or deep venous drainage [9]. AVM-associated aneurysms are typically considered rare, but in one series were seen 27% of cases suggesting that they may not be

N. Shimony, G. Jallo (eds.), *Pediatric Neurosurgery Board Review*,
https://doi.org/10.1007/978-3-031-23687-7_10

as rare as previously thought [11]. The re-bleeding rate for previously ruptured AVMs is approximately 4.5% [6] but may be as high as 6–15.8% in the first year [5, 12, 13].

Diagnosis

Initial diagnosis is often made with CTA or MRA, but digital subtraction angiography (DSA) remains the gold standard for definitive diagnosis and characterization of the lesion. Compared to DSA, CTA and MRI have an 87% and 80% sensitivity rate for diagnosis of a ruptured AVM in the setting of intraparenchymal hemorrhage [14]. DSA has a low procedural complication rate close to 0% and a 0.4% post-procedural complication rate [15]. DSA provides important information about angioarchitectural characteristics of the AVM, not as well delineated on other imaging modalities including flow rate, arterial feeder anatomy, detection of associated aneurysms, early venous drainage, venous drainage patterns, and venous outflow stenosis [16]. Characteristics of the AVM may change over time, and DSA may need to be delayed or repeated days to weeks after hemorrhage. Pressure from the clot may obscure AVM anatomy, and as the clot resorbs, the small feeding vessels or other characteristics not previously seen may become evident [17]. These characteristics are important for planning treatment including endovascular embolization and surgical resection [18].

Genetics

AVMs may be sporadic or related to known hereditary conditions predisposing individuals to multiple AVMs. Multiple hereditary diseases with a wide range of germline and somatic mutations have been reported along with their associated genes including hereditary hemorrhagic telangiectasia (HHT), cerebral cavernous malformation syndrome (CCM), and capillary malformation-arteriovenous malformation syndrome (CM-AVM). Some of the most common and well-described hereditary syndromes with their associated genes are listed here and in Table 10.1: HHT1 (ENG), HHT2 (ACVRL1), JP/HHT (MADH4), CCM1 (KRIT1), CCM2 (MGC4607), CCM3 (PDCD10), CM-AVM1 (RASA1), and CM-AVM2 (EPHB4).

HHT is an autosomal dominant disorder with a high penetrance and variable expressivity [19]. Patients with HHT may present with capillary vascular malformations, AVMs, and/or AVFs. HHT patients with AVMs are more likely to have multiple lesions that are supratentorial and superficial, and small (<3 cm), with low Spetzler-Martin grades (SM grades I–III) [20–23]. Brain AVMs are more common in HHT1 than HHT2 patients occurring at a rate of 13.4% and 2.4%, respectively [22]. In 75 patients with HHT and brain vascular malformations, Krings et al. found that 60% had HHT1 (endoglin) mutations. In another study of 109 patients with HHT and brain AVMs with available genotype information, 69% had HHT1, 17% had HHT2, and 2% had JP/HHT [24]. Twenty-three percent of those patients had multiple brain AVMs, 27% had history of rupture, and 17% had a seizure disorder. Patients with hereditary HHT should be screened with MRI [25], and approximately 60% of brain AVMs are discovered this way [26]. If no lesions are seen on initial screening imaging studies, follow-up imaging is typically delayed at least 5 years given a low reported rate of de novo lesion development [27]. The rate of rupture in patients with HHT is estimated at approximately 1% per year [26]. Although this finding suggests a lower rate of rupture for hereditary AVMs compared to sporadic brain AVMs, these patients are screened at a higher rate leading to a selection bias that may underestimate the relative risk of hereditary AVMs. The recent genetic definition of CM-AVM2, as hereditary mutations in EPHB4, has demonstrated additional genetic linkage related to brain AVMs [28] (Table 10.2).

Treatment

Treatment approach is typically based on both AVM location and anatomy and with the primary goal of obliteration of the lesion. Partially treated AVMs may have a higher risk of rupture [29]. Therefore, if treatment is planned success

Table 10.1 Hereditary forms of brain vascular malformations and their associated genes, chromosomes, mutations, and clinical presentations

Disease	Gene	Protein	Genetic locus	Vascular lesions/presentation	OMIM	Identified mutations[a]	Missense/ nonsense[a]
HHT1	ENG	Endoglin	9q34	Telangiectasias, AVMs (brain, lungs, liver, GI)	131195	>450	151
HHT2	ACVRL1	ALK1	12q13	Telangiectasias, AVMs (brain, lungs, liver, GI)	601284	>400	253
JP/HHT	MADH4	SMAD4	18q21	Colorectal polyps, telangiectasias, AVMs (brain, lungs, liver, GI)	600993	>100	54
CM-AVM1	RASA1	RAS p21	5q14.3	CMs (skin, brain, heart), AVMs, AVFs, VOGM, lymphedema, Parkes Weber syndrome	139150	>100	43
CM-AVM2	EPHB4	EPH receptor B4	7q22.1	CMs (skin, brain, heart), AVMs, AVFs, VOGM, lymphedema	600011	>60	>3
CCM1	KRIT1	Krev interaction trapped	7q21.2	CCMs (brain, spinal cord), hemangiomas	604214	>300	68
CCM2	MGC4607	Malcavernin	7p13	CCMs (brain, spinal cord), hemangiomas	607929	>90	21
CCM3	PDCD10	Programmed cell death 10	3p26.1	CCMs (brain, spinal cord), hemangiomas	609118	>70	17

HHT Hereditary hemorrhagic telangiectasia, *JP* juvenile polyposis, *CM-AVM* capillary malformation-arteriovenous malformation, *CCM* cerebral cavernous malformation, *AVM* Arteriovenous malformations, *AVF* arteriovenous fistula, *CM* capillary malformation, *VOGM* Vein of Galen Malformation, *HGMD* Human gene mutation database, *OMIM* Online Mendelian Inheritance in Man catalog number

[a] Data from HGMD: hgmd.cf.ac.uk

Table 10.2 Somatic mutations in brain vascular malformations. Reported somatic mutations associated with brain vascular malformations including oncogenes and chromatin-modifier genes associated with AVMs, VOGMs, and CCMs

Gene	Protein	Genetic locus	Associated lesions/syndromes	Reported mutation	References (First author, Journal, Year)
KRAS	Kirsten rat sarcoma viral oncogene homolog	12q12.1	AVM [144, 145], bladder cancer [146], lung cancer [147], gastric cancer [148], leukemia [149], cardiofaciocutaneous syndrome 2 [150]	p.G12D [144, 145] p.G12V1 [144, 145]	Nikolaev, NEJM, 2018 [144]; Goss, PlosONE, 2019 [145]
BRAF	Murine sarcoma viral oncogene homolog B1	7q34	AVM [145, 151], lung adenocarcinoma [152], colorectal cancer [153], melanoma [154], lymphoma [155], cardiofaciocutaneous syndrome 1 [150], Noonan syndrome [156]	p.V600E [145] p.Q636X [145]	Al-Olabi, J Clin Invest, 2018 [151]; Goss, PlosONE, 2019 [145]
MAP2K1	Mitogen-activated protein kinase kinase 1	15q22.31	AVM [151, 157], cardiofaciocutaneous syndrome 3 [158]	p.K57N [151] p.Q58_E62del [151] p.F53_Q58delinsL [151]	Couto, Am J Hum Genet, 2017 [157]; Al-Olabi, J Clin Invest, 2018 [151]
KEL	Kell blood group metalloendo-peptidase	7q34	VOGM [63]	p.Q321X p.G202S	Duran, Neuron, 2019 [63]
KMT2D	Lysine-specific methyltransferase 2D	12q13.12	Kabuki syndrome [159], VOGM [63]	p.C5230Y	Duran, Neuron, 2019 [63]
SMARCA2	SWI/SNF-related, matrix-associated, actin-dependent regulator of chromatin, subfamily a, member 2	9p24.3	Nicolaides-Baraitser syndrome [160], VOGM [63]	p.R855L	Duran, Neuron, 2019 [63]
SIRT1	Sirtuin 1	10q21.3	VOGM [63]	p.R341Afs*6	Duran, Neuron, 2019 [63]
KAT6A	Lysine acetyltransferase 6a	8p11.21	Arboleda-Tham syndrome [161], VOGM [63]	p.T478I	Duran, Neuron, 2019 [63]
CLDN14	Claudin 14	21q22.13	Autosomal recessive deafness [162], VOGM [63]	p.A113P p.V143M	Duran, Neuron, 2019 [63]
PIK3CA	Phosphatidylinositol 3-kinase, catalytic, alpha	3q26.32	Meningioma [163], CCM [163]	p.H1047R	Peyre, NEJM, 2021 [163]
AKT	AKT serine/threonine kinase	14q32.33	Meningioma [163], CCM [163], Cowden syndrome [164]	p.E17K	Peyre, NEJM, 2021 [163]

AVM Arteriovenous malformations, *AVF* arteriovenous fistula, *CCM* cerebral cavernous malformation, *GI* Gastrointestinal, *VOGM* Vein of Galen Malformation if predicate on removing the lesion from circulation while preserving normal blood flow to the brain. A combination of surgery, radiation, and endovascular embolization may be used to treat the lesion depending on location, accessibility, and angioarchitecture [30, 31].

Hemorrhagic AVMs or symptomatic lesions should be considered for treatment. AVM-associated aneurysms that have ruptured or demonstrated enlargement over time should also be considered for treatment. Partial resection or endovascular embolization may increase the risk of AVM rupture, although there may be rationale for embolization of a specific aneurysm within the nidus if associated with bleeding [29, 32]. There is no protection against AVM rupture risk during the latency period after radiation therapy. In one study, rupture risk during the 2-year latency period after gamma knife stereotactic radiosurgery (SRS) was higher for larger AVMs and older patients but lower when higher doses of radiation were used [33]. In addition, hemorrhage may occur after the latency period in non-obliterated AVMs after SRS [33]. In a recent study of 189 pediatric patients with brain AVMs, the authors found a 2% rate of periprocedural stroke or death [34]. The authors conclude that an individualized, multidisciplinary approach to management can result in a safe and effective treatment of pediatric AVMs [34].

Treatment of unruptured, asymptomatic AVMs remains controversial, but careful analysis suggests that the preponderance of data largely supports intervention in the pediatric population. The ARUBA trial in 2014 was the first randomized controlled trial to compare medical management with intervention for unruptured AVMs. The study enrolled 226 patients 18 years or older and was stopped early by an independent data safety monitoring committee [35]. At the time of analysis, 73 patients had not completed treatment and 7 crossed over from the medical arm to the treatment arm. The primary outcome of stroke or death occurred in 30% of patients in the treatment arm and 10% in the medical arm. Treatment included 5% surgery, 32% embolization, 33% radiotherapy, and 30% multimodal therapy. The authors quoted complication rates from a meta-analysis of 29% for surgery, 25% for embolization, and 13% for radiotherapy [36]. However, rates of severe complications in that study, such as symptomatic stroke and death, were only 7.4% for surgery, 6.6% for embolization, and 5.1% for radiosurgery—much lower than in the ARUBA trial. Furthermore, the rates of surgical treatment in the study were low, limiting the applicability to surgical patients. The benefits of surgical resection of AVMs should be measured over the lifetime of the patient since annual rupture risk accrues over time. Follow-up in the ARUBA trial was only 31 months on average, which may not be long enough to see the benefits of resection [37]. Finally, the study is not applicable to pediatric patients given the differences in lifespan, aneurysm etiology, and risk factors in the pediatric AVM population [38].

Outcomes

Obliteration rates for treated brain AVMs in a large meta-analysis were 96% for surgical resection, 38% for stereotactic radiosurgery, and 13% for embolization [36]. Winkler et al. reported complete angiographic obliteration in 73% of low-grade lesions (SM grades I–III) and 45% of high-grade lesions in their pediatric cohort [34]. Following SRS in 101 pediatric patients with unruptured brain AVMs, Chen et al. reported a 2% annual risk of morbidity and mortality, which appeared to plateau after 10 years post-treatment [39]. Ma et al. studied seizure outcomes in a pediatric group of patients with brain AVMs [40]. Of 198 patients, 32% had seizures prior to treatment, and good seizure outcome (Engel class I) was achieved in 74% of these patients [40]. Complete AVM obliteration and short duration of seizure disorder prior to treatment were independent predictors of good seizure outcome [40].

Arteriovenous Fistulas (AVFs)

Background

Arteriovenous fistulas are characterized by a direct connection between arteries and veins without intervening capillaries or nidus. The arterial supply of dural AVFs (dAVFs) is derived from dural arteries and meningeal branches, often involving the extracranial circulation and commonly occurring at the transverse-sigmoid junction, cavernous sinus, superior sagittal sinus, anterior cranial fossa, or tentorium [41].

Pial AVFs (pAVFs) are rare lesions characterized by pial or cortical arterial feeders with direct connection to a single draining vein and no intervening nidus. They account for approximately 1.6% of intracranial vascular malformations and were previously described as a fistulous type of AVM [42] but subsequently considered distinct from AVMs and dAVFs due to their unique angioarchitectural features, natural history, and treatment options [43, 44]. Unlike AVMs they do not have a distinct nidus, and unlike dAVFs their blood supply is derived from one or more feeding cortical or pial artery and not from dural or meningeal branches. The natural history of untreated pAVFs is poor, with reported mortality rates as high as 63% [44].

Classification

Several classification schemes have been reported for dAVFs including the Borden-Shucart classification [45], Cognard classification [46], and Zipfel classification [47]. The Borden classification is the simplest and most commonly used [41]. Dural AVFs are distinguished based on the characteristics of their venous drainage, cortical venous reflux (CVR). Borden type I dAVFs drain into a dural venous sinus without CVR. Borden type II lesions drain into a dural venous sinus with retrograde flow causing CVR and are more aggressive with an increased risk of hemorrhage. Borden type III dAVFs drain directly into cortical veins causing CVR and are the most aggressive (Fig. 10.1; Table 10.3). In the Cognard classification, types I and IIa do not demonstrate CVR and are considered lower risk, while type IIa drains into a dural sinus and has CVR, and type III drains directly into a cortical vein causing CVR (Fig. 10.1; Table 10.3).

Genetics and Pathogenesis

Pial AVFs have been associated with HHT [48] and RASA1 mutations in CM-AVM1 [49]. Therefore, genetic screening may be indicated, particularly in patients with multiple pAVFs [49].

Dural AVFs are also often observed following trauma and craniotomy [41]. This may be due to hypoxia-induced upregulation of angiogenic factors including hypoxia-inducible factor-1 (HIF-1) and VEGF [50]. Venous sinus thrombosis is another proposed driver of dAVF, although this has not been observed in prospective studies of venous thrombosis cohorts [51].

Treatment

Surgery, embolization, or a combination of both are the mainstays of treatment for pAVFs [44, 52–55]. Radiosurgery may be a rare option for some dAVFs, but is not used to treat pAVFs because of the risk of rupture during the latency period and difficulty targeting pAVFs [56].

Outcomes and Follow-Up

Age is a critical determinant of outcome for pediatric patients with AVFs. Overall, 72% of patients older than 2 years have a good clinical outcome, while younger children suffer higher complication rates and more frequently require additional multiple procedures [57]. Treatment of dAVFs and pAVFs is effective, with high rates of complete obliteration and good outcomes reported [49, 58].

Procedural complication rates have been reported in up to 60% of cases with major complications including stroke and death in the range of ~11% [57, 59]. These risks are directly related to patient age with children under 1 year experiencing complication rates of up to 85%, while older patients >2 years of age experience complication rates closer to 33% [57, 59]. Following treatment of AVFs, patients should be monitored

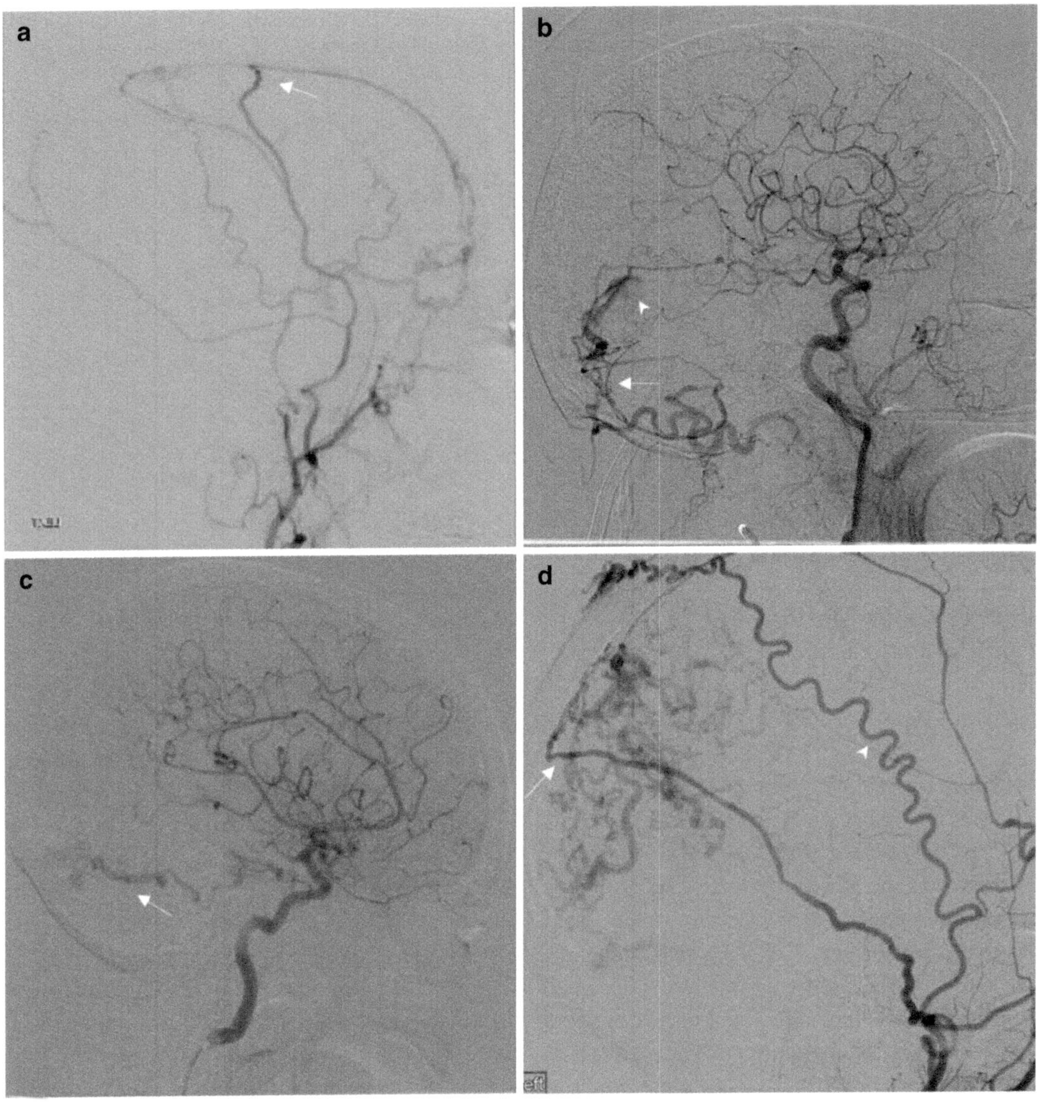

Fig. 10.1 (**a**) Left external carotid injection demonstrates a Borden type I and Cognard type I dural AVF with branches from the left middle meningeal artery draining into the superior sagittal sinus with antegrade flow (arrow). (**b**) A left common carotid artery injection demonstrates a Borden type II and Cognard type IIa + b dAVF with transosseous supply from the left occipital artery to the transverse sinus with retrograde flow into the straight sinus (arrowhead) and associated cortical venous reflux (arrows). (**c**) Right internal carotid artery injection demonstrates a right tentorial Borden type III, Cognard type III dAVF with arterial feeders from the right artery of Bernasconi and Cassinari, and the petrous branch of the right middle meningeal artery draining into cortical veins (arrow) of the right cerebellar hemisphere. (**d**) Left external carotid artery injection demonstrates a Borden type III and Cognard type IV dAVF with bilateral posterior auricular artery feeders draining directly into cortical veins (arrow) with retrograde venous flow, cortical venous reflux, and venous ectasia, ultimately connected to the right transverse sinus. There are also arterial feeders from the left STA which appears enlarged on angiography (arrowhead)

Table 10.3 Borden and Cognard classification schemes for intracranial dural AV fistulas. Adapted from Reynolds et al., 2017 [41], and Nerva et al., in Dumont, Lanzino, and Sheehan, 2017 [165]

Borden	*Cognard*	Venous drainage	Direction of flow	Cortical venous reflux (CVR)	Others
I	*I*	Dural venous sinus	*Antegrade*	No CVR	
	IIa	Dural venous sinus	*Retrograde*	No CVR	
II	*IIb*	Dural venous sinus	*Antegrade*	**With CVR**	
	IIa + b	Dural venous sinus	*Retrograde*	**With CVR**	
III	*III*	**Directly into cortical veins**	*Retrograde*	**With CVR**	
	IV	**Directly into cortical veins**	*Retrograde*	**With CVR**	With venous ectasia
	V	Directly into spinal perimedullary veins			

for development of hydrocephalus, which may be a result of venous thrombosis, altered venous outflow, or deranged CSF dynamics.

Vein of Galen Malformations (VOGMs)

Background

VOGMs are high-flow arteriovenous shunts of the developing choroidal system that drain into the median prosencephalic vein, the embryonic precursor of the vein of Galen. VOGMs are the most common and severe neonatal brain vascular malformation [60, 61]. They are congenital, high-flow lesions characterized by fistulous connection between the choroidal arteries and a persistent embryonic median prosencephalic vein (MPV) of Markowski, the embryonic precursor to the vein of Galen. During normal development, choroidal and subependymal arteries are connected to the MPV through an intervening capillary network. Direct, persistent connection of choroidal arteries to the MPV defines VOGMs [62]. Lasjaunias defined two types of VOGMs, the choroidal type with numerous feeding vessels from the choroidal arteries and an "interposed network before opening into [a] large venous pouch" [62] and a mural type with fewer vessels of larger caliber and "direct arteriovenous fistulas to the wall of the MPV" [62]. Choroidal VOGMs are more common and more severe, whereas mural VOGMs are better tolerated with fewer cardiac symptoms and higher clinical scores [63].

Clinical Features

Neonates may present with high-output cardiac failure, hydrocephalus, or brain hemorrhage, often in association with congenital heart defects [61]. In a series of 55 VOGMs, Duran et al. reported that 62% of cases were diagnosed before the first month of life, 62% of patients presented with high-output cardiac failure, 64% had macrocephaly, 60% had hydrocephalus, and 49% had prominent face and/or scalp vasculature [63].

Presentation

VOGM may be diagnosed prenatally on fetal ultrasound or may be present with congestive heart failure in the neonate. The Bicêtre neonatal evaluation score, proposed by Lasjaunias in 2006 [62], is a clinical score that stratifies prognosis and helps guide treatment decisions (Table 10.4). Patients with a score of less than 8 have severe systemic manifestations and a poor prognosis. Unless their score improves with medical management in the critical care unit, intervention is unlikely to improve their outcome. Neonates with a score between 8 and 12 are most likely to benefit from emergent embolization in order to prevent progression of systemic manifestations. A score of greater than 12 suggests the neonate is stable enough to delay treatment and continue medical management of their cardiopulmonary insufficiency. The score may vary from 1 day to the next in response to, or failure of, medical management and should be monitored closely.

Table 10.4 Bicêtre neonatal evaluation score. The total score out of 21 helps guide treatment decisions. A score of <8 suggests a poor prognosis, and the patient is unlikely to benefit from treatment. A score of 8–12 is most likely to benefit from emergent embolization. A score of 12–21 suggests the neonate is stable enough to delay treatment and continue medical management until at least 5 months of age unless the score drops to less than 12 in the interim [62] (Adapted from Lasjaunias et al., 2006 [62])

Points	Cardiac	Cerebral	Respiratory	Hepatic	Renal
5	Normal	Normal	Normal	–	–
4	Overload, no treatment required	Subclinical, isolated EEG abnormalities	Tachypnea, finishes bottle	–	–
3	Congestive heart failure, stable with treatment	Nonconvulsive, intermittent neurologic signs	Tachypnea, does not finish bottle	Normal	Normal
2	Congestive heart failure, not stable with treatment	Isolated convulsion	Assisted ventilation, normal SaO2, FiO2 < 25%	Hepatomegaly, normal function	Transient anuria
1	Ventilator support required	Seizures	Assisted ventilation, normal SaO2, FiO2 > 25%	Moderate or transient hepatic insufficiency	Oligura requiring treatment
0	Resistant to medical therapy	Permanent neurologic deficit	Assisted ventilation, desaturation	Coagulopathy, elevated liver enzymes	Anuria

Treatment for infants who maintain a score of 12–21 should be delayed until approximately 5 months, when Lasjaunias suggests the "balance best the maximum efficacy of embolization against the minimum risk of cerebral maturation delay [62]." In a large meta-analysis, treatment of neonates was associated with increased complications compared to treatment of infants [64]. In the interim patients who do not respond to ICU management, experience failure to thrive, or progressive symptoms should be treated. More recently, with advances in fetal imaging, biomarkers on fetal and neonatal MRI have also been used to predict clinical decompensation. Particularly associated with the physiologic stresses and changes surrounding birth, the narrowest medio-lateral diameter of the draining venous sinus is associated with the likelihood for neonatal clinical decompensation and need for intervention [65].

Hydrocephalus and macrocrania are the most common presenting symptoms in infants who were not previously diagnosed [64]. Hydrocephalus may develop due to elevated venous pressure and loss of the transmural gradient that normally drives CSF resorption [62]. Thrombosis or stenosis of deep draining veins such as the jugular bulb may contribute to elevated venous pressures as well [62, 66, 67]. Treatment of the VOGM typically resolves the hydrocephalus due to resolution of the pressure gradient [62, 64]. CSF shunting prior to treatment of the VOGM is dangerous and may increase the risk of intracranial hemorrhage, seizures, or other neurologic deficits [62]. Most patients will not require further CSF diversion after treatment or if they do it may only be for several months until CSF dynamics improve. In some cases, endoscopic third ventriculostomy is a durable option that can avoid the need for a shunt [62]. Other signs and symptoms include dilated scalp veins, proptosis, and neurocognitive delay [68].

Genetics

VOGMs have been reported in congenital cases of CM-AVM1 (RASA1 mutations) and CM-AVM2 (EPHB4 mutations), accounting for approximately 30% of VOGMs [63, 69]. CM-AVM is transmitted with incomplete penetrance and variable expressivity, with first-degree relatives of affected offspring with VOGMs often having only mild cutaneous vascular lesions [28, 63, 70]. Additionally, two cases of VOGM associated with HHT have been reported [71, 72]. Duran and colleagues identified additional damaging mutations in KEL, CLDN14, and intolerant chromatin modifier genes KMT2D, SMARCA2, SIRT1, and KAT6A, representing newly associated genetic mutations that may drive the disease process [73] (see Table 10.2).

Treatment

Endovascular therapy is the mainstay of treatment for VOGMs. Surgical clipping of the fistulous connection led to unacceptably high mortality rates of greater than 50% [74]. More than 60% of patients who undergo endovascular embolization of their VOGM have good long-term clinical outcomes, and this may be higher in well-selected patients and appropriate ICU management [64]. Arterial embolization of feeding arteries via transfemoral access in most cases. In some cases, due to the contrast dose limitations in neonates, serial embolization separated by several days to a week may be required [75, 76]. The goal of initial embolization is not complete obliteration of the lesion but adequate control of the arteriovenous shunt to prevent worsening cerebral and systemic complications. Complete disappearance of the VOGM may be achieved at follow-up despite persistent flow at the end of embolization [62, 77]. Venous embolization may be required in lesions with innumerable feeding vessels or otherwise difficult to treat lesions. Venous embolization has been associated with an increased risk of hemorrhage, but satisfactory results have also been reported [62].

Outcomes

In the Bicêtre series of 216 patients who underwent endovascular treatment, 74% were neurologically normal at follow-up, and 15% had moderate neurocognitive delay [62]. The Bicêtre admission and outcome score are graded from 0 (death) to 5 (normal) based on neurological and non-neurological symptoms and can be used for long-term follow-up and evaluation of patients with VOGMs [62] (see Table 10.5). Lasjaunias and the Bicêtre neurologists recommend the Denver test and Brunet-Lezine tests for neurocognitive evaluation and long-term follow-up [62, 76].

Table 10.5 Bicêtre admission and outcome score used for short- and long-term follow-up of patients with vein of Galen malformations (Adapted from Lasjaunias et al., 2006 [62])

Score	Neurologic status	Systemic condition
5	Normal	
4	Minimal neurologic signs	Asymptomatic enlargement of the cardiac silhouette
5	Transient neurologic signs	Asymptomatic cardiac overload under treatment
2	Permanent minor neurologic signs/ symptoms, cognitive delay of <20%, normal school nonpermanent neurologic symptoms under treatment	Normal school with support, congestive heart failure stabilized with treatment
1	Severe neurologic deficits, cognitive delay of >20% specialized school	Congestive heart failure unstable despite treatment
0	Death	–

However, even large series can be subject to referral bias or selection bias. With more established treatment paradigms, care for VOGM has tended to concentrate at referral centers, and recent series have more thoroughly captured the burden of disease, including those patients not considered for treatment. However, even recent experiences at national referral centers in Europe find that late termination of pregnancy, fetal death, or neonatal death may reach 55% [78–80]. Morbidity is particularly concentrated in the children who have neonatal decompensation, with severe long-term neurocognitive deficits in 50% of children who require neonatal treatment, compared to 30% of children who are stable for several months before elective treatment [78–80].

Dural Sinus Malformations (DSMs)

Background

Dural sinus malformations (DSMs) are a distinct entity within the subgroup of pediatric dural arteriovenous shunts (DAVS). DSMs are rare disorders, with only a few small case series reported

[81–85]. DSMs are divided into two types, and they are high-flow arteriovenous shunts with large venous dural lakes that involve the posterior sinuses with or without the torcular or a single-hole mural arteriovenous fistula involving the jugular bulb and sigmoid sinus [81, 83].

Clinical Characteristics

DSMs are a rare disease with a dural sinus malformation (DSM) high mortality rate [83]. They are high-flow lesions diagnosed prenatally on ultrasound or present with macrocrania, seizures, hydrocephalus, intracranial hemorrhage, or congestive heart failure (see Table 10.6). Barbosa et al. reported the largest series of 30 DSMs and found a 2:1 ratio of male-to-female patients, the majority of which were diagnosed prenatally or in the perinatal period [83]. Only 27% of cases were diagnosed in infants over 1 year of age. Early torcular thrombosis before adequate venous drainage through the cavernous sinus, or cavernous sinus capture, was highly correlated with poor neurologic outcome. In fact, only 29% of patients with torcular involvement had a favorable neurologic outcome, while 81% of patients without torcular involvement had a favorable outcome [83].

Treatment

Barbosa et al. reported that 47% of patients in their series were managed conservatively and 53% underwent endovascular embolization [83]. Conversely, 64% of the patients who did not undergo intervention had irreversible poor neurologic outcome, while 19% of patients who underwent embolization had unfavorable neurologic outcomes suggesting a role for intervention in these cases [83]. They found that patients with DSMs that do not involve the torcula and have a patent dural sinus malformation (DSM) cavernous sinus that drains the Sylvian veins, absence of jugular bulb dysmaturation and absence of reflux had the most favorable neurologic outcomes and benefited the most from endovascular intervention [83]. Their treatment of choice was partial endovascular transarterial embolization of mural feeders that supplied the shunt [83].

Table 10.6 Clinical presentations of dural sinus malformations. Data from Barbosa et al., 2013 [83]

Clinical features	% (of 30 patients)
Macrocrania	76.7%
Intracranial hemorrhage	26.7%
Hydrocephalus	26.7%
Seizures	23.3%
Psychomotor delay	23.3%
Congestive heart failure	20.0%

Cerebral Proliferative Angiopathy (CPA)

Background

Cerebral proliferative angiopathy (CPA) is an arteriovenous malformation of the brain characterized by a diffuse vascular network with normal intervening brain parenchyma and a moderate to slow arteriovenous shunt often involving multiple lobes or an entire hemisphere [86]. While CPA shares some similarities with AVMs, CPA has distinct angioarchitectural, pathological, and clinical characteristics [86].

Imaging Characteristics

CPA is a non-focal vascular malformation with a large, diffuse, dense vascular network with normal intervening parenchyma, often involving multiple lobes. Most frequently the frontal and temporal lobes are involved, but the whole hemisphere may be affected in up to 73% of cases [87], including rare cases of bilateral hemispheric disease [86, 87]. There are no dominant feeding arteries, and there draining veins are small in relation to the size of the lesion [86, 87].

There is an absence of dominant feeders on angiography in all cases [86]. Counterintuitively, approximately one third of cases have proximal artery stenosis of the ICA, MCA, or ACA [86, 87]. "Puddling" of contrast within capillary ectasias is characteristic [86]. Venous congestion and delayed venous drainage of distant brain parenchyma may be seen [86].

CPA causes severe oligemia, ischemia, and impaired vascular reserve. Fierstra et al. recruited four patients with CPA and measured BOLD signal in a 3T MRI machine while titrating the end-tidal PCO2 to measure cerebrovascular reactivity (CVR) and found severely limited cerebrovascular reserve [88]. Ducreux et al. and Vargas and Castillo reported similar findings with MR perfusion demonstrating increased time to peak and decreased relative cerebral blood flow and relative cerebral blood volume in brain parenchyma surrounding the lesion [89, 90]. Similar findings with single-photon emission computed tomography (SPECT) were reported by Kimiwada et al. [91].

Clinical Features

In Lasjaunias' large series of brain vascular malformations, CPA was diagnosed in 1.2% of all 4058 cases [62]. Overall, 67% of patients with CPA were young females with an average age of 22 years [86].

Although structural features of CPA may resemble brain AVMs, the clinical presentation and natural history diverge from other AVMs that are seen more commonly. Seizures were the presenting symptom in 45% of cases, while 41% had severe headaches, 16% had stroke-like symptoms or other neurologic deficits, and only 12% presented with hemorrhage [86]. Patients who present with hemorrhage are more likely to have recurrent hemorrhages compared to patients with AVMs [86, 87, 92]. Although only 12–18% of patients with CPA present with intracranial hemorrhage [86, 87] compared to approximately 50% for AVMs [93], the rate of recurrent hemorrhage in CPA is significantly higher, estimated at approximately 67% [86, 87] compared to 4.5% for AVMs [12, 13].

The natural history of CPA is not well understood. Aggressive lesions causing recurrent hemorrhage and death [94, 95] have been reported, as well as cases of conservative management with good outcomes [91, 96]. The only angiographic risk factor for initial development of intracranial hemorrhage was proximal artery stenosis [86, 97]. TIA, stroke-like symptoms, and seizures are common and related to the ischemic nature of the disease [86, 98].

Genetics and Pathophysiology

Cerebral ischemia may be an angiogenic factor in proliferation of the lesion [89, 90]. Up to 70% of CPA lesions involve a watershed zone, which may support this theory of ischemic/oligemic induced proliferation [87]. The rarity of the disorder has a limited genetic study to date.

Treatment

Conservative management has been reported with mixed results [98]. Some groups have treated patients with either antiepileptic drugs, acetazolamide, or supportive management with good results [91, 99, 100], while others have reported progression of disease, intracranial hemorrhage, and death [94, 95, 101]. Due to normal intervening brain parenchyma, surgery and neurointerventional radiosurgery may cause permanent neurological deficits [86]. Lasjaunias et al. reported partial embolization for the treatment of intractable headaches and epilepsy with good results [86, 102]. In two patients, they performed multiple burr holes for indirect revascularization with good results at 3–5 years of follow-up [86]. Indirect revascularizations including encephalomyosynangiosis and encephaloduroarteriosynangiosis have been reported by several groups [94, 103–106] and reviewed by Somji et al. [98] but in general is a very rarely used approach reserved for extreme circumstances.

CPA is a rare disease with only 95 cases reported in the literature [87]. The heterogeneity of the natural history of the disease and small number of case reports and case series in the literature limit the data available to direct treatment decisions. Conservative management has been reported in some cases with good results, while partial embolization or indirect revascularization may be an option for patients with severe or intractable symptoms. Radiosurgery and direct revascularization have not been well described for the treatment of CPA. Consequently, most management of this unusual condition remains on a case-by-case basis [98].

Cerebral Cavernous Malformations (CCMs)

Background

Cerebral cavernous malformations (CCMs, cavernous angiomas, hemangiomas, cavernomas) are slow-flow vascular lesions of the central nervous system composed of a compact nidus of thin-walled sinusoidal vessels without intervening parenchyma. They are well-circumscribed unencapsulated masses with an irregular “mulberry” appearance. Calcifications may be present, both grossly and microscopically. Cysts containing old hemorrhage products may develop, and surrounding parenchyma may be gliotic with hemosiderin stains causing a green, yellow, or brown discoloration [107].

Epidemiology

Disease prevalence is approximately 0.16–0.6% [108, 109], with an estimated annual incidence of 0.56 per 100,000 [110]. CCMs occur sporadically, in a familial form, or may develop de novo including after radiation therapy [111]. Twenty-eight percent [112] to 47% [113] of CCMs are asymptomatic lesions found incidentally. Symptomatic patients present with intracranial hemorrhage (35–62%), seizures (20–35%), or focal neurologic deficit without evidence of recent hemorrhage (15%) [112, 114]. Multiple CCMs occur in approximately 10–30% of cases but are characteristic of patients with familial disease [109, 113]. Patients with multiple lesions should be considered for genetic screening, and first-degree relatives or family members with neurologic symptoms including headaches should be considered for screening MRI studies [115]. Familial CCMs have an autosomal dominant inheritance pattern with incomplete penetrance, and the diagnosis can be confirmed by genetic testing for loss-of-function mutations in CCM1 (KRIT1), CCM2 (MGC4607), or CCM3 (PDCD10) [116, 117].

Presentation

In pediatric patients, the annual risk of hemorrhage is approximately 0.5% for incidental CCMs [114]. Prior hemorrhage is a statistically significant risk factor for subsequent hemorrhage, and the annual rate of a subsequent hemorrhage is approximately 11% [114] and is the highest in the first 2–3 years after hemorrhage [114, 118]. Developmental venous anomalies (DVAs) are often associated with CCMs and were recently reported in 38% of 731 cases [119]. Patients with spinal CMs and familial CCMs do not usually present with associated DVAs [120]. The impact of associated DVAs on bleeding or re-bleeding risk has been debated with conflicting reports in the literature. During a 5-year follow-up, Chen et al. found a decreased risk of symptomatic ICH and no difference in re-hemorrhage rate in patients with CCM and an associated DVA compared to those without [119]. When a DVA is present and surgery is indicated, the DVA should generally be preserved when possible to minimize the risk of venous infarction.

Imaging Characteristics

CMs are hyperdense on CT resembling a focus of blood products but may have mixed or minimal enhancement with contrast. On MRI they have a heterogeneous “popcorn” appearance with a surrounding T2 hypointense rim and blooming artifact on SWI. They typically do not enhance substantially with gadolinium. However, the commonly associated DVA, discussed later, is often visible on contrast-enhanced sequences.

Treatment

Surgical resection is typically indicated when CCMs present with symptoms and are located in non-eloquent cortex or spinal cord, and/or there is documented radiographic enlargement or hemorrhage [115, 121]. Lesions in eloquent cortex or in the brainstem may be observed even after an initial hemorrhage given the surgical risk associated with these hard-to-access lesions which require careful and thorough discussion with patients and their families to identify the appropriate risk-benefit tolerance for each patient. However, if a pattern of recurrent hemorrhage develops, surgical intervention is usually indicated. Deep lesions that are surgically inaccessible may be observed and treated symptomatically and/or referred for radiosurgery.

After microsurgical resection, CMs can recur if not excised completely and may be more likely to recur in familial or radiation-induced cases [107]. In 79 consecutive patients with CCMs in eloquent and deep supratentorial locations, complete resection was achieved in 96% and 98% of cases, respectively, with improved or unchanged neurologic status in 97% of patients at 6 months postoperatively [122]. In most patients, a postoperative MRI at 6 weeks to 6 months is used as a new baseline, and patients are typically followed with yearly MRIs for 2–5 years [107].

Outcomes

In a meta-analysis of 1226 cases, 75% of patients were seizure-free after microsurgical resection [123]. Indicators of a favorable outcome included CCM size <1.5 cm, single CCMs, medically controlled seizures, and the lack of secondarily generalized seizures [123]. In 168 patients, Baumann et al. reported an Engel class I rate of 70% (48% IA) 1 year after surgical resection [124]. Predictors for long-term disability include age ≥12 years, ≥2 preoperative hemorrhages, and poor preoperative neurologic status [125].

Developmental Venous Anomalies (DVAs)

Background

DVAs are the most common cerebral vascular malformation accounting for approximately 5–10% of intracranial lesions [126]. They are a collection of small veins draining normal brain parenchyma and converging into a dilated venous trunk that may reverse the typical deep or superficial drainage pattern of parenchyma [127] (Fig. 10.2).

Imaging Characteristics

On cross-sectional imaging, DVAs are best seen on contrast-enhanced CT or T1 MRI scans. SWI can show venous architecture and identify an enlarged draining vein and, if present, can help identify any associated CCM. Underlying white matter changes in adjacent brain parenchyma may be seen on T2-weighted or FLAIR sequences in approximately 7.8–12.5% of cases and may be due to venous hypertension, edema, and gliosis [127, 128].

Clinical Characteristics

DVAs are low-flow, low-resistance lesions that are typically benign and asymptomatic and do not warrant treatment [127, 129]. They may be isolated or associated with cerebral cavernous malformations (CCMs) [119]. When associated with CCMs, they should be preserved at the time of surgery [130]. They are thought to arise from errors in venous development prena-

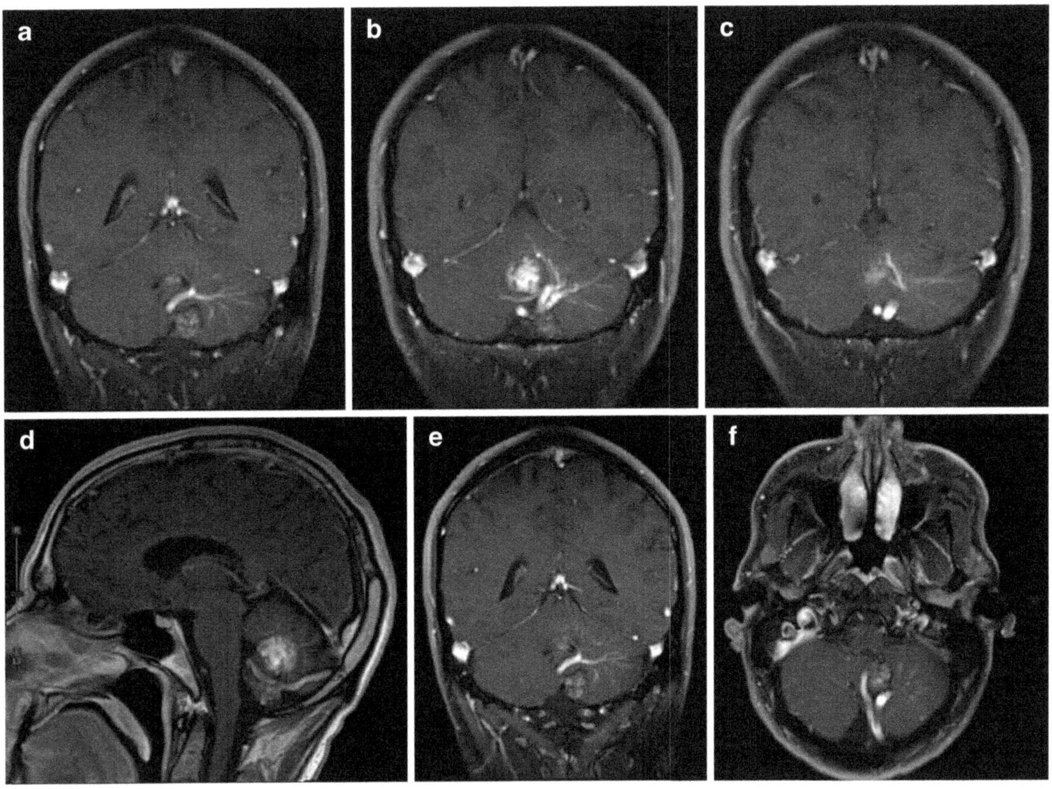

Fig. 10.2 (**a–c**) Anterior to posterior serial coronal slices of a midline cerebellar cavernous malformation with associated developmental venous anomaly (DVA) in the posterior fossa draining the left cerebellar hemisphere. The DVA has a classic "spoke-wheel pattern" and drains normal cerebellar parenchyma. Representative sagittal (**d**), coronal (**e**), and axial (**f**) slices are shown

tally, but their causal or secondary relationship to CCMs is unclear [127, 131]. Rarely, headaches, seizures, neurologic deficit, or hemorrhage may occur due to venous hypertension, and treatment may be indicated for symptomatic management, *developmental venous anomalies (DVAs)*, which may involve treatment of any upstream shunting pathology or downstream secondary pathophysiology such as hydrocephalus [132, 133]. Venous thrombosis has been reported in rare cases and required management with anticoagulation [134]. However, resection of DVAs has historically been associated with severe neurologic deficit, while their natural history is typically benign [129, 135].

Spinal Cord Vascular Malformations (SCVM)

Background

Spinal cord vascular malformations (SCVMs) are rare, with an estimated incidence of spinal arteriovenous shunts of 0.177 per 100,000 person-years [136]. Pediatric SCVMs are even more rare—in a series of 1168 spinal vascular malformations, only 72 (6.2%) occurred in children under 14 years of age [137]. SCVMs are a heterogeneous group of lesions that include cavernous malformations, arteriovenous malformations, spinal aneurysms, and spinal dural arteriovenous fistulas [137, 138]. Some SCVMs are associated with hereditary or syndromic conditions including hereditary hemorrhagic telangiectasia (Osler-Weber-Rendu disease), Klippel-Trenaunay disease, and Cobb syndrome [137–139].

Classification

Spinal arteriovenous shunts can be classified as extradural, intradural dorsal, intradural ventral, intramedullary, extradural-intradural, or conus medullaris AVMs [140, 141]. Juvenile or metameric AVMs are extradural-intradural lesions that may involve the muscle, bone, spinal cord, and nerve roots at a given dermatome or dermatomes [140].

Natural History

SCVMs may present with pain, myelopathy, or acute paralysis. Hemorrhage may occur within the spinal cord or subarachnoid spaces. Some series suggest a higher rate of spinal cord hemorrhage in pediatric patients compared to adults [138, 142]. Treatment often involves endovascular embolization or surgery, but rarely radiosurgery may be considered [143]. With treatment, recurrent hemorrhage is, rare and improvement may be seen in more than 70% of patients [138]. Incompletely treated lesions, however, may rebleed and cause neurologic decline [143].

Conclusion

Pediatric vascular malformations are a diverse group of lesions that require a thoughtful, tailored approach to treatment and management. Many pediatric vascular malformations are congenital and have a specific pathogenetic mechanism. It is important to carefully characterize the angioarchitectural features, biological behavior, clinical manifestations, treatment options, natural history, and outcomes when evaluating a pediatric vascular malformation. Arteriovenous shunting may be common in high-flow lesions and in some may be life-threatening. The risk of rupture, re-rupture, seizure, or other associated neurologic deficits are important factors to consider in determining treatment options. Surgery, radiosurgery, endovascular embolization, or conservative management are common treatment options, but certain lesions may be best managed with one modality or another. In some cases, the natural history of the disease may be more benign than the treatment itself. In others, surgical or endovascular intervention must be undertaken emergently to save the patient's life.

Review Questions

1. What is the rate of re-rupture for a hemorrhagic AVM in the first year?
   A. 2–4%
   B. 6–15%
   C. 18–27%
   D. 36–42%

   Answer: **B**—The re-rupture rate in the first year after initial presentation of a ruptured AVM ranges from 6 to 15.8% [13]. Although, the overall rate of re-hemorrhage for AVMs is 4.5% [6], the rate is higher during the first year after initial hemorrhage. Furthermore, the rate is highest in the first month after rupture and decreases with time from initial hemorrhage [166]. Approximately 66% of AVMs that re-rupture in the first year are associated with intranidal or perinidal aneurysms [13]. Additionally, the morbidity and mortality associated with re-rupture is higher than that associated with initial hemorrhage [13].

   The rate of hemorrhage for unruptured AVMs is approximately 2-4% [6, 4, 35].
2. What feature is *NOT* associated with AVM rupture risk?
   A. Deep AVM location
   B. Associated aneurysm
   C. Exclusively deep venous drainage
   D. Size >3 cm
   E. Prior hemorrhage

   Answer: **D**—Gross and Du 2013 performed a meta-analysis of nine studies including, patients and looked at risk factors for rupture risk in AVMs. They found that "prior hemorrhage (HR 3.2, 95% CI 2.1–4.3), deep AVM location (HR 2.4, 95% CI 1.4–3.4), exclusively deep venous drainage (HR 2.4, 95% CI 1.1–3.8), and associated aneurysms (HR 1.8, 95% CI 1.6–2.0) were statistically significant risk factors for hemorrhage." [6] Interestingly, age, gender and size of the AVM were not associated with rupture risk.

3. Which gene is implicated in the pathogenesis of AVMs in hereditary hemorrhagic telangiectasia type I (HHT1)?
   A. KRIT1
   B. EPHB4
   C. ENG
   D. PDCD10
   E. ALK1

   Answer: **C**—HHT1 is associated with mutations in endoglin (ENG). Endoglin codes for a component of the transforming growth factor-beta (TGFB) receptor complex which is highly expressed by endothelial cells and binds TGFB1 [167]. Patients with HHT who develop intracranial AVMs experience a rupture rate of approximately 1.02% per-year [26].

   KRIT1 is associated with CCM1, EPHB4 is associated with CM-AVM2, PDCD10 is associated with CCM3, and ALK1 is associated with HHT2.

4. A 12 year old girl presents with headaches and first time seizure. She is otherwise healthy, takes no medications and denies any known drug allergies. Her parents state that she was playing with her brother when she developed sudden jerking movements of the right arm which then generalized to full body convulsions with loss of consciousness. The episode lasted 2–3 min and the patient suffered from grogginess, disorientation and mild right sided weakness that slowly improved over the course of 1–2 h. In the Emergency department she has no focal neurologic deficits, but endorses mild to moderate headaches 3–4/10 improved with Tylenol. CT of the head demonstrates a 2 × 3 cm left frontoparietal hemorrhage. What is the most likely diagnosis? Describe the initial management of this patient.
   A. Arteriovenous malformation
   B. Pial arteriovenous fistula
   C. Cerebral proliferative angiopathy
   D. Cavernous malformation

   Answer: **A**—AVMs are the most common cause of pediatric stroke and intracranial hemorrhage, and a child who presents with a new, fist-time seizure and an intracranial hemorrhage most likely has a ruptured AVM. It is important to note that the severity of the patients presentation can alter the treatment plan which has to be individually tailored. On initial evaluation a ruptured AVM should be considered high on the differential and a CT angiogram may be helpful in the acute setting to identify the presence of dilated vessels nidus and drainage pattern. Exclusively deep venous drainage or intranidal or perinidal aneurysms may encourage urgent or emergent treatment. Patients with good neurologic status and no high risk features on CTA can be managed conservatively for 1–2 weeks prior to intervention to allow the clot to resorb and improve the chance of successful resection. If no clear lesion is found, repeat imaging in 4–6 weeks with MRI should be performed to evaluate the hemorrhage cavity after the clot has cleared. Initial ICU management of a ruptured AVM includes the following:

   - Access: 2 Large bore IVs, arterial line, foley catheter, airway intubation if the patient is unable to protect his or her airway, and orogastric or nasogastric tube if intubated.
   - Blood pressure control: IV push labetolol or continuous IV nicardipine drip with goal of normotension for age.
   - ICP control: external ventricular drain if hydrocephalus (avoid over drainage of CSF to prevent re-rupture, often no more than 5 cc at a time), elevate the head of the bed.
   - Seizures: Anti-epileptic medication if concern for seizure.

5. A 4-year-old girl presents with sudden onset paraparesis. Spine MRI/MRA demonstrates a juvenile-type intradural-extradural AVM from thoracic vertebrae 8–10 and involving surrounding soft tissue, ribs and vertebral body. On secondary examination, multiple small, red dermal lesions were noted on the patient's skin. She underwent spinal angiography with Onyx embolization of epidural feeders and a large pedicle to the nidus involving the right T8-10 ribs and vertebral bodies. However, residual shunting was seen and the patient underwent a second embolization procedure with complete obliteration. She had persistent imbalance and gait impairment but significant improvement in strength and mobility and 2 year follow up. What syndrome is associated with this presentation?
   A. Parkes Weber syndrome
   B. Cobb syndrome
   C. Klippel Feil syndrome
   D. Foix-Alajouanine syndrome
   Answer: **B**—Cobb syndrome is a rare, non-hereditary, sporadic syndrome that presents with metameric, juvenile-type spinal AVMs and cutaneous lesions including vascular nevi [139, 168]. Other skin lesions may occur including port-wine stains, angiomas, angiolipomas and lymphangiomas [139]. In this case the presentation of a metameric spinal AVM with vascular nevi is consistent with a diagnosis of Cobb syndrome.

   Foix-Alajounaine syndrome is a rare cause of spinal AVMs that occurs in patients 50 years of age or older and presents with lower thoracolumbar radicular pain and slowly progressive paraplegia [169]. Parkes Weber syndrome presents with capillary malformations, venous malformation and arteriovenous malformations characteristically occurring in a limb and causing severe overgrowth of the affected appendage [170]. Parkes Weber syndrome is associated with RASA1 mutations and may be seen in patients with CM-AVM 1 [171]. Klippel-Feil syndrome is a congenital fusion of the upper cervical vertebral bodies and is not associated with spinal cord vascular malformations [172].

References

1. Perry A, Brat DJ. Practical surgical neuropathology: a diagnostic approach. Philadelphia: Churchill Livingstone/Elsevier; 2010.
2. Derdeyn CP, Zipfel GJ, Albuquerque FC, Cooke DL, Feldmann E, Sheehan JP, Torner JC. Management of brain arteriovenous malformations: a scientific statement for healthcare professionals from the American Heart Association/American Stroke Association. Stroke. 2017;48:e200–24.
3. Jordan LC, Kleinman JT, Hillis AE. Intracerebral hemorrhage volume predicts poor neurologic outcome in children. Stroke. 2009;40:1666–71.
4. Hernesniemi JA, Dashti R, Juvela S, Väärt K, Niemelä M, Laakso A. Natural history of brain arteriovenous malformations: a long-term follow-up study of risk of hemorrhage in 238 patients. Neurosurgery. 2008;63:823–9.
5. Can A, Gross BA, Du R. The natural history of cerebral arteriovenous malformations. Handb Clin Neurol. 2017;143:15–24.
6. Gross BA, Du R. Natural history of cerebral arteriovenous malformations: a meta-analysis. J Neurosurg. 2013;118:437–43.
7. Stapf C, Mast H, Sciacca RR, Choi JH, Khaw AV, Connolly ES, Pile-Spellman J, Mohr JP. Predictors of hemorrhage in patients with untreated brain arteriovenous malformation. Neurology. 2006;66:1350–5.
8. Kim H, Al-Shahi Salman R, McCulloch CE, Stapf C, Young WL. Untreated brain arteriovenous malformation: patient-level meta-analysis of hemorrhage predictors. Neurology. 2014;83:590–7.
9. Garzelli L, Shotar E, Blauwblomme T, Sourour N, Alias Q, Stricker S, Mathon B, Kossorotoff M, Gariel F, Boddaert N, et al. Risk factors for early brain AVM rupture: cohort study of pediatric and adult patients. Am J Neuroradiol. 2020;41:2358–63.
10. Redekop G, Terbrugge K, Montanera W, Wwillinsky R. Arterial aneurysms associated with cerebral arteriovenous malformations: classification, incidence, and risk of hemorrhage. J Neurosurg. 1998;89:539–46.
11. Platz J, Berkefeld J, Singer OC, Wolff R, Seifert V, Konczalla J, Güresir E. Frequency, risk of hemorrhage and treatment considerations for cerebral arteriovenous malformations with associated aneurysms. Acta Neurochir (Wien). 2014;156:2025–34.
12. Mast H, Young WL, Koennecke H-C, Sciacca RR, Osipov A, Pile-Spellman J, Hacein-Bey L, Duong H, Stein BM, Mohr JP. Risk of spontaneous haemorrhage after diagnosis of cerebral arteriovenous malformation. Lancet. 1997;350:1065–8.

13. Gross BA, Du R. Rate of re-bleeding of arteriovenous malformations in the first year after rupture. J Clin Neurosci. 2012;19:1087–8.
14. Gross BA, Frerichs KU, Du R. Sensitivity of CT angiography, T2-weighted MRI, and magnetic resonance angiography in detecting cerebral arteriovenous malformations and associated aneurysms. J Clin Neurosci. 2012;19:1093–5.
15. Lin N, Smith ER, Scott RM, Orbach DB. Safety of neuroangiography and embolization in children: complication analysis of 697 consecutive procedures in 394 patients. J Neurosurg Pediatr. 2015;16:432–8.
16. Mossa-Basha M, Chen J, Gandhi D. Imaging of cerebral arteriovenous malformations and dural arteriovenous fistulas. Neurosurg Clin N Am. 2012;23:27–42.
17. Elhadi AM, Zabramski JM, Almefty KK, Mendes GAC, Nakaji P, McDougall CG, Albuquerque FC, Preul MC, Spetzler RF. Spontaneous subarachnoid hemorrhage of unknown origin: hospital course and long-term clinical and angiographic follow-up. J Neurosurg. 2015;122:663–70.
18. Gross BA, Moon K, Mcdougall CG. Endovascular management of arteriovenous malformations. Handb Clin Neurol. 2017;143:59–68.
19. Borst AJ, Nakano TA, Blei F, Adams DM, Duis J. A primer on a comprehensive genetic approach to vascular anomalies. Front Pediatr. 2020;8:634.
20. Krings T, Ozanne A, Chng SM, Alvarez H, Rodesch G, Lasjaunias PL. Neurovascular phenotypes in hereditary haemorrhagic telangiectasia patients according to age. Review of 50 consecutive patients aged 1 day-60 years. Neuroradiology. 2005;47:711–20.
21. Krings T, Kim H, Power S, Nelson J, Faughnan ME, Young WL, terBrugge KG. Neurovascular manifestations in hereditary hemorrhagic telangiectasia: imaging features and genotype-phenotype correlations. AJNR Am J Neuroradiol. 2015;36:863–70.
22. Brinjikji W, Starke RM, Murad MH, Fiorella D, Pereira VM, Goyal M, Kallmes DF. Impact of balloon guide catheter on technical and clinical outcomes: a systematic review and meta-analysis. J Neurointerv Surg. 2018;10:335–9.
23. Bharatha A, Faughnan ME, Young WL, Terbrugge KG, Kim H, Pourmohamad T, Krings T, Bayrak-Toydemir P, Pawlikowska L, Mcculloch CE, et al. Brain arteriovenous malformation multiplicity predicts the diagnosis of hereditary hemorrhagic telangiectasia: quantitative assessment. Stroke. 2012;43:72–8.
24. Nishida T, Faughnan ME, Krings T, Chakinala M, Gossage JR, Young WL, Kim H, Pourmohamad T, Henderson KJ, Schrum SD, et al. Brain arteriovenous malformations associated with hereditary hemorrhagic telangiectasia: gene-phenotype correlations. Am J Med Genet A. 2012;158A:2829–34.
25. Faughnan ME, Mager JJ, Hetts SW, Palda VA, Lang-Robertson K, Buscarini E, Deslandres E, Kasthuri RS, Lausman A, Poetker D, et al. Second international guidelines for the diagnosis and management of hereditary hemorrhagic telangiectasia. Ann Intern Med. 2020;173:989–1001.
26. Kim H, Nelson J, Krings T, TerBrugge KG, McCulloch CE, Lawton MT, Young WL, Faughnan ME. Hemorrhage rates from brain arteriovenous malformation in hereditary hemorrhagic telangiectasia patients. Stroke. 2015;46:1362–4.
27. Latino GA, Al-Saleh S, Carpenter S, Ratjen F. The diagnostic yield of rescreening for arteriovenous malformations in children with hereditary hemorrhagic telangiectasia. J Pediatr. 2014;165:197–9.
28. Amyere M, Revencu N, Helaers R, Pairet E, Baselga E, Cordisco M, Chung W, Dubois J, Lacour J-P, Martorell L, et al. Germline loss-of-function mutations in EPHB4 cause a second form of capillary malformation-arteriovenous malformation (CM-AVM2) deregulating RAS-MAPK signaling. Circulation. 2017;136:1037–48.
29. Miyamoto S, Hashimoto N, Nagata I, Nozaki K, Morimoto M, Taki W, Kikuchi H. Posttreatment sequelae of palliatively treated cerebral arteriovenous malformations. Neurosurgery. 2000;46:589–94.
30. Darsaut TE, Guzman R, Marcellus ML, Edwards MS, Tian L, Do HM, Chang SD, Levy RP, Adler JR, Marks MP, et al. Management of pediatric intracranial arteriovenous malformations: experience with multimodality therapy. Neurosurgery. 2011;69:540–56.
31. Lee B-B, Do YS, Yakes W, Kim DI, Mattassi R, Hyon WS. Management of arteriovenous malformations: a multidisciplinary approach. J Vasc Surg. 2004;39:590–600.
32. Lv X, Wu Z, Li Y, Yang X, Jiang C. Hemorrhage risk after partial endovascular NBCA and ONYX embolization for brain arteriovenous malformation. Neurol Res (New York). 2012;34:552–6.
33. Karlsson B, Lax I, Söderman M. Risk for hemorrhage during the 2-year latency period following gamma knife radiosurgery for arteriovenous malformations. Int J Radiat Oncol Biol Phys. 2001;49:1045–51.
34. Winkler EA, Lu A, Morshed RA, Yue JK, Rutledge WC, Burkhardt J-K, Patel AB, Ammanuel SG, Braunstein S, Fox CK, et al. Bringing high-grade arteriovenous malformations under control: clinical outcomes following multimodality treatment in children. J Neurosurg Pediatr. 2020;26:1–10.
35. Mohr JP, Parides MK, Stapf C, Moquete E, Moy CS, Overbey JR, Salman RA-S, Vicaut E, Young WL, Houdart E, et al. Medical management with or without interventional therapy for unruptured brain arteriovenous malformations (ARUBA): a multicentre, non-blinded, randomised trial. Lancet (British Ed). 2014;383:614–21.
36. van Beijnum J, van der Worp HB, Buis DR, Salman RA-S, Kappelle LJ, Rinkel GJE, van der Sprenkel JWB, Vandertop WP, Algra A, Klijn CJM. Treatment of brain arteriovenous malformations: a systematic review and meta-analysis. JAMA. 2011;306:2011–9.

37. Russin J, Spetzler R. Commentary: the ARUBA trial. Neurosurgery. 2014;75:E96–7.
38. Vlak MH, Algra A, Brandenburg R, Rinkel GJ. Prevalence of unruptured intracranial aneurysms, with emphasis on sex, age, comorbidity, country, and time period: a systematic review and meta-analysis. Lancet Neurol. 2011;10:626–36.
39. Chen C-J, Lee C-C, Kano H, Kearns KN, Ding D, Tzeng S-W, Atik AF, Joshi K, Huang PP, Kondziolka D, et al. Radiosurgery for unruptured intervention-Naïve pediatric brain arteriovenous malformations. Neurosurgery. 2020;87:368–76.
40. Ma X, Tong X, Wu J, Cao Y, Wang S. Seizure control following treatment of brain arteriovenous malformations in pediatric patients. Childs Nerv Syst. 2016;32:2387–94.
41. Reynolds MR, Lanzino G, Zipfel GJ. Intracranial dural arteriovenous fistulae. Stroke. 2017;48:1424–31.
42. Yasargil MG. Microneurosurgery, Volume IIIA. AVM of the brain, history, embryology, pathological considerations, hemodynamics, diagnostic studies, microsurgical anatomy. 1987, Thieme, ISBN-10: 9780865772588.
43. Lasjaunias P, Manelfe C, Chiu M. Angiographic architecture of intracranial vascular malformations and fistulas-pretherapeutic aspects. Neurosurg Rev. 1986;9:253–63.
44. Newman CB, Hu YC, McDougall CG, Albuquerque FC. Balloon-assisted Onyx embolization of cerebral single-channel pial arteriovenous fistulas: technical note. J Neurosurg Pediatr. 2011;7:637–42.
45. Borden JA, Wu JK, Shucart WA. A proposed classification for spinal and cranial dural arteriovenous fistulous malformations and implications for treatment. J Neurosurg. 1995;82:166–79.
46. Cognard C, Gobin YP, Pierot L, Bailly A-L, Houdart E, Casasco A, Chiras J, Merland J-J. Cerebral dural arteriovenous fistulas: clinical and angiographic correlation with a revised classification of venous drainage. Radiology. 1995;194:671–80.
47. Zipfel GJ, Shah MN, Refai D, Dacey Ralph GJ, Derdeyn CP. Cranial dural arteriovenous fistulas: modification of angiographic classification scales based on new natural history data. Neurosurg Focus. 2009;26:E14.
48. Garcia-Monaco R, Taylor W, Rodesch G, Alvarez H, Burrows P, Coubes P, Lasjaunias P. Pial arteriovenous fistula in children as presenting manifestation of Rendu-Osler-Weber disease. Neuroradiology. 1995;37:60–4.
49. Walcott BP, Smith ER, Scott RM, Orbach DB. Pial arteriovenous fistulae in pediatric patients: associated syndromes and treatment outcome. J Neurointerv Surg. 2013;5:10–4.
50. Lawton MT, Jacobowitz R, Spetzler RF. Redefined role of angiogenesis in the pathogenesis of dural arteriovenous malformations. J Neurosurg. 1997;87:267–74.
51. Ferro JM, Coutinho JM, Jansen O, Bendszus M, Dentali F, Kobayashi A, van der Veen B, Miede C, Caria J, Huisman H, et al. Dural arteriovenous fistulae after cerebral venous thrombosis. Stroke. 2020;51:3344–7.
52. Hoh BL, Putman CM, Budzik RF, Ogilvy CS. Surgical and endovascular flow disconnection of intracranial pial single-channel arteriovenous fistulae. Neurosurgery. 2001;49:1351–64.
53. Zenteno M, Lee A, Satyarthee GD, Moscote-Salazar LR. Endovascular management of intracranial pial arteriovenous fistulas: experience of largest series at a single center over six years. J Neurosci Rural Pract. 2018;9:406–9.
54. Alurkar A, Karanam L, Nayak S, Ghanta R. Intracranial pial arteriovenous fistulae: diagnosis and treatment techniques in pediatric patients with review of literature. J Clin Imaging Sci. 2016;6:2.
55. Cuoco JA, Guilliams EL, Apfel LS, Marvin EA, Patel BM. Incidental pediatric high-flow nongalenic giant pial arteriovenous fistula. Neuropediatrics. 2021;52:65–8.
56. Jabbour P, Tjoumakaris S, Chalouhi N, Randazzo C, Gonzalez LF, Dumont A, Rosenwasser R. Endovascular treatment of cerebral dural and pial arteriovenous fistulas. Neuroimaging Clin N Am. 2013;23:625–36.
57. Hetts SW, Keenan K, Fullerton HJ, Young WL, English JD, Gupta N, Dowd CF, Higashida RT, Lawton MT, Halbach VV. Pediatric intracranial nongalenic pial arteriovenous fistulas: clinical features, angioarchitecture, and outcomes. AJNR Am J Neuroradiol. 2012;33:1710–9.
58. Walcott BP, Smith ER, Scott RM, Orbach DB. Dural arteriovenous fistulae in pediatric patients: associated conditions and treatment outcomes. J Neurointerv Surg. 2013;5:6–9.
59. Kraneburg UM, Nga VDW, Ting EYS, Hui FKH, Lwin S, Teo C, Chou N, Yeo TT. Intracranial pial arteriovenous fistula in infancy: a case report and literature review. Childs Nerv Syst. 2014;30:365–9.
60. Long DM, Seljeskog EL, Chou SN, French LA. Giant arteriovenous malformations of infancy and childhood. J Neurosurg. 1974;40:304–12.
61. Duran D, Karschnia P, Gaillard JR, Karimy JK, Youngblood MW, DiLuna ML, Matouk CC, Aagaard-Kienitz B, Smith ER, Orbach DB, et al. Human genetics and molecular mechanisms of vein of Galen malformation. J Neurosurg Pediatr. 2018;21:367–74.
62. Lasjaunias PL, Chng SM, Sachet M, Alvarez H, Rodesch G, Garcia-Monaco R. The management of vein of Galen aneurysmal malformations. Neurosurgery. 2006;59:S184–94.
63. Duran D, Zeng X, Jin SC, Choi J, Nelson-Williams C, Yatsula B, Gaillard J, Furey CG, Lu Q, Timberlake AT, et al. Mutations in chromatin modifier and ephrin signaling genes in vein of Galen malformation. Neuron. 2019;101:429–443.e4.
64. Brinjikji W, Krings T, Murad MH, Rouchaud A, Meila D. Endovascular treatment of vein of Galen malformations: a systematic review and meta-analysis. AJNR Am J Neuroradiol. 2017;38:2308–14.

65. Arko L, Lambrych M, Montaser A, Zurakowski D, Orbach DB. Fetal and neonatal MRI predictors of aggressive early clinical course in vein of Galen malformation. AJNR Am J Neuroradiol. 2020;41:1105–11.
66. Chang D, Babadjouni R, Nisson P, Chan JL, Quintero-Consuegra M, Toscano JF, Gonzalez NR. Transvenous pressure monitoring guides endovascular treatment of vein of Galen malformation: a technical note. Pediatr Neurosurg. 2021;56:401–6.
67. Quisling RG, Mickle JP. Venous pressure measurements in vein of Galen aneurysms. AJNR Am J Neuroradiol. 1989;10:411–7.
68. Hoang S, Choudhri O, Edwards M, Guzman R. Vein of Galen malformation. Neurosurg Focus. 2009;27:E8.
69. Zeng X, Hunt A, Jin SC, Duran D, Gaillard J, Kahle KT. EphrinB2-EphB4-RASA1 signaling in human cerebrovascular development and disease. Trends Mol Med. 2019;25:265–86.
70. Revencu N, Boon LM, Mendola A, Cordisco MR, Dubois J, Clapuyt P, Hammer F, Amor DJ, Irvine AD, Baselga E, et al. RASA1 mutations and associated phenotypes in 68 families with capillary malformation-arteriovenous malformation. Hum Mutat. 2013;34:1632–41.
71. Chida A, Shintani M, Wakamatsu H, Tsutsumi Y, Iizuka Y, Kawaguchi N, Furutani Y, Inai K, Nonoyama S, Nakanishi T. ACVRL1 gene variant in a patient with vein of Galen aneurysmal malformation. J Pediatr Genet. 2013;2:181–9.
72. Tsutsumi Y, Kosaki R, Itoh Y, Tsukamoto K, Matsuoka R, Shintani M, Nosaka S, Masaki H, Iizuka Y. Vein of Galen aneurysmal malformation associated with an endoglin gene mutation. Pediatrics. 2011;128:e1307–10.
73. Kundishora A, Zeng X, Duran D, Allocco AA, Choi J, Jin SC, Conine SB, Nelson-Williams C, Gaillard J, Furey CG, et al. Exome sequencing defines the molecular pathogenesis of vein of Galen malformation. Neurosurgery. 2019;66:310.
74. Hoffman HJ, Chuang S, Hendrick EB, Humphreys RP. Aneurysms of the vein of Galen. Experience at The Hospital for Sick Children, Toronto. J Neurosurg. 1982;57:316–22.
75. Sato S, Niimi Y, Mochizuki T, Shima S, Inoue T, Kawamata T, Okada Y. Umbilical vessel catheter retro-exchange technique (U-RET) for repeat use of the umbilical artery for neonatal vascular intervention: technical note. Interv Neuroradiol. 2021;28(4):386–90. https://doi.org/10.1177/15910199211041445.
76. Lasjaunias P. Vascular diseases in neonates, infants and children: interventional neuroradiology management. Berlin, Heidelberg: Springer; 1997.
77. Lasjaunias P, Rodesch G, Terbrugge K, Pruvost P, Devictor D, Comoy J, Landrieu P. Vein of Galen aneurysmal malformations: report of 36 cases managed between 1982 and 1988. Acta Neurochir (Wien). 1989;99:26–37.
78. Paladini D, Deloison B, Rossi A, Chalouhi GE, Gandolfo C, Sonigo P, Buratti S, Millischer AE, Tuo G, Ville Y, et al. Vein of Galen aneurysmal malformation (VGAM) in the fetus: retrospective analysis of perinatal prognostic indicators in a two-center series of 49 cases. Ultrasound Obstet Gynecol. 2017;50:192–9.
79. Gopalan V, Rennie A, Robertson F, Kanagarajah L, Toolis C, Bhate S, Ganesan V. Presentation, course, and outcome of postneonatal presentations of vein of Galen malformation: a large, single-institution case series. Dev Med Child Neurol. 2018;60: 424–9.
80. Lecce F, Robertson F, Rennie A, Heuchan A, Lister P, Bhate S, Bhattacharya J, Brew S, Kanagarajah L, Kuczynski A, et al. Cross-sectional study of a United Kingdom cohort of neonatal vein of Galen malformation. Ann Neurol. 2018;84:547–55.
81. Lasjaunias P, Magufis G, Goulao A, Piske R, Suthipongchai S, Rodesch R, Alvarez H. Anatomoclinical aspects of dural arteriovenous shunts in children: review of 29 cases. Interv Neuroradiol. 1996;2:179–91.
82. Morita A, Meyer FB, Nichols DA, Patterson MC. Childhood dural arteriovenous fistulae of the posterior dural sinuses: three case reports and literature review. Neurosurgery. 1995;37: 1193–200.
83. Barbosa M, Mahadevan J, Weon YC, Yoshida Y, Ozanne A, Rodesch G, Alvarez H, Lasjaunias P. Dural Sinus Malformations (DSM) with Giant Lakes, in neonates and infants. Review of 30 consecutive cases. Interv Neuroradiol. 2003;9:407–24.
84. Albright AL, Latchaw RE, Price RA. Posterior dural arteriovenous malformations in infancy. Neurosurgery. 1983;13:129–35.
85. Garcia-Monaco R, Rodesch G, Terbrugge K, Burrows P, Lasjaunias P. Multifocal dural arteriovenous shunts in children. Childs Nerv Syst. 1991;7:425–31.
86. Lasjaunias PL, Landrieu P, Rodesch G, Alvarez H, Ozanne A, Holmin S, Zhao W-Y, Geibprasert S, Ducreux D, Krings T. Cerebral proliferative angiopathy: clinical and angiographic description of an entity different from cerebral AVMs. Stroke. 2008;39:878–85.
87. Yamaki VN, Solla DJF, Telles JPM, Liem GLJ, da Silva SA, Caldas JGMP, Teixeira MJ, Paschoal EHA, Figueiredo EG. The current clinical picture of cerebral proliferative angiopathy: systematic review. Acta Neurochir (Wien). 2020;162:1727–33.
88. Fierstra J, Spieth S, Tran L, Conklin J, Tymianski M, Ter Brugge KG, Fisher JA, Mikulis DJ, Krings T. Severely impaired cerebrovascular reserve in patients with cerebral proliferative angiopathy: clinical article. J Neurosurg Pediatr. 2011;8:310–5.
89. Ducreux D, Petit-Lacour MC, Marsot-Dupuch K, Bittoun J, Lasjaunias P. MR perfusion imaging in a case of cerebral proliferative angiopathy. Eur Radiol. 2002;12:2717–22.

90. Vargas MC, Castillo M. Magnetic resonance perfusion imaging in proliferative cerebral angiopathy. J Comput Assist Tomogr. 2011;35:33–8.
91. Kimiwada T, Hayashi T, Shirane R, Tominaga T. 123I-IMP-SPECT in a patient with cerebral proliferative angiopathy: a case report. J Stroke Cerebrovasc Dis. 2013;22:1432–5.
92. Ochoa A, Mantese B, Requejo F. Hemorrhagic cerebral proliferative angiopathy in two pediatric patients: case reports. Childs Nerv Syst. 2021;38:789.
93. Lawton MT, Rutledge WC, Kim H, Stapf C, Whitehead KJ, Li DY, Krings T, terBrugge K, Kondziolka D, Morgan MK, et al. Brain arteriovenous malformations. Nat Rev Dis Primers. 2015;1:15008.
94. Liu P, Lv X, Lv M, Li Y. Cerebral proliferative angiopathy: clinical, angiographic features and literature review. Interv Neuroradiol. 2016;22:101–7.
95. Maekawa H, Terada A, Ishiguro T, Komiyama M, Lenck S, Renieri L, Krings T. Recurrent periventricular hemorrhage in cerebral proliferative angiopathy: case report. Interv Neuroradiol. 2018;24: 713–7.
96. Kumar S, Srivastava T, Tejwani S, Khilnani K. Cerebral proliferative angiopathy with papilledema. Clin Neurol Neurosurg. 2015;139:12–5.
97. Mansmann U, Meisel J, Brock M, Rodesch G, Alvarez H, Lasjaunias P. Factors associated with intracranial hemorrhage in cases of cerebral arteriovenous malformation. Neurosurgery. 2000;46:272–80.
98. Somji M, McEachern J, Silvaggio J. Cerebral revascularization in cerebral proliferative angiopathy: a systematic review. Neurosurg Focus. 2019;46:E11.
99. Srivastava T, Mathur T, Jain R, Sannegowda RB. Cerebral proliferative angiopathy: a rare clinical entity with peculiar angiographic features. Ann Indian Acad Neurol. 2013;16:674–5.
100. Kumar S, Sharma M, Srivastava T, Sinha VD. Infratentorial hemorrhagic cerebral proliferative angiopathy: a rare presentation of a rare disease. Asian J Neurosurg. 2015;10:240–2.
101. Gold JJ, Crawford JR. Acute hemiparesis in a child as a presenting symptom of hemispheric cerebral proliferative angiopathy. Case Rep Neurol Med. 2013;2013:920853–9.
102. Meisel HJ, Mansmann U, Alvarez H, Rodesch G, Brock M, Lasjaunias P. Effect of partial targeted N-butyl-cyano-acrylate embolization in brain AVM. Acta Neurochir (Wien). 2002;144:879–88.
103. Ellis MJ, Armstrong D, Dirks PB. Large vascular malformation in a child presenting with vascular steal phenomenon managed with pial synangiosis. J Neurosurg Pediatr. 2011;7:15–21.
104. Kono K, Terada T. Encephaloduroarteriosynangiosis for cerebral proliferative angiopathy with cerebral ischemia. J Neurosurg. 2014;121:1411–5.
105. Sakata H, Fujimura M, Sato K, Niizuma K, Endo H, Tominaga T. Development of abnormal hemispheric vascular networks mimicking cerebral proliferative angiopathy in a child originally diagnosed with deep-seated arteriovenous fistula. J Stroke Cerebrovasc Dis. 2016;25:e200–4.
106. Puerta P, Guillén A, Muchart J, González V, Ferrer E. Cerebral proliferative angiopathy in a child. Pediatr Neurosurg. 2017;52:214–6.
107. Smith ER, Scott RM. Cavernous malformations. Neurosurg Clin N Am. 2010;21:483–90.
108. Morris Z, Whiteley WN, Longstreth WT, Weber F, Lee Y-C, Tsushima Y, Alphs H, Ladd SC, Warlow C, Wardlaw JM, et al. Incidental findings on brain magnetic resonance imaging: systematic review and meta-analysis. BMJ. 2009;339:194–550.
109. Al-Holou WN, O'Lynnger TM, Pandey AS, Gemmete JJ, Thompson BG, Muraszko KM, Garton HJL, Maher CO. Natural history and imaging prevalence of cavernous malformations in children and young adults: clinical article. J Neurosurg Pediatr. 2012;9:198–205.
110. Al-Shahi R, Bhattacharya JJ, Currie DG, Papanastassiou V, Ritchie V, Roberts RC, Sellar RJ, Warlow CP. Prospective, population-based detection of intracranial vascular malformations in adults: the Scottish Intracranial Vascular Malformation Study (SIVMS). Stroke. 2003;34:1163–9.
111. Gastelum E, Sear K, Hills N, Roddy E, Randazzo D, Chettout N, Hess C, Cotter J, Haas-Kogan DA, Fullerton H, et al. Rates and characteristics of radiographically detected intracerebral cavernous malformations after cranial radiation therapy in pediatric cancer patients. J Child Neurol. 2015;30:842–9.
112. Horne MA, Flemming KD, Su I-C, Stapf C, Jeon JP, Li D, Maxwell SS, White P, Christianson TJ, Agid R, et al. Clinical course of untreated cerebral cavernous malformations: a meta-analysis of individual patient data. Lancet Neurol. 2016;15:166–73.
113. Al-Shahi RS, Hall JM, Horne MA, Moultrie F, Josephson CB, Bhattacharya JJ, Counsell CE, Murray GD, Papanastassiou V, Ritchie V, et al. Untreated clinical course of cerebral cavernous malformations: a prospective, population-based cohort study. Lancet Neurol. 2012;11:217–24.
114. Gross BA, Du R, Orbach DB, Scott RM, Smith ER. The natural history of cerebral cavernous malformations in children. J Neurosurg Pediatr. 2016;17:123–8.
115. Akers A, Al-Shahi Salman R, Awad IA, Dahlem K, Flemming K, Hart B, Kim H, Jusue-Torres I, Kondziolka D, Lee C, et al. Synopsis of guidelines for the clinical management of cerebral cavernous malformations: consensus recommendations based on systematic literature review by the Angioma Alliance Scientific Advisory Board Clinical Experts Panel. Neurosurgery. 2017;80: 665–80.
116. Riant F, Bergametti F, Ayrignac X, Boulday G, Tournier-Lasserve E. Recent insights into cerebral cavernous malformations: the molecular genetics of CCM. FEBS J. 2010;277:1070–5.
117. Cavalcanti DD, Kalani MYS, Martirosyan NL, Eales J, Spetzler RF, Preul MC. Cerebral cavernous malformations: from genes to proteins to disease. J Neurosurg. 2012;116:122–32.

118. Barker FG 2nd, Amin-Hanjani S, Butler WE, Lyons S, Ojemann RG, Chapman PH, Ogilvy CS. Temporal clustering of hemorrhages from untreated cavernous malformations of the central nervous system. Neurosurgery. 2001;49:15–25.
119. Chen B, Herten A, Saban D, Rauscher S, Radbruch A, Schmidt B, Zhu Y, Jabbarli R, Wrede KH, Kleinschnitz C, et al. Hemorrhage from cerebral cavernous malformations: the role of associated developmental venous anomalies. Neurology. 2020;95:e89–96.
120. Petersen TA, Morrison LA, Schrader RM, Hart BL. Familial versus sporadic cavernous malformations: differences in developmental venous anomaly association and lesion phenotype. AJNR Am J Neuroradiol. 2010;31:377–82.
121. Smith ER, Michael Scott R. Surgical treatment of cavernous malformations in children. 2011;135–42.
122. Chang EF, Gabriel RA, Potts MB, Berger MS, Lawton MT. Supratentorial cavernous malformations in eloquent and deep locations: surgical approaches and outcomes: clinical article. J Neurosurg. 2011;114:814–27.
123. Englot DJ, Han SJ, Lawton MT, Chang EF. Predictors of seizure freedom in the surgical treatment of supratentorial cavernous malformations: clinical article. J Neurosurg. 2011;115:1169–74.
124. Baumann CR, Acciarri N, Bertalanffy H, Devinsky O, Elger CE, Lo Russo G, Cossu M, Sure U, Singh A, Stefan H, et al. Seizure outcome after resection of supratentorial cavernous malformations: a study of 168 patients. Epilepsia. 2007;48:559–63.
125. Li D, Hao S-Y, Tang J, Xiao X-R, Jia G-J, Wu Z, Zhang L-W, Zhang J-T. Surgical management of pediatric brainstem cavernous malformations. J Neurosurg Pediatr. 2014;13:484–502.
126. Brinjikji W, El-Rida El-Masri A, Wald JT, Lanzino G. Prevalence of developmental venous anomalies increases with age. Stroke. 2017;48:1997–9.
127. Pearl M, Gregg L, Gandhi D. Cerebral venous development in relation to developmental venous anomalies and vein of Galen aneurysmal malformations. Semin Ultrasound CT MRI. 2011;32:252–63.
128. Santucci GM, Leach JL, Ying J, Leach SD, Tomsick TA. Brain parenchymal signal abnormalities associated with developmental venous anomalies: detailed MR imaging assessment. AJNR Am J Neuroradiol. 2008;29:1317–23.
129. Lasjaunias P, Burrows P, Planet C. Developmental venous anomalies (DVA): the so-called venous angioma. Neurosurg Rev. 1986;9:233–42.
130. San Millán Ruíz D, Yilmaz H, Gailloud P. Cerebral developmental venous anomalies: current concepts. Ann Neurol. 2009;66:271–83.
131. Wurm G, Schnizer M, Fellner FA. Cerebral cavernous malformations associated with venous anomalies: surgical considerations. Neurosurgery. 2007;61:358–90.
132. Pereira VM, Geibprasert S, Krings T, Aurboonyawat T, Ozanne A, Toulgoat F, Pongpech S, Lasjaunias PL. Pathomechanisms of symptomatic developmental venous anomalies. Stroke. 2008;39:3201–15.
133. Okahara M, Kiyosue H, Mori H, Tanoue S, Sainou M, Nagatomi H. Anatomic variations of the cerebral arteries and their embryology: a pictorial review. Eur Radiol. 2002;12:2548–61.
134. Kiroglu Y, Oran I, Dalbasti T, Karabulut N, Calli C. Thrombosis of a drainage vein in developmental venous anomaly (DVA) leading venous infarction: a case report and review of the literature. J Neuroimaging. 2011;21:197–201.
135. Im S-H, Han MH, Kwon BJ, Ahn JY, Jung C, Park S-H, Oh CW, Han DH. Venous-predominant parenchymal arteriovenous malformation: a rare subtype with a venous drainage pattern mimicking developmental venous anomaly. J Neurosurg. 2008;108:1142–7.
136. Murai S, Hiramatsu M, Suzuki E, Ishibashi R, Takai H, Miyazaki Y, Takasugi Y, Yamaoka Y, Nishi K, Takahashi Y, et al. Trends in incidence of intracranial and spinal arteriovenous shunts: hospital-based surveillance in Okayama, Japan. Stroke. 2021;52:1455–9.
137. Du J, Ling F, Chen M, Zhang H. Clinical characteristic of spinal vascular malformation in pediatric patients. Childs Nerv Syst. 2008;25:473–8.
138. Rodesch G, Hurth M, Alvarez H, Ducot B, Tadie M, Lasjaunias P. Angio-architecture of spinal cord arteriovenous shunts at presentation. Clinical correlations in adults and children. The Bicêtre experience on 155 consecutive patients seen between 1981-1999. Acta Neurochir (Wien). 2004;146:217–26.
139. Pal P, Ray S, Chakraborty S, Dey S, Talukdar A. Cobb syndrome: a rare cause of paraplegia. Ann Neurosci. 2015;22:191–3.
140. Kim LJ, Spetzler RF. Classification and surgical management of spinal arteriovenous lesions: arteriovenous fistulae and arteriovenous malformations. Neurosurgery. 2006;59:S195–201.
141. Spetzler RF, Detwiler PW, Riina HA, Porter RW. Modified classification of spinal cord vascular lesions. J Neurosurg. 2002;96:145–56.
142. Rodesch G, Pongpech S, Alvarez H, Zerah M, Hurth M, Sebire G, Lasjaunias P. Spinal cord arteriovenous malformations in a pediatric population children below 15 years of age the place of endovascular management. Interv Neuroradiol. 1995;1:29–42.
143. Cho W-S, Wang K-C, Phi JH, Lee JY, Chong S, Kang H-S, Han MH, Kim S-K. Pediatric spinal arteriovenous malformations and fistulas: a single institute's experience. Childs Nerv Syst. 2016;32:811–8.
144. Nikolaev SI, Vetiska S, Bonilla X, Boudreau E, Jauhiainen S, Rezai Jahromi B, Khyzha N, DiStefano PV, Suutarinen S, Kiehl T-R, et al. Somatic activating KRAS mutations in arteriovenous malformations of the brain. N Engl J Med. 2018;378:250–61.
145. Goss JA, Huang AY, Smith E, Konczyk DJ, Smits PJ, Sudduth CL, Stapleton C, Patel A, Alexandrescu S, Warman ML, et al. Somatic mutations in intracranial arteriovenous malformations. PLoS One. 2019;14:e0226852.
146. Grimmond SM, Raghavan D, Russell PJ. Detection of a rare point mutation in Ki-ras of a human bladder

cancer xenograft by polymerase chain reaction and direct sequencing. Urol Res. 1992;20:121–6.
147. Nakano H, Yamamoto F, Neville C, Evans D, Mizuno T, Perucho M. Isolation of transforming sequences of two human lung carcinomas: structural and functional analysis of the activated c-K-ras oncogenes. Proc Natl Acad Sci U S A. 1984;81:71–5.
148. Lee KH, Lee JS, Suh C, Kim SW, Kim SB, Lee JH, Lee MS, Park MY, Sun HS, Kim SH. Clinicopathologic significance of the K-ras gene codon 12 point mutation in stomach cancer. An analysis of 140 cases. Cancer. 1995;75:2794–801.
149. Bollag G, Adler F, elMasry N, McCabe PC, Conner EJ, Thompson P, McCormick F, Shannon K. Biochemical characterization of a novel KRAS insertion mutation from a human leukemia. J Biol Chem. 1996;271:32491–4.
150. Niihori T, Aoki Y, Narumi Y, Neri G, Cavé H, Verloes A, Okamoto N, Hennekam RCM, Gillessen-Kaesbach G, Wieczorek D, et al. Germline KRAS and BRAF mutations in cardio-facio-cutaneous syndrome. Nat Genet. 2006;38:294–6.
151. Al-Olabi L, Polubothu S, Dowsett K, Andrews KA, Stadnik P, Joseph AP, Knox R, Pittman A, Clark G, Baird W, et al. Mosaic RAS/MAPK variants cause sporadic vascular malformations which respond to targeted therapy. J Clin Invest. 2018;128:1496–508.
152. Naoki K, Chen T-H, Richards WG, Sugarbaker DJ, Meyerson M. Missense mutations of the BRAF gene in human lung adenocarcinoma. Cancer Res. 2002;62:7001–3.
153. Rajagopalan H, Bardelli A, Lengauer C, Kinzler KW, Vogelstein B, Velculescu VE. Tumorigenesis: RAF/RAS oncogenes and mismatch-repair status. Nature. 2002;418:934.
154. Brose MS, Volpe P, Feldman M, Kumar M, Rishi I, Gerrero R, Einhorn E, Herlyn M, Minna J, Nicholson A, et al. Mutations in human lung cancer and melanoma. Cancer Res. 2002;62:6997–7000.
155. Lee JW, Yoo NJ, Soung YH, Kim HS, Park WS, Kim SY, Lee JH, Park JY, Cho YG, Kim CJ, et al. BRAF mutations in non-Hodgkin's lymphoma. Br J Cancer. 2003;89:1958–60.
156. Sarkozy A, Carta C, Moretti S, Zampino G, Digilio MC, Pantaleoni F, Scioletti AP, Esposito G, Cordeddu V, Lepri F, et al. Germline BRAF mutations in Noonan, LEOPARD, and cardiofaciocutaneous syndromes: molecular diversity and associated phenotypic spectrum. Hum Mutat. 2009;30:695–702.
157. Couto JA, Huang AY, Konczyk DJ, Goss JA, Fishman SJ, Mulliken JB, Warman ML, Greene AK. Somatic MAP2K1 mutations are associated with extracranial arteriovenous malformation. Am J Hum Genet. 2017;100:546–54.
158. Kang H, Jha S, Deng Z, Fratzl-Zelman N, Cabral WA, Ivovic A, Meylan F, Hanson EP, Lange E, Katz J, et al. Somatic activating mutations in MAP2K1 cause melorheostosis. Nat Commun. 2018;9:1390.
159. Ng SB, Bigham AW, Buckingham KJ, Hannibal MC, McMillin MJ, Gildersleeve HI, Beck AE, Tabor HK, Cooper GM, Mefford HC, et al. Exome sequencing identifies MLL2 mutations as a cause of Kabuki syndrome. Nat Genet. 2010;42:790–3.
160. Van Houdt JKJ, Nowakowska BA, Sousa SB, van Schaik BDC, Seuntjens E, Avonce N, Sifrim A, Abdul-Rahman OA, van den Boogaard M-JH, Bottani A, et al. Heterozygous missense mutations in SMARCA2 cause Nicolaides-Baraitser syndrome. Nat Genet. 2012;44:445–9, S1.
161. Arboleda VA, Lee H, Dorrani N, Zadeh N, Willis M, Macmurdo CF, Manning MA, Kwan A, Hudgins L, Barthelemy F, et al. De novo nonsense mutations in KAT6A, a lysine acetyl-transferase gene, cause a syndrome including microcephaly and global developmental delay. Am J Hum Genet. 2015;96:498–506.
162. Wilcox ER, Burton QL, Naz S, Riazuddin S, Smith TN, Ploplis B, Belyantseva I, Ben-Yosef T, Liburd NA, Morell RJ, et al. Mutations in the gene encoding tight junction claudin-14 cause autosomal recessive deafness DFNB29. Cell. 2001;104:165–72.
163. Peyre M, Miyagishima D, Bielle F, Chapon F, Sierant M, Venot Q, Lerond J, Marijon P, Abi-Jaoude S, Le Van T, et al. Somatic PIK3CA mutations in sporadic cerebral cavernous malformations. N Engl J Med. 2021;385:996–1004.
164. Orloff MS, He X, Peterson C, Chen F, Chen J-L, Mester JL, Eng C. Germline PIK3CA and AKT1 mutations in Cowden and Cowden-like syndromes. Am J Hum Genet. 2013;92:76–80.
165. Dumont AS, Lanzino G, Sheehan JP. Brain arteriovenous malformations and arteriovenous fistulas. New York: Thieme Medical Publishers; 2017.
166. Halim AX, Johnston SC, Singh V, McCulloch CE, Bennett JP, Achrol AS, Sidney S, Young WL. Longitudinal risk of intracranial hemorrhage in patients with arteriovenous malformation of the brain within a defined population. Stroke. 2004;35:1697–702.
167. Ríus C, Smith JD, Almendro N, Langa C, Botella LM, Marchuk DA, Vary CP, Bernabéu C. Cloning of the promoter region of human endoglin, the target gene for hereditary hemorrhagic telangiectasia type 1. Blood. 1998;92:4677–90.
168. Ighani M, Aboulafia AJ. Cobb syndrome (cutaneomeningospinal angiomatosis). BMJ Case Rep. 2018;2018:bcr2018225208.
169. Mishra R, Kaw R. Foix-Alajouanine syndrome: an uncommon cause of myelopathy from an anatomic variant circulation. South Med J. 2005;98:567–9.
170. Stefanov-Kiuri S, Fernandez-Heredero A. Images in clinical medicine. Parkes Weber syndrome. N Engl J Med. 2014;371:2114.
171. Revencu N, Boon LM, Mulliken JB, Enjolras O, Cordisco MR, Burrows PE, Clapuyt P, Hammer F, Dubois J, Baselga E, et al. Parkes Weber syndrome, vein of Galen aneurysmal malformation, and other fast-flow vascular anomalies are caused by RASA1 mutations. Hum Mutat. 2008;29:959–65.
172. Frikha R. Klippel-Feil syndrome: a review of the literature. Clin Dysmorphol. 2020;29:35–7.

Pediatric Epilepsy Surgery

11

Oguz Cataltepe

Introduction

Epilepsy is one of the most common neurological disorders in pediatric age group. The overall incidence of epilepsy in children is estimated about 30–80 cases per 100,000 children per year [1, 2]. Pediatric epilepsy is concerning not only or seizures but also for frequently associated other disabilities. High rates of comorbid learning disabilities, mental retardation, developmental delay, psychiatric/behavioral difficulties, and psychosocial problems are seen almost half of the children with epilepsy. Therefore, the goal of treatment in pediatric epilepsy patients is not limited with seizure control. The primary goal in the management of these children is seizure control and eliminating anti-epileptic medications if feasible. The related benefits are to prevent the potential harmful consequences of uncontrolled seizures secondary to persistent interictal electrographic activities and adverse effects of anti-epileptic drugs (AEDs) which may cause developmental stagnation or decline in young children as well as permanent cognitive, behavioral, and psychosocial problems [3–6].

Today, despite of major advances and improvements in the diagnostic techniques and newer AEDs, still, approximately 20% of children with epilepsy continue to suffer from medically intractable epilepsy. Surgical management of epilepsy is often the single remaining treatment option for these children [3–9].

Surgical management of epilepsy is a quite complex and multidisciplinary process, and it necessitates a well-coordinated, collaborative relationship between the medical and surgical teams. Pediatric epileptologists, epilepsy surgeons, neuropsychologists, neuroradiologists, nuclear medicine team, neurophysiologists, specialized long term EEG/Video nursing and EEG technologists with special expertise in the management of pediatric patients staying in dedicated pediatric epilepsy monitoring units are needed to provide a safe and effective pediatric epilepsy surgery service [6, 7].

Pediatric epilepsy surgery is an established treatment option in well-selected candidates and it has been performed in many specialized centers today, despite of initial hesitancy for surgical interventions in pediatric epilepsy patients. Pediatric epilepsy surgery helps to improve the overall outcome of this young patient group by providing not only seizure reduction and freedom but also resulting in improved behavior, quality of life, language, and cognitive function [7–11].

O. Cataltepe (✉)
Department of Neurological Surgery, University of Massachusetts Chan Medical School and Medical Center, Worcester, MA, USA
e-mail: oguz.cataltepe@umassmemorial.org

N. Shimony, G. Jallo (eds.), *Pediatric Neurosurgery Board Review*,
https://doi.org/10.1007/978-3-031-23687-7_11

Epilepsy Surgery in Children

Surgical management of pediatric and adult epilepsy patients has many common features as well as many significant differences. Pediatric epilepsy patients suffer from very diverse group of epileptic disorders associated with different electrophysiological and semiological characteristics compared to adult patients. Pediatric epilepsy patients frequently have age-related developmental and psychosocial problems that must be taken into account when considering surgery. Among pediatric epilepsy patients, infants and young children especially constitute a challenging subset. Awareness of age-related characteristics and special issues in this very young patient group is an important prerequisite for ensuring good surgical outcomes [1, 3–9, 11–14]. This point was nicely described by the "Subcommission for Pediatric Epilepsy Surgery of International League Against Epilepsy (ILAE)" report:

> "…neurobiological aspects of epilepsy are unique to children, especially the young, and as such require specific pediatric epilepsy expertise. Collectively these features justify the unique approach necessary for dedicated pediatric epilepsy surgery centers…" [5].

Special Considerations for Pediatric Epilepsy Surgery

There are a certain group of pediatric epilepsy syndromes amenable to surgery such as infantile spasms, multi-lobar/hemispheric syndromes such as Rasmussen encephalitis and Sturge-Weber syndrome [1, 3, 4]. Some of these are exclusively seen in children and rarely or never occur in adults and they have their own unique diagnostic and surgical challenges. Again, some of the pediatric epilepsy syndromes seen in infants and young children are much more then seizure disorders and their natural course can even be catastrophic because of the associated cognitive and severe developmental delay or regression. These cases are problematic, and their management requires a great deal of expertise.

The neuropathologic substrate of epilepsy and its observed frequency in children constitutes another significant difference from adults. For example, while cortical malformations are the most common neuropathologic substrate in epilepsy surgery cases among children (23–78%), mesial temporal sclerosis (MTS) in children is seen much less frequently than in adults [1, 4, 5, 8, 13, 15–17]. The clinical and electrophysiological spectrum and presentation of seizures are often quite heterogeneous and wide ranging in childhood. Electrophysiological findings associated with intractable seizures in children can be quite atypical and poorly defined compared with the relatively well-defined clinical and electrophysiological characteristics seen in adults [5, 13].

Most commonly seen seizure onset locations are also different in children. Epileptogenic zones in children are frequently extratemporal in location and cover large cortical areas, including the eloquent cortex. Therefore, these children are frequently quite challenging cases both for diagnostic work up and for surgical planning.

The age of the pediatric epilepsy patients is also a very significant topic to consider during the surgical work up and planning because of its effect on multiple fronts including the feasibility of certain preoperative assessment techniques and tests (such as WADA test), surgical indications, the timing of surgery, surgical approaches (such as feasibility of awake surgery and cortical mapping), and also for outcome measures. Rapid brain maturation during early infancy and childhood plays a major role in the complex evolution of clinical seizure semiology as well as peculiar EEG and neuroimaging findings. All these characteristics make a significant aspect of decision-making process in pediatric epilepsy surgery [5, 13].

Timing of surgery is another significant topic because of harmful and sometimes catastrophic effects of ongoing seizures on the developing brain of young children. This aspect of pediatric epilepsy constitutes a major concern, and early surgical intervention is considered in some infants to prevent this downward spiral secondary to frequent clinical seizures. Ongoing seizures, continuous postictal state and ongoing interictal epileptiform discharges may cause an irritable, dysfunctional cortex and, possibly, secondary epileptogenesis in young children. Consequently, intractable seizures and their deleterious effect on the developing brain may result in mental retardation, debilitating behavioral problems, aggression, attention deficit disorder, and hyperactivity. Therefore, pediatric epilepsy team must not only consider seizures when making decisions regarding epilepsy surgery, but also consider the potentially harmful effects of seizures on the developing brain.

There is another significant characteristic in young children who are considered as a candidate for epilepsy surgery: functional plasticity potential of a young brain [9]. Young children have a significant capacity for reorganization of neurological function and much greater potential for recovery following epilepsy surgery [10]. This is especially evident in the speedy recovery of speech-related functions in young children and it constitutes a remarkable asset of early childhood. Therefore, the functional plasticity and higher potential for recovery of the young brain needs to be considered when making presurgical assessments and surgical decisions is pediatric epilepsy patients [5].

The definition of medical intractability in children is also somewhat different compared to adult patients. Because many types of pediatric epilepsy syndromes are inherently medically refractory, there is no need to "prove" medical intractability in some pediatric epileptic disorders as opposed to adults. As we briefly mentioned above, considering the brain plasticity in children is a significant factor on the timing of surgery and delaying surgical treatment just to prove intractability is not a good idea in some cases. The potential for significant recovery is highest during the period of high synaptic and dendritic density (ages 3–7 years), when the plasticity of the brain peaks [17]. Surgery performed within this time frame may help hasten recovery, and anticipated postoperative impairments may be milder. Therefore, among well-selected patients, early surgical intervention may prevent the negative cognitive, psychosocial, and developmental effects of seizures.

Accumulating data shows the positive effect of epilepsy surgery on clinical outcome of pediatric epilepsy patients. It is not only the seizure control enhanced in these patients, but the behavioral, cognitive, and developmental domains of life also show considerable improvement [2–4]. Thus, early surgical intervention helps children with epilepsy to develop without further psychosocial harm and, in many cases, to maximize their developmental potential.

Special Epilepsy Syndromes of Childhood

Infantile hemispheric epilepsy This is a term used for a group of congenital disorders characterized with intractable partial seizures and hemiparesis secondary to hemispheric insults. The underlying lesion might be extensive cortical dysplasia, hemimegalencephaly, porencephalic cyst or cortical damage secondary to perinatal cerebrovascular events. The patients typically present with severe intractable seizures within the first few months of life and clinical picture progresses with hemiparesis between ages of 3 and 6 months [6, 7, 14, 18, 19].

Infantile spasms Typically presents with myoclonic seizures at the age of 3–11 months and frequently progress with profound mental retardation. Typical triad includes epileptic spasms in clusters, hypsarrhythmia in interictal EEG and the arrest or deterioration of psychomotor development. Underlying structural abnormalities such as cortical dysplasia or perinatal ischemic injuries may or may not be determined [6, 7, 14, 18, 19].

Lennox-Gastaut Syndrome The patient presents with frequent, intractable generalized tonic and atypical absence seizures, pronounced mental retardation and typical slow spike-wave pattern on interictal EEG. It is generally accepted as generalized seizure disorder and surgical options are limited with corpus callosotomy and vagus nerve stimulator placement [6, 7, 14, 18].

Sturge-Weber Syndrome (SWS) SWS is characterized by facial and ipsilateral cerebral angiomatosis which might also be associated with medically intractable epilepsy with very frequent seizures and progressive neurological deficits. Early surgery in patients with severe, frequent intractable seizures and progressive hemiparesis leads to the best outcome by ensuring maximal recovery and avoiding cognitive decline. Depending on the extent of cortical involvement, limited cortical resection or hemispherectomy might be considered [6, 7, 14, 18].

Rasmussen's encephalopathy It is caused by chronic localized encephalitis characterized by intractable focal epilepsy associated with "Epilepsia partialis continua" and slowly progressing neurological deficits affecting the opposite side of the body. The causative factors are unknown. Typically presents with infrequent partial seizures at the age of 1–14 years, with a peak at around 6 years of age. It is thought as an immune-mediated encephalitis but no specific autoantibodies was found. Chronic inflammation may spread to the entire hemisphere and clinical symptomatology may progress with gradually increasing seizures, progressive hemiparesis, and cognitive decline. Multilobar resections or functional hemispherectomy constitute the surgical management options [6, 7, 14, 18, 20–22].

Neuronal Migrational Disorders (NMD) NMD constitutes a large group of congenital structural lesions which frequently cause medically intractable seizures. They represent broad variety developmental abnormalities including focal cortical dysplasia, schizencephaly, lissencephaly, and grey matter heterotopias. Epileptogenic area frequently is larger than seen in MRI and determining the extent of epileptogenic zone might be challenging and may necessitates invasive monitoring [6, 7, 14, 18, 23, 24].

Neuropathology of Pediatric Epilepsy

Identifying the nature of underlying pathological process of the epilepsy is critical to define the most appropriate medical and surgical management plan [15–17]. There are a group of lesions that frequently cause medically intractable epilepsy in children (*see* Table 11.1). The detailed information on these pathologies can be found in other sources seen in References section.

Table 11.1 Neuropathological substrates in pediatric epilepsy

Malformations of cortical development
Abnormal neuronal and glial proliferation or differentiation
Focal cortical dysplasia
Tuberous sclerosis complex
Hemimegalencephaly
Abnormal neuronal migration
Lissencephaly
Subcortical band heterotopia
Periventricular nodular heterotopia
Abnormal cortical organization
Polymicrogyria
Schizencephaly
Neoplastic lesions
Glioneuronal tumors
Dysembryoplastic neuroepithelial tumor
Ganglion cell tumors
Ganglioglioma
Gangliocytoma
Glial tumors
Oligodendroglioma
Diffuse astrocytoma
Pleomorphic xanthoastrocytoma
Hamartomas
Glioneuronal and glial hamartomas
Hypothalamic hamartomas
Meningoangiomatosis
Mesial temporal sclerosis
Vascular malformations
Arteriovenous malformations (AVM)
Cavernous angiomas
Sturge-Weber syndrome
Acquired lesions
Ischemic stroke
Porencephalic cyst
Traumatic lesions
Inflammatory lesions
Infections
Noninfectious or autoimmune lesions
Rasmussen's encephalitis
Autoimmune encephalitis

Preoperative Assessment

The primary goals of the preoperative assessment in epilepsy patients are determining whether or not the patient is a surgical candidate and, if so, what the most appropriate surgical approach is. Selecting the surgical candidates and surgical approach mainly depend upon the etiology of seizures, location of epileptogenic focus, and its relations with the eloquent cortex. Therefore, preoperative assessment of epilepsy patients necessitates obtaining extensive data from multiple modalities to locate the epileptogenic focus and to determine its functional correlates. The work up for the selection process of surgical candidates start with description of seizure semiology, basic routine EEG and MRI studies and then progress to quite complex studies such as magnetoencephalography, PET, SPECT and neuropsychological tests as well as more invasive procedures in some cases (*see* Table 11.2). Preoperative assessment process can be defined as Phase 1 (noninvasive presurgical evaluation) and Phase 2 (invasive diagnostic studies) based on the modalities involving. Then selected surgical candidates proceed for Phase 3 which is the surgical intervention. There are three goals during Phase 1 and 2; lateralizing and localizing the epileptogenic focus, documenting the functional correlates of the epileptogenic focus, and determining the most appropriate surgical approach to have the maximal seizure control without causing a new neurological deficit. Invasive monitoring techniques (Phase 2) are needed when the epileptogenic zone cannot be determined with noninvasive techniques and/or when seizure onset zone is adjacent to the eloquent cortex. In these cases, cortical stimulation and mapping will be needed to define the feasibility and safety of cortical excision covering the epileptogenic focus [5, 7, 12, 17, 24–27].

Table 11.2 Preoperative assessment

Past medical history, including perinatal events
Seizure types and semiology (clinical manifestations of the seizures)
Physical and neurological examination
Neurophysiological data
Routine EEG (interictal data)
Continuous video-EEG monitoring in Epilepsy Monitoring Unit (EMU)
EEG (interictal and ictal data)
Video (documenting seizure semiology)
Magnetoencephalography (MEG)
Structural imaging
Brain MRI with epilepsy protocol (3 T or 7 T)
Functional imaging
Functional MRI (fMRI)
SPECT (interictal and ictal)
PET (interictal)
Neuropsychological testing
Invasive tests
Intracarotid amobarbital procedure (WADA test)
Invasive intracranial monitoring
Subdural strip and grid
Stereoelectroencephalography
Electrocorticography
Cortical stimulation and mapping

Seizure Semiology The clinical manifestations of seizures vary based on the location of the epileptogenic focus and detailed video documentation of seizure semiology has a great value for the epilepsy team to develop a working hypothesis for lateralization and localization of the seizure onset zone. For example, oral and hand automatisms are seen mostly in temporal lobe seizures but dystonia and other motor automatisms are more common in frontal lobe seizures. However, although seizure semiology is very supportive to localize the epileptogenic zone, it is certainly not a definitive information. It can be even misleading at times because of a very fast propagation potential of electrical discharges during the seizures [18, 26, 27].

Neuropsychological Tests Although it might be difficult to apply in young children, when it is feasible, neuropsychological assessment of verbal and non-verbal communication skills provides valuable adjunctive information for the lateralization and even localization of the epileptogenic region as well as determining the hemispheric dominance of speech and memory functions. WADA test (intra-arterial amobarbital test) is also a very helpful technique to lateralize speech and memory dominance; however, its application in children is quite limited because of its invasive nature (catheter angiography) and necessity for full cooperation of the patient during the speech and memory function assessment testing after amobarbital injection.

Neuroimaging Studies

Magnetic Resonance Imaging MRI is a critical study for detecting structural abnormalities in the brain and for surgical planning. Appreciation of some developmental abnormalities in the brain, such as cortical dysplasia might be quite subtle and difficult to see on MRI. Special MRI sequences with epilepsy protocol, volumetric studies and using a higher resolution (3 T or 7 T) MRI machine might be helpful in these cases. Functional MRI is also a powerful non-invasive method to map the functional cortical areas in relation to epileptogenic or lesional zones and to lateralize the hemispheric dominance; however, the application of fMRI during preoperative evaluation is frequently not feasible in young children [18, 27–29].

SPECT and PET Both SPECT and PET have important role in the identification of epileptogenic zone by using radiotracers and detecting the alterations of the metabolism based on cerebral blood flow changes in the epileptogenic region. Cerebral blood flow increases in epileptogenic zone during seizures and Ictal SPECT can be very useful in detecting the hyperperfused epileptogenic focus. On the other hand, PET can be useful by reliably demonstrating the region of hypometabolism corresponding the epileptogenic zone during the interictal phase [28, 29].

Noninvasive Electrophysiological Techniques

Electroencephalography (EEG) Although one of the oldest diagnostic techniques, EEG is still the most critical test for localizing epileptogenic focus and for the surgical planning. Even routine EEG may document interictal electrographic abnormalities and gives us a valuable input about the lateralization and potentially localization of the epileptogenic activities. However, most critical information comes from ictal EEG recordings, and this is only possible with long-term EEG/Video monitoring (LTM) in dedicated epilepsy monitoring units. Therefore, LTM is the cornerstone of presurgical evaluation of epilepsy patients. It provides valuable data to localize the seizure onset zone by documenting both clinical characteristics of seizures (semiology) and the location of initial electroencephalographic changes during the seizure onset [18, 26].

Magnetoencephalography (MEG) Although it is not widely available, MEG is a very valuable technique to localize both epileptogenic and eloquent cortices by measuring the magnetic fields associated with the intracellular current flows. It helps to identify the smaller and deep-seated epileptogenic focus noninvasively. It is especially helpful as a complementary study to EEG [18, 24].

Invasive Electrophysiological Techniques

Invasive intracranial monitoring techniques are needed in more complex cases when the localizing the epileptogenic zone is not successful with noninvasive techniques. In some cases, the information obtained with noninvasive monitoring techniques might be inconclusive, discordant, or insufficient for precise localization of epileptogenic zone. Invasive monitoring techniques are also very helpful if the epileptogenic zone is intimately involved to the functionally critical cortical areas. In these cases, invasive monitoring techniques are helpful not just to localize the epileptogenic zone and perform extraoperative cortical stimulation studies, but also to further delineate and map the boundaries of the epileptogenic zone and its relations with the eloquent cortex.

Intracranial monitoring can be done either by using subdural strip and grid electrodes or depth electrodes and it may be needed in pediatric epilepsy patients both with temporal and extratemporal lobe epilepsy [28, 30, 31].

Subdural strip and grid electrodes These are thin, silastic sheets, with varying number of embedded multiple electrode contacts. Subdural strips are single row of contact electrodes (1 × 4, 1 × 6, 1 × 8, etc.) and subdural grid electrodes are larger plates of rectangular arrays with several parallel rows of contact electrodes (2 × 4, 4 × 8, 8 × 8, etc.). Both strips and grids are laid over the cortical surfaces. Subdural strips can be placed through burr holes, but subdural grids can only be placed through appropriate size craniotomy flaps. They are ideal to lateralize and localize the epileptogenic cortical areas and also to perform extraoperative cortical stimulation and mapping. However, they have limited capacity to document the electrographical activities in deeper structures and larger networks extending beyond the cortex under these electrodes [32].

Depth electrodes Depth electrodes are thin, tubular, multicontact electrode arrays and they are placed using stereotactic equipment and techniques. They are especially valuable when the suspicious epileptogenic areas are deep seated, such as hippocampus, cingulum, insula, etc. They can be used in addition to subdural strip and grid electrodes or they can be used alone as in stereo-electroencephalography technique [31–35].

Stereoelectroencephalography (SEEG) SEEG is an invasive monitoring method to define the anatomical boundaries of the cortical and subcortical epileptogenic zones using multiple depth electrodes. Numbers of the depth electrodes are determined based on the preoperative hypothesis (unilateral, bilateral, perisylvian, etc.) and the extent of the network that will be explored. Multiple depth electrodes, generally 6–15 electrodes, are used in SEEG cases. These electrodes are strategically placed based on a precise hypothesis of the anatomical location of the epileptogenic zone and probable propagation pathways. SEEG provides a 3-dimensional recording of cortical and subcortical brain regions and helps to map the anatomo-electro-clinical network to identify the epileptogenic zone, to document its functional correlates and to guide the surgical approach in each case [31, 33–35].

Awake Surgery and Electrocorticography

Awake surgery is not feasible in young children and it is quite uncommon even in older children. In principle, awake surgery can be considered if the functional cortex is adjacent or intimately involve to the epileptogenic zone. The goal is briefly mapping the functional areas (speech and motor) over the exposed cortex after the craniotomy using cortical stimulation techniques. After mapping of the eloquent cortex is completed, excision of the epileptogenic zone is performed by protecting the eloquent cortex and performing the excision while testing the patient's speech and motor functions during the excision. Electrocorticography technique can be used under general anesthesia in some cases, such as cortical dysplasia, to document and map the abnormal electrographical activities and tailoring the extent of the resection by including irritable cortex.

Surgical Procedures

Some surgical procedures, such as hemispheric or multilobar resections, disconnections, or multistage resections, are performed much more commonly in pediatric epilepsy patients than in adults. Table 11.3 shows the frequency of pediatric epilepsy surgery procedures performed in three large centers [3].

Here we will review the surgical procedures performed in epilepsy patients by grouping them as resective, disconnective, ablation and neuromodulation procedures.

Table 11.3 Commonly performed pediatric epilepsy surgery procedures

Cleveland Clinic (Wyllie, 1998)
Temporal 53%, Extratemporal 35%, Hemispherectomy 12%
UCLA (Mathern, 1999)
Temporal 20%, Extratemporal 46%, Hemispherectomy 34%
Great Ormond Street Hospital, London (Cross, 2000)
Temporal 44%, Extratemporal 25%, Hemispherectomy 32%, Others 13%

Resective Procedures

The goal in excisional surgical procedures in epilepsy patients is to obtain optimal resection of epileptogenic tissue while preserving eloquent cortex. When it is feasible, it may help to decrease the seizure frequency significantly and even provides seizure-free outcome in many cases. However, this is a complex process and not every patient is a candidate for resective surgical procedures and even if the patient is a candidate, resective surgery may not be feasible when the epileptogenic zone involves the eloquent cortex.

The first step in surgical planning in these cases is to define the boundaries of epileptogenic zone and eloquent cortex. Then epilepsy surgery team tries to determine potential risks of surgical resection, long-term recovery chance of possible functional losses by considering the role of brain plasticity in children. If the risk for functional loss is high, then the other surgical approaches such as disconnection and neuromodulation techniques can be considered. Risks of resective surgical procedures are intimately related to the anatomical location of the surgical site as well as cerebral dominance.

Temporal lobe resections Although temporal lobe epilepsy is much more common in adults, it also constitutes about 30% of surgical cases in children with epilepsy. Surgical approach in temporal lobe epilepsy might be tailored to keep the resection limited with the boundaries of the epileptogenic zone such as tailored resection in focal cortical dysplasia and selective amygdalohippocampectomy in patients with hippocampal sclerosis, or excision might a performed as a standard anteromesial temporal lobectomy when the patient has a larger epileptogenic network in the temporal lobe. Potential risks in these cases may involve homonymous superior quadrantanopia, speech difficulties, word finding difficulties, and memory dysfunction which depends on hemispheric dominance and the extent of the cortical excision [36–41].

Extratemporal resection Extratemporal seizures are seen more commonly in children and extratemporal procedures are performed quite frequently in children. Extratemporal epilepsy is characterized with earlier onset and more frequent daily seizures. Developmental abnormalities such as cortical dysplasia and low-grade tumors are the most common pathological substrates in pediatric epilepsy surgery patients. Extratemporal location presents significant diagnostic and surgical challenges to the epilepsy team. Intimately connected widespread neural pathways covering quite large cortical areas and very fast spread of the discharges make the task of locating the epileptogenic zone and defining its boundaries very challenging. This patient group frequently needs more extensive work-up including invasive monitoring and functional neuroimaging studies. Surgical complications are dependent on the functional characteristics and extent of resection areas and closely related to involvement of paracentral, supplementary sensorimotor, and visual cortical areas, while the degree of neurological deficit is dependent on the anatomical boundaries of the surgical excision. For example, while resection of hand sensory-motor cortex causes severe and permanent fine-motor deficits, resection of non-dominant primary face area may not cause a permanent deficit because of bilateral innervation of facial muscles. Again, resection of supplementary sensorimotor area leads to transient contralateral neglect and/or weakness with various degree of mutism. However, these findings are almost always resolve within days or weeks, while occipital resections may produce contralateral homonymous hemianopsia which might be permanent [26, 42–44].

Lesionectomy Some epilepsy patients have distinct structural lesions such as tumor or vascular malformations. In these cases, dual surgical goals are excision of the lesion and seizure freedom. Therefore, surgical planning in these cases necessitates defining the epileptogenic zone around the lesion and then extending surgical resection to include the surrounding epileptogenic zone around the lesion. Inevitably, the critical components of this approach are the accessibility of the lesion and its relations with the eloquent cortex. Based on Phase 1 preoperative work up results, some lesional cases might be candidates for a simple lesionectomy without excision of surrounding cortex, but some others might necessitate further work-up such as invasive intracranial monitoring and even awake surgery techniques [7, 15, 32, 37, 39].

Multilobar/resections and anatomical hemispherectomy Although anatomical multilobar excisional procedures and hemispherectomy have been gradually replaced by disconnective procedures such as anterior/posterior quadrantotomy and hemispherotomy, they are still used in some cases such as Rasmussen's syndrome, large porencephalic cysts and Sturge-Weber syndrome. These patients generally have frequent, severely debilitating, and medically intractable seizures arising from a structurally abnormal hemisphere or very large cortical areas and they are not candidates for more restrictive excisional surgeries. The typical surgical candidates for these procedures are the patients with already established hemiparesis, absent fine finger and foot movements but preserved proximal extremity movements such as shoulder, elbow and with the ability to walk. The other hemisphere is frequently structurally and functionally normal in these patients. Anatomical hemispherectomy aims the removal of the entire hemisphere with or without sparing basal ganglia. It is a quite old surgical technique and historically associated with high complication rates. Therefore, a further modification of this technique was later developed by Rasmussen and named as functional hemispherectomy. Functional hemispherectomy can be defined as anatomically limited but functionally complete hemispherectomy technique. It includes resection of paracentral cortical region and mesial temporal structures but the remaining frontal and parieto-occipital lobes are left in place by fully disconnecting their entire white matter tracts as well as corpus callosum. Further modifications of this technique were developed later by gradually decreasing the amount of cortical excision and evolved to a mainly disconnective surgical technique: "hemispherotomy" [45–48].

Disconnective Procedures

Disconnective procedures aim to disconnect the epileptogenic cortical areas from remaining cortex to prevent spread of seizures to the other parts of the brain. This disconnection can be limited with just corpus callosum (callosotomy) or it can include the entire hemisphere (hemispherotomy) as we described above.

Corpus callosotomy The purpose of corpus callosotomy is to prevent the spread of the epileptogenic discharges to the opposite hemisphere by altering the propagation pathways. The surgical candidates typically have generalized epilepsy arising from multiple areas bilaterally and present with severely disabling, frequent and multiple types of seizures, particularly drop attacks. The procedure can be performed with different techniques including craniotomy/interhemispheric approach and endoscopic approach. Corpus callosum is frequently sectioned as 1/2 or 2/3 anterior disconnection by preserving the splenium and might be associated with or without anterior commissurotomy. This type of partial callosotomy is very frequently effective. However, in some cases full callosotomy might be needed by extending the callosal disconnection to remaining splenium as a second step for a better seizure control. There are several complications related to this procedure including "disconnection syndrome" associated with decreased spontaneity of speech, dysarthria, force grasping on the non-dominant side, antagonism in basic manual tasks and deficits in visual and tactile transfer functions, especially when the splenium is also transected. Nowadays, corpus callosotomy is largely replaced by vagus nerve stimulator placement procedures and rarely performed anymore [46].

Multiple subpial transection This procedure, although rarely performed, is a surgical alternative when the epileptogenic zone overlaps the eloquent cortex. Subpial cortical transection lines were created to disconnect lateral neural connections within the epileptogenic area in the eloquent cortex. It is developed to prevent lateral spread of the epileptogenic discharges over the cortex in a cortical area while leaving the columnar circuitry and central projections of the cortex intact. Although it is not widely used surgical technique, it has been used successfully in well-selected and carefully mapped cases such as Landau-Kleffner syndrome, epilepsia partialis continua originating from eloquent cortex.

Hemispherotomy This technique is historically evolved from functional hemispherectomy technique as we summarized above, and it aims to disconnect the entire hemisphere from the remaining half with no or very limited cortical excision. There are several hemispherotomy techniques including Vertical parasagittal hemispherotomy (Delalande, 1992), Perisylvian transventricular hemispherotomy (Schramm, 1995), Peri-insular hemispherotomy (Villemure 1995), Transsylvian hemispheric deafferentation (Schramm, 2001), and endoscope-assisted hemispherotomy (Chandra, 2015). Regardless of technical differences in these approaches, all of them aim to minimize the amount of resection while obtaining complete white matter disconnection of the entire hemisphere. Disconnections are performed either through transventricular or interhemispheric working windows and include full corpus callosotomy, anterior and posterior commissurotomy, frontobasal disconnection, occipitobasal disconnection, perysylvian disconnection through superior and inferior circular sulci, amygdalohippocampectomy or hippocampotomy. Almost all hemispherotomy techniques provide high rate of seizure-free outcome with significantly low complications rates compare to anatomical hemispherectomy [45].

Multilobar disconnection A complete disconnection of multilobar epileptogenic zone might be needed for seizure control in some patients. For example, if the patient has sub-hemispheric epilepsy covering a large area anterior to motor cortex, anterior peri-insular quadrantotomy might be an appropriate alternative to protect the residual motor functions. The surgery here aims to perform anterior callosotomy, intrafrontal white matter disconnection and frontobasal disconnection through a suprainsular window. On the other hand, if the epileptogenic zone is larger and located in the temporo-parieto-occipital region, then posterior peri-insular quadrantotomy might be the appropriate surgical approach. In these cases, the aim is performing posterior perisylvian and intraparietal disconnection of the parieto-occipital lobes and posterior callosotomy along posterior hippocampotomy using the infrainsular window [45, 48].

Neuromodulation and Ablation Procedures

Vagus Nerve Stimulation (VNS) VNS has been used in the treatment of intractable epilepsy since 1988 and it is proven as an effective adjunct in the treatment of intractable epilepsy when the patients are not candidates for resective or disconnective surgeries. It has a generator which is implanted in a subcutaneous pocket on the chest and connected electrodes with three coils to wrap around the left vagus nerve. It is a safe, well-tolerated procedure even for young children and provides up to 50% seizure reduction [49, 50].

Responsive Neurostimulation (RNS) RNS is a relatively new (FDA approval in 2013) closed-loop cortical stimulator and the stimulation is delivered only in response to the patient's recorded seizure activity through the connected intracranial electrodes of the system. The electrodes (currently two electrodes; depth and/or strip electrodes) are stereotactically placed into previously determined two epileptogenic target areas in the brain and they are connected to an implanted stimulator device in the skull which continually senses electrocorticographic data and responds accordingly. It provides up to 60% seizure reduction [51].

Stereotactic laser ablation MRI-guided laser interstitial therapy is a minimally invasive surgical treatment option which may be helpful in some epilepsy patients. It is especially helpful in the treatment of hypothalamic hamartoma and constitutes an alternative in the surgical management of periventricular heterotopia, focal cortical dysplasia, and mesial temporal sclerosis [54].

Conclusion

Pediatric epilepsy surgery is a well-established management option in the treatment of medically intractable seizures in children. However, children, especially young children and infants, still represent anatomically and physiologically unique patient population, and epilepsy in young children is not a fixed but an evolving and complex process. Therefore, the selection of young patients for epilepsy surgery stays as a challenging endeavor and needs to be handled with great care and expertise. There are many surgical treatment options to choose and surgical outcome in well-selected cases is very satisfactory and similar to that obtained in the adults. Epilepsy surgery may be a definitive treatment not just for seizure control but also for preventing long-term harmful effects of seizures on children's cognitive and motor development.

Questions

1. Eight-year-old female patient with medically intractable seizures for 2 years. Her typical seizure starts with lip smacking and associated with hand automatisms and staring. It ends in 1–3 min and seizures happen 1–3 times a month. She does not remember the events. EEG shows interictal sharp waves on the right temporal region and MRI shows a 1 cm in diameter lesion in the right temporal pole. MRI findings are suggestive for a cavernoma and no other clear-cut abnormality is noted in the brain. What is the most appropriate management plan?
   (a) Invasive monitoring with depth electrodes
   (b) Vagus nerve stimulator placement
   (c) No surgery, radiological observation
   (d) Biopsy
   (e) Lesionectomy with excision of surrounding hemosiderin rim
2. Sixteen-year-old male patient with medically intractable seizures within the last 4 years. He previously had seizures as a toddler and placed on seizure medications with good response. He had no seizure for 3 years and medications are discontinued. He was seizure free for 2 years and then started to have seizures again. He has different type of seizures. Most of the seizures are generally 2–3 min and start with gaging and associated with salivation, sometimes vomiting. It may progress to generalized tonic-clonic seizures at times. He also describes brief aura-like events associated with anxiety feeling and sweating profusely. He had long-term scalp EEG/Video monitoring which showed that interictal epileptogenic activities are mainly located left mesial temporal and left perisylvian region but there are also independent spikes on the right hippocampus. Five seizures were captured during EEG/Video monitoring. His seizure onset was located in the left anterior-mid temporal region in all seizures, except one seizure which was originated from the right mid-temporal region. His MRI showed subtle cortical thickening in the left posterior insular cortex and Flair hyperintense right hippocampus. SPECT and PET study results were not localizing. What is the most appropriate next step in the management of this patient?
   (a) Not a surgical candidate, findings are suggestive for bilateral seizure onset
   (b) Vagus nerve stimulator placement
   (c) Antero-mesial temporal lobectomy on the left side
   (d) Invasive monitoring with subdural grid covering the left temporal/perisylvian region
   (e) Bilateral exploration with SEEG depth electrodes

3. Which of these surgical procedures is used for curative purposes and with a high chance of seizure-free outcome?
   (a) Anteromesial temporal lobectomy in a patient with mesial temporal sclerosis
   (b) Corpus callosotomy in a patient with drop attacks
   (c) Lesionectomy in a patient with Rasmussen's disorder
   (d) Vagus nerve stimulator placement
   (e) Responsive neurostimulator placement
4. Which surgical procedure is a disconnection procedure
   (a) Selective amygdalohippocampectomy
   (b) Multilobar excision
   (c) Responsive neurostimulator placement
   (d) Hemispherotomy
   (e) Anterior temporal lobectomy
5. Which of these tests has been used in the Phase 2 assessment of the epilepsy patients
   (a) EEG
   (b) MRI
   (c) Functional MRI
   (d) SEEG
   (e) PET

Answers

1. (e)
2. (e)
3. (a)
4. (d)
5. (d)

References

1. Guerrini R. Epilepsy in children. Lancet. 2006;367:499–524.
2. Camfield P, Camfield C. Epidemiology of intractable epilepsy in children. In: Cataltepe O, Jallo G, editors. Pediatric epilepsy surgery. New York: Thieme; 2019. p. 21–7.
3. Cross JH. Epilepsy surgery in childhood. Epilepsia. 2002;43(Suppl 3):65–70.
4. Spencer S, Huh L. Outcomes of epilepsy surgery in adults and children. Lancet Neurol. 2008;7:525–37.
5. Cross JH, Jayakar P, Nordli D, Delalande O, Duchowny M, Wieser HG, et al. International League Against Epilepsy, Subcommission for Paediatric Epilepsy Surgery; Commissions of Neurosurgery and Paediatrics. Proposed criteria for referral and evaluation of children for epilepsy surgery: recommendations of the Subcommission for Paediatric Epilepsy Surgery. Epilepsia. 2006;47:952–9.
6. Wyllie E. Catastrophic epilepsy in infants and children: identification of surgical candidates. Epileptic Disord. 1999;1:261–4.
7. Duchowny M. Epilepsy surgery in children. Curr Opin Neurol. 1995;8:112–6.
8. Wyllie E, Comair YG, Kotagal P, Bulacio J, Bingaman W, Ruggieri P. Seizure outcome after epilepsy surgery in children and adolescents. Ann Neurol. 1998;44:740–8.
9. Stafstrom CE, Lynch M, Sutula TP. Consequences of epilepsy in the developing brain: implications for surgical management. Semin Pediatr Neurol. 2000;7:147–57.
10. Depositario-Cabacar DT, Riviello JJ, Takeoka M. Present status of surgical intervention for children with intractable seizures. Curr Neurol Neurosci Rep. 2008;8:123–9.
11. Green JR, Pootrakul A. Surgical aspects of the treatment of epilepsy during childhood and adolescence. Ariz Med. 1982;39:35–8.
12. Obeid M, Wyllie E, Rahi AC, Mikati MA. Approach to pediatric epilepsy surgery: state of the art, part I: general principles and presurgical workup. Eur J Paediatr Neurol. 2008;30:1–13.
13. Shewmon DA, Shields WD, Chugani HT, Peacock WJ. Contrasts between pediatric and adult epilepsy surgery: rationale and strategy for focal resection. J Epilepsy. 1990;3(Suppl):141–55.
14. Saneto RP, Wyllie E. Surgically treatable epilepsy syndromes in infancy and childhood. In: Miller JW, Silbergeld DL, editors. Epilepsy surgery. New York: Taylor and Francis; 2006. p. 121–41.
15. Smith TW. Surgical neuropathology of pediatric epilepsy surgery. In: Cataltepe O, Jallo G, editors. Pediatric epilepsy surgery. New York: Thieme; 2019. p. 26–46.
16. Thom M, Blumcke I, Aronica E. Long-term epilepsy-associated tumors. Brain Pathol. 2012;22(3):350–79.
17. Adelson PD. Temporal lobectomy in children with intractable seizures. Pediatr Neurosurg. 2001;34:268–77.
18. Duchowny M, Cross JH. Preoperative evaluation in children for epilepsy surgery. Handb Clin Neurol. 2012;108:676–85.
19. Oguni H. Infantile and childhood-onset catastrophic epilepsy syndromes. In: Cataltepe O, Jallo G, editors. Pediatric epilepsy surgery. New York: Thieme; 2019. p. 60–9.
20. Shields WD. Catastrophic epilepsy in childhood. Epilepsia. 2000;41(Suppl 2):S2–6.
21. Rasmussen T. Hemispherectomy for seizures revisited. Can J Neurol Sci. 1983;10:71–8.
22. Varadkar S, Bien CG, Kruse CA, et al. Rasmussen's encephalitis: clinical features, pathobiology, and treatment advances. Lancet Neurol. 2014;13(2):195–205.

23. Andermann F, Palmini AL. Neuronal migration disorders. In: Luders H, editor. Epilepsy surgery. New York: Raven Press; 1993. p. 203–11.
24. Aronica E, Becker AJ, Spreafico R. Malformations of cortical development. Brain Pathol. 2012;22(3):380–401.
25. Grinenko O, Najm I. Focal cortical dysplasia: histopathology, neuroimaging, and electroclinical presentation. In: Cataltepe O, Jallo G, editors. Pediatric epilepsy surgery. New York: Thieme; 2019. p. 404–13.
26. Akman CI, Riviello JJ. Intractable epilepsy in children and selection of surgical candidates. In: Cataltepe O, Jallo G, editors. Pediatric epilepsy surgery. New York: Thieme; 2019. p. 81–91.
27. Fogarasi A. Clinical semiology in preoperative assessment. In: Cataltepe O, Jallo G, editors. Pediatric epilepsy surgery. New York: Thieme; 2019. p. 92–102.
28. Jayakar P, Dunoyer C, Dean P, et al. Diagnostic utility of invasive EEG for epilepsy surgery: indications, modalities, and techniques. Epilepsia. 2016;57(11):1735–47.
29. Murphy MA, O'Brien TJ, Morris K, Cook MJ. Multimodality image-guided surgery for the treatment of medically refractory epilepsy. J Neurosurg. 2004;100(3):452–62.
30. Jayakar P, Hyslop A, Miller I. Invasive electrophysiological monitoring. In: Cataltepe O, Jallo G, editors. Pediatric epilepsy surgery. New York: Thieme; 2019. p. 127–33.
31. Noviawaty I, Chauvel P. Stereoelectroencephalograph y. In: Cataltepe O, Jallo G, editors. Pediatric epilepsy surgery. New York: Thieme; 2019. p. 145–52.
32. Cataltepe O, Pilitsis J. Implantation of strip, grid and depth electrodes for invasive intracranial monitoring. In: Cataltepe O, Jallo G, editors. Pediatric epilepsy surgery. New York: Thieme; 2019. p. 313–22.
33. McGovern RA, Gonzalez-Martinez JA. Stereoelec troencephalography in children: methodology and surgical technique. In: Cataltepe O, Jallo G, editors. Pediatric epilepsy surgery. New York: Thieme; 2019. p. 323–32.
34. Gonzalez-Martinez J, Mullin J, Bulaco J, Gupta A, Enatsu R, Najm I, Bingaman W, Wyllie E, Lachhwani D. Stereoelectroencephalography in children with adolescents with difficult to-localize refractory focal epilepsy. Neurosurgery. 2014;75(3):258–68.
35. Cardinale F, Casaceli G, Raneri F, Miller J, Lo Russo G. Implantation of stereoelectroencephalography electrodes: a systematic review. J Clin Neurophysiol. 2016;33(6):490–502.
36. Rasmussen T. Surgical aspects. In: Lee RG, editor. Topics in child neurology. New York: Spectrum Publications; 1977. p. 143–57.
37. Falconer MA. Place of surgery for temporal lobe epilepsy during childhood. Br Med J. 1972;2:631–5.
38. Duchowny M, Levin B, Jayakar P, Resnick T, Alvarez L, Morrison G, et al. Temporal lobectomy in early childhood. Epilepsia. 1992;33:298–303.
39. Cataltepe O, Turanli G, Yalnizoglu D, Topcu M, Akalan N. Surgical management of temporal lobe tumor related epilepsy in children. J Neurosurg. 2005;102(Suppl 3):280–7.
40. Cardinale F, d'Orio P, Rizzi M. Surgical management of MRI-negative temporal lobe epilepsy. In: Cataltepe O, Jallo G, editors. Pediatric epilepsy surgery. New York: Thieme; 2019. p. 376–85.
41. Cascino GD, Sharbrough FW, Trennerry MR. Extratemporal cortical resections and lesionectomies. Epilepsia. 1994;35:1085–90.
42. Perry MS, Duchowny M. Surgical management of intractable childhood epilepsy: curative and palliative procedures. Semin Pediatr Neurol. 2011;18(3):195–202.
43. Roland JL, Smyth M. Surgical management of MRI-negative extratemporal lobe epilepsy. In: Cataltepe O, Jallo G, editors. Pediatric epilepsy surgery. New York: Thieme; 2019. p. 481–8.
44. Cataltepe O. Hemispherectomy and hemispherotomy techniques in pediatric epilepsy surgery. In: Cataltepe O, Jallo G, editors. Pediatric epilepsy surgery. New York: Thieme; 2019. p. 497–505.
45. Graham D, Tisdall MM, Gill D. Corpus callosotomy outcomes in pediatric patients: a systematic review. Epilepsia. 2016;57(7):1053–68.
46. Cossu G, Messerer M, Lebon S, Pralong E, Seeck M, Daniel RT. Anterior peri-insular quadrantotomy. In: Cataltepe O, Jallo G, editors. Pediatric epilepsy surgery. New York: Thieme; 2019. p. 459–64.
47. Uribe R, Jallo GI, Hoffman J. Multifocal epilepsy and multilobar resections. In: Cataltepe O, Jallo G, editors. Pediatric epilepsy surgery. New York: Thieme; 2019. p. 506–9.
48. Englot DJ, Chang EF, Auguste KI. Vagus nerve stimulation for epilepsy: a meta-analysis of efficacy and predictors of response. J Neurosurg. 2011;115(6):1248–55.
49. Roland JL, Limbrick DD, Smyth MD. Vagal nerve stimulation. In: Cataltepe O, Jallo G, editors. Pediatric epilepsy surgery. New York: Thieme; 2019. p. 613–8.
50. Woodward EE, Shimony N, Jallo G. Cortical and deep brain stimulation. In: Cataltepe O, Jallo G, editors. Pediatric epilepsy surgery. New York: Thieme; 2019. p. 619–24.
51. Curry DJ, Gadgil N. Stereotactic laser ablation for hypothalamic hamartoma. In: Cataltepe O, Jallo G, editors. Pediatric epilepsy surgery. New York: Thieme; 2019. p. 640–4.

Management of Pediatric Patient with Neurofibromatosis

12

Chelsea Kotch and Michael J. Fisher

Introduction

Neurofibromatosis type 1 and neurofibromatosis type 2 are distinct disorders characterized by the development of central and peripheral nervous system tumors. Neurofibromatosis type 1 (NF1) is one of the most common inherited genetic conditions worldwide, affecting approximately 1 in 3000 people and impacting all sexes and races equally [1]. Neurofibromatosis type 2 (NF2) has an incidence of 1 in 33,000 and classically presents by the age of 30 years with bilateral vestibular schwannomas. While promising novel therapies are arising for the management of NF-associated neoplasms, surgical management remains an important aspect of therapy. Multidisciplinary medical and surgical care is necessary for all patients with NF and NF-associated neoplasms, given the range and severity of manifestations and symptoms. Further, it is essential that clinicians and surgeons alike be aware of the management options and complications observed in these complex disorders.

C. Kotch (✉) · M. J. Fisher
Division of Oncology, Department of Pediatrics, Children's Hospital of Philadelphia and University of Pennsylvania Perelman School of Medicine, Philadelphia, PA, USA
e-mail: KOTCHC@chop.edu; FISHERM@chop.edu

Neurofibromatosis Type 1

Neurofibromatosis type 1 is the most common genetic cancer predisposition syndrome and has a variety of manifestations, including predisposition to benign and malignant tumors. NF1 is an autosomal dominant disorder and occurs due to an inherited or de novo germline mutation in one of two alleles of the *NF1* gene. Approximately half of pathogenic *NF1* mutations are sporadic and more than 2800 different pathogenic variants have been described [2, 3]. The *NF1* gene, located on chromosome 17q11, encodes for the tumor suppressor protein neurofibromin. Neurofibromin is expressed in most tissues and in high levels in the nervous system, and is a negative regulator of the Ras/mitogen activated protein kinase pathway [4]. Tumors typically develop in the setting of bi-allelic inactivation of the *NF1* gene due to a second somatic loss of function mutation, resulting in loss of neurofibromin expression and unregulated cell proliferation.

Diagnosis

The diagnosis of NF1 may be made from clinical criteria or the identification of a pathogenic germline mutation and associated clinical features. The National Institutes of Health (NIH) Consensus Conference held in 1987 identified the original clinical diagnostic criteria for NF1,

N. Shimony, G. Jallo (eds.), *Pediatric Neurosurgery Board Review*,
https://doi.org/10.1007/978-3-031-23687-7_12

which were subsequently revised in 2021 (*see* Table 12.1) [5]. Symptoms of NF1 typically present during childhood, with nearly all patients meeting the diagnostic criteria by 8 years of age [6]. Given that NF1 affects nearly every organ system in the body, patients may present with a variety of findings (*see* Table 12.2). Regardless of inheritance pattern or pathogenic variant, penetrance is approximately 100% by the third decade of life. However, there is significant variability in the manifestation of NF1, even amongst members of the same family [7].

Table 12.1 Diagnostic criteria for neurofibromatosis type 1

Two or more of the following findings in a child who does not have a parent with NF1 OR
1 or more in the child of a parent who meets diagnostic criteria for NF1:

- 6 or more café-au-lait macules >5 mm in diameter in prepubertal patients and >15 mm in post-pubertal patients
- Freckling in axillary or inguinal region.
- 2 or more neurofibromas of any type or 1 plexiform neurofibroma
- Optic pathway glioma
- ≥2 iris Lisch nodules or ≥2 choroidal abnormalities
- Osseous lesion (sphenoid dysplasia, pseudarthrosis of long bone, tibial bowing)
- Heterozygous pathogenic NF1 variant with variant allele fraction of 50% in normal tissue

[a]Adapted from [5]

Table 12.2 Manifestations of neurofibromatosis type 1 by organ system

Tumors of the nervous system	Low grade glioma, high grade glioma, plexiform neurofibroma, malignant peripheral nerve sheath tumor
Skeletal system	Scoliosis, tibial dysplasia, long bone pseudarthrosis, sphenoid wing dysplasia
Endocrine	Precocious or delayed puberty, short stature
Vascular	Primary and secondary hypertension, vasculopathy, congenital heart disease
Skin	Café au lait macules, axillary and inguinal freckling, juvenile xanthogranuloma, cutaneous neurofibroma, pruritis
Ophthalmologic	Lisch nodules, choroidal abnormalities
Neurologic/ neurocognitive	Macrocephaly, focal T2 hyperintensities, developmental delay including speech, learning deficits, attention deficit hyperactivity disorder, social skills issues

Manifestations and Management by System

Cutaneous

Cutaneous findings in NF1 commonly include multiple café-au-lait macules (CALM), skinfold freckling, and cutaneous neurofibromas. Less frequently observed findings include juvenile xanthogranulomas and nevus anemicus [8]. CALM are usually the first presenting sign of NF1, with classic lesions appearing as well-demarcated tan to dark brown patches (*see* Fig. 12.1). Of note, up to 20% of healthy individuals will have an isolated CALM. In NF1, CALM may increase in number or size throughout childhood and greater than 6 CALM is one of the diagnostic criteria of NF1 (*see* Table 12.1). Skinfold freckling occurs in up to 90% of patients by 7 years of age [8]. Cutaneous neurofibromas (CN) are another common finding in NF1 and may occur anywhere on the body. CN arise from nerves within the epidermis and dermis and present as superficial, soft small nodules. CN do not undergo malignant transformation and typically arise during puberty.

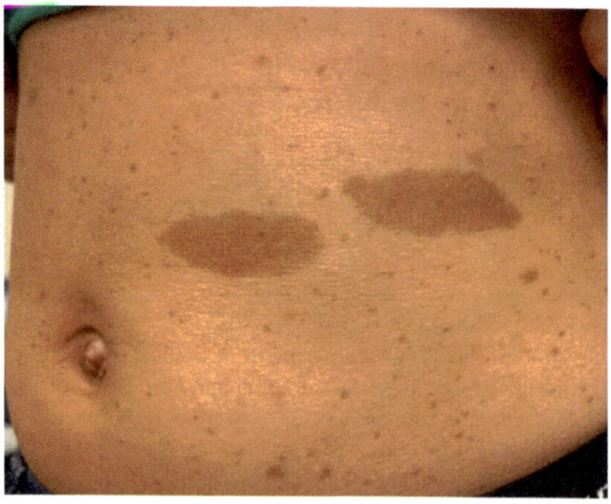

Fig. 12.1 Café-au-lait macules

CN may be targeted by laser therapy or removed surgically if they cause discomfort, or their location is bothersome to the patient. Disadvantages of removal include regrowth of tumor, development of new tumors, and risk of scarring [9].

Skeletal

Skeletal abnormalities observed in patients with NF1 may include scoliosis (dystrophic and non-dystrophic), macrocephaly, short stature, dysplasia of the long bone or sphenoid wing, and pseudarthrosis. The incidence of scoliosis in NF1 reported in the literature ranges between 10 and 60% [10, 11]. Management is dependent on the degree of curvature, age of patient, and progression [1]. Dysplasia of the long bones occurs in up to 4% of patients, with the tibia most frequently affected [7]. Tibial dysplasia may result in obvious bowing on physical examination. Patients with dysplasia are at risk for pathologic fractures with abnormal healing, resulting in pseudarthrosis. If dysplasia is diagnosed, patients should be referred to a pediatric orthopedic surgeon for prevention and management of potential fractures. In addition, up to 40% of patients with NF1 may have a diagnosis of macrocephaly [1]. Sphenoid wing dysplasia occurs in up to 7% of patients with NF1 and rarely may be associated with temporal lobe herniation into the orbital cavity due to complete or partial absence of the greater wing of the sphenoid. Management of this complication is surgical and includes repair of the anterior skull base [12].

Ophthalmologic

Lisch nodules are small, asymptomatic hyperpigmented hamartomas of the iris and are one of the diagnostic criteria for NF1. These are identified by slit-lamp examination and typically develop in children between 5 and 10 years of age [4, 13]. Choroidal abnormalities occur in 82–100% of adults and over 70% of children with NF1 [14, 15]. These abnormalities are undetectable on conventional ophthalmologic examination, but appear as bright, patchy nodules on infrared fundus autofluorescence and irregular hyperreflective choroidal foci on optical coherence tomography. Neither lisch nodules nor choroidal abnormalities impact visual acuity or cause visual disturbances. An ophthalmology evaluation is required for all patients with suspected NF1 to evaluate for Lisch nodules and/or choroidal abnormalities, as these are one of the NF1 diagnostic criteria, in addition to assess for signs of optic pathway glioma.

Vascular

Patients with NF1 are at increased risk of hypertension and vasculopathy compared to the general population. NF1 vasculopathy affects vessels of different sizes, and renal artery stenosis is the most common vasculopathy observed. The prevalence of cerebral arteriopathy is approximately 2.5–6%, with abnormalities including narrowed or stenotic vessels, aneurysms, and moyamoya syndrome (*see* Fig. 12.2) [16]. At present, there are no evidence-based guidelines for screening children with NF1 with imaging for vascular disease [17]. Rather, screening should include annual neurological examination (to evaluate for focal neurologic findings) and blood pressure monitoring, as hypertension may be the initial sign of renal artery stenosis. Imaging is prompted by symptoms or exam findings and may include doppler ultrasound or CT angiography to evaluate for renal artery stenosis or magnetic resonance imaging/angiography (MRI/MRA) to evaluate for cerebrovascular disease.

A subset of patients with NF1-arteriopathy will develop moyamoya syndrome (MMS). MMS is a chronic progressive vaso-occlusive disorder of the cerebral vasculature with a predilection for the distal branches of the internal carotid arteries. The prevalence of MMS in patients with NF1 is approximately 0.6%. The pathophysiology is unknown; however, it is postulated that alteration of neurofibromin function in blood vessels may result in proliferation of vascular smooth muscle cells [18]. In addition, prior intracranial radiation is associated with increased risk for development and severity of disease [19]. Patients may

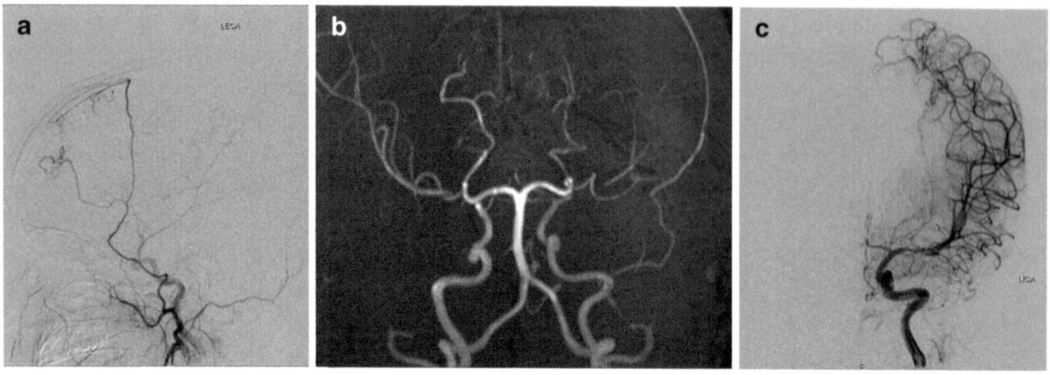

Fig. 12.2 Bilateral tortuous internal carotid arteries in a patient with neurofibromatosis type 1 on magnetic resonance angiography (**b**) and interventional angiogram (**a**, **c**). Imaging reveals bilateral A1 and M1 narrowing with non-visualization of the anterior cerebral arteries (**b**), significant left external carotid artery synangiosis to anterior cerebral artery distribution (**a**), and significant hypoperfusion of the left anterior carotid artery anterior distribution on angiography (**c**)

be asymptomatic or present with headache, seizures, or intracranial hemorrhage. The diagnosis is made with cerebral angiography, with a classic "puff of smoke" appearance due to the formation of abnormal intracranial collateral vessels. Although MMS can cause significant neurologic morbidity due to stroke, there are currently no imaging guidelines for the screening of asymptomatic patients. The treatment of MMS is primarily surgical and is indicated with the onset of clinical symptoms or concerns for ischemia. Surgical revascularization methods, such as pial synangiosis, appear safe and protective against future stroke and neurologic complications [20]. Patients may also receive aspirin therapy, at the discretion of neurology or neurosurgery guidance.

Neurologic

The non-neoplastic neurologic manifestations of NF1 include seizures, headaches, focal areas of signal intensity on brain MRI, hydrocephalus, neurocognitive and behavioral deficits, and social skills issues such as autism spectrum disorder. Patients with NF1 are at increased risk for seizures, occurring in up to 7% of patients, with focal seizures representing the predominant seizure type. Seizures are often related to intracranial pathology, however, may occur in the absence of an inciting lesion. Any patient with NF1 and new-onset seizure should undergo brain MRI given the risk of development of intracranial neoplasm, even in the setting of previously normal neuroimaging. Patients with NF1 who develop epilepsy may require more aggressive medical management than the general population and may ultimately be candidates for epilepsy surgery [21].

Focal areas of signal intensity (FASI), previously called "unidentified bright objects," are bright areas on T2-weighted MRI occurring in up to 90% of pediatric patients with NF1. These lesions are most frequently identified in the basal ganglia, cerebellum, thalamus, and brainstem. FASI typically increase in size and number in childhood and regress during adolescence. Although they can be challenging to distinguish from low-grade glioma, FASI typically do not cause mass effect and lack contrast-enhancement. In addition, FASI do not appear to be correlated with neurologic deficits or tumor development [22, 23]. FASI that are typical in appearance do not require routine radiographic surveillance.

Patients with NF1 are also at increased risk for the development of obstructive hydrocephalus in the setting of aqueductal stenosis or optic pathway, midbrain, or thalamic gliomas [24]. Thus, there should be a low threshold for intracranial imaging with the onset of signs or symptoms concerning for increased intracranial pressure.

MRI with gadolinium is the diagnostic modality of choice in the evaluation of hydrocephalus, particularly given the heightened concern for potential obstruction in the setting of tumor. Treatment of symptomatic hydrocephalus in NF1 may be directed towards the etiology or the hydrocephalus itself, with craniospinal fluid diversion, chemotherapy, and/or surgical debulking.

Benign and Malignant Neoplasms of Neurofibromatosis Type 1

Plexiform Neurofibroma

Plexiform neurofibromas (PN) are histologically benign peripheral nerve sheath tumors that affect up to 50% of patients with NF1. PN arise from nerves throughout the entire body and usually involve multiple nerve fascicles. They are multicellular tumors, composed of Schwann cells, perineural cells, fibroblasts, mast cells, macrophages, and collagen and are often highly vascular [25]. The growth of PN varies between patients and even among a patient's multiple tumors. Overall, younger age is associated with more rapid tumor growth, whereas most PN in adults are no longer growing or grow slowly. PN may be asymptomatic or cause significant morbidity such as pain, disfigurement, and loss of function, and may be life-threatening when they impinge on vital structures such as the airway (see Fig. 12.3).

PN may transform to atypical plexiform neurofibroma or malignant peripheral nerve sheath tumor (MPNST). Atypical PN are defined on histopathologic examination by nuclear atypia, increased mitotic indices, and loss of the classic neurofibroma architecture, and are molecularly characterized by loss of *CDKN2A/B*. Atypical PN may be pre-malignant, as they have a higher risk for the development of MPNST compared to classic PN. However, all PN, regardless of the presence of atypia, are at risk to undergo transformation to MPNST, which occurs in up to 13% of patients with NF1 [26]. Rapid growth of a PN or worsening pain may be an indication of malignant transformation and should prompt evaluation.

MRI is the gold standard diagnostic imaging modality for PN and should be performed using short tau inversion recovery (STIR) sequences, a fat suppression technique which provides optimal visualization of PN. Intravenous contrast is not required. At present, screening imaging to detect PN is not recommended. Imaging is usually prompted by concerns identified by history or physical examination. For known PN, there is no current standard of care for frequency of surveillance imaging to monitor for tumor growth, and intervals vary widely. Finally, a biopsy to confirm the diagnosis of PN is not necessary unless clinical or imaging findings are concerning for malignant transformation.

Most PN do not require treatment, but rather should be observed at the time of diagnosis. Treatment is considered for tumors that are causing morbidity (e.g., severe pain, significant disfigurement, or functional impairment) or are progressing and associated with impending morbidity. The decision to treat is complex and often guided by symptoms as opposed to tumor size, as small tumors may cause significant morbidity while large PN may be asymptomatic. Until recently, treatment options for PN were limited to surgical resection or debulking. The main goals of resection include to restore function, ameliorate pain, and/or reduce significant disfigurement. However, surgical resections are often limited to incomplete debulking due to the infiltrative nature of these tumors and attempts at resection are associated with risks of worsening of pain and functional impairment. To date, there are no prospective studies of surgical outcomes after resection of PN; however, the largest retrospective series suggests that complete excision of tumor is accomplished in only 15% of cases [27]. Radiation therapy is avoided for PN given the baseline risk of malignancy in NF1, in addition to the risk of malignant transformation of these tumors [28]. If treatment is warranted, the selection of medical versus surgical intervention should be guided by a multi-disciplinary team of neurofibromatosis clinicians and surgeons.

There have been recent significant advances in the medical management of PN. Targeted inhibition of the mitogen-activated protein kinase

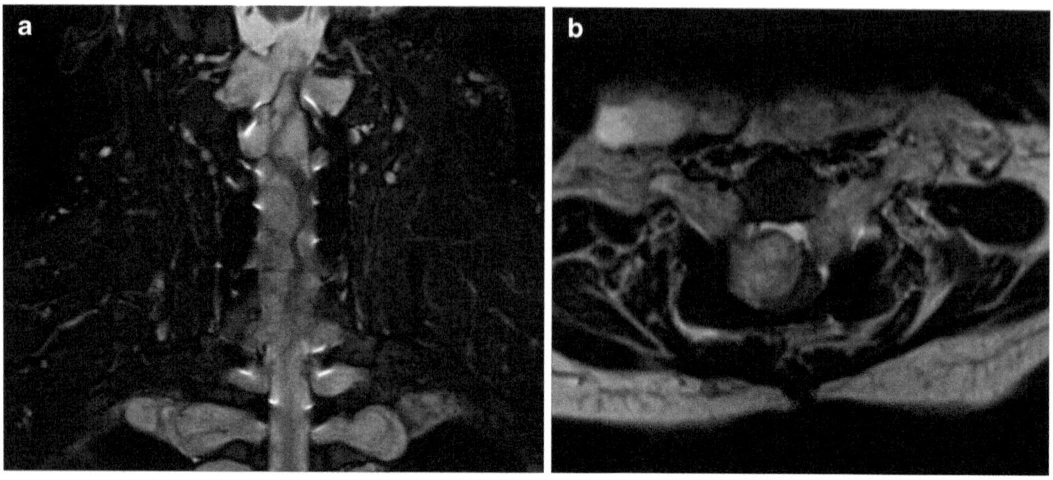

Fig. 12.3 Multiple paraspinal plexiform neurofibromas with intradural extension and spinal cord compression at T1 visualized on coronal short tau inversion recovery (**a**) and T2 turbo spin echo transverse (**b**) sequences

(MAPK) kinase (MEK) has been explored as a therapeutic option. In a groundbreaking phase 2 clinical trial of the MEK inhibitor selumetinib for children with NF1 and inoperable symptomatic PN, 68% had a partial response, in addition to improvements in function and quality of life [29]. On the basis of this trial, selumetinib was approved by the Food and Drug Administration for the treatment of symptomatic, inoperable PN in children with NF1. Other MEK inhibitors, including mirdametinib and binimetinib, have also demonstrated efficacy in recent or ongoing clinical trials for children or adults with PN [30, 31]. Common side effects observed with MEK inhibitors include rash, paronychia, diarrhea, abdominal pain, and elevations of aminotransferases and creatine kinase. Careful monitoring for ophthalmologic toxicity and change in cardiac function is required. At present, there are still outstanding questions on the duration and durability of treatment, as well as the long-term toxicities of these agents. In addition to MEK inhibitors, a multi-receptor tyrosine kinase inhibitor, cabozantinib, has also demonstrated efficacy in clinical trials of adolescents and adults with PN with reduction of tumor size and pain [25]. Ongoing studies are evaluating cabozantinib for the treatment of PN in children.

Malignant Peripheral Nerve Sheath Tumors

MPNST are aggressive soft tissue tumors that occur in 8–13% of patients with NF1. The overall survival is poor, with current 5-year estimates between 20 and 50% [26]. The majority of NF1-associated MPNST develop in preexisting PN due to malignant transformation [26]. Importantly, the diagnosis of MPNST can only be made by pathologic evaluation, and the detection of MPNST within a PN can be challenging given the risk of sampling error. Fluorodeoxyglucose (FDG) positron emission tomography (PET) is a sensitive and specific imaging tool to aid in the detection of MPNST and/or targeting of biopsy, as MPNST are more likely to be FDG-avid [32]. Diffusion weighted and dynamic contrast enhanced MRI sequences are also being explored to help with MPNST detection [33]. As with other sarcomas, MPNST are commonly staged with the American Joint Commission on Cancer staging system. Features associated with poor prognosis include large tumor size (>5 cm), deep location, and presence of metastases [34]. The most common sites of metastases include lung, liver, brain, and bone; thus, CT chest should be obtained upon histologic confirmation of MPNST in addition to full body PET if not previously obtained. Gross total surgical resection with wide negative margins is the gold standard intervention, as incompletely resected tumors portend a worse prognosis [26]. The role of adjuvant radiation therapy for MPNST is debated and is often utilized for MPNST with high-risk features, incomplete resections, or prior to surgery in some cases. The role of chemotherapy for MPNST remains undetermined as well, as these tumors appear to have intermediate sensitivity to classic chemotherapy agents. However, adjuvant chemotherapy is often utilized in an attempt to reduce tumor burden prior to resection and for treatment of undetected micro-metastases [35]. Targeted therapies for MPNST based on preclinical mouse models are presently under evaluation in clinical trials. In summary, all efforts should be made to achieve gross total resection with wide negative margins if the intent of therapy is curative.

Low Grade Glioma

Children with NF1 are at risk for developing low grade glioma both (LGG) within and extrinsic to the optic pathway. The optic pathway is the most common location followed by the brainstem. These tumors are typically not biopsied, as most are indolent and do not require therapy. Recent molecular characterization confirmed that most of NF1-LGG are pilocytic astrocytoma with no additional molecular alterations beyond the loss of both *NF1* alleles; thus, routine biopsy of typically appearing LGG in children with NF1 is not indicated. However, there are a small percentage of NF1-LGG in children that have unexpected findings, although this is rare for LGG in the optic pathway or hypothalamus [36]. Thus, it may be reasonable to consider biopsy for tumors outside of the optic pathway or hypothalamus which are unresponsive to standard chemotherapy, or those tumors with atypical features on MRI.

Optic pathway glioma (OPG) occur in up to 20% of patients with NF1 at a median age of diagnosis of 4.6 years (see Fig. 12.4) [1]. OPG often follow an indolent course and at least half of patients with NF1-OPG will never require therapy. The primary indications for therapy include a decline in visual acuity or visual fields. In fact, radiographic progression and visual acuity often do not correlate, thus initiation of therapy may not occur with radiographic progression alone [37].

Surgical excision is usually contraindicated in NF1-OPG, due to the risks of visual worsening with both biopsy and resection. Surgery may be considered for unilateral optic nerve tumors associated with complete loss of vision and painful or disfiguring proptosis. Other indications may include partial tumor debulking or fenestration of cystic components when these cause mass effect on surrounding brain structures. Overall, interventions for NF1-OPG should be implemented primarily based on functional impact, such as vision, rather than radiographic changes, as the goal of therapy is visual preservation.

Approximately 5–10% of children with NF1 will develop a non-optic pathway LGG [38]. In children, these occur most frequently in the brainstem. The mean age of diagnosis for brainstem glioma in NF1 is approximately 7 years [39]. As with OPG, many of these tumors remain asymptomatic and do not require treatment. If symptoms develop, they are often related to cranial nerve palsies or obstructive hydrocephalus in the setting of stenosis of the aqueduct.

If treatment is indicated for NF1-LGG either within or extrinsic to the optic pathway, initial therapy is usually carboplatin-based chemotherapy. In a large Children's Oncology Group study, carboplatin and vincristine was associated with a 5-year progression free survival of 69%. Second-line chemotherapy regimens include weekly vinblastine monotherapy, which has demonstrated efficacy with low toxicity in children with NF1-LGG [40]. While there are other chemotherapy regimens effective for LGG, most are avoided in patients with NF1 because of the concern of alkylator-induced secondary leukemia.

MEK inhibitors have been explored for the treatment of NF1-LGG. Selumetinib demonstrated clinical activity in early phase clinical trials for recurrent NF1-LGG with a response rate of 40% and 2-year progression free survival of 96% [41]. An ongoing Children's Oncology Group study (NCT03871257) is evaluating if selumetinib is an equivalent option to standard chemotherapy for the treatment of chemotherapy-naïve NF1-LGG. Everolimus, an inhibitor of the mammalian target of rapamycin pathway, also demonstrated efficacy for patients with recurrent/progressive NF1-LGG, with 68% of subjects demonstrating either response or stable disease in a phase 2 clinical trial [42]. In contrast, sorafenib, a multi-target (including RAF) small molecule tyrosine kinase inhibitor, was stopped early due to unexpected accelerated tumor growth [43]. As with other NF1-associated tumors, radiation therapy for NF1-LGG is avoided due to the increased risk of secondary malignancies and vasculopathy such as moyamoya syndrome [19].

High Grade Glioma

Patients with NF1 are also at increased risk for the development of high-grade gliomas compared to the general population, with an increasing incidence with age. NF1-associated high-grade gliomas demonstrate mutations in the *TP53*, *ATRX*, and *CDKN2A* genes, however they typically lack the *IDH* and *histone H3* mutations commonly observed in non-NF1 malignant gliomas [44]. Currently, surgical resection and radiation are the mainstays of therapy; however, there is variability in approach to treatment across institutions. There is ongoing interest in the potential use of combinations of novel molecular agents such as MEK inhibitors and possible CDK4/6 inhibitors for the treatment of NF1-associated high-grade gliomas, however, prospective clinical trials have yet to be implemented [45].

Screening of Patients with Neurofibromatosis Type 1

Screening recommendations for patients with a diagnosis of NF1 have been proposed based on manifestations most likely to occur at different ages. Children with NF1 should be followed at least annually by a provider experienced in the management of patients with neurofibromatosis. Based on the risk of developing optic pathway glioma, children with suspected or diagnosed NF1 should undergo ophthalmologic screening at least annually. Preferably, this examination is performed by an ophthalmologist experienced in the evaluation of patients with NF1. In addition, due to the potential involvement of NF1-associated gliomas with the hypothalamus, annual screening for changes in linear growth and pubertal development is recommended. The use of imaging as screening for

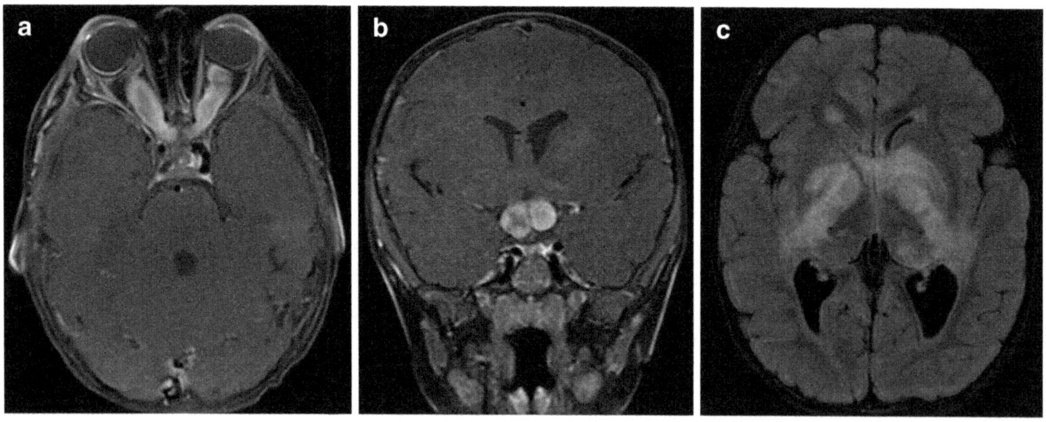

Fig. 12.4 Optic pathway glioma of the bilateral optic nerves on axial T1 post-gadolinium (**a**), chiasm/hypothalamus on coronal T1 post-gadolinium with fat suppression (**b**) and posterior pathway including optic tract/radiations on axial T2 fluid attenuated inversion recovery (**c**) sequences

OPG is controversial, and the Optic Pathway Task Force recommended against routine MRI [46]. There are currently no recommendations for routine imaging for the detection or monitoring of asymptomatic PN; thus, imaging should be guided by the onset of signs and symptoms. Patients should also be monitored at least annually for the development of hypertension, which may be primary or secondary in etiology. Congenital heart disease has a greater incidence in patients with NF1 than the general population, thus children with NF1 and a cardiac murmur should be evaluated with echocardiography [1]. Overall, many advances have been made in the management of children with NF1 and the clinical assessment and management of NF1-associated neoplasms should be performed by an experienced multidisciplinary team.

Neurofibromatosis Type 2

Neurofibromatosis type 2 is an autosomal dominant tumor predisposition syndrome characterized by the development of bilateral vestibular schwannomas. NF2 is caused by a loss of function mutation on the *NF2* gene, located on chromosome 22q12. Approximately 50% of cases result from hereditary transmission of pathogenic mutations, with the remaining mutations occurring de novo. Mutations in *NF2* result in loss of production of merlin, a tumor suppressor protein that functions in multiple signaling pathways including the phosphoinositol-3 kinase (PI3K)/Akt/mTOR, Raf/MEK/ERK, NF-kB, and Hippo pathways. In contrast to NF1, genotype-phenotype associations have been more commonly identified in NF2, with more severe phenotypes observed with truncating (frameshift or nonsense) mutations [47]. NF2 typically presents in young adults; however, up to 18% of newly diagnosed patients may be less than 15 years of age [48]. Earlier presentation of NF2 appears to be associated with poorer prognosis [49].

Diagnosis

There are two main diagnostic criteria systems for NF2 (National Institutes of Health and Manchester). The Manchester criteria are the most widely used and were updated recently (*see* Table 12.3) [50, 51]. NF2 typically presents in adulthood with hearing loss related to vestibular schwannoma. However, in childhood, the most commonly identified initial features of NF2 are meningiomas and ocular abnormalities (retinal hamartomas and epiretinal membranes) [52]. In addition, presenting symptoms may be due to non-cranial schwannoma or mononeuropathy without definitive tumor burden, leading to challenges or delay in diagnosis [53]. Current limitations in the diagnostic criteria for NF2 also include significant overlap in features of NF2 and schwannomatosis and the spontaneous occurrence of bilateral vestibular schwannomas in patients over the age of 50 years unrelated to NF2. Ongoing revisions to the criteria will likely be published in the future.

Genetic testing is an important aspect of the management of patients with NF2, particularly as it relates to counseling around transmission to offspring. An abnormality in *NF2* will be detected with molecular testing of leukocytes in over 90% of patients with affected family members. When

Table 12.3 Neurofibromatosis type 2 revised Manchester diagnostic criteria

Bilateral vestibular schwannoma <70 years of age OR one of the following combinations:

- First-degree relative with NF2 and unilateral vestibular schwannoma <70 years of age
- First-degree relative with NF2 and any 2 of: meningioma, cataract, ependymoma, schwannoma, cerebral calcification
- Unilateral vestibular schwannoma and any 2 of: meningioma, cataract, ependymoma, schwannoma, cerebral calcification
- Multiple meningiomas (2 or more) with any 2 of: unilateral vestibular schwannoma, cataract, ependymoma, schwannoma, cerebral calcification
- Constitutional pathogenic *NF2* gene variant in blood or identical in 2 tumors

[a]Adapted from [51]

a mutation has been identified in an individual, targeted mutational testing can be performed on family members to screen for presence of the mutation [40]. However, in a subset of patients, molecular screening may not identify a pathogenic mutation, such as in the setting of mosaicism. In mosaic disease, only a subset of cells contains the abnormal *NF2* gene leading to an insufficient proportion of circulating mutated cells for detection of the mutation. In cases of suspected mosaicism, tumor analysis may be necessary to identify the pathogenic mutation [54].

Manifestations and Management by System

Dermatologic

Patients with NF2 may have dermatologic findings that are more subtle than those found in NF1 (see Table 12.4). Signs can include plaque-like dermal schwannomas, nodular dermal schwannomas, and hyperpigmented macules. Approximately 70% of adult patients with NF2 have cutaneous lesions, the most frequent being the plaque-like schwannomas [55].

Ophthalmologic

Patients with NF2 can develop a variety of ophthalmologic complications and up to 80% of patients will develop cataracts. The most frequently observed type of cataract in NF2 are posterior subcapsular lenticular opacities, which are usually asymptomatic and rarely require removal. Juvenile cortical wedge cataracts can be observed shortly after birth; these cataracts may be associated with amblyopia requiring intervention [56]. Patients may also develop visual complaints due to the development of retinal hamartomas or optic nerve damage due to meningioma.

Table 12.4 Manifestations of neurofibromatosis type 2 by organ system

Tumors of the nervous system	Schwannoma, meningioma, ependymoma
Skin	Plaque-like dermal schwannomas, nodular dermal schwannomas, café au lait macules
Ophthalmologic	Cataracts, epiretinal membranes, retinal hamartomas
Neurologic/neurocognitive	Neuropathy

Neurologic

Peripheral neuropathy is a common complaint in patients with NF2, often presenting as a mononeuropathy in children and polyneuropathy in adults. The etiology is unclear; however, it may be due to local compression of nerves from Schwann cell proliferation. Patients may require treatment with neuropathic pain medications if symptoms impact quality of life or daily function (Table 12.4) [56].

Benign and Malignant Neoplasms of Neurofibromatosis Type 2

Vestibular Schwannoma

Schwannomas are slow-growing tumors, comprised of proliferations of neoplastic Schwann cells of the peripheral nervous system. The most common intracranial tumor in patients with NF2 is the vestibular schwannoma (VS), developing in over 95% of people affected. VS arise from the vestibular branches of the vestibulocochlear nerve and most patients present with hearing loss and tinnitus. Patients may also develop cranial neuropathies in the setting of brainstem compression if mass effect is significant. On MRI, these tumors typically appear isointense on T1-weighted images and heterogeneously intense on T2-weighted, with enhancement on post-gadolinium T1 sequences (*see* Fig. 12.5) [56].

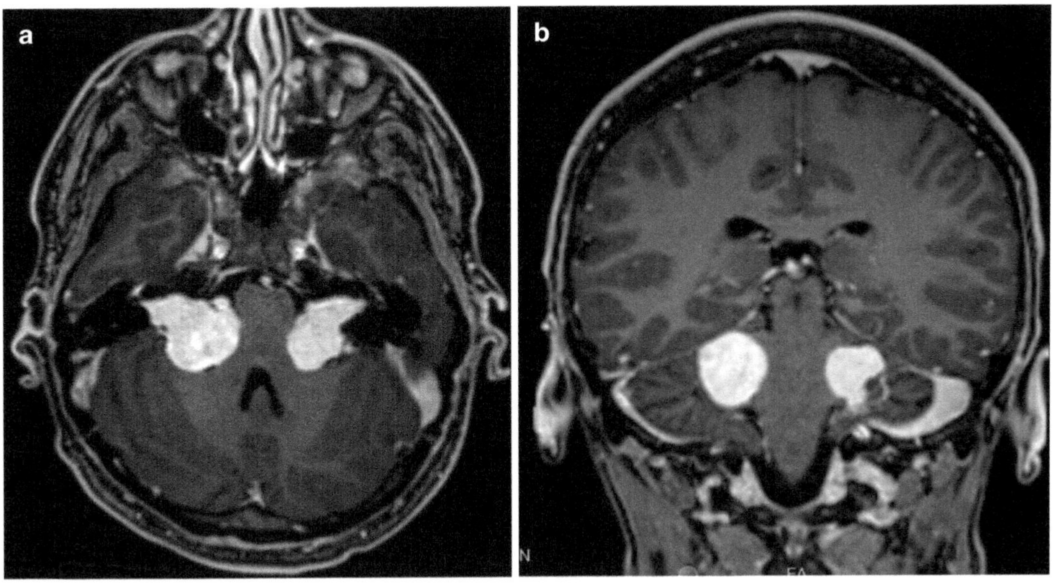

Fig. 12.5 Bilateral vestibular schwannoma visualized on magnetic resonance imaging in a pediatric patient with neurofibromatosis type 2 (**a**) axial T2 turbo inversion recovery magnitude on left and (**b**) coronal T1 post-gadolinium on right)

Treatment options for newly diagnosed VS include observation, surgery, radiation, and chemotherapy with bevacizumab. The mainstay of management of VS is surgical, with the goal of intervention to conserve function (primarily hearing) and quality of life. The decision to pursue surgical intervention for VS requires comprehensive evaluation and consideration of patient age, hearing, neurologic status, and size of tumor. The risks of surgical resection include worsened tinnitus, hearing loss or deafness, and facial nerve damage; therefore, the risks and benefits of surgery must be considered. In both pediatric and adult patients, there is no consensus as to when to pursue surgery. In adults, tumors less than 3 cm may be monitored for growth and/or hearing loss. If a VS is greater than 3 cm in size without adjacent compression of vital structures, surgical intervention may be warranted to protect the brainstem and facial nerve from subsequent compression. Surgical intervention may be urgently indicated if a patient with large bilateral VS presents with obstructive hydrocephalus or symptoms of brainstem dysfunction [57]. Similar recommendations based on tumor size have not been established for pediatric patients. As with other tumor predisposition syndromes, radiation therapy carries significant risks in patients with NF2, such as secondary malignancies, vascular complications, and ipsilateral hearing loss; thus, utilization of radiation therapy in children with NF2 should be deferred if feasible [53].

Medical therapies for VS are lacking and there is no approved systemic therapy. Clinical trials exploring the use of lapatinib, sorafenib, and everolimus have not shown to result in an improvement in hearing. Bevacizumab, a monoclonal antibody against vascular endothelial growth factor (VEGF), is a non-FDA approved therapy which has demonstrated hearing improvement in 36–45% and reduction of tumor volume in 32–43% of patients with VS [58–60]. However, hearing improvement and tumor response appear to be less common in pediatric than adult patients across multiple studies, but pediatric patients do experience some clinical benefit from bevacizumab, specifically with improvement in quality-of-life measures (tinnitus) and stabilization of disease [58, 60]. Thus, while pediatric patients may derive benefit, there remains uncertainty on the optimal use of bevacizumab in children with NF2 and VS. Studies of other targeted medical therapies for NF2-associated VS are ongoing, including several studies evaluating focal adhesion kinase 1 inhibitors based on promising efficacy in preclinical models [61, 62]; these studies include a Neurofibromatosis Clinical Trials Consortium study of crizotinib (NCT04283669) and a multi-institutional trial of brigatinib (NCT04374305).

Non-vestibular Schwannoma

Non-VS are common in NF2 and can occur along the cranial nerves, spinal nerve roots, and peripheral nerves. The preferred initial management of these tumors is observation unless the non-VS causes significant symptoms such as pain or impending functional decline due to compression of adjacent structures. If therapy is required, surgical management is preferred, with radiation therapy generally avoided [63].

Meningioma

Meningiomas are the second most frequent tumor type encountered in patients with NF2 and arise from the meninges surrounding the brain and spinal cord. *NF2*-mutated intracranial meningiomas occur in approximately half of adults with NF2 and may be multiple in number, whereas spinal meningiomas are diagnosed in approximately 20% of patients. Intracranial meningiomas tend to develop at a younger age than sporadic, non-NF associated meningioma. Meningiomas are typically low-grade, slow growing tumors; however, they can progress to high-grade lesions. Symptoms of meningioma may include seizure and neurologic deficits due to mass effect [42]. The optimal intervention for symptomatic or growing intracranial meningioma is surgical resection. The appearance of tumor-associated edema on MRI may suggest a more aggressive meningioma and should prompt expedited surgical intervention. The timing of surgical resection for spinal meningioma is not well established; however, intervention prior to symptoms may be considered to prevent the onset of compression and neurologic deficits.

Medical therapy for meningioma is limited. Inhibitors of the VEGF pathway have demonstrated variable activity in small, non-randomized studies [64]. Ongoing prospective studies of medical therapies include basket trials of brigatinib (NCT04374305) and selumetinib (NCT03095248) for progressive NF2-associated tumors including meningioma, as well as several trials evaluating histone deacetylase inhibitors (NCT02282917, NCT05130866). Radiation therapy is typically reserved for atypical, anaplastic, or recurrent meningioma due to the risk of secondary malignancy [57].

Ependymoma

Ependymomas arise from proliferations of neoplastic ependymal cells of the ventricles and spinal cord. Between 30 and 50% of patients with NF2 will be diagnosed with spinal or intracranial ependymoma, with the majority of ependymoma occurring along the cervical spinal cord or cervico-medullary junction. Patients with NF2 may develop multiple spinal ependymomas, resulting in a "string of pearls" appearance along the spinal cord on MRI [65].

Spinal ependymoma may be myxopapillary or subependymal (WHO grade I) and exhibit an indolent growth pattern, with tumor progression in a minority of patients. Due to the expectation of indolent growth, the management of NF2-associated spinal ependymomas has historically been conservative; thus, observation and radiographic surveillance is a reasonable initial approach for asymptomatic spinal cord ependymomas given the risk of morbidity with resection. Tumors with progressive growth or onset of symptoms should be considered for excision. Further, bevacizumab has been reported to be a potential surgery-sparing agent in patients with high operative risk, particularly for cystic lesions; however, tumor shrinkage has not been consistently described [66]. Prospective studies of medical therapies for spinal ependymoma are required to optimize management of these tumors.

While rarely reported, most intracranial ependymomas in NF2 are classic histology (WHO grade II) and may present at a younger age than spinal ependymoma [67]. The standard of care for intracranial ependymoma in pediatric patients is best possible resection followed by radiation therapy; however, a recent Children's Oncology Group study suggests that adding maintenance chemotherapy after radiation is warranted for the subgroup of patients who achieve a gross total resection [68]. It is unknown whether this improvement in survival outcomes applies to the population of patients with NF2-associated ependymoma.

Screening for Patients with NF2

A child of a parent with NF2 has a 50% risk of inheriting a pathogenic mutation for NF2; thus, children of a parent with NF2 should undergo screening for NF2 soon after birth. Ophthalmologic complications of NF2, such as cataracts, can affect vision in childhood, hence annual ophthalmology screening should be initiated within the first year of life for suspected (offspring) as well as confirmed cases of NF2. When the diagnosis of NF2 is established, at a minimum, a patient should undergo annual examination with a neuro-oncologist or neurologist, as well as an annual audiology evaluation of pure-tone thresholds and word recognition score. Imaging screening for VS should begin at 10 years of age with brain MRI (including high resolution imaging through the internal auditory canals) and continue every 2 years for patients less than 20 years of age with no evidence of tumor. Those with high-risk genotypes may require earlier screening. Surveillance spinal MRI is also recommended every 2–3 years beginning at 10 years of age and is often performed in conjunction with brain imaging. For patients with newly diagnosed tumor, such as VS or spinal ependymoma, where observation is the most appropriate initial management, serial MRI is typically obtained every 6–12 months. More frequent observation may be warranted for patients with atypical imaging findings or symptomatic progression [53].

Summary

In review, neurofibromatosis type 1 and type 2 are complex and distinct tumor predisposition syndromes affecting multiple organ systems. Children who are diagnosed with these conditions should be followed by a physician familiar with the surveillance and management of neurofibromatosis. Initial management of most newly diagnosed neurofibromatosis-associated tumors is close observation with surveillance imaging, as well as assessment of the functional impact of the tumors. While promising novel therapies such as MEK inhibitors are changing the management of a subset of NF1-associated tumors, and bevacizumab offers some benefit to patients with NF2 and VS, the mainstay of therapy for many of these tumors remains surgical. Surgeons should be aware of the indications and contraindications for biopsy and intervention based on underlying diagnosis and tumor type.

Board Style Questions

1. A 3-year-old female with café au lait macules presents with visual acuity of the right eye with a Snellen equivalent of 20/40. MRI of the brain demonstrates a T2-weighted hyperintense lesion of the right optic nerve and chiasm with minimal enhancement on T1-weighted post-gadolinium images. What is the next best step in management?
   A. Observation
   B. Biopsy of mass to determine pathologic diagnosis and next steps in treatment

C. Referral to neuro-oncology for initiation of chemotherapy
D. Referral to initiate radiation therapy

2. An 18-year-old male falls off a trampoline and experiences loss of consciousness. Non-contrast head CT obtained in the Emergency Department demonstrates a left cerebellopontine angle mass with mild mass effect on the adjacent cerebellum, as well as a smaller right cerebellopontine angle mass. The patient denies prior tinnitus or change in hearing. MRI demonstrates a 2.8 × 2.3 cm extra-axial enhancing mass on the left and a 1.9 × 1.1 cm mass on the right. Both lesions protrude into the porus acousticus resulting in mild expansion. The next step in evaluation is:
   A. Consult ophthalmology to evaluate for Lisch nodules
   B. Audiogram
   C. Retro-sigmoid biopsy and/or resection of mass
   D. Referral to initiate radiation therapy
3. A 7-year-old female with neurofibromatosis type 1 presents with a plexiform neurofibroma extending from the upper mediastinum to the right axilla and down to the distal humerus that has progressed and has associated weakness of the distal upper extremity. The most appropriate next step in therapy is:
   A. Continue radiologic observation with STIR sequences on MRI
   B. Biopsy of the growing portion of the tumor
   C. Surgical resection of the tumor
   D. Referral to neuro-oncology for initiation of carboplatin-based chemotherapy
   E. Referral to neuro-oncology for initiation of selumetinib
4. A 16-year-old male presents with intermittent tinnitus. MRI is obtained which demonstrates bilateral vestibular schwannomas. Audiology is consulted; word recognition is 98% on the right and 95% on the left. MRI obtained 1 year later demonstrates that the VS on right has grown by 2 mm but is stable in size on the left. Word recognition is now 98% on the right and 68% on the left. The patient has no other change in neurologic examination. What is the next step?
   A. Observation with shorter interval follow up MRI
   B. Surgical resection of growing VS
   C. Surgical resection of VS associated with hearing decline
   D. Referral to neuro-oncology for initiation of bevacizumab

Answer Key

1. A
2. B
3. E
4. D

References

1. Miller DT, et al. Health supervision for children with neurofibromatosis type 1. Pediatrics. 2019;143(5):e20190660.
2. Koczkowska M, et al. Clinical spectrum of individuals with pathogenic NF1 missense variants affecting p.Met1149, p.Arg1276, and p.Lys1423: genotype-phenotype study in neurofibromatosis type 1. Hum Mutat. 2020;41(1):299–315.
3. Wimmer K, et al. Spectrum of single- and multiexon NF1 copy number changes in a cohort of 1,100 unselected NF1 patients. Genes Chromosomes Cancer. 2006;45(3):265–76.
4. Ly KI, Blakeley JO. The diagnosis and management of neurofibromatosis type 1. Med Clin North Am. 2019;103(6):1035–54.
5. Legius E, et al. Revised diagnostic criteria for neurofibromatosis type 1 and Legius syndrome: an international consensus recommendation. Genet Med. 2021;23(8):1506–13.
6. DeBella K, Szudek J, Friedman JM. Use of the national institutes of health criteria for diagnosis of neurofibromatosis 1 in children. Pediatrics. 2000;105(3 Pt 1):608–14.
7. Jett K, Friedman JM. Clinical and genetic aspects of neurofibromatosis 1. Genet Med. 2010;12(1):1–11.
8. Boyd KP, Korf BR, Theos A. Neurofibromatosis type 1. J Am Acad Dermatol. 2009;61(1):1–14; quiz 15–6.

9. Chamseddin BH, Le LQ. Management of cutaneous neurofibroma: current therapy and future directions. Neurooncol Adv. 2020;2(Suppl 1):i107–16.
10. Jaremko JL, et al. Whole-body MRI in neurofibromatosis: incidental findings and prevalence of scoliosis. Skelet Radiol. 2012;41(8):917–23.
11. Well L, et al. Phenotyping spinal abnormalities in patients with Neurofibromatosis type 1 using whole-body MRI. Sci Rep. 2021;11(1):16889.
12. Lotfy M, et al. Reconstruction of skull base defects in sphenoid wing dysplasia associated with neurofibromatosis I with titanium mesh. Clin Neurol Neurosurg. 2010;112(10):909–14.
13. Lubs ML, et al. Lisch nodules in neurofibromatosis type 1. N Engl J Med. 1991;324(18):1264–6.
14. Yasunari T, et al. Frequency of choroidal abnormalities in neurofibromatosis type 1. Lancet. 2000;356(9234):988–92.
15. Viola F, et al. Choroidal abnormalities detected by near-infrared reflectance imaging as a new diagnostic criterion for neurofibromatosis 1. Ophthalmology. 2012;119(2):369–75.
16. Rea D, et al. Cerebral arteriopathy in children with neurofibromatosis type 1. Pediatrics. 2009;124(3):e476–83.
17. Kaas B, et al. Spectrum and prevalence of vasculopathy in pediatric neurofibromatosis type 1. J Child Neurol. 2013;28(5):561–9.
18. Hamilton SJ, Friedman JM. Insights into the pathogenesis of neurofibromatosis 1 vasculopathy. Clin Genet. 2000;58(5):341–4.
19. Ullrich NJ, et al. Moyamoya following cranial irradiation for primary brain tumors in children. Neurology. 2007;68(12):932–8.
20. Koss M, et al. Moyamoya syndrome associated with neurofibromatosis Type 1: perioperative and long-term outcome after surgical revascularization. J Neurosurg Pediatr. 2013;11(4):417–25.
21. Ostendorf AP, Gutmann DH, Weisenberg JL. Epilepsy in individuals with neurofibromatosis type 1. Epilepsia. 2013;54(10):1810–4.
22. Salman MS, et al. Cerebellar radiological abnormalities in children with neurofibromatosis type 1: part 1—clinical and neuroimaging findings. Cerebellum Ataxias. 2018;5:14.
23. Ferner RE, et al. MRI in neurofibromatosis 1. The nature and evolution of increased intensity T2 weighted lesions and their relationship to intellectual impairment. J Neurol Neurosurg Psychiatry. 1993;56(5):492–5.
24. Roth J, Constantini S, Cinalli G. Neurofibromatosis type 1-related hydrocephalus: causes and treatment considerations. Childs Nerv Syst. 2020;36(10):2385–90.
25. Fisher MJ, et al. Cabozantinib for neurofibromatosis type 1-related plexiform neurofibromas: a phase 2 trial. Nat Med. 2021;27(1):165–73.
26. Widemann BC. Current status of sporadic and neurofibromatosis type 1-associated malignant peripheral nerve sheath tumors. Curr Oncol Rep. 2009;11(4):322–8.
27. Prada CE, et al. Pediatric plexiform neurofibromas: impact on morbidity and mortality in neurofibromatosis type 1. J Pediatr. 2012;160(3):461–7.
28. Bhatia S, et al. Subsequent neoplasms after a primary tumor in individuals with neurofibromatosis type 1. J Clin Oncol. 2019;37(32):3050–8.
29. Gross AM, et al. Selumetinib in children with inoperable plexiform neurofibromas. N Engl J Med. 2020;382(15):1430–42.
30. Weiss BD, et al. NF106: a neurofibromatosis clinical trials consortium phase II trial of the MEK inhibitor mirdametinib (PD-0325901) in adolescents and adults with NF1-related plexiform neurofibromas. J Clin Oncol. 2021;39(7):797–806.
31. Mueller S, et al. NFB-17. MEK inhibitor binimetinib shows clinical activity in children with neurofibromatosis type 1-associated plexiform neurofibromas: a report from PNOC and the NF clinical trials consortium. Neuro-Oncology. 2020;22(Suppl 3):iii420–1.
32. Ferner RE, et al. [18F]2-fluoro-2-deoxy-D-glucose positron emission tomography (FDG PET) as a diagnostic tool for neurofibromatosis 1 (NF1) associated malignant peripheral nerve sheath tumours (MPNSTs): a long-term clinical study. Ann Oncol. 2008;19(2):390–4.
33. Ahlawat S, et al. Imaging biomarkers for malignant peripheral nerve sheath tumors in neurofibromatosis type 1. Neurology. 2019;93(11):e1076–84.
34. Martin E, et al. A nationwide cohort study on treatment and survival in patients with malignant peripheral nerve sheath tumours. Eur J Cancer. 2020;124: 77–87.
35. Zehou O, et al. Chemotherapy for the treatment of malignant peripheral nerve sheath tumors in neurofibromatosis 1: a 10-year institutional review. Orphanet J Rare Dis. 2013;8:127.
36. Fisher MJ, et al. Integrated molecular and clinical analysis of low-grade gliomas in children with neurofibromatosis type 1 (NF1). Acta Neuropathol. 2021;141(4):605–17.
37. Campen CJ, Gutmann DH. Optic pathway gliomas in neurofibromatosis type 1. J Child Neurol. 2018;33(1):73–81.
38. Costa, A.A. and D.H. Gutmann, Brain tumors in Neurofibromatosis type 1. Neurooncol Adv, 2019. 1(1): vdz040.
39. Mahdi J, et al. A multi-institutional study of brainstem gliomas in children with neurofibromatosis type 1. Neurology. 2017;88(16):1584–9.
40. Bouffet E, et al. Phase II study of weekly vinblastine in recurrent or refractory pediatric low-grade glioma. J Clin Oncol. 2012;30(12):1358–63.
41. Fangusaro J, et al. Selumetinib in paediatric patients with BRAF-aberrant or neurofibromatosis type 1-associated recurrent, refractory, or progressive low-grade glioma: a multicentre, phase 2 trial. Lancet Oncol. 2019;20(7):1011–22.
42. Ullrich NJ, et al. A phase II study of continuous oral mTOR inhibitor everolimus for recurrent, radiographic-progressive neurofibromatosis

type 1-associated pediatric low-grade glioma: a Neurofibromatosis Clinical Trials Consortium study. Neuro Oncol. 2020;22(10):1527–35.
43. Karajannis MA, et al. Phase II study of sorafenib in children with recurrent or progressive low-grade astrocytomas. Neuro Oncol. 2014;16(10):1408–16.
44. D'Angelo F, et al. The molecular landscape of glioma in patients with Neurofibromatosis 1. Nat Med. 2019;25(1):176–87.
45. Packer RJ, et al. Implications of new understandings of gliomas in children and adults with NF1: report of a consensus conference. Neuro Oncol. 2020;22(6):773–84.
46. Listernick R, et al. Optic pathway gliomas in children with neurofibromatosis 1: consensus statement from the NF1 Optic Pathway Glioma Task Force. Ann Neurol. 1997;41(2):143–9.
47. Selvanathan SK, et al. Further genotype—phenotype correlations in neurofibromatosis 2. Clin Genet. 2010;77(2):163–70.
48. Evans DG. Neurofibromatosis type 2: genetic and clinical features. Ear Nose Throat J. 1999;78(2):97–100.
49. Baser ME, et al. Predictors of the risk of mortality in neurofibromatosis 2. Am J Hum Genet. 2002;71(4):715–23.
50. Smith MJ, et al. Revisiting neurofibromatosis type 2 diagnostic criteria to exclude LZTR1-related schwannomatosis. Neurology. 2017;88(1):87–92.
51. Evans DG, et al. Identifying the deficiencies of current diagnostic criteria for neurofibromatosis 2 using databases of 2777 individuals with molecular testing. Genet Med. 2019;21(7):1525–33.
52. Gaudioso C, et al. Neurofibromatosis 2 in children presenting during the first decade of life. Neurology. 2019;93(10):e964–7.
53. Evans DGR, et al. Cancer and central nervous system tumor surveillance in pediatric neurofibromatosis 2 and related disorders. Clin Cancer Res. 2017;23(12):e54–61.
54. Evans DG, et al. Mosaicism in neurofibromatosis type 2: an update of risk based on uni/bilaterality of vestibular schwannoma at presentation and sensitive mutation analysis including multiple ligation-dependent probe amplification. J Med Genet. 2007;44(7):424–8.
55. Evans DG. Neurofibromatosis type 2 (NF2): a clinical and molecular review. Orphanet J Rare Dis. 2009;4:16.
56. Coy S, et al. An update on the CNS manifestations of neurofibromatosis type 2. Acta Neuropathol. 2020;139(4):643–65.
57. Blakeley JO, et al. Consensus recommendations for current treatments and accelerating clinical trials for patients with neurofibromatosis type 2. Am J Med Genet A. 2012;158A(1):24–41.
58. Morris KA, et al. Bevacizumab in neurofibromatosis type 2 (NF2) related vestibular schwannomas: a nationally coordinated approach to delivery and prospective evaluation. Neurooncol Pract. 2016;3(4):281–9.
59. Blakeley JO, et al. Efficacy and biomarker study of bevacizumab for hearing loss resulting from neurofibromatosis type 2-associated vestibular schwannomas. J Clin Oncol. 2016;34(14):1669–75.
60. Plotkin SR, et al. Multicenter, prospective, phase II and biomarker study of high-dose bevacizumab as induction therapy in patients with neurofibromatosis type 2 and progressive vestibular schwannoma. J Clin Oncol. 2019;37(35):3446–54.
61. Chang LS, et al. Brigatinib causes tumor shrinkage in both NF2-deficient meningioma and schwannoma through inhibition of multiple tyrosine kinases but not ALK. PLoS One. 2021;16(7):e0252048.
62. Troutman S, et al. Crizotinib inhibits NF2-associated schwannoma through inhibition of focal adhesion kinase 1. Oncotarget. 2016;7(34):54515–25.
63. Jordan JT, Plotkin SR. Neurofibromatoses. Hematol Oncol Clin North Am. 2022;36(1):253–67.
64. Nunes FP, et al. Bevacizumab treatment for meningiomas in NF2: a retrospective analysis of 15 patients. PLoS One. 2013;8(3):e59941.
65. Plotkin SR, et al. Spinal ependymomas in neurofibromatosis Type 2: a retrospective analysis of 55 patients. J Neurosurg Spine. 2011;14(4):543–7.
66. The response of spinal cord ependymomas to bevacizumab in patients with neurofibromatosis Type 2. J Neurosurg Spine. 2017;26(4):474–82.
67. Kresbach C, et al. Neurofibromatosis type 2 predisposes to ependymomas of various localization, histology, and molecular subtype. Acta Neuropathol. 2021;141(6):971–4.
68. Smith A, et al. EPEN-54. ACNS0831, phase III randomized trial of post-radiation chemotherapy in patients with newly diagnosed ependymoma ages 1 TO 21 years. Neuro-Oncology. 2020;22(Suppl 3):iii318–9.

Management of Pediatric Patient with Non-NF Phakomatosis

13

Rita Snyder and Howard L. Weiner

Introduction

Neurocutaneous syndromes, or "phakomatoses" are a group of disorders caused by mutations in tumor suppressor genes with prominent manifestations in the skin and nervous systems. Patients may present from infancy to late adulthood, and frequently require neurosurgical care at some point during their lifetimes. Therefore, a basic understanding of underlying pathogenesis, symptomatology, medical and surgical indications and interventions is beneficial for the practicing neurosurgeon. The following chapter focuses on the following non-neurofibromatosis neurocutaneous syndromes with prominent CNS manifestations: Tuberous Sclerosis Complex (TSC), Von Hippel Lindau (VHL), and Sturge-Weber syndrome (SWS).

R. Snyder
Baylor College of Medicine, Houston, TX, USA
e-mail: Rita.Snyder@bcm.edu

H. L. Weiner (✉)
Neurosurgery, Texas Children's Hospital, Houston, TX, USA

Neurosurgery, Baylor College of Medicine, Houston, TX, USA
e-mail: hlweiner@texaschildrens.org

Tuberous Sclerosis Complex

Epidemiology and Etiology

First coined in 1880 by Bourneville, Tuberous Sclerosis Complex (TSC) is the second most common neurocutaneous disorder, affecting 1 in 6000 to 10,000 births [1]. TSC is autosomal dominant with near complete penetrance, variable expressivity and wide range of severity with no predilection for gender or race [2, 3]. One-third of cases are familial and have equal distribution of TSC1 and TSC2 mutations. The other two-thirds occur either from spontaneous mutations or mosaicism. TSC2 mutations are 4 times more likely in these cases [4].

The two major genes involved are TSC1, located on chromosome 9q34, and TSC2, located on chromosome 16p13. TSC1 encodes hamartin, while TSC2 encodes tuberin [2]. The two form a complex with protein TBC1D7 (Tre2-Bub2-Cdc16 1 domain family, member 7) to maintain RHEB protein (Ras Homolog Enriched in Brain) in the inactive state. RHEB serves to activate the mTOR (mechanistic target of rapamycin) pathway, a key component for cell growth. Inadequate suppression results in unregulated cell division, and the subsequent radiographic and clinical characteristics of this condition.

Clinical Presentation

Patients with TSC often present with neurologic manifestations early in life. Of children with TSC,

N. Shimony, G. Jallo (eds.), *Pediatric Neurosurgery Board Review*,
https://doi.org/10.1007/978-3-031-23687-7_13

50% present with seizures, and 10–25% with epileptic spasms prior to 1 year of age [4]. Epileptic spasms typically occur around sleep-wake transitions and appear as symmetric flexion or extension of the neck and limbs. Hypsarrhythmia, a pattern of highly disorganized brain activity on EEG, may or may not be present.

Cutaneous hallmarks of the disease are prevalent, and include facial angiofibromas, hypomelanotic macules ("Ash leaf spots"), connective tissue nevi ("Shagreen patches"), and nontraumatic ungual or periungual fibromas (*see* Fig. 13.1). Facial angiofibromas occur in 75% of patients and are often found in a malar distribution across the bridge of the nose and cheeks. Cardiac rhabdomyomas which are often detected on prenatal ultrasound leading to early diagnosis, typically regress during childhood. Renal cysts and benign angiomyolipomas may result in hypertension and renal failure. Retinal astrocytic hamartomas, pigmentary changes, palpebral angiofibromas, and colobomas can also develop and are typically asymptomatic. Lymphangioleiomyomatosis (LAM), a progressive process involving cystic degeneration of lung parenchyma is seen in up to 80% of women with TSC by age 40, but may also develop in 10% of men (*see* Fig. 13.1). Rarely, malignancies such as renal cell carcinoma and clear cell lung cancer develop [4]. Conversely, sclerotic bone lesions incidentally found on screening imaging may raise concern for malignancy; however, these are very common in patients with TSC and rarely require intervention [5].

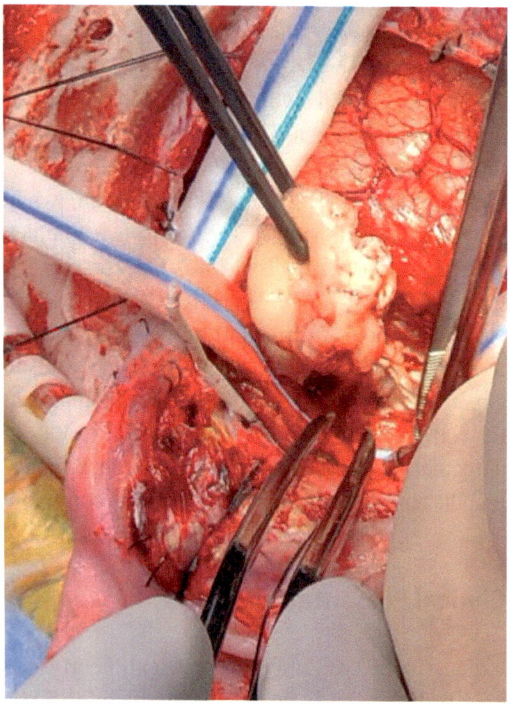

Fig. 13.1 Intraoperative photo displaying gross appearance of cortical tuber resection

The 11 major and 7 minor diagnostic criteria for TSC are listed below. The classic triad of seizures, mental retardation and facial angiofibromas occurs in less than one-third of cases [1]. "Definite" diagnosis, according to the recent 2021 Tuberous Sclerosis Complex Consensus Group, requires two major criteria, one major criterion and two minor, or the presence of a TSC1 or TSC2 pathogenic mutation confirmed on genetic testing [5]. As 10–25% of TSC patients lack a mutation in these genes, a normal gene result does not necessarily rule out the disease [5].

Major Criteria

- Hypomelanotic macule (Ash leaf spots), three or more, at least 5 mm in diameter
- Angiofibroma, three or more (formerly known as adenoma sebaceum) or fibrous cephalic plaque
- Nontraumatic ungual or periungual fibroma
- Connective Tissue Nevus (Shagreen patch)
- Multiple retinal hamartomas
- Multiple cortical tubers and/or radial migration lines
- Subependymal nodule, two or more
- Subependymal giant cell astrocytoma
- Cardiac rhabdomyoma
- Lymphangiomyomatosis
- Angiomyolipoma, two or more

Minor Criteria

- Dental enamel pits, three or more
- Sclerotic bone lesions
- Intraoral fibromas, two or more
- Nonrenal hamartomas
- Retinal achromic patch
- "Confetti" skin lesions
- Multiple renal cysts

Investigation

Astrocytic hamartomas, or cortical tubers, develop in up to 80% of patients with TSC, and consist of focal hypertrophic lesions consisting of large and fibrillary astrocytes [4]. Tubers may present throughout the cerebral cortex and rarely found infratentorially [6]. Classification is based on their radiographic appearance into A, B and C types. Type C are believed to harbor intra-tuber epileptogenic zones, unlike types A and B which are thought to propagate seizures over a broader network area [7, 8]. One study comparing MRI characteristics and seizure burden found cumulative volume of type B tubers correlated with early-onset epilepsy [9]. Radiographic characteristics of these groups are described below in Table 13.1.

Neurologic manifestations are the leading cause of morbidity and mortality. It is estimated

Table 13.1 Neuroradiographic features of TSC [6]

Feature	Imaging characteristics	Example
Subependymal nodules	Wall of lateral ventricle Hyperintense on T1-MRI Iso- to hyperintense on T2 and FLAIR prior to calcification 90% are calcified by adulthood Variable enhancement	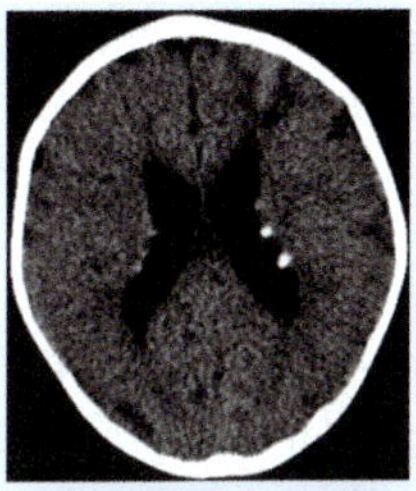
Subependymal giant cell astrocytoma	Wall of lateral ventricles, typically within caudo-thalamic groove (Frassanito) Iso- to hypointense on T1 Iso- to hyperintense on T2 High choline: creatinine ratio, low NAA:creatinine ratio on MR spectroscopy Contrast-enhances	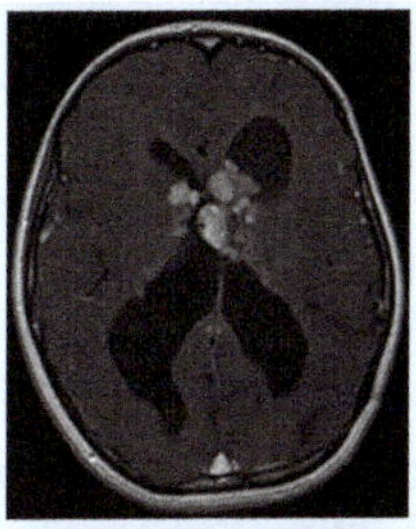
Cortical tuber	Triangular configuration with apex pointing towards ventricle Hypointense on T1, hyperintense on T2 and FLAIR (*opposite intensity pattern in infants due to lack of myelination*) *Type A:* isointense T1W, hyperintense T2W/FLAIR, no increased value on ADC *Type B:* hypointense T1W, hyperintense T2W/FLAIR, increased ADC value *Type C:* hypointense T1W, hypointense central area with hyperintense rim on T2W/FLAIR, increased ADC value 10% contrast-enhance	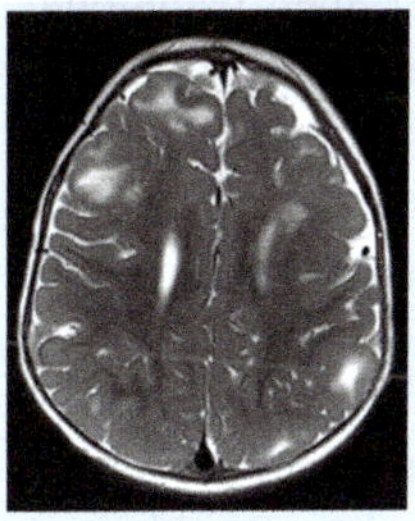
Cerebral white matter radial migration lines	Thin, straight T1 hypo- to isointense and T2 hyperintense lines extending from periventricular white matter to the cortex	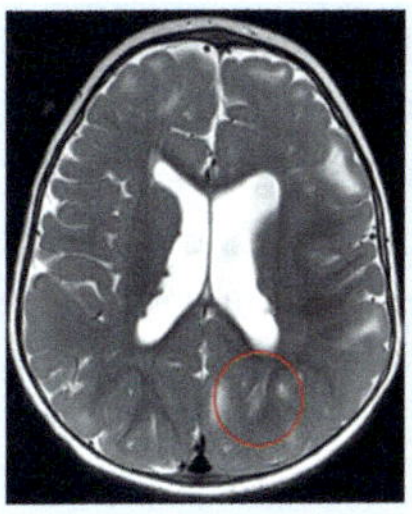

that between 85 and 96% of symptomatic TSC patients suffer from epilepsy, 80% of which first occur within 3 years of life [10]. Behavioral and cognitive dysfunction are seen in 40–50% of patients [2]. In 90% of individuals, cognitive, behavioral, psychiatric or academic disorders, otherwise known as TSC-associated neuropsychiatric disorders (TAND) are present [4]. Intellectual disability is seen in 45%, and up to 50% have autism spectrum disorder (Sahin). History of epileptic spasms, refractory epilepsy, early age at seizure onset, and TSC2 mutation have been found to correlate with a worse cognitive outcome [11]. Deficits in long-term and working memory in even normal IQ TSC patients have been found to bear resemblance to early subcortical dementia, similar to that seen in Huntington's or Parkinson's disease. Volumetric changes in radiologic normal gray matter, including the thalamus, prefrontal gray, and caudate predict performance in these areas [10].

In addition to cortical tubers, subependymal nodules are present in 90% of patients with TSC and are located along the walls of the lateral ventricles [4]. SENs are closely related to the caudate nucleus and develop exclusively along its margin [12]. Subependymal giant cell astrocytomas (SEGAs) are thought to arise from SENs; however, their pathological mechanism remains undetermined. SEGAs arise almost exclusively within the caudothalamic groove, the rare exception being various intraparenchymal locations noted in case reports [12–17]. Size greater than 2 cm and younger age at onset are predictive of accelerated growth [18, 19]. Average age at presentation is 11 years [18]. SEGAs are classified as World Health Organization grade I astrocytic neoplasms, although some argue a mixed neuronal-glial classification would be more appropriate given the presence of neuronal elements [20]. In cases with obstructive hydrocephalus, surgical resection and/or cerebrospinal fluid diversion is recommended, as rapid neurologic deterioration and worsening seizures may occur.

Treatment Paradigm

Surveillance

Patients with TSC are recommended to have MRI brain imaging performed every 1–3 years to assess for the presence or enlargement of SEGAs at least until age 25 [3]. Development may still occur after this age as well but is much less common. Patients who are unable to report symptoms due to cognitive or behavioral disability may benefit from more frequent or continued screening. Recent guidelines recommend gadolinium be reserved only for growing lesions or if suspicion for SEGA exists [5]. Baseline EEG is recommended at time of diagnosis, as well as comprehensive screening for TAND as early intervention may improve functional outcomes. Involvement of the skin and eyes warrants annual physical examinations, and biannual check-ups if dental signs are present. A baseline screening EKG is recommended, and an echocardiogram every 1–3 years for monitoring cardiac rhabdomyomas until regression is confirmed. Abdominal MRI is performed every 1–3 years with annual blood pressure and GFR measurement. Screening low-dose radiation chest CT is performed in all females and symptomatic males aged 18 and older. Annual pulmonary function test and high-resolution chest radiographs are recommended depending on the presence of lung involvement [5].

Medical Management

Antiepileptics are the preferred initial treatment for seizure control. While there is strong evidence for the use of vigabatrin for as first-line therapy for infantile spasms, with ACTH being second-line, subsequent AED management remains at the discretion of the prescriber [3, 4]. Unfortunately, over 60% of patients will go on to develop medically refractory epilepsy [11].

Medical therapies have also shown recent promise targeting the mTOR cell growth signaling pathway which is responsible for the manifestations of TSC. Sirolimus was first approved by the FDA in 1999 to prevent kidney transplant host rejection. Everolimus, a subsequent analog, achieved FDA approval in 2010 for the treatment of SEGAs following two prospective trials which showed reduction in tumor volume or growth cessation in all treated patients [6]. Compared to its predecessor, Everolimus is more readily absorbed in the digestive tract and has a shorter time course to steady state kinetics and elimination. In addition to the treatment of SEGAs, Everolimus has also been applied for the treatment of TSC-associated medically refractory epilepsy [20]. A recent randomized double-blind controlled trial showed significant benefit with 18.4% average reduction in seizure burden with low dose, and 34.9% reduction with high dose treatment [21]. This led to FDA approval in 2018 for its use as an adjunctive therapy in partial-onset refractory seizures for children older than 2 years. Many second generation mTOR inhibitors have been developed since and are currently under investigation for clinical use.

Pre-operatively, mTOR inhibitors have been used to shrink larger lesions, improve brain-tumor interphase, and decrease tumor vascularity [22]. The use of Everolimus in lieu of urgent surgery as well as to relieve symptoms from obstructive hydrocephalus have been reported [23, 24]. However, the consensus opinion remains that mTOR inhibitors should be reserved for asymptomatic growing lesions, patients with mild symptoms, or those who are not surgical candidates [5]. One single-center study demonstrated a marked reduction in the rate of SEGA surgeries following the introduction of mTOR inhibitors to clinical practice [25]. However, 64% of the 11 treated patients suffered treatment-related side effects, including oral ulcers and irregular menstruation. Given the need for lifelong medical therapy in the absence of gross total resection, risks and benefits of medical therapy alone versus surgical resection must be weighed on a case-by-case basis.

Surgical Management of SEGAs

Surgery is indicated for SEGA resection if clinical symptoms resulting from obstructive hydrocephalus occur, if the tumor in question is at least 2 cm in diameter with evidence of ventriculomegaly, or if growth is documented on serial imaging [26]. In cases where surgery is contraindicated due to patient factors, or the likelihood of achieving total resection is low, mTOR inhibitors may be used instead. SEGAs arising near the internal capsule are treated non-operatively given the significant risk of postoperative deficits with excessive manipulation [27]. Surgery may still be considered if tumor size is the precluding factor, pending tumor response to mTOR inhibition therapy and patient/family preference. Given their periventricular location, surgical approaches include transcortical-transventricular, interhemispheric-transcallosal, and endoscopic techniques. Any approach selected should enable initial gross total resection, as subtotally resected tumors have a predictably high recurrence rate [19]. Tumor size >2 cm, narrow ventricles, presence of calcification and increased vascularity are relative contraindications to an endoscopic approach, however, the smaller incision and degree of cortical exposure of the latter is favorable when conditions are appropriate [26, 28]. SEGAs >3 cm demonstrate a high rate of recurrence, however this may vary from center to center based on surgeon experience [29]. Laser interstitial thermal therapy has been employed as a less invasive alternative treatment modality; however, given its novelty, long-term outcome data remains undefined (Northrup). Authors reporting its successful use mention the possible exacerbation of obstructive hydrocephalus from postoperative edema, warranting placement of a ventriculostomy catheter prior to ablation in select cases [30].

Operative Pearls for SEGAs [27]

- Establish margins of the tumor anteriorly, medially, and posteriorly
- Protect veins
  - The thalamostriate vein is typically displaced inferiorly and posteriorly. It is important to avoid damage to this structure as injury can result in a venous infarct of the ipsilateral basal ganglia
  - The caudate vein is usually stretched across the surface of the lesion, take care and attempt to preserve it
  - The septal vein is usually medial to the tumor, and is easily dissected free

- Identify and protect the fornix early on, using a cottonoid patty to prevent blunt injury
- Work medially first, dissecting tumor away from the fornix and septum
- Identify the attachment to the caudate nucleus and protect the normal surrounding structures with cottonoid patties
- Truncate the tumor at the attachment point, and resect the remaining portion using microscissors or an ultrasonic aspirator
- The choroid plexus is typically superiorly displaced and may be divided and coagulated without adverse effect
- Place an external ventriculostomy drain at the conclusion of the case

Surgical Management of Refractory Epilepsy

Historically, surgical intervention for TSC-refractory epilepsy was limited to resection of a single, dominant, epileptogenic tuber. For multicentric cases, non-ablative palliative techniques such as corpus callosotomy or hemispherectomy were utilized [31]. This practice has drastically changed in recent years due to increased understanding of the focal nature of TSC-associated epilepsy, and the development of multi-staged surgical approaches. While traditional resective surgery consists of two parts, an invasive diagnostic monitoring period followed by surgical resection of the identified seizure foci, given the frequent multiplicity and close proximity of tubers, resection of a primary focus may unmask additional foci nearby. A novel three-stage surgical approach was created to address this phenomenon, where an additional post-operative monitoring period is performed, and subsequent resection completed as needed [32]. This technique has been found to grant greater likelihood of meaningful seizure control, and improved cognitive outcomes for children [33, 34]. Remarkably, four of the five children in the original hallmark study describing this method were seizure-free following intervention, despite originally being considered inoperable [32, 33].

Additional technological advances have also contributed to advancing the management paradigm of TSC. 7 Tesla (T) MRI machines are able to reveal smaller tubers which may lie occult on 1.5 T and 3.0 T studies. Stereotactic EEG and MRI-guided laser interstitial therapy (MRIgLITT) may be used to treat lesions in previously inaccessible areas deep within the brain. Approved by the FDA for neurosurgical applications since 2007, MRIgLITT has been employed in the treatment of drug-resistant epilepsy including TSC since 2010. While further study comparing MRIgLITT to open surgery is needed, seizure reduction rate has been found to be comparable to open resection in at least one small case series [35].

If a patient is not a candidate for resective surgery, neuromodulation may offer attractive effective treatment alternatives. Vagal nerve stimulation (VNS) has shown successful seizure reduction rates across a broad range of seizure etiologies, over 50% in 50–90% of patients [8]. Another FDA-approved neuromodulatory strategy is responsive neurostimulation (RNS), which can simultaneously monitor and address seizure activity using a combination of up to four grid and/or depth electrodes. Additional leads may be implanted during the initial surgery and the configuration adjusted following further data collection, granting remarkable flexibility and personalization with this approach [36]. A recent case series involving five patients with TSC reported greater than 50% seizure reduction at 1 year; no serious adverse events were observed. Of note, the RNS system achieved MRI-conditional rating for 1.5 T full-body imaging, enabling patients to undergo continued recommended screening following implantation [36].

Operative Pearls for Cortical Tuber Resection

- Tubers are expanded gyri which may be resected en bloc using subpial dissection (*see* Fig. 13.1) using an ultrasonic aspirator
- Multi-stage approaches involve placement of subdural or depth electrodes at the conclusion of the case, with the patient returning to the EMU postoperatively for additional invasive monitoring
- If adjacent foci are identified by this post-resection monitoring period, a subsequent resection may be indicated, followed by routine postoperative care

Other Treatment for Refractory Epilepsy

First employed for the treatment of refractory epilepsy in the 1920s, the ketogenic diet has afforded benefit for a variety of epileptic etiologies. While its exact mechanism is not fully understood, low carbohydrate intake and elevated fat and protein consumption mimic a state of starvation where the body uses ketones rather than glucose as a primary source of energy. The traditional ketogenic diet involves a 4:1 ratio of fat to carbohydrate and protein. A less restrictive, modified-Atkins diet affords the benefits of not requiring an initial fasting period, allows unlimited protein and fat intake, and does not restrict calories or fluids. Randomized controlled trials have shown improvement in seizure burden across a wide variety of seizure types and etiologies using these dietary regimens, including infantile spasms and TSC-associated epilepsy [37–39]. In one study of 12 children at various ages with TSC, all but one had a 50% reduction in their seizure burden after 6 months [40].

Another rising alternative therapy for epilepsy, Cannabidiol, or "Epidiolex" achieved FDA-approval in 2018 for refractory seizures associated with Lennox-Gastaut syndrome, Dravet syndrome, and TSC in patients older than 1 year of age. A recent phase III clinical trial in TSC patients, including patients <2 years of age, revealed significant reduction of seizures when Epidiolex was added to patients' antiepileptic drug regimen compared to placebo alone. Treatment achieved 48% decrease in seizure events, versus 26.5% with placebo. Low (25 mg/kg/day) and high (50 mg/kg/day) dosing of Epidiolex were found to be equally effective. Overall, the safety profile was deemed acceptable, and no long-term side effects were noted [41].

Multidisciplinary Approach

Given the multitude of disease manifestations of this disease, a multidisciplinary team approach is required. The TSC Alliance, an international nonprofit organization, has sought to help patients and their families locate high-quality care via designation of TSC Clinics and Centers of Excellence. TSC clinics may be categorized as provisional or established, with provisional requiring re-accreditation annually, and established clinics once every 3 years. TSC clinics can provide essential services for the diagnosis and management of TSC, including access to specialists in neurology, nephrology, genetics, psychiatry/psychology and/or developmental pediatrics, cardiology, ophthalmology, and dermatology. Adult clinics must also have pulmonology services available. There must be at least one clinic day per month dedicated to treating TSC patients, and a TSC Clinic Coordinator available as a point of contact for patients and their families. For a center to be considered a Center of Excellence, it must also be adept in managing advanced cases and have multiple days per month dedicated to the treatment of TSC patients. Involvement in clinical trials is highly recommended (TSCalliance.org). There are currently 63 designated TSC clinics worldwide, 10 of which are located outside the US (Jerusalem, Canada, India, and Mexico), and 13 TSC Centers of Excellence in total [42].

Von Hippel-Lindau Disease

Epidemiology and Etiology

In 1904, ophthalmologist Eugene von Hippel first identified the condition of retinal angiomatosis. In 1921, pathologist Arvid Lindau published a case series of patients with retinal and cerebellar tumors, proposing a common genetic origin [43]. Von-Hippel Lindau (VHL) disease was subsequently termed in 1936, and its causative genetic mutation successfully isolated 60 years later [44]. Occurring in 1 in 36,000 newborns, VHL is caused by germline, autosomal-dominant mutations affecting the VHL tumor suppressor gene on chromosome 3p25 [44, 45]. Eighty percent of patients have an affected parent, and penetrance is 90% by age 65 [3, 46]. The end product of the intact VHL gene inhibits a protein called Hypoxia-Inducible Factor-Alpha (HIF-α) via ubiquitination in response to low availability of oxygen [47]. Without this inhibitory check, multiple downstream target genes related to angiogenesis and proliferation are upregulated, including vascular endothelial growth factor (VEGF), glutaminase 1 (GLUT1), transforming growth factor-beta (TGF-B), platelet-derived growth factor (PDGF) and erythropoietin (EPO) [43, 46]. VHL also plays a role in ECM turnover and microtubule stability [46]. Despite increased understanding of pathophysiology and management strategies, life expectancy remains well below that of the normal population at 40–52 years [48].

Clinical Presentation

Retinal hemangioblastomas (otherwise known as retinal angiomas) are the most common clinical manifestation of VHL and may lead to retinal detachment and vision loss. CNS hemangioblastomas occur in 60–80% of patients with VHL; 40% occur between the ages of 15 and 40 [43]. Hydrocephalus is more common in children than adults, and presenting symptoms are typically more acute and severe [49]. Given the low incidence of hemangioblastomas in children (1 per 1,000,000), diagnosis warrants genetic testing [50]. Infratentorial lesions may also present with symptoms from increased intracranial pressure or truncal ataxia [44, 45]. Spinal hemangioblastomas can result in a variety of symptoms, including hypesthesia, hyperreflexia, dysesthesia, bowel/bladder dysfunction, spasticity, proprioceptive deficits, and weakness [51]. Abdominal, flank pain and renal dysfunction may portend renal cysts, hemangioblastomas, or carcinoma. Renal cell carcinoma (RCC) has a lifetime risk of 70% in this population and is arguably the most common cause of mortality. RCC brain metastasis occurs in 2–17% of cases and portends a poor prognosis with median survival of 10 months [52].

Audiovestibular dysfunction, including vertigo, tinnitus, and hearing loss in VHL patients should prompt a thorough investigation of endolymphatic sac tumors (ELSTs). ELSTs are noted in 10–17% of patients with VHL and may occur bilaterally. These are slow-growing, World Health Organization grade I tumors which have been found to present as early as 15 years of age, but more commonly present in the fifth to sixth decades of life [43, 53]. Symptoms can occur suddenly or gradually. Rarely, drop metastases may be present [53].

Pheochromocytomas and paragangliomas, neoplasms which arise from chromaffin cells of the sympathetic nervous system, usually present with symptoms such as headaches, palpitations and diaphoresis, nausea, or abdominal pain. These occur in 10–17% of VHL patients. Mean age of diagnosis is 28 years [3, 43]. Other manifestations include pancreatic cysts, neuroendocrine tumors and cystadenomas, hepatic cysts, and epididymal or broad ligament papillary cystadenomas. These are often asymptomatic; however, malignant transformation is possible and may result in abdominal pain, gastrointestinal obstruction, or constitutional symptoms such as unexplained weight loss and fatigue.

Investigation

Hemangioblastomas of the brain and spinal cord enhance avidly due to their highly vascular nature. Spinal cord hemangioblastomas typically occur within the cervical or thoracic segments and may be intramedullary and/or extramedullary [51]. The vast majority (>90%) occur within the dorsal spine. T2-weighted and FLAIR sequences are helpful in delineating edema from syrinx. Intracranial hemangioblastomas are typically found within the cerebellum but may occur supratentorially as well. In VHL, multiple lesions may be present. Solid portions are T1 isointense and hyperintense on T2, with high signal on ADC (apparent diffusion coefficient) MRI sequences.

Endolymphatic sac tumors are located within the petrous bone, posterior to the vestibular apparatus and medial to the mastoid air cells. CT imaging is often useful to reveal erosive changes, but lesions may be occult on CT and MRI. Involvement of the otic capsule, internal auditory canal, vestibular aqueduct, jugular bulb, hypotympanum, semicircular canals, and sigmoid sinus may be present. Larger tumors can extend into the posterior or middle fossa. ELSTs demonstrate heterogenous enhancement on T1-weighted and FLAIR MRI sequences. Intralabyrinthine hemorrhage may also be present as intrinsic T1 hyperintensity [53].

Treatment

Surveillance

Annual ophthalmic examinations are recommended to screen for retinal angiomas, as well as yearly MRI brain and spine every 1–3 years to check for interval development of hemangioblastomas [3]. Renal cell carcinoma screening is completed using abdominal MRI or ultrasound obtained every year after age 16. Annual urine or plasma studies to assess for elevated catecholamine metabolites screens for possible pheochromocytoma or paraganglioma is recommended [45]. Hearing evaluations are performed every 2–3 years [3].

Medical Treatment

Small series and case reports have reported promising effects of tyrosine kinase inhibitors and various immunotherapy agents for central CNS hemangioblastomas. Due to lack of large-scale studies, treatment remains primarily surgical and palliative [54]. Recent FDA-approval of belzutifan for adult patients with von Hippel-Lindau disease may lead to future changes to the standard of care. This selective small molecule inhibitor of HIF-2α showed a 63% response rate in 24 patients with VHL-associated hemangioblastomas and was well-tolerated [55, 56]. Future work will continue to determine long-term efficacy and characterize the safety profile of this and other targeted immunotherapy agents [57].

In cases of pheochromocytoma, several medications common to neurosurgical practice are contraindicated, including corticosteroids, metoclopramide, prochlorperazine, morphine, tramadol, and naloxone. A hypertensive patient with VHL warrants careful work-up prior to administering these medications which could precipitate a hypertensive crisis if present.

Surgical Treatment

As previously mentioned, prior to any surgical intervention, it is critical to rule out the presence of a chromaffin tumor, as a catecholamine surge may result in hypertensive emergency and dangerous cardiac arrhythmias. Screening may be performed with plasma and 24-h urine screening for catecholamines and metanephrines [58]. Patients with pheochromocytomas are treated with alpha-adrenergic blockage for 1–2 weeks prior to surgery. Beta-blockers may safely be used subsequently thereafter without the risk of congestive heart failure due to unopposed alpha-adrenergic stimulation. The definitive treatment for pheochromocytoma is surgical resection.

Multiple hemangioblastomas throughout the CNS is common in VHL. Tumor growth is intermittent and unpredictable, and most patients present initially with multiple lesions. Surgery is typically reserved only for symptomatic lesions [51, 59, 60]. Complete resection reliably prevents recurrence [51]. Given their highly vascular nature, preoperative embolization is recommended for cranial lesions but not spinal, given the risk of post-embolization edema [49, 60, 61]. Spinal hemangioblastomas typically occur near the dorsal root entry zone and lend themselves to a posterolateral approach. Ventral tumors may be accessed posteriorly via a midline myelotomy, although some authors support an anterior approach via corpectomy. Ventral and intramedullary location has been associated with worse functional outcome in a multivariate analysis [51].

Early surgery for ELSTs can preserve hearing and reduce audiovestibular dysfunction [44]. Surgical approaches are dependent upon size and morphology of the tumor, as well as whether hearing preservation is an objective of surgery. Preoperative embolization through the inferior tympanic artery, a tributary of the ascending pharyngeal artery, or the stylomastoid artery, which arises from the posterior auricular branch, may be performed. Hearing preservation following surgery is common; however, patients should be counseled on the possibility of hearing loss and persistence of audiovestibular symptoms.

Vertigo, tinnitus, and aural fullness may continue following resection and require additional medical management. Finally, in patients which may qualify for cochlear implantation, preservation of the otic capsule and cochlea is crucial. Radiation therapy has been employed for residual disease and unresectable tumors with mixed results but is generally considered to be less effective than surgery [53, 62–64].

Operative Pearls for Hemangioblastoma Resection

- Smaller circulating blood volume in pediatric patients and high vascularity of tumors warrant consideration of preoperative embolization for intracranial lesions
- Ultrasonography is helpful to confirm tumor location prior to dural opening in addition to frameless stereotaxy
- Careful circumferential dissection and coagulation of arterial feeders via microsurgical dissection limits bleeding; avoid internal debulking
- Identification of arterial feeders
  - Intraoperative indocyanine green angiography may be used to differentiate arterial feeders from draining veins [65]
  - Temporary arterial occlusion with spinal evoked potentials can help to distinguish tumor vasculature from spinal arteries [65]
- The cyst wall is generally not neoplastic (it does not enhance) and need not be resected in most cases

Multidisciplinary Approach

VHL is a disorder which requires teamwork amongst a multitude of specialist care. Genetic counseling is also highly encouraged. Several informative and networking resources for patients and their families are available through the VHL Family Alliance. An international nonprofit organization, this organization seeks to fund research, promote awareness, and help coordinate care for patients living with VHL and their families (vhl.org) [66].

Sturge-Weber Syndrome

Epidemiology and Etiology

First described in 1860, Sturge-Weber Syndrome, otherwise known as encephalofacial angiomatosis, is the third most prevalent neurocutaneous disorder. SWS is caused by a spontaneous, single-nucleotide mutation in the GNAQ (G protein subunit alpha Q) gene located on chromosome 9 [67, 68]. The condition occurs in approximately 3 of every 1000 newborns and affects both genders equally. The severity of the syndrome and extent of involvement correlates with the timing of the mutation to have occurred during development, with earlier occurrence resulting in greater extent of disease [68].

Clinical Presentation

Typically, patients present at birth with a unilateral capillary malformation in the distribution of the ophthalmic branch of the trigeminal nerve, referred to as a "port-wine stain" [67, 68]. Any newborn with this finding has a 15–50% risk of developing SWS, depending on the size and extent of the lesion. A unilaterally enlarged and/or injected eye due to increased vascularity may also be apparent. However, it is important to note that in 10% of cases, the brain may be the only organ affected. Presentation is these cases may occur later in childhood, with hand or visual gaze preference and failure to meet developmental milestones. Seizures are nearly universal in patients with SWS, and 80–93% of patients with this condition will develop epilepsy, typically focal in nature, within the first 2 years of life [69]. Glaucoma, most frequent in infancy and young adulthood, is also common, occurring in 30–70% of patients. Mental retardation occurs in 50% of children. Headaches and transient ischemic attacks are also frequent, resulting in temporary hemiparesis or visual field deficits [70].

Investigation

Imaging may be initially benign as the characteristic pial angioma may not be present until as late as 2 years of age. Progressive hemispheric atrophy and pial enhancement becomes more apparent with time. As leptomeningeal angiomas grow, chronic ischemia and cortical atrophy ensues due to vascular insufficiency. By age 2, "tram-track" calcifications within the cortices are present. Enlargement of the ipsilateral choroid plexus and dilation of transparenchymal veins may also occur; polymicrogyria may or may not be present [71]. Other notable radiographic findings include ventricular enlargement, cerebral or cerebellar overgrowth, thickening of the corpus callosum and optic nerve sheaths, and Chiari I malformation. Interestingly, patients with earlier and larger areas of cortical hypometabolism on FDG-PET imaging were found to have higher IQs, suggesting superior cortical reorganization in cases with severe rather than mild damage from ischemic changes. Extensive EEG abnormalities were associated with higher degree of mental retardation however [72].

Treatment Paradigm

Surveillance

Annual ophthalmic examinations are recommended to screen for glaucoma. Additional assessments for endocrine abnormalities such as growth hormone deficiency and central hypothyroidism are also indicated [68].

Medical Treatment

There are no direct medical treatments available for SWS, however, low-dose aspirin (3–5 mg/kg/day) may be beneficial in helping to prevent ischemic events. Known side effects include nosebleeds and gingival bleeding; however, therapy is generally well-tolerated and safe for children as early as 1 month of age [73]. Antiepileptics are the initial strategy for addressing seizures, and 40% of patients obtain seizure control with traditional therapies [70]. However, refractoriness commonly occurs with disease progression, prompting consideration of surgical treatment. Some support the use of antiepileptics and aspirin for patients with bilateral lesions even if patients are asymptomatic, as these children are at higher risk for epilepsy and cognitive impairment.

Surgical Treatment

Depending on the severity of symptoms and the extent of disease, surgical excision of seizure foci may involve focal cortical resection, lobectomy, or hemispherotomy [74]. Hemispherotomy success rates for seizure control range from 44 to 100% [69]. The most active epileptogenic areas are usually cortical areas surrounding angiomatous territory; complete resection of these lesions is more likely to result in good seizure control [70, 75]. In cases of bilateral involvement, earlier onset of seizures is typical [76]. These patients were historically considered to be inoperable, however, long-term control of seizures and improved quality of life have been reportedly achieved following functional hemispherotomies [77]. Timing of surgical intervention remains a subject of debate, as some believe improved cortical plasticity and seizure control at an earlier age will afford developmental benefit, while others fear that early intervention may potentially do more harm than good [70]. Given the rarity of this disease and limited available data, study results must be interpreted cautiously. Reports vary considerably, as some cite no difference in developmental outcome with early surgery [78] others report improved seizure control rates, cognitive development [69, 79, 80], and higher IQ [81] when surgery is performed earlier, while others found older age at time of surgery was positively correlated with seizure reduction [82]. Of note, in cases of unilateral or bilateral involvement, all patients who did not have seizures were of normal intelligence. Therefore, it may be reasonably concluded that seizures are the main contributing factor for cognitive impairment. A cycle of poorly controlled seizures, increased oxygen demand, subsequent ischemia, and further cortical deterioration and seizure activity is likely the major contributing factor of progressive developmental and cognitive decline. Therefore, early surgical intervention at <1 year of age may be indicated for refractory seizures.

The original anatomic hemispherectomy described by Dandy in the early 1920s was associated with several significant long-term complications, including superficial cerebral hemosiderosis, which occurred in up to a third of all patients postoperatively [83]. The functional hemispherotomy developed by Rasmussen in the 1980s was developed to avoid these complications by surgically disconnecting the diseased brain but preserving most of the tissue in situ. Several variations have been developed since, with varying degrees of tissue resection. The transsylvian-transventricular technique developed by Schramm in 2002 reduced surgical exposure, operative time, and blood loss in comparison to earlier methods [84]. Techniques aiming to further diminish perioperative risks and morbidity continue to be developed, including endoscopic assisted, extraventricular, and MRIgLITT approaches [85–87].

Operative Pearls for Transsylvian-Transventricular Functional Hemispherotomy

- The anterior border of the craniotomy should overlay the limen insulae, the superior border the corpus callosum, the inferior border approximately 0.5 cm below the ascending M1 branch (slightly over temporal operculum), and the posterior border the level of the pulvinar nucleus [88]
- Abundant diploic veins within the bone can cause substantial bleeding, use wax liberally to limit blood loss
- The frontal and parietal operculum may be resected using bipolar cautery and an ultrasonic aspirator for direct access to the frontal horn of the lateral ventricle, versus widely splitting the Sylvian fissure
- After the frontal horn of the lateral ventricle is entered, take care to identify and preserve the cingulate gyrus as well as the anterior cerebral pericallosal arteries
- Follow the pericallosal arteries rostral to the level of the anterior communicating artery to help identify the rostral-most aspect of the callosotomy
- Use frameless stereotaxy throughout to confirm accuracy and completeness of the callosotomy anteriorly and posteriorly
- Use sub-pial technique using an ultrasonic aspirator for resection of mesial temporal lobe structures, identifying and preserving the third cranial nerve, posterior cerebral artery, optic nerve, internal carotid artery, and middle and anterior cerebral arteries
- Place an external ventriculostomy drain prior to closure

Multidisciplinary Approach

SWS patients often require a variety of subspecialty care, including ophthalmology, neurology, developmental pediatrics, physical medicine and rehabilitation, dermatology, and neurosurgery. The Sturge-Weber Foundation is a non-profit organization which helps to educate and support patients and families, serving as a resource for establishing this network of care. It also seeks to educate governmental agencies, healthcare professionals, and the general populace of this disease, and opportunities to forward treatment options (sturge-weber.org) [89].

Conclusion

Management of Tuberous Sclerosis Complex, Von-Hippel Lindau Disease, and Sturge-Weber Syndrome requires an understanding of the underlying pathophysiology, diagnostic and radiographic manifestations, clinical symptomatology, and treatment indications and modalities. Active surveillance, multidisciplinary approaches, and evidence-based practices have greatly improved outcomes for children with these phakomatoses in recent years. Collaborative efforts of dedicated, non-profit, international organizations pertaining to awareness, education, and research serve patients and their families as medical and surgical treatments continue to be developed and advanced.

Questions

1. What percentage of patients with TSC will develop medically intractable epilepsy, defined as poor seizure control despite the use of two or more antiepileptics?
2. What percentage of patients with Sturge-Weber Syndrome present with isolated brain involvement?
3. Which phakomatoses commonly presents with retinal angiomas? Which causes glaucoma? Which causes retinal hamartomas?
4. What is the genetic mutation responsible for the development of TSC? VHL? SWS?
5. Which vein is typically displaced inferiorly and posteriorly by SEGA tumors?

Answers

1. Sixty percent of TSC patients will develop medically refractory epilepsy
2. Ten percent of SWS patients have isolated brain involvement, and do not present with the characteristic facial hemangioma, otherwise known as a "port-wine stain."
3. VHL patients commonly present with retinal angiomas. Glaucoma may be present in patients with SWS. TSC patients may have retinal hamartomas.
4. The genetic mutation responsible for the development of TSC involves the tuberin or hamartin genes, located on chromosome 9q34 and 16p13 respectfully. VHL results from an autosomal dominant mutation of the VHL tumor suppressor gene on chromosome 3p25. SWS arise from a single-nucleotide spontaneous point mutation of the GNAQ gene, located on chromosome 9.
5. Thalamostriate vein.

References

1. Cruess AF, Sharma S. Tuberous sclerosis and the eye in Ryan's retina. 6th ed. Elsevier; 2018. p. 2438–45.
2. Satpathy RK. Tuberous sclerosis. In: Ferri's clinical advisor 2021. 2021. p. 1404.e2–e5. https://doi.org/10.1016/B978-0-323-71333-7.00936-X.
3. Sahin M, Ullrich N, Srivastava S, Pinto A. Neurocutaneous syndromes. In: Nelson textbook of pediatrics. 2020. p. 3140–50.e1. https://doi.org/10.1016/B978-0-323-52950-1.00614-3.
4. Randle SC. Tuberous sclerosis complex: a review. Pediatr Ann. 2017;46(4):e166–71. https://doi.org/10.3928/19382359-20170320-01.
5. Northrup H, Aronow ME, Bebin EM, Bissler J, Darling TN, de Vries PJ, Frost MD, Fuchs Z, Gosnell ES, Gupta N, Jansen AC, Jóźwiak S, Kingswood JC, Knilans TK, McCormack FX, Pounders A, Roberds SL, Rodriguez-Buritica DF, Roth J, Sampson JR, Sparagana S, Thiele EA, Weiner HL, Wheless JW, Towbin AJ, Krueger DA. International Tuberous Sclerosis Complex Consensus Group. Updated international tuberous sclerosis complex diagnostic criteria and surveillance and management recommendations. Pediatr Neurol. 2021;123:50–66. https://doi.org/10.1016/j.pediatrneurol.2021.07.011. Epub 2021 Jul 24. PMID: 34399110.
6. Manoukian SB, Kowal DJ. Comprehensive imaging manifestations of tuberous sclerosis. Am J Roentgenol (1976). 2015;204(5):933–43. https://doi.org/10.2214/AJR.13.12235.
7. Gallagher A, Grant EP, Madan N, Jarrett DY, Lyczkowski DA, Thiele EA. MRI findings reveal three different types of tubers in patients with tuberous sclerosis complex. J Neurol. 2010;257(8):1373–81. https://doi.org/10.1007/s00415-010-5535-2.
8. Treiber JM, Curry DJ, Weiner HL, Roth J. Epilepsy surgery in tuberous sclerosis complex (TSC): emerging techniques and redefinition of treatment goals. Childs Nerv Syst. 2020;36(10):2519–25. https://doi.org/10.1007/s00381-020-04715-2.
9. Jesmanas S, Norvainytė K, Gleiznienė R, Šimoliūnienė R, Endzinienė M. Different MRI-defined tuber types in tuberous sclerosis complex: quantitative evaluation and association with disease manifestations. Brain Dev (Tokyo. 1979). 2018;40(3):196–204. https://doi.org/10.1016/j.braindev.2017.11.010.
10. Ridler K, Suckling J, Higgins N, de Vries P, Stephenson C, Bolton P, Bullmore E. Neuroanatomical correlates of memory deficits in tuberous sclerosis complex. Cereb Cortex (New York, N.Y. 1991). 2006;17(2):261–71. https://doi.org/10.1093/cercor/bhj144.
11. Chu-Shore CJ, Major P, Camposano S, Muzykewicz D, Thiele EA. The natural history of epilepsy in tuberous sclerosis complex. Epilepsia (Copenhagen). 2010;51(7):1236–41. https://doi.org/10.1111/j.1528-1167.2009.02474.x.
12. Katz JS, Milla SS, Wiggins GC, Devinsky O, Weiner HL, Roth J. Intraventricular lesions in tuberous sclerosis complex: a possible association with the caudate nucleus: clinical article. J Neurosurg Pediatr. 2012;9(4):406–13. https://doi.org/10.3171/2011.12.PEDS11418.

13. Katz JS, Frankel H, Ma T, Zagzag D, Liechty B, Zeev BB, Tzadok M, Devinsky O, Weiner HL, Roth J. Unique findings of subependymal giant cell astrocytoma within cortical tubers in patients with tuberous sclerosis complex: a histopathological evaluation. Childs Nerv Syst. 2017;33(4):601–7. https://doi.org/10.1007/s00381-017-3335-z.
14. Işik U, Dinçer A, Sav A, Ozek MM. Basal ganglia location of subependymal giant cell astrocytomas in two infants. Pediatr Neurol. 2010;42:157–9.
15. Dashti SR, Robinson S, Rodgers M, Cohen AR. Pineal region giant cell astrocytoma associated with tuberous sclerosis. Case report. J Neurosurg. 2005;102(3 Suppl):322–5.
16. Bollo RJ, Berliner JL, Fischer I, Miles DK, Thiele EA, Zagzag D, et al. Extraventricular subependymal giant cell tumor in a child with tuberous sclerosis complex. Case report. J Neurosurg Pediatr. 2009;4:85–90.
17. Arca G, Pacheco E, Alfonso I, Duchowny MS, Melnick SJ. Characteristic brain magnetic resonance imaging (MRI) findings in neonates with tuberous sclerosis complex. J Child Neurol. 2006;21:280–5.
18. Frassanito P, Noya C, Tamburrini G. Current trends in the management of subependymal giant cell astrocytomas in tuberous sclerosis. Childs Nerv Syst. 2020;36(10):2527–36. https://doi.org/10.1007/s00381-020-04889-9.
19. Kotulska K, Borkowska J, Mandera M, Roszkowski M, Jurkiewicz E, Grajkowska W, Bilska M, Jóźwiak S. Congenital subependymal giant cell astrocytomas in patients with tuberous sclerosis complex. Childs Nerv Syst. 2014;30(12):2037–42. https://doi.org/10.1007/s00381-014-2555-8.
20. MacKeigan JP, Krueger DA. Differentiating the mTOR inhibitors everolimus and sirolimus in the treatment of tuberous sclerosis complex. Neuro Oncol (Charlottesville, VA). 2015;17(12):1550–9. https://doi.org/10.1093/neuonc/nov152.
21. French JA, Lawson JA, Yapici Z, Ikeda H, Polster T, Nabbout R, Curatolo P, de Vries PJ, Dlugos DJ, Berkowitz N, Voi M, Peyrard S, Pelov D, Franz DN. Adjunctive everolimus therapy for treatment-resistant focal-onset seizures associated with tuberous sclerosis (EXIST-3): a phase 3, randomised, double-blind, placebo-controlled study. Lancet (British Edition). 2016;388(10056):2153–63. https://doi.org/10.1016/S0140-6736(16)31419-2.
22. Jiang T, Du J, Raynald, Wang J, Li C. Presurgical administration of mTOR inhibitors in patients with large subependymal giant cell astrocytoma associated with tuberous sclerosis complex. World Neurosurg. 2017;107:1053.e1–6.
23. Arroyo MS, Krueger DA, Broomall E, Stevenson CB, Franz DN. Acute management of symptomatic subependymal giant cell astrocytoma with everolimus. Pediatr Neurol. 2017;72:81–5.
24. Moavero R, Carai A, Mastronuzzi A, et al. Everolimus alleviates obstructive hydrocephalus due to subependymal giant cell astrocytomas. Pediatr Neurol. 2017;68:59–63.
25. Tomoto K, Fujimoto A, Inenaga C, Okanishi T, Imai S, Ogai M, Fukunaga A, Nakamura H, Sato K, Obana A, Masui T, Arai Y, Enoki H. Experience using mTOR inhibitors for subependymal giant cell astrocytoma in tuberous sclerosis complex at a single facility. BMC Neurol. 2021;21(1):139. https://doi.org/10.1186/s12883-021-02160-5.
26. Jóźwiak S, Mandera M, Młynarski W. Natural history and current treatment options for subependymal giant cell astrocytoma in tuberous sclerosis complex. Semin Pediatr Neurol. 2015;22(4):274–81. https://doi.org/10.1016/j.spen.2015.10.003.
27. Harter DH, Bassani L, Rodgers SD, Roth J, Devinsky O, Carlson C, Wisoff JH, Weiner HL. A management strategy for intraventricular subependymal giant cell astrocytomas in tuberous sclerosis complex: clinical article. J Neurosurg Pediatr. 2014;13(1):21–8. https://doi.org/10.3171/2013.9.PEDS13193.
28. Rodgers SD, Bassani L, Weiner HL, Harter DH. Stereotactic endoscopic resection and surgical management of a subependymal giant cell astrocytoma: case report. J Neurosurg Pediatr. 2012;9(4):417–20. https://doi.org/10.3171/2011.12.PEDS11349.
29. Fohlen M, Ferrand-Sorbets S, Delalande O, Dorfmüller G. Surgery for subependymal giant cell astrocytomas in children with tuberous sclerosis complex. Childs Nerv Syst. 2018;34(8):1511–9. https://doi.org/10.1007/s00381-018-3826-6.
30. Dadey DYA, Kamath AA, Leuthardt EC, Smyth MD. Laser interstitial thermal therapy for subependymal giant cell astrocytoma: technical case report. Neurosurg Focus. 2016;41(4):E9. https://doi.org/10.3171/2016.7.FOCUS16231.
31. Cuddapah VA, Thompson M, Blount J, Li R, Guleria S, Goyal M. Hemispherectomy for hemimegalencephaly due to tuberous sclerosis and a review of the literature. Pediatr Neurol. 2015;53(5):452–5. https://doi.org/10.1016/j.pediatrneurol.2015.06.020.
32. Bauman JA, Feoli E, Roberts DW, Madsen JR, Romanelli P, Doyle WK, Devinsky O, Weiner HL, Humphreys RP, Telfeian A, Sutton LN, Berger MS. Multistage epilepsy surgery: safety, efficacy, and utility of a novel approach in pediatric extratemporal epilepsy. Comment. Neurosurgery. 2005;56(2):318–34.
33. Weiner HL, Carlson C, Ridgway EB, Zaroff CM, Miles D, LaJoie J, Devinsky O. Epilepsy surgery in young children with tuberous sclerosis: results of a novel approach. Pediatrics (Evanston). 2006;117(5):1494–502. https://doi.org/10.1542/peds.2005-1206.
34. Romanelli P, Najjar S, Weiner HL, Devinsky O. Epilepsy surgery in tuberous sclerosis: multistage procedures with bilateral or multilobar foci. J Child Neurol. 2002;17(9):689–92. https://doi.org/10.1177/088307380201700907.
35. Tovar-Spinoza Z, Carter D, Ferrone D, Eksioglu Y, Huckins S. The use of MRI-guided laser-induced thermal ablation for epilepsy. Childs Nerv Syst. 2013;29(11):2089–94. https://doi.org/10.1007/s00381-013-2169-6.

36. McDermott DS, Mirro EA, Fetrow K, Burdette DE, Chen S, Hopp J, Masel T, Johnson EA, Elefant FMK, Le S, Patra SE, Brown M, Haneef Z. Brain-responsive neurostimulation for the treatment of adults with epilepsy in tuberous sclerosis complex: a case series. Epilepsia Open. 2021;6(2):419–24. https://doi.org/10.1002/epi4.12481.
37. Neal EG, Chaffe H, Schwartz RH, Lawson MS, Edwards N, Fitzsimmons G, Whitney A, Cross JH. The ketogenic diet for the treatment of childhood epilepsy: a randomised controlled trial. Lancet Neurol. 2008;7(6):500–6. https://doi.org/10.1016/S1474-4422(08)70092-9.
38. Lambrechts DAJE, de Kinderen RJA, Vles JSH, de Louw AJA, Aldenkamp AP, Majoie HJM. A randomized controlled trial of the ketogenic diet in refractory childhood epilepsy. Acta Neurol Scand. 2018;137(1):152–4.
39. Sharma S, Tripathi M. Ketogenic diet in epileptic encephalopathies. Epilepsy Res Treat. 2013;2013:652052–5. https://doi.org/10.1155/2013/652052.
40. Kossoff EH, Thiele EA, Pfeifer HH, McGrogan JR, Freeman JM. Tuberous sclerosis complex and the ketogenic diet. Epilepsia. 2005;46(10):1684–6. https://doi.org/10.1111/j.1528-1167.2005.00266.x. PMID: 16190943.
41. Thiele EA, Bebin EM, Bhathal H, Jansen FE, Kotulska K, Lawson JA, O'Callaghan FJ, Wong M, Sahebkar F, Checketts D, Knappertz V. Add-on cannabidiol treatment for drug-resistant seizures in tuberous sclerosis complex: a placebo-controlled randomized clinical trial. JAMA Neurol. 2021;78(3):285–92. https://doi.org/10.1001/jamaneurol.2020.4607.
42. TSC Clinics. TSC Alliance. https://www.tscalliance.org.
43. Pope JC. Chapter 39—Renal dysgenesis and cystic disease of the kidney. In: Campbell-Walsh-Wein urology. 12th ed. Elsevier Inc.; 2021. p. 741–75.e6. https://doi.org/10.1016/B978-0-323-54642-3.00039-2.
44. Findeis-Hosey JJ, McMahon KQ, Findeis SK. Von Hippel–Lindau disease. J Pediatr Genet (Birmingham, AL). 2016;5(2):116–23. https://doi.org/10.1055/s-0036-1579757.
45. Maher ER, Kaelin J. von Hippel-Lindau disease. Medicine (Baltimore). 1997;76(6):381–91. https://doi.org/10.1097/00005792-199711000-00001.
46. Krasnick BA, Goedegebuure SP, Fields R. Chapter 29—Tumor biology and tumor markers. In: Sabiston textbook of surgery. 21st ed. Elsevier Inc.; 2022. p. 656–86. https://doi.org/10.1016/B978-0-323-64062-6.00029-3.
47. Ordookhanian C, Kaloostian PE, Ghostine SS, Spiess PE, Etame AB. Management strategies and outcomes for VHL-related craniospinal hemangioblastomas. J Kidney Cancer VHL. 2017;4(3):37–44. https://doi.org/10.15586/jkcvhl.2017.90.
48. Wilding A, Ingham SL, Lalloo F, Clancy T, Huson SM, Moran A, et al. Life expectancy in hereditary cancer predisposing diseases: an observational study. J Med Genet. 2012;49:264.
49. Cheng J, Liu W, Hui X, Zhang S, Ju Y. Pediatric central nervous system hemangioblastomas: different from adult forms? A retrospective series of 25 cases. Acta Neurochir. 2017;159(9):1603–11. https://doi.org/10.1007/s00701-017-3275-0.
50. Klingler J-H, Glaesker S, Bausch B, Urbach H, Krauss T, Jilg CA, Steiert C, Puzik A, Neumann-Haefelin E, Kotsis F, Agostini H, Neumann HPH, Beck J. Hemangioblastoma and von Hippel-Lindau disease: genetic background, spectrum of disease, and neurosurgical treatment. Childs Nerv Syst. 2020;36(10):2537–52. https://doi.org/10.1007/s00381-020-04712-5.
51. Mehta GU, Asthagiri AR, Bakhtian KD, Auh S, Oldfield EH, Lonser RR. Functional outcome after resection of spinal cord hemangioblastomas associated with von Hippel-Lindau disease: clinical article. J Neurosurg Spine. 2010;12(3):233–42. https://doi.org/10.3171/2009.10.SPINE09592.
52. Juloori A, Miller JA, Parsai S, Kotecha R, Ahluwalia MS, Mohammadi AM, Murphy ES, Suh JH, Barnett GH, Yu JS, Vogelbaum MA, Rini B, Garcia J, Stevens GH, Angelov L, Chao ST. Overall survival and response to radiation and targeted therapies among patients with renal cell carcinoma brain metastases. J Neurosurg. 2020;132(1):188–96. https://doi.org/10.3171/2018.8.JNS182100.
53. Wick CC, Manzoor NF, Semaan MT, Megerian CA. Endolymphatic sac tumors. Otolaryngol Clin N Am. 2015;48(2):317–30. https://doi.org/10.1016/j.otc.2014.12.006.
54. Gläsker S, Vergauwen E, Koch CA, Kutikov A, Vortmeyer AO. Von Hippel-Lindau disease: current challenges and future prospects. Onco Targets Ther. 2020;13:5669–90. https://doi.org/10.2147/OTT.S190753.
55. Choueiri TK, Bauer TM, Papadopoulos KP, Plimack ER, Merchan JR, McDermott DF, Michaelson MD, Appleman LJ, Thamake S, Perini RF, Zojwalla NJ, Jonasch E. Inhibition of hypoxia-inducible factor-2α in renal cell carcinoma with belzutifan: a phase 1 trial and biomarker analysis. Nat Med. 2021;27(5):802–5. https://doi.org/10.1038/s41591-021-01324-7.
56. FDA Approves Belzutifan for Cancers Associated with von Hippel-Lindau Disease. https://www.fda.gov/drugs/resources-information-approved-drugs/fda-approves-belzutifan-cancers-associated-von-hippel-lindau-disease.
57. Romero D. Belzutifan has potential in RCC. Nat Rev Clin Oncol. 2021;18(6):322. https://doi.org/10.1038/s41571-021-00517-w. PMID: 33931768.
58. Gayle JA, Rubin R, Kaye AD. Pheochromocytoma. In: Anesthesiology. Springer International Publishing; 2017. p. 183–9. https://doi.org/10.1007/978-3-319-50141-3_26.
59. Ammerman JM, Lonser RR, Dambrosia J, Butman JA, Oldfield EH. Long-term natural history of hemangioblastomas in patients with von Hippel-Lindau disease: implications for treatment. J Neurosurg. 2006;105(2):248–55. https://doi.org/10.3171/jns.2006.105.2.248.

60. Oppenlander ME, Spetzler RF. Advances in spinal hemangioblastoma surgery. World Neurosurg. 2010;74(1):116–7. https://doi.org/10.1016/j.wneu.2010.04.018.
61. Sayyahmelli S, Aycan A, Erginoglu U, Başkaya MK. Spinal hemangioblastomas: clinical presentation, radiology, and treatment. Contemp Neurosurg. 2019;41(9):1–5. https://doi.org/10.1097/01.CNE.0000558612.20449.66.
62. Asthagiri AR, Mehta GU, Zach L, Li X, Butman JA, Camphausen KA, Lonser RR. Prospective evaluation of radiosurgery for hemangioblastomas in von Hippel-Lindau disease. Neuro Oncol (Charlottesville, VA). 2010;12(1):80–6. https://doi.org/10.1093/neuonc/nop018.
63. Carlson ML, Thom JJ, Driscoll CL, Haynes DS, Neff BA, Link MJ, Wanna GB. Management of primary and recurrent endolymphatic sac tumors. Otol Neurotol. 2013;34(5):939–43. https://doi.org/10.1097/MAO.0b013e31828680da.
64. Ferreira MAT, Feiz-Erfan I, Zabramski JM, Spetzler RF, Coons SW, Preul MC. Endolymphatic sac tumor: unique features of two cases and review of the literature. Acta Neurochir. 2002;144(10):1047–53. https://doi.org/10.1007/s701-002-8293-x.
65. Takeshima Y, Tanaka Y, Hironaka Y, Shida Y, Nakase H. Visualization of vascular structure of spinal hemangioblastoma using intraoperative indocyanine green videoangiography and temporary feeder occlusion. Eur Spine J. 2015;24(S4):585–9. https://doi.org/10.1007/s00586-014-3755-3.
66. About VHLA. The VHL Alliance. https://www.vhl.org.
67. Shirley MD, Tang H, Gallione CJ, Baugher JD, Frelin LP, Cohen B, North PE, Marchuk DA, Comi AM, Pevsner J. Sturge–Weber syndrome and Port-Wine stains caused by somatic mutation in GNAQ. N Engl J Med. 2013;368(21):1971–9. https://doi.org/10.1056/NEJMoa1213507.
68. Comi A. Current therapeutic options in Sturge-Weber syndrome. Semin Pediatr Neurol. 2015;22(4):295–301. https://doi.org/10.1016/j.spen.2015.10.005. Epub 2015 Nov 11. PMID: 26706016; PMCID: PMC4943027.
69. Bourgeois M, Crimmins DW, De Oliveira RS, Arzimanoglou A, Garnett M, Roujeau T, Di Rocco F, Sainte-Rose C. Surgical treatment of epilepsy in Sturge–Weber syndrome in children. J Neurosurg. 2007;106(1):20–8. https://thejns.org/pediatrics/view/journals/j-neurosurg-pediatr/106/1/article-p20.xml. Accessed 2 Aug 2021.
70. Di Rocco C, Tamburrini G. Sturge–Weber syndrome. Childs Nerv Syst. 2006;22:909. https://doi.org/10.1007/s00381-006-0143-2.
71. Gunny R, Saunders DE, Argyropoulou MI. Paediatric neuroradiology. In: Grainger & Allison's diagnostic radiology. Vol. 76. p. 1984–2045.
72. Lee HW. Multidiscipline immunotherapy-based rational combinations for robust and durable efficacy in brain metastases from renal cell carcinoma. Int J Mol Sci. 2021;22(12):6290. https://doi.org/10.3390/ijms22126290. PMID: 34208157; PMCID: PMC8230742.
73. Lance EI, Sreenivasan AK, Zabel TA, Kossoff EH, Comi AM. Aspirin use in Sturge-Weber syndrome: side effects and clinical outcomes. J Child Neurol. 2013;28(2):213–8. https://doi.org/10.1177/0883073812463607.
74. Shekhtman Y, Kim I, Riviello JJ Jr, Milla SS, Weiner HL. Focal resection of leptomeningeal angioma in a rare case of Sturge-Weber syndrome without facial nevus. Pediatr Neurosurg. 2014;49(2):99–104. https://doi.org/10.1159/000357357.
75. Arzimanoglou AA, Andermann F, Aicardi J, Sainte-Rose C, Beaulieu M-A, Villemure J-G, Olivier A, Rasmussen T. Sturge-Weber syndrome: indications and results of surgery in 20 patients. Neurology. 2000;55(10):1472–9. https://doi.org/10.1212/WNL.55.10.1472.
76. Bebin EM, Gomez MR. Prognosis in Sturge-Weber disease: comparison of unihemispheric and bihemispheric involvement. J Child Neurol. 1988;3(3):181–4. https://doi.org/10.1177/088307388800300306.
77. Tuxhorn IE, Pannek HW. Epilepsy surgery in bilateral Sturge-Weber syndrome. Pediatr Neurol. 2002;26(5):394–7. https://doi.org/10.1016/S0887-8994(01)00414-3.
78. Carson BS, Javedan SP, Freeman JM, Vining EPG, Zuckerberg AL, Lauer JA, Guarnieri M. Hemispherectomy: a hemidecortication approach and review of 52 cases. J Neurosurg. 1996;84(6):903–11. https://doi.org/10.3171/jns.1996.84.6.0903.
79. Hoffman HJ, Hendrick EB, Dennis M, et al. Hemispherectomy for Sturge-Weber syndrome. Childs Brain. 1979;5:233–48.
80. Oakes J. The natural history of patients with the Sturge-Weber syndrome. Pediatr Neurosurg. 1992;18(5–6):287–90. https://doi.org/10.1159/000120677.
81. Ogunmekan AO, Hwang PA, Hoffman HJ. Sturge-Weber-Dimitri disease. Role of hemispherectomy in prognosis. Can J Neurol Sci. 1989;16:78.
82. Kossoff EH, Buck C, Freeman JM. Outcomes of 32 hemispherectomies for Sturge-Weber syndrome worldwide. Neurology. 2002;59(11):1735–8. https://doi.org/10.1212/01.WNL.0000035639.54567.5C.
83. Rasmussen T. Hemispherectomy for seizures revisited. Can J Neurol Sci. 1983;10(2):71–8. https://doi.org/10.1017/S0317167100044668.
84. Schramm J, Kral T, Clusmann H. Transsylvian keyhole functional hemispherectomy. Neurosurgery. 2001;49(4):891–901. https://doi.org/10.1097/00006123-200110000-00021.
85. Wagner K, Vaz-Guimaraes F, Camstra K, Lam S. Endoscope-assisted hemispherotomy: translation of technique from cadaveric anatomical feasibility study to clinical implementation. J Neurosurg Pediatr. 2018;23(2):1–186. https://doi.org/10.3171/2018.8.PEDS18349.
86. Giordano F, Spacca B, Barba C, Mari F, Pisano T, Guerrini R, Genitori L. Vertical extraventricular func-

tional hemispherotomy: a new variant for hemispheric disconnection. Technical notes and results in three patients. Childs Nerv Syst. 2015;31(11):2151–60. https://doi.org/10.1007/s00381-015-2788-1.
87. Chua MMJ, Bushlin I, Stredny CM, Madsen JR, Patel AA, Stone S. Magnetic resonance imaging–guided laser-induced thermal therapy for functional hemispherotomy in a child with refractory epilepsy and multiple medical comorbidities. J Neurosurg Pediatr. 2021;27(1):30–5. https://doi.org/10.3171/2020.6.PEDS20455.
88. Binder DK, Schramm J. Transsylvian functional hemispherectomy. Childs Nerv Syst. 2006;22(8):960–6. https://doi.org/10.1007/s00381-006-0131-6.
89. Our Mission and Vision. The Sturge-Weber Foundation. https://sturge-weber.org.

14 Management of Spasticity

Rebecca Reynolds, Casey Ryan, and S. Hassan A. Akbari

What Is Spasticity?

To understand *spasticity*, it is important to first understand hypertonia [1]. Hypertonia is the perceived heightened resistance against an externally imposed, regular movement about a joint. Hypertonia can be caused by spasticity, dystonia, or rigidity, as well as a combination of these movement disorders in unison. In addition to tone, movement disorders are also subclassified by their kinetics: hyperkinetic, isokinetic, and negative or hypokinetic. This distinction is helpful for differentiating disorders of spasticity from dystonia.

In 2003, a taskforce focused on the classification and definition of disorders causing hypertonia in children published a review that delineates the definitions of spasticity, dystonia, and rigidity [2]. The purpose of the consensus statement was to facilitate the diagnosis of complex pediatric movement disorders and highlight the appropriate management options for each of the different clinical entities.

R. Reynolds · S. H. A. Akbari (✉)
Division of Pediatric Neurosurgery, Johns Hopkins University School of Medicine, Johns Hopkins All Children's Hospital, St. Petersburg, FL, USA
e-mail: rreyno26@jhmi.edu; sakbari3@jhmi.edu

C. Ryan
Department of Neurosurgery, University of South Florida, Tampa, FL, USA
e-mail: caseyryan1@usf.edu

Differentiating Spasticity and Dystonia

Spasticity, as defined by the taskforce, "is a velocity-dependent resistance of a muscle to stretch" [3]. It has one or both of the following signs: (1) increasing resistance to externally imposed movement with increasing speed of stretch, which varies with the direction of joint movement and/or (2) increasing resistance to externally imposed movement above a threshold speed or joint angle [2].

It is important to be able to identify spasticity from hypertonic dystonia as they are managed differently [3]. To simplify, the two entities can be distinguished in terms of their kinetics. Spasticity is isokinetic, where dystonia is hyperkinetic. In other words, spasticity does not cause increases in the amount of movement whereas movement disorders with dystonic features (like dystonic CP) increase the amount of movement in response to passive motion. Both spasticity and dystonia are the result of simultaneous contractions of agonist and antagonist muscle groups, but these opposing contractions tend to occur to a greater extent and are more pronounced in dystonia than spasticity. Spasticity is velocity-dependent and fluctuates with a patient's current state including the degree of movement, level of alertness, pain, and anxiety. Hypertonic dystonia is a sustained contraction opposing passive motion.

N. Shimony, G. Jallo (eds.), *Pediatric Neurosurgery Board Review*,
https://doi.org/10.1007/978-3-031-23687-7_14

Cerebral Palsy and Spasticity: Classification

In 2005, the Executive Committee for the Definition of Cerebral Palsy defined cerebral palsy (CP) as a "group of disorders of the development of movement and posture, causing activity limitation, that are attributed to non-progressive disturbances that occurred in the developing fetal or infant brain" [4]. Abnormal motor behavior is a core feature of CP, which is characterized by the inability to coordinate movements and muscle tone. This includes spasticity.

CP is a heterogenous group of disorders that has developed numerous classification schemes over the years [5]. Ingram [6] and Hagberg [7] classified CP based on anatomy, clinical presentation, and severity to guide diagnosis. The four different types of CP are described in Table 14.1.

The spastic type of CP can be further divided into four subgroups based on involved anatomy: diplegia, hemiplegia, triplegia, and bilateral hemiplegia or tetraplegia. Spastic diplegia affects the bilateral lower limbs more than the upper limbs. Spastic hemiplegia involves an upper and lower extremity on one side of the body. Spastic triplegia typically affects the bilateral legs and one arm. Bilateral hemiplegia, also known as spastic tetraplegia or spastic quadriplegia, shows a predominance for the upper limbs but involves all four limbs. These classifications have implications for neurosurgical management discussed later in the chapter.

Table 14.1 Types of cerebral palsy

Type	Description
Spastic	Characterized by enhanced muscle tension, hyperreflexia, and pathological reflexes
Dyskinetic	Characterized by involuntary, uncontrolled, repetitive movements Muscle tension tends to change over time, either increased or decreased
Ataxic	Characterized by loss of motor coordination, with ataxia and trembling Predominantly lowered muscle tension
Mixed	Characterized by having more than one of the above types due to multiple areas of brain injury

Etiologies of Spasticity

In general, spasticity in children can be the result of any process that harms the developing upper motor neurons within a child's central nervous system [8]. The most common cause of spasticity is cerebral palsy, which results from an injury to the central nervous system during fetal development to 2 years of age [9]. Other causes of spasticity include asphyxia before birth, hypoxia of the brain before/during/after birth, stroke, birth trauma during delivery, and non-accidental head trauma in infancy. Prematurity and low birth weight are also significant risk factors in the development of spasticity [9, 10].

Epidemiology

Spasticity is a common problem that affects quality of life and can be challenging to treat [9]. The most common cause of spasticity, CP, has an estimated prevalence of 2.5 of 1000 live births [10] with an incidence of approximately 300,000 individuals less than 18 years of age. It is thought that the incidence of CP may be increasing due to improving survival of premature and low-birth weight infants—a known risk factor of CP [9–11]. Of note, this is an underestimate of the true disease burden because acquired spasticity after severe traumatic brain injury, stroke, and other intracranial insult is also a contributing factor that is largely unmeasured [10].

Of note, spasticity that occurs with CP may improve over time but should not get worse [10]. Practitioners may believe spasticity is getting worse when in fact the patient is developing increasing muscle strength, worsening contractures, or may be misdiagnosed. Generally, children with CP spasticity are diagnosed at 1 year of life or later, have worsening manifestations during their second and third years of life, and then gradually improve over time. Nelson and Ellenberg showed that almost two-thirds of spastic diplegic children will outgrow their motor symptoms of CP by the age of 7 [12]. Similarly, in children that have a head injury with resultant spasticity, the spasticity tends to improve or even resolve with time [10]. It is, therefore, critical to understand the natural history of spasticity when considering management of the disorder.

Pathology/Pathophysiology

Muscle tone is modulated by competing signals: descending inhibitory impulses from the basal ganglia and excitatory afferent signals from the muscle spindles to the spinal cord via type Ia afferents. The inhibitory signals are mediated through gamma-aminobutyric acid (GABA) [1]. The excitatory signals are mediated via excitatory neurotransmitters, including glutamate and aspartate. These inputs modulate the behavior of the alpha motor neurons, which in turn set the tone of the resting muscle. In Sanger's review of the Pathophysiology of Pediatric Movement Disorders, there is a simplified depiction of the interaction of the descending and afferent impulses into the motoneuron pools affecting the signal to the muscle [1]. Clarified by Filloux, spasticity is not the result of one leg of the system faltering, but a combination of decreased cortical input into descending tracts (reticulospinal and corticospinal) due to upper motor neuron damage that results in a disruption and reduction of the normal reflex arcs present within the grey matter of the spinal cord [13]. This results in the potential sensitization of the arc that impacts the regulation of the agonist and antagonist muscle groups. Consistently over the years, it has been proposed that the pathophysiology of spasticity includes a combination of the loss of a variety of types of inhibition: reciprocal Ia inhibition, presynaptic inhibition, recurrent inhibition, group II afferent inhibition, and Golgi tendon organ inhibition [3]. The exact mechanism, however, is not well elucidated, and the level of different tract's involvement and regulation may vary depending on the specific pathology and patient entity.

Of note, spasticity that occurs in childhood has a unique pathophysiology compared to spasticity that occurs in the adult population. The co-activation of agonist and antagonistic muscle groups seen in childhood spasticity seems to be related to early central nervous system injury and its predilection for reorganizing descending white matter projections [14, 15]. Table 14.2 lists potential lesions and etiologies of spasticity.

Table 14.2 Lesions that cause spasticity

Localization	Pathology
Descending spinal tracts	Spinal cord injury, syringomyelia
Midbrain/pons	Fetal injuries (often fatal), trauma
Internal capsule	Stroke, multiple sclerosis
Periventricular white matter	Prematurity
Motor or premotor cortex	Stroke, encephalitis, trauma

Lesion localization can impact the presentation as well as severity of disease. Spinal cord injuries that result in spasticity tend to be more severe since they have a more potent disruption of the descending tracts that carry inhibitory impulses. Spinal cord injury resulting in spasticity is also more frequently associated with painful muscle spasms compared to spasticity from lesions affecting the upper motor neurons of the cerebrum. If a muscle remains spastic for a prolonged period, a muscular contracture can develop. A contracture is a permanent shortening of the muscle and its tendon. This does not improve regardless of treatment of spasticity, although preventative measures such as casting and splinting exist.

Clinical Features and Grading

Generally, children with spasticity will have muscle stiffness, tightness, and pain. Patients often tend to have other motor impairments that impact their function including weakness, which is not directly due to spasticity. Certain muscle groups tend to be affected more than others including flexors in the upper extremity, extensors in the distal lower extremity, and internal rotators. This contributes to the pathognomonic posture of a child with spastic quadriplegia: flexion at the elbow and wrist joints, flexion at the hips, internal rotation of the legs, and extension at the ankle [16]. That being said, every child is different and presentation can vary widely.

There are three current grading scales: the Ashworth (and Modified Ashworth) scales (*see* Table 14.3) [17, 18], the Tardieu scale (*see* Table 14.4) [19], and the Gross Motor Function Classification System (GMFCS; *see* Table 14.5) [20]. The Ashworth scale provides a subjective grading of resistance to passive muscle stretch, has been validated over time with much research, and has undergone modifications to enhance its ability to describe and quantify the severity of spasticity. The Tardieu Scale is used less commonly but is thought to provide a potentially more precise analysis of spasticity. The Tardieu scale differs from the Ashworth scale in that it utilizes joint angle measurements at three specified velocities and grades the muscle's reaction to stretch.

The GMFCS was designed to better understand a child's activity and participation levels while including metrics from the World Health Organization's classification of functioning, disability, and health [20, 21]. The scale utilizes not only gross motor function but those functions that are specifically self-initiated including sitting and walking. These are classified into five graded levels from Level 1 being independent movement to level 5 requiring complete assistance. The GMFCS also scales for age-appropriate functions.

Table 14.3 Modified Ashworth Scale (MAS)

Score	Description
0	No increase in muscle tone
1	Slight increase in muscle tone, described as the catch and release
1+	Slight increase in muscle tone, described as a catch followed by minimal resistance
2	Marked increase in muscle tone, with perseveration of passive movement
3	More considerable increase in muscle tone associated with difficulty of passive motion
4	Affected muscle(s) rigid, fixed in flexion or extension

Table 14.4 Tardieu Scale

Score	Description (quality of muscle reaction)
0	No resistance through course of passive motion
1	Slight resistance through course of passive motion, without a clear catch at a precise angle
2	Clear catch at precise angle that interrupts passive movement and is then followed by a release
3	Fatigable clonus (<10 s with maintained pressure) at a precise angle
4	Persistent clonus (>10 s with maintained pressure) at a precise angle
5	Immobile joint
	Joint angles
R1	Angle that muscle reaction is elicited[a]
R2	Angle of full range of passive motion
	Velocity definitions
V1	Slow, slower than the natural drop of a limb segment to gravity
V2	Regular, equal to the speed of the limb segment falling with gravity
V3	Fast, faster than the rate of drop of a limb segment due to gravity

[a] Joint angles for the Tardieu Scale are defined as the angle measured relative to the position of minimal stretch from the corresponding angle zero. Corresponding angle zero for all joints except for the hip is the natural resting anatomic position of the joint, i.e., ankle = 90°. The hip is measured from midline

Table 14.5 Gross Motor Function Classification Scale (GMCFS)

Score	Description
Level I	Walks without limitations in all settings, can climb stairs without assist. Performs gross motor skills, but speed, balance, and coordination may be impacted
Level II	Walks with limitations in most settings, can climb stairs with railing assist. Long distances and balancing on uneven surfaces or in crowded/confined spaces may pose difficulty. Maintain limited gross motor skills
Level III	Walks using a hand-hand mobility device in most indoor settings and can climb stairs with a railing with supervision or assistance
Level IV	Self-mobility with limitations; may use powered mobility. May walk at home/familiar settings with physical assistance of body support. In most other settings, transported via manual wheelchair or powered mobility
Level V	Transported in a manual wheelchair in all settings. Limited in ability support head and trunk postures antigravity and control leg and arm movements

Diagnostic Studies

Although there is no pathognomonic imaging finding that predicts or diagnoses spasticity, there are associated generalized findings depending on the type of spasticity [10]. Periventricular leukomalacia on MRI is most likely to be seen with spastic diplegia. Children with spastic quadriplegia are more likely to have diffuse multifocal, cystic encephalomalacia involving both cortex and white matter on MRI with varying levels of cerebral atrophy. Other diagnostic testing modalities that can be used include H-reflex excitability curves, electromyograms, and gait analysis. However, these tests can be resource-intensive and are not used consistently.

Spasticity Treatment

Given spasticity's multifactorial etiology, there are a number of different approaches to management. The goal of spasticity treatment is to prevent contractures from forming, which often cause pain, decrease mobility, and reduce a patient's or caretaker's ability to perform activities of daily living (ADLs). Treatment traditionally starts with a single approach and evolves into a complicated, multifaceted regimen over time that is often optimized by pediatric neurologists, developmental pediatricians, and physical medicine and rehabilitation specialists. Pediatric neurosurgeons are frequently consulted once a patient's tone and spasticity has become refractory to medical therapy for consideration of surgical intervention: selective dorsal rhizotomy or baclofen pump insertion.

First-line treatment of spasticity generally consists of non-invasive measures such as physical and occupational therapy as well as splinting and/or orthotics. The type of therapy that a child receives will depend upon his/her ability to participate in active exercises in addition to passive range of motion. Orthoses and splints can be a useful treatment regimen to help prevent contractures from forming. Treatment often starts with aggressive 24-h splinting and is relaxed over time as spasticity improves. Serial casting at the discretion of orthopedic surgery is useful to help lengthen muscles. The classic example is a child who walks on their toes due to gastrocnemius hyperactivity, and serial casting provides the opportunity to lengthen the muscles enough to fit in foot or ankle orthoses.

Other relatively non-invasive measures include oral medications and injections. A brief overview of the mechanism of activity for medications often used for spasticity treatment can be found in Table 14.6 [23].

Oral spasticity medications can be divided into those with a central or peripheral mechanism of action. There is only one peripherally acting

Table 14.6 Medical treatments for spasticity

	Mechanism of action	Side effects
Centrally acting drugs – Baclofen – Clonidine – Tizanidine – Benzodiazepines – Gabapentin	– GABA B agonist – Alpha 2 agonist – Alpha 2 agonist – GABA A agonist – Voltage gated calcium channel blockade	Lethargy, dizziness Hypotension, bradycardia Sedation, hypotension, long QT Sedation, tolerance/dependence Sedation, tremor, nystagmus
Peripherally acting drugs – Dantrolene	– Calcium blockade at the sarcoplasmic reticulum	Generalized muscle weakness, liver failure
Intramuscular injections – Botulinum toxin – Phenol/alcohol	– Inhibits Acetylcholine release @ NMJ – Protein denaturation	Flaccid paralysis, anticholinergic (dry mouth/constipation) Dysesthesia, tissue necrosis [22]
Intrathecal injection – Baclofen	– GABA B agonist	Lethargy, dizziness, hypotonia

medication, which is why the treatment of spasticity with oral medications is fraught with side effects. Centrally acting medications possess the ability to cross the blood-brain barrier, which enables their treatment of the spastic nervous system, but unfortunately means that they are not selective. Centrally acting medications include baclofen, clonidine, tizanidine, benzodiazepines, and gabapentin. There is one peripherally acting medication—dantrolene—which does not possess the central sedating side effects of the other medications, but is also non-selective and thus can carry unwanted side effects of systemic muscle weakness.

Intramuscular injections can provide a meaningful adjunct or replacement to oral therapies, especially if patients are experiencing significant systemic drug side effects. Botulinum toxin (or botox) is produced by the bacteria Clostridium botulinum and is administered directly into skeletal muscle. These injections are generally repeated every 3–4 months if the treatment is beneficial in improving range of motion [24]. Another injection modality is phenols, which are injected into peripheral nerves to cause chemical neurolysis. Phenols are non-selective for motor neurons and as a result, motor and sensory nerves can be compromised. It is not typically used in patients with preserved sensation [22].

While all of the aforementioned therapies are good options to improve the care of patients with spasticity and increase their range of motion, their effects on quality of life have offered mixed results [25, 26]. Surgical treatment of spasticity has shown sustained improvement in function and quality of life in these patients [27–29]. Surgical options include baclofen pump insertion and selective dorsal and/or ventral rhizotomy.

Intrathecal Baclofen Pump

As discussed earlier, baclofen crosses the blood-brain barrier; however, intrathecal delivery provides superior symptom management for patients with severe spasticity that is refractory to oral medications and also causes fewer side effects due to direct delivery to the central nervous system. Patients are considered candidates for a baclofen pump if their spasticity remains difficult to control despite the less invasive measures. A baclofen pump, when placed in the cervical spinal canal, is the only surgical treatment that can lower upper extremity tone and thus is often the surgical option for patients with spastic quadriplegia. Prior to insertion, a baclofen trial is completed via lumbar puncture with physical therapy evaluations pre- and post-injection to assess for improvement in spasticity and/or function and to monitor for adverse events such as somnolence or respiratory depression. The standard dose is 50 mcg of baclofen per injection in pediatric patients with an option for 25 mcg for very small or young children [30]. If patients tolerate the procedure well, then a baclofen pump implantation is pursued. If patients do not see improvement, a 75 mcg dose is often tried in another sitting. Baclofen pumps are inserted with the pump typically in the right or left lower quadrant of the abdomen with care given to keep ample proximity away from other common concomitant abdominal devices such as a gastrostomy tube. The pump is also situated away from the rib cage and the iliac crest, and patient size may preclude pump placement. The intrathecal catheter is tunneled subcutaneously from the back after it is inserted in the intrathecal space under direct fluoroscopy. The catheter tip is typically placed in the mid to lower thoracic region for lower extremity spasticity control and can be safely placed in the cervical region to control spastic quadriplegia [31].

After a pump insertion or replacement, patients are commonly kept overnight to monitor for signs or symptoms of baclofen toxicity. No dose modifications are typically made within the first 24 h of implantation due to system equilibration of the new drug. The common initial daily dose is double that of the patient's trial dose, averaged over the course of the day. This is then titrated up over time with no more than 5–15% interval change at any one visit. The average daily dose in pediatric patients is 300–400 mcg/day, but ranges widely. Depending on the child's daily usage and the pump size (20 or 40 mL), the need for clinic return for pump refill and ultimately pump replacement for end of battery life will be determined. The average battery life is around 7 years.

Baclofen overdose is possible if the pump is not calibrated correctly. There is no antidote for baclofen overdose and so the pump must be dialed down or turned off while the patient is monitored closely for respiratory compromise. Baclofen withdrawal symptoms typically include tachycardia, hypertension, fevers, and increased tone, and may become fatal. It is treated with a combination of oral baclofen and benzodiazepines. If it is secondary to pump malfunction, then oral baclofen often reaches insufficient concentrations in the cerebrospinal fluid and urgent pump revision needs to be considered [32].

Selective Dorsal Rhizotomy

An increasingly popular alternative to baclofen pumps for definitive spasticity control is a selective dorsal rhizotomy (SDR). It offers the benefit of no implantable device; thus, it removes the need for pump refills, replacements, and troubleshooting concerns for malfunction. However, it is primarily a surgery to benefit the lower extremities and is thus better suited for spastic diplegia. The underlying premise of the operation is to break the hyperactive motor reflex arc that is seen in upper motor neuron disease by selectively cutting approximately 2/3 of each abnormal sensory root. SDR is an ideal option for children with normal or near-normal intelligence and spasticity that predominantly affects their legs with little to no presence in their arms, specifically spastic diplegia. Children need to be able to participate in aggressive daily therapy after the procedure to obtain maximum benefit in terms of reduced tone and gained function. This includes an extensive stay in inpatient rehabilitation. Additional qualifiers include younger children typically between ages 2 and 8, GMFCS scores 1–3, spasticity without dystonia, those with periventricular leukomalacia on brain imaging, and the ability to isolate joint movement proximally in the lower extremities [33]. Given the complexity of the assessment, a multidisciplinary clinic that employs a developmental pediatrician, neurologist, neurosurgeon, orthopedist, and/or physical therapists are often the best resources for identifying children that are most likely to benefit from the procedure.

The surgical technique for an SDR varies, but the essential elements include a single-level laminectomy at the conus or multilevel laminectomies to visualize exiting dorsal nerve roots. Intraoperative neuromonitoring is commonly used to stimulate and identify nerve function once the dura is opened. A fraction of the dorsal nerve roots, typically 2/3, are sectioned with care to preserve anal sphincter and bladder function. Postoperatively, patients will experience an initial setback in their lower extremity function due to prior reliance on hypertonicity for movement, which is why early and aggressive physical therapy is important to retrain muscles for their desired range of motion. Postoperative complications are limited and can include cerebrospinal fluid leakage, low-pressure headaches, incontinence (typically temporary), and lower extremity weakness. There is a suggested increased propensity for scoliosis in the future, although this has not been fully studied and may be related to the extent of laminectomies performed [34].

There is also a surgical option for nonambulatory patients and caregivers who wish to avoid an implant. Severe spasticity can lead to contractures, joint dislocations, and skin breakdown. A combined selective dorsal and ventral root rhizotomy is a palliative procedure that aims to facilitate daily care by the patient's caregivers and improve pain associated with hypertonicity. By sectioning ventral and dorsal nerve roots, the goal is not to facilitate patient gait, but to prevent secondary injuries from hypertonicity. Complications are similar to that of the SDR.

Questions

1. Which of the following criteria would make a child a LESS favorable selective dorsal rhizotomy candidate?
   (a) Child who is 4 years old.
   (b) Child with GMFCS 5.
   (c) Child with cerebral palsy and spastic diplegia

(d) Child who is a toe-walker with increased tone.
(e) Child with periventricular leukomalacia on MRI.

2. A child with spastic quadriplegia undergoes a baclofen trial. Soon after the trial, she experiences rapid decline in mentation and requires intubation for respiratory support. The ICU team is asking you what should be the most appropriate next step. You state:
   (a) Give flumazenil to reverse the clinical picture.
   (b) Continue supportive therapy. The patient should wake up in the next several days.
   (c) Give diazepam to reverse the clinical picture.
   (d) Watch for tachycardia, fever, and increasing tone, as these are signs of baclofen withdrawal.
   (e) Continue supportive therapy. The patient should wake up in the next several hours.
3. You are consenting a family for placement of an intrathecal baclofen pump. As part of the discussion, you state that the pump will need to be refilled periodically. Typically, the child will be on a regular schedule for refills, but the child's parents should also watch for all of the following signs and symptoms of pump malfunction leading to overdose EXCEPT:
   (a) Worsening tone
   (b) Tachycardia
   (c) Fever
   (d) Hypotension
   (e) Pump alarm
4. The primary mechanism of action of baclofen includes:
   (a) GABA_B agonist
   (b) GABA_A inhibition
   (c) Blockade in the sarcoplasmic reticulum
   (d) Alpha_2 agonist
   (e) Inhibition of acetylcholine release at the neuromuscular junction
5. You are a surgeon who has started to perform a selective dorsal rhizotomy on a 4-year-old child. You have opened the dura and identified the conus. As you begin to section nerves in conjunction with the help of the neuro-monitoring tech, they report a significant decrease in left vastus lateralis, tibialis anterior, and gastrocnemius EMG signal. Your next response is:
   (a) Ask anesthesia to increase the MAP.
   (b) Ask anesthesia to drop the head of the bed to reduce CSF egress.
   (c) Ask the neuromonitoring technologist to check their leads.
   (d) You are not concerned and continue the case. There is often crossover of muscle innervation in spastic patients.
   (e) You continue the case, but tell the parents at the end of the case that you are concerned that their child will have a worse-than-expected deficit.

Answers
1. (b)
2. (e)
3. (d)
4. (a)
5. (d)

References

1. Sanger TD. Pathophysiology of pediatric movement disorders. J Child Neurol. 2003;18(Suppl 1):S9–S24.
2. Sanger TD, Delgado MR, Gaebler-Spira D, Hallett M, Mink JW, Task Force on Childhood Motor Disorders. Classification and definition of disorders causing hypertonia in childhood. Pediatrics. 2003;111(1):e89–97.
3. Smyth MD, Peacock WJ. The surgical treatment of spasticity. Muscle Nerve. 2000;23(2):153–63.
4. Bax M, Goldstein M, Rosenbaum P, et al. Proposed definition and classification of cerebral palsy, April 2005. Dev Med Child Neurol. 2005;47(8):571–6.
5. Sadowska M, Sarecka-Hujar B, Kopyta I. Cerebral palsy: current opinions on definition, epidemiology, risk factors, classification and treatment options. Neuropsychiatr Dis Treat. 2020;16:1505.
6. Balf C, Ingram T. Problems in the classification of cerebral palsy in childhood. Br Med J. 1955;2(4932):163.

7. Hagberg B, Hagberg G, Olow I. The changing panorama of cerebral palsy in Sweden 1954-1970. Acta Paediatr. 1975;64(2):193–200.
8. Shamsoddini A, Amirsalari S, Hollisaz M-T, Rahimnia A, Khatibi-Aghda A. Management of spasticity in children with cerebral palsy. Iran J Pediatr. 2014;24(4):345.
9. Mandigo CE, Anderson RC. Management of childhood spasticity: a neurosurgical perspective. Pediatr Ann. 2006;35(5):354–62.
10. Albright AL, Pollack IF, Andelson PD. Principles and practice of pediatric neurosurgery. Thieme; 2015.
11. O'Shea TM, Preisser JS, Klinepeter KL, Dillard RG. Trends in mortality and cerebral palsy in a geographically based cohort of very low birth weight neonates born between 1982 to 1994. Pediatrics. 1998;101(4):642–7.
12. Nelson KB, Ellenberg JH. Children who 'outgrew' cerebral palsy. Pediatrics. 1982;69(5):529–36.
13. Filloux FM. Neuropathophysiology of movement disorders in cerebral palsy. J Child Neurol. 1996;11(Suppl 1):S5–S12.
14. Brouwer B, Ashby P. Do injuries to the developing human brain alter corticospinal projections? Neurosci Lett. 1990;108(1–2):225–30.
15. Brouwer B, Ashby P. Altered corticospinal projections to lower limb motoneurons in subjects with cerebral palsy. Brain. 1991;114(3):1395–407.
16. Trompetto C, Marinelli L, Mori L, et al. Pathophysiology of spasticity: implications for neurorehabilitation. Biomed Res Int. 2014;2014:354906.
17. Bohannon RW, Smith MB. Interrater reliability of a modified Ashworth scale of muscle spasticity. Phys Ther. 1987;67(2):206–7.
18. Ashworth B. Preliminary trial of carisoprodol in multiple sclerosis. Practitioner. 1964;192:540–2.
19. Gracies JM, Burke K, Clegg NJ, et al. Reliability of the Tardieu Scale for assessing spasticity in children with cerebral palsy. Arch Phys Med Rehabil. 2010;91(3):421–8.
20. Palisano R, Rosenbaum P, Walter S, Russell D, Wood E, Galuppi B. Development and reliability of a system to classify gross motor function in children with cerebral palsy. Dev Med Child Neurol. 1997;39(4):214–23.
21. Compagnone E, Maniglio J, Camposeo S, et al. Functional classifications for cerebral palsy: correlations between the gross motor function classification system (GMFCS), the manual ability classification system (MACS) and the communication function classification system (CFCS). Res Dev Disabil. 2014;35(11):2651–7.
22. Ryan S. D'Souza, Nafisseh S. Warner. Phenol nerve block. StatPearls Publishing. https://www.ncbi.nlm.nih.gov/books/NBK525978/. Published 2022. Updated 30 Apr 2022. Accessed 22 Aug 2022.
23. Chang E, Ghosh N, Yanni D, Lee S, Alexandru D, Mozaffar T. A review of spasticity treatments: pharmacological and interventional approaches. Crit Rev Phys Rehabil Med. 2013;25(1–2):11–22.
24. Schwabe AL. Botulinum toxin in the treatment of pediatric upper limb spasticity. Semin Plast Surg. 2016;30(1):24–8.
25. Wong C, Westphall I, Michelsen JS. Measuring effects on pain and quality of life after abobotulinum toxin a injections in children with cerebral palsy. Toxins (Basel). 2022;14(1):43.
26. Datta Gupta A, Visvanathan R, Cameron I, Koblar SA, Howell S, Wilson D. Efficacy of botulinum toxin in modifying spasticity to improve walking and quality of life in post-stroke lower limb spasticity—a randomized double-blind placebo controlled study. BMC Neurol. 2019;19(1):96.
27. Robins JMW, Boyle A, McCune K, Lodh R, Goodden JR. Quality of life after selective dorsal rhizotomy: an assessment of family-reported outcomes using the CPQoL questionnaire. Childs Nerv Syst. 2020;36(9):1977–83.
28. Park TS, Dobbs MB, Cho J. Evidence supporting selective dorsal rhizotomy for treatment of spastic cerebral palsy. Cureus. 2018;10(10):e3466.
29. Kraus T, Gegenleitner K, Svehlik M, Novak M, Steinwender G, Singer G. Long-term therapy with intrathecal baclofen improves quality of life in children with severe spastic cerebral palsy. Eur J Paediatr Neurol. 2017;21(3):565–9.
30. Boster AL, Bennett SE, Bilsky GS, et al. Best practices for intrathecal baclofen therapy: screening test. Neuromodulation. 2016;19(6):616–22.
31. McCall TD, MacDonald JD. Cervical catheter tip placement for intrathecal baclofen administration. Neurosurgery. 2006;59(3):634–40; discussion 634–40.
32. Watve SV, Sivan M, Raza WA, Jamil FF. Management of acute overdose or withdrawal state in intrathecal baclofen therapy. Spinal Cord. 2012;50(2):107–11.
33. Nicolini-Panisson RD, Tedesco AP, Folle MR, Donadio MVF. Selective dorsal rhizotomy in cerebral palsy: selection criteria and postoperative physical therapy protocols. Rev Paul Pediatr. 2018;36(1):9.
34. Abbott R. The selective dorsal rhizotomy technique for spasticity in 2020: a review. Childs Nerv Syst. 2020;36(9):1895–905.

Management of Brachial Plexus Injury Across Different Age Groups

15

Jesse A. Stokum, Daniel Lubelski, and Allan Belzberg

Introduction

Epidemiology and Pathophysiology

Pediatric brachial plexus palsy (BPP) is primarily due to obstetrical BPP (OBPP). OBPP occurs in 1.6–2.9 per 1000 full-term births [1, 2], although its incidence appears to be decreasing [3], perhaps due to increasing rates of cesarean-section. A significant number of patients with OBPP are left with a permanent life-altering palsy, which causes substantial emotional and economic hardship [4].

In OBPP, distraction of shoulder away from the head during delivery can result in a stretch injury to the brachial plexus. These distractive forces are usually caused by shoulder dystocia, which increases the risk of OBPP by ~100-fold [5]. Gestational weight is strongly associated with OBPP [1, 2, 6], and birthweights of >4500 g increase the risk of OBPP by 14- to 45-fold [1, 5]. Instrumented vaginal delivery is also associated with increased risk of OBPP [2, 5]. The incidence of OBPP is much higher (~175-fold) in patients with breech delivery versus vertex delivery [7, 8]. In patients with breech delivery, OBPP is more likely to be bilateral, occurs more often in children with lower birthweight, and is more likely to include nerve root avulsions [7, 8]. While injuries such as clavicular fracture are often reported to be associated with OBPP, they may represent associated injuries rather than causative factors [9]. While cesarean section is highly protective, 0.2 births per 1000 via cesarean section still result in BPP [5]. So-called intrauterine maladaptation is thought to account for these injuries, wherein forces are exerted upon the brachial plexus during uterine contractions [9].

Neonates can present with BPP from other causes. Familial forms exist, although the precise genetic etiology remains unknown [9]. Uterine malformations, congenital varicella syndrome, osteomyelitis of the vertebral body or humerus, exostosis of the first rib, and trauma can cause a BPP in this age group [9]. Placental insufficiency may potentially cause hypoperfusion and malformation of the brachial plexus during development [10].

Older children can also present with brachial plexus injuries, mostly from motor vehicle accidents. However, non-obstetrical traumatic pediatric brachial plexus injuries are rare, occurring in only 0.1% of pediatric multitrauma patients [11]. Therefore, this chapter will focus primarily upon management of OBPP.

J. A. Stokum
Department of Neurosurgery, University of Maryland School of Medicine, Baltimore, MD, USA
e-mail: JStokum@som.umaryland.edu

D. Lubelski · A. Belzberg (✉)
Department of Neurosurgery, Johns Hopkins University School of Medicine, Baltimore, MD, USA
e-mail: dlubelski@jhmi.edu; abelzbe1@jhmi.edu

N. Shimony, G. Jallo (eds.), *Pediatric Neurosurgery Board Review*,
https://doi.org/10.1007/978-3-031-23687-7_15

Classification and Functional Scoring of OBPP

Patients with OBPP are classified based upon the anatomical and functional extent of their injuries [12]. While a comprehensive review [13] is beyond the scope of this chapter, the most common systems are described here.

The Narakas classification organizes patients into four groups [14], each distinguished by the number of involved spinal nerve roots. Group 1, Erb's palsy, includes injury to the C5 and C6 nerve roots and weakness of shoulder abduction, external rotation, and elbow flexion. Group 2, the extended Erb's palsy, involves injury to the C5, C6, and C7 nerve roots, resulting in weakness of wrist and elbow extension in addition to the weakness experienced by group 1. Group 3, a total BPP without a Horner's syndrome, involves injury to the C5 through T1 nerve roots and total paralysis of the affected arm. Group 4, a total BPP with a Horner's syndrome, usually involves nerve root avulsion(s). The Narakas classification does not include Klumpke's palsy, a syndrome of isolated hand weakness caused by injury to the lower nerve roots. Klumpke's palsy is rare, only occurring in ~0.6% of all patients with OBPP [15].

There exist three major functional scoring systems. First, the Mallet score is a five-grade score (grades I through V) of shoulder function where five key movements are scored [16]. While the Mallet score is widely used, it cannot be applied to infants since it requires that the examinee follows commands [12]. Second, the more recently published active movement scale (AMS) includes 15 separate movements of the upper extremity, which are individually assigned a grade from 0 to 7, and then summated to produce a total limb motion score with a maximum score of 105 [12]. The AMS can be applied to infants and does not require the examinee to follow commands [12]. Third, The Toronto Test is comprised of a subset of the movements contained in the AMS that were selected based upon their ability to identify patients with OBPP who might spontaneously improve without surgery [17]. A score of <3.5 indicates a potential need for surgery [17]. While all three scoring systems have been validated and are reproducible [18], the Mallet score does not correlate well with the AMS and Toronto Test and therefore they should not be used interchangeably [12].

Natural History of OBPP

Rates of Spontaneous Recovery

The natural history of OBPP has been difficult to accurately assess, as reviewed elsewhere [19]. This gap in knowledge has led to a widespread misconception that more than 90% of patients with OBPP will undergo spontaneous recovery [19]. This assumption may have hindered surgical referral in the past. There are several important population studies that have revealed a more accurate natural history of OBPP. In one study from Sweden, 98 children with OBPP and regular follow-up were identified from 38,749 live births. 21.8% (approximately 1 in 5) of these children still had weakness at 10–12 years of age [20]. In a second study from Malmö, 48 children with OBPP were identified from 25,736 live births. 25% (1 in 4) of these children had a persistent, functionally limiting palsy at 10 years [21]. Finally, a study from a single medical center identified 19 children with OBPP and regular follow-up from 8258 live births. 21.1% (approximately 1 in 5) of these children still had weakness at greater than 26 months [22]. A recent systematic review largely corroborated these findings, concluding that ~20–30% of patients with OBPP suffer from persistent palsies [19].

In patients with OBPP that do exhibit spontaneous improvement, strength will usually improve within ~4 months [23]. Rarely, improvement can still occur within 2 years, after which further improvement is unlikely [23, 24]. Earlier improvement, particularly within 1 month, is associated with more complete recovery, whereas recovery after 4 months is associated with permanent deficits [21, 25].

Not all movements are equally likely to spontaneously recover after OBPP. Interestingly, children with OBPP rarely fail to eventually recover at least antigravity elbow flexion, even in cases where elbow flexion does not return by 3 months of age [26–29]. In contrast, patients with persistent palsies often suffer from long-term shoulder weakness, particularly in external rotation [28, 29]. For example, one study reported that only ~55% of patients with a persistent palsy spontaneously recovered good shoulder function (Mallet score of IV or greater) without surgical intervention [27]. Hand function is also unlikely to recover spontaneously in children with injuries to lower nerve roots [30]. One study showed that those in Narakas groups 3 and 4 spontaneously recover useful hand function in only 45.7% and 29.6% of cases, respectively [14].

Deformities of the upper extremity are common in patients with OBPP. Shoulder contractures and osseus deformities occur in ~50% and 33% of patients with OBPP, respectively [31]. Paresis of the shoulder external rotators and abductors lead to unopposed action of the internal rotators and adductors. With prolonged muscle imbalance, a medial rotation contracture forms, and posterior subluxation and dislocation of the glenohumeral joint can occur [32].

Prognostication

Patients with more severe axonotmetic or neurotmetic injuries, who have little potential for spontaneous recovery should be identified early as potential surgical candidates. Therefore, prognostication of (lack of) spontaneous recovery is of critical importance. Notably, prognostication is very difficult at early ages since injuries of different severities can present with identical signs and symptoms [33].

Several key prognostic factors have been identified. First, the number of injured nerve roots, usually summarized by the patient's Narakas group, is strongly correlated with potential for recovery [14, 21]. For example, a meta-analysis of 24 studies showed that at 6 months, 65% of those in Narakas groups I and II had complete recovery, whereas only 14% of those in Narakas groups III and IV had complete recovery [34]. Second, the time-to-recovery for biceps strength has been shown to predict recovery, and has been commonly used to identify surgical candidates, as discussed in later sections. Specifically, a return of biceps strength to at least antigravity within 3 months is associated with full recovery, whereas later recovery of biceps is associated with lower downstream Mallet scores [25]. Notably, a group of patients that do not recover biceps antigravity strength by 3 months still go on to mount full recovery, leading some clinicians to argue against the sole use of bicep strength [17]. Third, neurophysiological measurements have been shown to predict recovery and could potentially supplement physical examination [35]. Finally, clinical signs of avulsion injury, such as a Horner's syndrome or hemidiaphragm paralysis, strongly portend poor spontaneous recovery [36, 37], and nearly always indicate a need for early surgical intervention.

Initial Management and Workup

Initial Evaluation and Management of OBPP

Within 2–3 weeks of birth, all patients with OBPP should be referred to a multidisciplinary team comprised of a peripheral nerve surgeon, physiotherapists, and occupational therapists. An initial visit should include a detailed history, including obstetrical history, birth complications, birth related injuries, and maternal risk factors. An initial physical examination should be conducted using a standardized strength scoring system. Active exercises, passive stretches, and sensory stimulation should be performed daily if possible and can help to prevent laterality bias or neglect, muscle atrophy, joint deformity, and contracture which can limit functional recovery even in context of good neuronal regeneration [38]. Stretching exercises are particularly important and can be conducted at home by the caregiver [39]. Splinting may be necessary in cases of unopposed action of the triceps, or to bring a drop-wrist into a more functional position. Botulinum toxin injections may be deployed to help combat contractures [40].

Role for Imaging and Electrophysiology

Magnetic resonance imaging (MRI) and CT myelography can be obtained in patients with OBPP to identify nerve root avulsion. MRI and CT myelography exhibit a sensitivity and specificity of ~60–80% and ~70–100% for the detection of nerve root avulsion injury in OBPP [41–43].

While electrophysiology has a well-established role in the workup of adult patients with peripheral nerve injuries, electrophysiology does not occupy a major role in OBPP. In adults, a denervated muscle typically shows absent motor unit potentials and denervation activity on EMG. In contrast, in OBPP, a paretic muscle may show present motor unit potentials and absent denervation activity. Various explanations have been suggested to account for this phenomenon [33]. Therefore, electromyography is not typically obtained in patients with OBPP [44]. Furthermore, unlike MRI and CT myelography, electrophysiological testing is not particularly sensitive for the detection of pre-ganglionic avulsion injury (~31% sensitivity and 90% specificity) [45].

Nerve Surgery for OBPP

General Principles

Historically, nerve surgery for OBPP was first reported by Kennedy in 1903 [46] and later popularized by practitioners like Alain Gilbert [47]. Nerve surgery is indicated for the 20–30% of OBPP patients with severe axonotmetic or neurotmetic injuries that are unlikely to spontaneously improve with time. Unfortunately, in the United States, only 3.3% of OBPP patients undergo nerve surgery [48], suggesting that many additional patients could benefit from surgical intervention.

The goal of surgery in OBPP to the upper plexus is complete repair, with restoration of function to elbow flexion, shoulder abduction, and external rotation. The goal of surgery in pan-plexal injuries is to restore useful hand movement, which has better success rates in the pediatric population with OBPP versus the adult population [49, 50]. If indicated, nerve surgery should be performed as soon as possible to prevent muscle atrophy, which can limit the outcome. Usually, surgery is offered between 3 and 9 months.

Surgical Criteria

The largest challenge in OBPP surgery is selection of surgical candidates. Surgery may entail resection of the injured nerve segment, whereupon any potential for spontaneous recovery is lost. Therefore, surgical candidacy should be reserved for the 20–30% of children with OBPP who will not mount a spontaneous recovery. Identification of this cohort at early ages is challenging and controversial.

In cases of a total BPP, particularly when clinical signs of nerve root avulsion are present, most practitioners endorse offering surgery early at ~3 months of age. For the remaining patients with OBPP, one of two major approaches are typically used to identify surgical patients.

In one system popularized by Gilbert, if biceps function is absent at 3 months of age, then patients are offered surgery [51]. Even through most patients with OBPP exhibit recovery in elbow flexion, absence of biceps function at 3 months is believed to represent a sentinel exam finding that portends poor recovery. In one study, the positive predictive value of elbow flexion at 3 months was 88% [20]. Some have critiqued this strategy's focus on a single muscle group to guide treatment of the entire plexus and its potential to lead to surgery for patients that may eventually spontaneously recover. For example, in one study, the authors found that elbow flexion at 3 months did not accurately predict outcome in 12.8% of cases [17]. Some have suggested adding electrophysiological studies [35] or additional muscles [17] to improve predictive power.

In an alternative system popularized by Clarke [52, 53], upper extremity strength is assessed at 3 months of age using the Toronto Test. If patients exhibit a score of less than 3.5 at this time or exhibit signs or symptoms of nerve root avulsion, they are offered surgery. Otherwise, at 9 months the "Cookie Test" is performed, which entails testing whether children can bring a cookie to the mouth without flexing the neck more than 45° with their arm at the side. Failure of the Cookie Test suggests need for surgery.

Surgical Technique

Surgical management of OBPP can consist of either primary repair, wherein innervation is restored to the target musculature, and/or secondary surgeries such as muscle transfer, tendon transfer, and orthopedic surgery. Primary repair consists of neuroma excision with nerve grafting, and/or nerve transfer. Historically, primary repair most often consisted of graft reconstruction. However, there has been growing interest in nerve transfer as an alternative approach. Nerve transfer results in a shorter gap that reinnervating axons must traverse to meet their target, which would theoretically lead to faster recovery and less muscular atrophy. Notably, in 2015, the International Federation of Societies for Surgery of the Hand Committee reviewed the role of nerve transfer in OBPP surgery, concluding that while the data supporting transfer was promising, further evidence was needed, and that nerve grafting should be performed when possible [54]. They outline four indications for nerve transfer: (1) inadequate proximal nerve root availability, possibly due to avulsion injury, (2) failure of primary graft reconstruction, (3) late patient presentation, and (4) isolated strength deficits, with recovery of all but one movement.

During surgery, the brachial plexus is usually exposed via a supraclavicular approach, with careful preservation of the phrenic nerve and division of the anterior scalene muscle [55]. More distal lesions may require additional infraclavicular approach [55]. The nerve roots and trunks are then exposed. Typically, a neuroma-in-continuity of the upper trunks is encountered [33]. Neurolysis is performed, and the anatomy is identified. Of note, neurolysis is not recommended as a solitary treatment and is inferior to nerve grafting [49]. Next, the neuroma is resected unless fascicular structure is intact on microscopic examination. If the lesion is postganglionic, the defect is then repaired with nerve grafting, usually using the sural nerves [55]. If the lesion is pre-ganglionic, then grafting is not performed, and nerve transfer can be considered.

The role of intraoperative electrophysiology differs between adult BPP and OBPP. In adult patients or older children with a brachial plexus injury in continuity, the decision whether to neurolyse versus reconstruct with graft is guided by intraoperative electrophysiology. In these patients, the presence of a nerve action potential (NAP) across an injured segment indicates preservation of at least 3000–4000 myelinated axons and a >90% rate of recovery with neurolysis alone [56]. In contrast to adults, intraoperative NAP is not usually applied to OBPP patients since the presence of a NAP across an injured segment does not correlate well with functional recovery [57, 58]. The inability to objectively measure regenerative potential with electrophysiology represents a major barrier to offering earlier nerve reconstruction. Currently, visual inspection, intraoperative histology, and preoperative functional testing are the sole means in which to judge the severity of nerve injury in OBPP.

If indicated, nerve transfers can be considered. A nerve transfer requires sacrifice of a donor nerve or the coaptation of fascicles of a nerve, which are transected and transferred onto the end (end-to-end) or side (end-to-side) of the target nerve. While many different nerve transfers have been explored in adults, only a subset has been translated to OBPP patients. Numerous terminal brachial plexus nerves can be reconstructed using intercostal nerve transfer [59]. Musculocutaneous innervation to biceps can be repaired with transfer of pectoral nerves, median nerve fascicles, ulnar nerve fascicles, phrenic nerve, or hypoglossal nerve transfer, although the morbidity associated with phrenic nerve and hypoglossal nerve transfer usually precludes its use [60–64]. The axillary nerve can be repaired using a triceps nerve [65]. The suprascapular nerve can be reinnervated with the spinal accessory nerve [66]. Interestingly, in cases of avulsion of the upper trunk, the contralateral C7 nerve root can be extended with the ipsilateral ulnar nerve, tunneled across the midline, and transferred to the distal end of the avulsed trunk [67]. These patients rarely show deficits resulting from harvest from the contralateral C7 nerve root, although synchronous activity of the arms may occur. Finally, various end-to-side nerve transfers have been performed to supplement nerve grafting [68].

Outcomes After Surgery

Unfortunately, there currently exists no randomized controlled trial that demonstrates the effectiveness of surgical graft repair vs nonsurgical treatment. A few single center series are noteworthy and together comprise grade IV evidence in support of nerve repair surgery in select patients with OBPP, as reviewed elsewhere [30, 69]. In one 2009 study, 92 patients that underwent neuroma resection and grafting were compared with 16 that underwent neurolysis only [49]. All patients were selected using Clarke's criteria, as discussed above. At 4 years follow-up, a greater proportion of grafted patients had functionally useful function (defined as AMS scores of 6 or 7) in multiple AMS movements, with all patients recovering elbow flexion. No changes in AMS scores were noted in patients who underwent neurolysis only. In a second 2000 study, 31 patients with OBPP and no recovery of elbow flexion at 3 months were either treated with therapy/neurolysis or taken for graft repair [70]. While none of the patients treated with neurolysis or therapy alone achieved a good result, defined by a Mallet score of at least IV, 70% of the grafted patients did. Finally, in another 2000 study of 247 patients with OBPP, patients treated with surgical graft repair exhibited greater range of motion in the ipsilateral shoulder compared to those treated nonsurgically [71].

After brachial plexus graft repair, elbow flexion recovers well in most cases, with ~80–90% of patients recovering at least antigravity function [72–74]. Recovery of shoulder function is less certain, with 65–80% recovery of shoulder abduction and 20–50% recovery of external rotation [72, 74–76]. Interestingly, unlike in adults, where recovery of useful hand function after lower plexus injuries is highly unlikely, repair of lower plexus injuries in OBPP yields useful hand function in 60–97% of cases [50, 75, 77, 78].

There is growing evidence to support the use of nerve transfers in OBPP. Spinal accessory nerve to suprascapular nerve transfer can be conducted to improve shoulder function, with ~14% of patients exhibiting greater than 20° of external rotation at follow-up [74]. Compared to graft repair, most studies show similar outcome between graft reconstruction versus nerve transfer for suprascapular nerve repair [66, 74, 79, 80]. Transfer of ulnar fascicles (Oberlin's transfer), median nerve fascicles, intercostal nerves, or median pectoral nerve to the biceps branch of the musculocutaneous nerve can be conducted to improve biceps function with overall good results. OBPP patients treated with Oberlin's transfer show good recovery of bicep function (MRC $\geq$ 3) in ~70–80% of patients [61, 81], with some groups reporting superior recovery of supination versus graft repair [82]. Median nerve fascicle transfer to biceps nerve has been shown to lead to a good result (AMS bicep score $\geq$ 6) in 90% of patients (24511548). Intercostal and medial pectoral nerve transfer to biceps nerve also results in good outcome in 80–90% of patients, with one study showing no statistical difference in response rate between these two transfers [64, 83–85]. Contralateral C7 transfer is relatively uncommon, but its use has been applied for both upper and lower trunk reconstruction. In one study, contralateral C7 to ipsilateral median and musculocutaneous nerve resulted in 77% patients with good (MRC $\geq$ 3) biceps function and 55% with good wrist and finger flexion [86]. In this study, 33% had "considerable" synchronous arm movement. In a second study, contralateral C7 was used to repair the injured ipsilateral lower trunk. All patients had return of hand sensation in the ulnar distribution; however only one patient had return of ulnar intrinsic movement [87]. Parenthetically, while end-to-side transfer has been explored in patients with OBPP, the evidence does not yet support its widespread application [68, 72].

Secondary Surgery for OBPP

Secondary surgeries, comprised of various tendon or muscle transfers or osteotomies, are deployed in patients who either have undergone primary repair of the brachial plexus and have residual deficits, or as a primary strategy in patients that have not undergone nerve reconstruction. Shoulder function can be improved with tendon and muscle transfers such as the Hoffer procedure, where the latissimus dorsi and teres major muscles are transferred to the posterior rotator cuff to improve external rotation [88]. Rotational osteotomy of the humerus can also be performed to improve external rotation [89]. Elbow flexion can be improved by the Steindler procedure [90], where medial epicondylar flexor muscles are transferred to the medial humerus, or through gracilis free flap transfer [91]. Finally, wrist extension and pronation can be improved through transfer of brachialis muscle or gracilis transfer [92, 93].

Summary

Pediatric brachial plexus palsy (BPP) is primarily due to obstetrical BPP (OBPP) and occurs in 1.6–2.9 per 1000 full-term births mostly due to shoulder dystocia during vaginal delivery. While many patients with OBPP recover spontaneously, ~20–30% of patients suffer from persistent palsies. OBPP is classified based on the number of injured nerve roots, functional impairment, and whether the injury is pre- or post-ganglionic. All patients with OBPP should be referred to a multidisciplinary team for physical therapy, family support, and surgical evaluation. Surgery is offered to patients that have low likelihood for spontaneous recovery. Surgical candidates are usually identified using one of two major systems, either absence of biceps function at 3 months, or using the AMS score and cookie test at 3 and 9 months, respectively. Nerve repair usually consists of excision of a neuroma-in-continuity followed by sural nerve graft reconstruction and/or distal nerve transfers. After nerve surgery, elbow flexion recovers in 80–90% of patients, shoulder abduction in 65–80% of patients, shoulder external rotation in 20–50% of patients, and useful hand function in 60–97% of patients. Similar recovery rates have been reported after nerve grafting versus transfer, however experts currently recommend graft reconstruction when possible.

Questions

1. The incidence of brachial plexus injury at birth is
   (a) 1–3%
   (b) 4–6%
   (c) 0.1–0.3%
   (d) >10%
2. Risks for plexus injury at birth including all the following except
   (a) Birthweight > 4500 g
   (b) Breech delivery
   (c) Vaginal delivery with instruments
   (d) Caesarean section
3. What lack of muscle group function at 3 months portends to surgical exploration?
   (a) Deltoid
   (b) Biceps
   (c) Triceps
   (d) Wrist flexion
4. Following brachial plexus nerve surgery, elbow flexion recovers in % of children?
   (a) 20–30%
   (b) 40–50%
   (c) 60–70%
   (d) 80–90%

Answers

1. (c)
2. (d)
3. (b)
4. (d)

References

1. Bager B. Perinatally acquired brachial plexus palsy—a persisting challenge. Acta Paediatr. 1997;86:1214–9.
2. Dawodu A, Sankaran-Kutty M, Rajan TV. Risk factors and prognosis for brachial plexus injury and clavicular fracture in neonates: a prospective analysis from the United Arab Emirates. Ann Trop Paediatr. 1997;17:195–200.
3. Chauhan SP, Blackwell SB, Ananth CV. Neonatal brachial plexus palsy: incidence, prevalence, and temporal trends. Semin Perinatol. 2014;38:210–8.
4. Louden E, Allgier A, Overton M, Welge J, Mehlman CT. The impact of pediatric brachial plexus injury on families. J Hand Surg Am. 2015;40:1190–5.
5. Foad SL, Mehlman CT, Ying J. The epidemiology of neonatal brachial plexus palsy in the United States. J Bone Joint Surg Am. 2008;90:1258–64.
6. Eng GD, Binder H, Getson P, O'Donnell R. Obstetrical brachial plexus palsy (OBPP) outcome with conservative management. Muscle Nerve. 1996;19:884–91.
7. Tan KL. Brachial palsy. J Obstet Gynaecol Br Commonw. 1973;80:60–2.
8. Tada K, Tsuyuguchi Y, Kawai H. Birth palsy: natural recovery course and combined root avulsion. J Pediatr Orthop. 1984;4:279–84.
9. Alfonso DT. Causes of neonatal brachial plexus palsy. Bull NYU Hosp Jt Dis. 2011;69:11–6.
10. Jain V, Sebire NJ, Talbert DG. Kaiser Wilhelm syndrome: obstetric trauma or placental insult in a historical case mimicking Erb's palsy. Med Hypotheses. 2005;65:185–91.
11. Dorsi MJ, Hsu W, Belzberg AJ. Epidemiology of brachial plexus injury in the pediatric multitrauma population in the United States. J Neurosurg Pediatr. 2010;5:573–7.
12. Greenhill DA, Lukavsky R, Tomlinson-Hansen S, Kozin SH, Zlotolow DA. Relationships between 3 classification systems in brachial plexus birth palsy. J Pediatr Orthop. 2017;37:374–80.
13. Chang KW, Justice D, Chung KC, Yang LJ. A systematic review of evaluation methods for neonatal brachial plexus palsy: a review. J Neurosurg Pediatr. 2013;12:395–405.
14. Al-Qattan MM, El-Sayed AA, Al-Zahrani AY, Al-Mutairi SA, Al-Harbi MS, Al-Mutairi AM, Al-Kahtani FS. Narakas classification of obstetric brachial plexus palsy revisited. J Hand Surg Eur Vol. 2009;34:788–91.
15. al-Qattan MM, Clarke HM, Curtis CG. Klumpke's birth palsy. Does it really exist? J Hand Surg Br. 1995;20:19–23.
16. Mallet J. [Obstetrical paralysis of the brachial plexus. II. Therapeutics. Treatment of sequelae. Priority for the treatment of the shoulder. Method for the expression of results]. Rev Chir Orthop Reparatrice Appar Mot. 1972;58(Suppl 1):166–8.
17. Michelow BJ, Clarke HM, Curtis CG, Zuker RM, Seifu Y, Andrews DF. The natural history of obstetrical brachial plexus palsy. Plast Reconstr Surg. 1994;93:675–80; discussion 681.
18. Bae DS, Waters PM, Zurakowski D. Reliability of three classification systems measuring active motion in brachial plexus birth palsy. J Bone Joint Surg Am. 2003;85:1733–8.
19. Pondaag W, Malessy MJ, van Dijk JG, Thomeer RT. Natural history of obstetric brachial plexus palsy: a systematic review. Dev Med Child Neurol. 2004;46:138–44.
20. Annika J, Paul U, Anna-Lena L. Obstetric brachial plexus palsy—a prospective, population-based study of incidence, recovery and long-term residual impairment at 10 to 12 years of age. Eur J Paediatr Neurol. 2019;23:87–93.
21. Sjoberg I, Erichs K, Bjerre I. Cause and effect of obstetric (neonatal) brachial plexus palsy. Acta Paediatr Scand. 1988;77:357–64.
22. Jackson ST, Hoffer MM, Parrish N. Brachial-plexus palsy in the newborn. J Bone Joint Surg Am. 1988;70:1217–20.
23. Jahnke AH Jr, Bovill DF, McCarroll HR Jr, James P, Ashley RK. Persistent brachial plexus birth palsies. J Pediatr Orthop. 1991;11:533–7.
24. Adler JB, Patterson RL Jr. Erb's palsy. Long-term results of treatment in eighty-eight cases. J Bone Joint Surg Am. 1967;49:1052–64.
25. Waters PM. Comparison of the natural history, the outcome of microsurgical repair, and the outcome of operative reconstruction in brachial plexus birth palsy. J Bone Joint Surg Am. 1999;81:649–59.
26. Hems TEJ, Savaridas T, Sherlock DA. The natural history of recovery of elbow flexion after obstetric brachial plexus injury managed without nerve repair. J Hand Surg Eur Vol. 2017;42:706–9.
27. Smith NC, Rowan P, Benson LJ, Ezaki M, Carter PR. Neonatal brachial plexus palsy. Outcome of absent biceps function at three months of age. J Bone Joint Surg Am. 2004;86:2163–70.
28. Hulleberg G, Elvrum AK, Brandal M, Vik T. Outcome in adolescence of brachial plexus birth palsy. 69 individuals re-examined after 10-20 years. Acta Orthop. 2014;85:633–40.
29. Lagerkvist AL, Johansson U, Johansson A, Bager B, Uvebrant P. Obstetric brachial plexus palsy: a prospective, population-based study of incidence, recovery, and residual impairment at 18 months of age. Dev Med Child Neurol. 2010;52:529–34.
30. Pondaag W, Malessy MJA. Evidence that nerve surgery improves functional outcome for obstetric brachial plexus injury. J Hand Surg Eur Vol. 2021;46:229–36.
31. Hoeksma AF, Ter Steeg AM, Dijkstra P, Nelissen RG, Beelen A, de Jong BA. Shoulder contracture and osseous deformity in obstetrical brachial plexus injuries. J Bone Joint Surg Am. 2003;85:316–22.
32. Al-Qattan MM. Classification of secondary shoulder deformities in obstetric brachial plexus palsy. J Hand Surg Br. 2003;28:483–6.
33. Malessy MJ, Pondaag W, van Dijk JG. Electromyography, nerve action potential, and compound motor action potentials in obstetric brachial plexus lesions: validation in the absence of a "gold standard". Neurosurgery. 2009;65:A153–9.

34. Foad SL, Mehlman CT, Foad MB, Lippert WC. Prognosis following neonatal brachial plexus palsy: an evidence-based review. J Child Orthop. 2009;3:459–63.
35. Bisinella GL, Birch R, Smith SJ. Neurophysiological prediction of outcome in obstetric lesions of the brachial plexus. J Hand Surg Br. 2003;28:148–52.
36. El-Sayed AA. The prognostic value of concurrent Horner syndrome in extended Erb obstetric brachial plexus palsy. J Child Neurol. 2014;29:1356–9.
37. Yoshida K, Kawabata H. The prognostic value of concurrent phrenic nerve palsy in newborn babies with neonatal brachial plexus palsy. J Hand Surg Am. 2015;40:1166–9.
38. Yang LJ. Neonatal brachial plexus palsy—management and prognostic factors. Semin Perinatol. 2014;38:222–34.
39. Murphy KM, Rasmussen L, Hervey-Jumper SL, Justice D, Nelson VS, Yang LJ. An assessment of the compliance and utility of a home exercise DVD for caregivers of children and adolescents with brachial plexus palsy: a pilot study. PM R. 2012;4:190–7.
40. Basciani M, Intiso D. Botulinum toxin type-A and plaster cast treatment in children with upper brachial plexus palsy. Pediatr Rehabil. 2006;9:165–70.
41. Grahn P, Poyhia T, Sommarhem A, Nietosvaara Y. Clinical significance of cervical MRI in brachial plexus birth injury. Acta Orthop. 2019;90:111–8.
42. Chow BC, Blaser S, Clarke HM. Predictive value of computed tomographic myelography in obstetrical brachial plexus palsy. Plast Reconstr Surg. 2000;106:971–7; discussion 978–9.
43. Somashekar D, Yang LJ, Ibrahim M, Parmar HA. High-resolution MRI evaluation of neonatal brachial plexus palsy: a promising alternative to traditional CT myelography. AJNR Am J Neuroradiol. 2014;35:1209–13.
44. Grossman JA. Early operative intervention for birth injuries to the brachial plexus. Semin Pediatr Neurol. 2000;7:36–43.
45. Smith BW, Chang KWC, Yang LJS, Spires MC. Comparative accuracies of electrodiagnostic and imaging studies in neonatal brachial plexus palsy. J Neurosurg Pediatr. 2018;23:119–24.
46. Kennedy R. SUTURE of the BRACHIAL PLEXUS in BIRTH PARALYSIS of the UPPER EXTREMITY. Br Med J. 1903;1:298–301.
47. Gilbert A, Tassin JL. [Surgical repair of the brachial plexus in obstetric paralysis]. Chirurgie. 1984;110:70–5.
48. Squitieri L, Steggerda J, Yang LJ, Kim HM, Chung KC. A national study to evaluate trends in the utilization of nerve reconstruction for treatment of neonatal brachial plexus palsy [outcomes article]. Plast Reconstr Surg. 2011;127:277–83.
49. Lin JC, Schwentker-Colizza A, Curtis CG, Clarke HM. Final results of grafting versus neurolysis in obstetrical brachial plexus palsy. Plast Reconstr Surg. 2009;123:939–48.
50. Pondaag W, Malessy MJ. Recovery of hand function following nerve grafting and transfer in obstetric brachial plexus lesions. J Neurosurg. 2006;105:33–40.
51. Meyer RD. Treatment of adult and obstetrical brachial plexus injuries. Orthopedics. 1986;9:899–903.
52. Clarke HM, Curtis CG. An approach to obstetrical brachial plexus injuries. Hand Clin. 1995;11:563–80; discussion 580–1.
53. Marcus JR, Clarke HM. Management of obstetrical brachial plexus palsy evaluation, prognosis, and primary surgical treatment. Clin Plast Surg. 2003;30:289–306.
54. Tse R, Kozin SH, Malessy MJ, Clarke HM. International Federation of Societies for Surgery of the Hand Committee report: the role of nerve transfers in the treatment of neonatal brachial plexus palsy. J Hand Surg Am. 2015;40:1246–59.
55. Chuang DC, Mardini S, Ma HS. Surgical strategy for infant obstetrical brachial plexus palsy: experiences at Chang Gung Memorial Hospital. Plast Reconstr Surg. 2005;116:132–42; discussion 143–4.
56. Tiel RL, Happel LT Jr, Kline DG. Nerve action potential recording method and equipment. Neurosurgery. 1996;39:103–8; discussion 108–9.
57. Konig RW, Antoniadis G, Borm W, Richter HP, Kretschmer T. Role of intraoperative neurophysiology in primary surgery for obstetrical brachial plexus palsy (OBPP). Childs Nerv Syst. 2006;22:710–4.
58. Pondaag W, van der Veken LP, van Someren PJ, van Dijk JG, Malessy MJ. Intraoperative nerve action and compound motor action potential recordings in patients with obstetric brachial plexus lesions. J Neurosurg. 2008;109:946–54.
59. El-Gammal TA, Abdel-Latif MM, Kotb MM, El-Sayed A, Ragheb YF, Saleh WR, Geith MA, Abdel-Ghaffar HS. Intercostal nerve transfer in infants with obstetric brachial plexus palsy. Microsurgery. 2008;28:499–504.
60. Luedemann W, Hamm M, Blomer U, Samii M, Tatagiba M. Brachial plexus neurotization with donor phrenic nerves and its effect on pulmonary function. J Neurosurg. 2002;96:523–6.
61. Noaman HH, Shiha AE, Bahm J. Oberlin's ulnar nerve transfer to the biceps motor nerve in obstetric brachial plexus palsy: indications, and good and bad results. Microsurgery. 2004;24:182–7.
62. Murison J, Jehanno P, Fitoussi F. Nerve transfer to biceps to restore elbow flexion and supination in children with obstetrical brachial plexus palsy. J Child Orthop. 2017;11:455–9.
63. Blaauw G, Sauter Y, Lacroix CL, Slooff AC. Hypoglossal nerve transfer in obstetric brachial plexus palsy. J Plast Reconstr Aesthet Surg. 2006;59:474–8.
64. Blaauw G, Slooff AC. Transfer of pectoral nerves to the musculocutaneous nerve in obstetric upper brachial plexus palsy. Neurosurgery. 2003;53:338–41; discussion 341–2.
65. O'Grady KM, Power HA, Olson JL, Morhart MJ, Harrop AR, Watt MJ, Chan KM. Comparing the efficacy of triple nerve transfers with nerve graft reconstruction in upper trunk obstetric brachial plexus injury. Plast Reconstr Surg. 2017;140:747–56.
66. Seruya M, Shen SH, Fuzzard S, Coombs CJ, McCombe DB, Johnstone BR. Spinal accessory

nerve transfer outperforms cervical root grafting for suprascapular nerve reconstruction in neonatal brachial plexus palsy. Plast Reconstr Surg. 2015;135:1431–8.
67. Lin H, Hou C, Chen D. Contralateral C7 transfer for the treatment of upper obstetrical brachial plexus palsy. Pediatr Surg Int. 2011;27:997–1001.
68. Pondaag W, Gilbert A. Results of end-to-side nerve coaptation in severe obstetric brachial plexus lesions. Neurosurgery. 2008;62:656–63; discussion 656–63.
69. Pondaag W, Malessy MJ. The evidence for nerve repair in obstetric brachial plexus palsy revisited. Biomed Res Int. 2014;2014:434619.
70. Xu J, Cheng X, Gu Y. Different methods and results in the treatment of obstetrical brachial plexus palsy. J Reconstr Microsurg. 2000;16:417–20; discussion 420–2.
71. Strombeck C, Krumlinde-Sundholm L, Forssberg H. Functional outcome at 5 years in children with obstetrical brachial plexus palsy with and without microsurgical reconstruction. Dev Med Child Neurol. 2000;42:148–57.
72. Mencl L, Waldauf P, Haninec P. Results of nerve reconstructions in treatment of obstetrical brachial plexus injuries. Acta Neurochir (Wien). 2015;157:673–80.
73. Terzis JK, Kokkalis ZT. Elbow flexion after primary reconstruction in obstetric brachial plexus palsy. J Hand Surg Eur Vol. 2009;34:449–58.
74. Pondaag W, de Boer R, van Wijlen-Hempel MS, Hofstede-Buitenhuis SM, Malessy MJ. External rotation as a result of suprascapular nerve neurotization in obstetric brachial plexus lesions. Neurosurgery. 2005;57:530–7; discussion 530–7.
75. Birch R, Ahad N, Kono H, Smith S. Repair of obstetric brachial plexus palsy: results in 100 children. J Bone Joint Surg Br. 2005;87:1089–95.
76. Malessy MJ, Pondaag W. Neonatal brachial plexus palsy with neurotmesis of C5 and avulsion of C6: supraclavicular reconstruction strategies and outcome. J Bone Joint Surg Am. 2014;96:e174.
77. Maillet M, Romana C. Complete obstetric brachial plexus palsy: surgical improvement to recover a functional hand. J Child Orthop. 2009;3:101–8.
78. Morrow BT, Harvey I, Ho ES, Clarke HM. Long-term hand function outcomes of the surgical management of complete brachial plexus birth injury. J Hand Surg Am. 2021;46:575–83.
79. Tse R, Marcus JR, Curtis CG, Dupuis A, Clarke HM. Suprascapular nerve reconstruction in obstetrical brachial plexus palsy: spinal accessory nerve transfer versus C5 root grafting. Plast Reconstr Surg. 2011;127:2391–6.
80. Smith BW, Chang KWC, Koduri S, Yang LJS. Nerve graft versus nerve transfer for neonatal brachial plexus: shoulder outcomes. J Neurosurg Pediatr. 2020;27:1–6.
81. Siqueira MG, Socolovsky M, Heise CO, Martins RS, Di Masi G. Efficacy and safety of Oberlin's procedure in the treatment of brachial plexus birth palsy. Neurosurgery. 2012;71:1156–60; discussion 1161.
82. Chang KWC, Wilson TJ, Popadich M, Brown SH, Chung KC, Yang LJS. Oberlin transfer compared with nerve grafting for improving early supination in neonatal brachial plexus palsy. J Neurosurg Pediatr. 2018;21:178–84.
83. Pondaag W, Malessy MJ. Intercostal and pectoral nerve transfers to re-innervate the biceps muscle in obstetric brachial plexus lesions. J Hand Surg Eur Vol. 2014;39:647–52.
84. Kawabata H, Shibata T, Matsui Y, Yasui N. Use of intercostal nerves for neurotization of the musculocutaneous nerve in infants with birth-related brachial plexus palsy. J Neurosurg. 2001;94:386–91.
85. Wellons JC, Tubbs RS, Pugh JA, Bradley NJ, Law CR, Grabb PA. Medial pectoral nerve to musculocutaneous nerve neurotization for the treatment of persistent birth-related brachial plexus palsy: an 11-year institutional experience. J Neurosurg Pediatr. 2009;3:348–53.
86. Lin H, Hou C, Chen D. Modified C7 neurotization for the treatment of obstetrical brachial plexus palsy. Muscle Nerve. 2010;42:764–8.
87. Vu AT, Sparkman DM, van Belle CJ, Yakuboff KP, Schwentker AR. Retropharyngeal contralateral C7 nerve transfer to the lower trunk for brachial plexus birth injury: technique and results. J Hand Surg Am. 2018;43:417–24.
88. Phipps GJ, Hoffer MM. Latissimus dorsi and teres major transfer to rotator cuff for Erb's palsy. J Shoulder Elb Surg. 1995;4:124–9.
89. Kirkos JM, Papadopoulos IA. Late treatment of brachial plexus palsy secondary to birth injuries: rotational osteotomy of the proximal part of the humerus. J Bone Joint Surg Am. 1998;80:1477–83.
90. Gilbert A, Valbuena S, Posso C. Obstetrical brachial plexus injuries: late functional results of the Steindler procedure. J Hand Surg Eur Vol. 2014;39:868–75.
91. El-Gammal TA, El-Sayed A, Kotb MM, Saleh WR, Ragheb YF, Refai O, Morsy MM. Free functioning gracilis transplantation for reconstruction of elbow and hand functions in late obstetric brachial plexus palsy. Microsurgery. 2015;35:350–5.
92. Bertelli JA. Brachialis muscle transfer to the forearm muscles in obstetric brachial plexus palsy. J Hand Surg Br. 2006;31:261–5.
93. Bahm J, Ocampo-Pavez C. Free functional gracilis muscle transfer in children with severe sequelae from obstetric brachial plexus palsy. J Brachial Plex Peripher Nerve Inj. 2008;3:23.

Management of Musculoskeletal Malformations

16

Mari Groves

Introduction

Musculoskeletal malformations encountered by pediatric neurosurgeons are frequently manifestations of complex congenital or developmental conditions resulting in neural compression, spinal instability, or spinal deformity. Given the unique anatomy of the pediatric spine and its potential for growth, management decisions are frequently multifaceted and difficult. Many musculoskeletal malformations arise in the context of a genetic condition which the pediatric neurosurgeon should be familiar with to anticipate a patient's response to treatment and course.

Management of musculoskeletal malformations in pediatric neurosurgery patients is a broad topic which frequently requires multidisciplinary care. Here, we briefly review the bony and soft tissue development of the spine and outline principles of management of craniovertebral junction abnormalities, Klippel-Feil syndrome, congenital and developmental spinal stenosis, pediatric lumbar disc herniation, and pediatric spondylolisthesis. We also provide a review of genetic conditions and issues which will be encountered by a pediatric neurosurgeon managing these patients.

M. Groves (✉)
Department of Neurosurgery, Johns Hopkins University, Baltimore, MD, USA
e-mail: mgroves2@jhmi.edu

Craniovertebral Junction Abnormalities

Embryology and Anatomy of the Craniovertebral Junction

The craniovertebral junction (CVJ) consists of the clivus and caudal occipital bone, atlas, and axis. These structures are formed primarily through endochondral ossification from the four occipital sclerotomes and first and second cervical sclerotomes. During this process, a cartilaginous matrix is formed and subsequently populated with osteoblasts, osteoclasts, bone marrow cells, and vasculature to form bone [1].

The fourth occipital and first and second cervical sclerotomes contribute to the formation of the CVJ. Each of these sclerotomes divides into a centrum, hypocentrum, and neural arch. The fourth occipital sclerotome is also referred to as the "proatlas." The proatlas hypocentrum will form the anterior tubercles of the clivus. The centrum will form the apical ligament and apex of the odontoid. The neural arch subdivides into a rostral division forming the occipital condyles and alar and cruciform ligaments and caudal division forming the posterior arch and lateral masses of the atlas. The first cervical sclerotome hypocentrum forms the anterior arch of the atlas, the centrum contributes to the odontoid process, and the neural arch contributes to postero-inferior portion of the posterior arch of the atlas. The

N. Shimony, G. Jallo (eds.), *Pediatric Neurosurgery Board Review*,
https://doi.org/10.1007/978-3-031-23687-7_16

second cervical sclerotome's hypocentrum involutes, the centrum forms the vertebral body of the axis, and the neural arch forms the posterior arch and facets of the axis [2].

The lateral masses of the atlas are present at birth, and the complete ring should form by 3 years [3]. The axis ossifies from six ossification centers: three ossification centers form the body and posterior arch, the tip of the dens is its own ossification center, and the dens proper is formed by paired ossification centers which will fuse by 3 months of age. At birth, a rudimentary cartilaginous disc separates the dens from the vertebral body of C2, termed the neurocentral synchondrosis. The dens begins to fuse to the body of the axis by age 4 and is complete by age 8, at which point the neurocentral synchondrosis is no longer visible [4]. The tip of the dens fuses to the rest of the odontoid process by age 12 [5].

Craniovertebral Junction Instability

The major contributors to stability at the craniovertebral junction are the bony, cup-shaped occipito-atlantal joints and associated capsular ligaments. The tectorial membrane and anterior and posterior atlanto-occipital membranes provide significant soft tissue support. The two major structures providing stability at the atlantoaxial joint are the bony odontoid process and transverse ligament. The alar and apical ligaments contribute to stability in minor ways [6]. Children have a relatively lax transverse ligament compared to adults and up to 5 mm of motion of C1 on C2 on lateral radiographs is considered normal [7].

CVJ abnormalities typically present in an insidious manner with brainstem, cervical spine, cranial nerve, cervical nerve root, or vascular dysfunction. Frequently, there is a history of antecedent trauma with subsequent progressive symptoms. A head tilt with neck and suboccipital pain and posterior fossa localizing signs can be present. Rarely, patients present with acute catastrophic neurologic injury or death [4]. Diagnosis is frequently made with lateral radiographs initially, followed by MRI and dynamic imaging to assess the biomechanics of the abnormality.

Down Syndrome and CVJ Abnormalities

Patients with Down Syndrome (DS) have a characteristic "rocker-bottom" shape of the atlanto-occipital joint with wide, flat occipital condyles interfacing with a flat C1 superior articulating surface which predisposes the joint to sliding and instability. Abnormalities of the atlas such as a bifid arch and dens are also frequently observed, further contributing to potential instability. Ligamentous laxity is also commonly observed in DS.

Screening has been recommended for patients with DS for participation in "high-risk" sports, prior to otolaryngological procedures (due to reports of atlantoaxial subluxation with positioning), and prior to anesthesia (due to concern for hyperextension injury with intubation). This is frequently done with lateral flexion/extension radiographs. The atlantodens interval (ADI) and neural canal width (NCW) are the most useful measurements to determine if the spinal cord is at risk with movement. If an ADI >4.5 mm or NCW is <14 mm is observed, cervical MRI is recommended to look for evidence of spinal cord injury (SCI) [8]. If greater than 10 mm of motion of the occipital condyle on C1 is observed on lateral radiographs, the joint is considered unstable and occipito-cervical fusion is recommended. The presence of an os odontoideum (discussed below) is also considered unstable. Routine CT scan for screening purposes is not recommended as biomechanically significant bony abnormalities are typically observed on lateral radiographs (Fig. 16.1) [8].

Os Odontoideum

Os odontoideum occurs when a circumferentially corticated separate ossicle of variable size is separated from a shortened odontoid body or process. The etiology of os odontoideum is likely post-traumatic, however, rare congenital causes have been reported [9]. Two types have been described: orthotopic and dystopic. An orthotopic os odontoideum describes an ossicle which is located in a normal anatomic position and

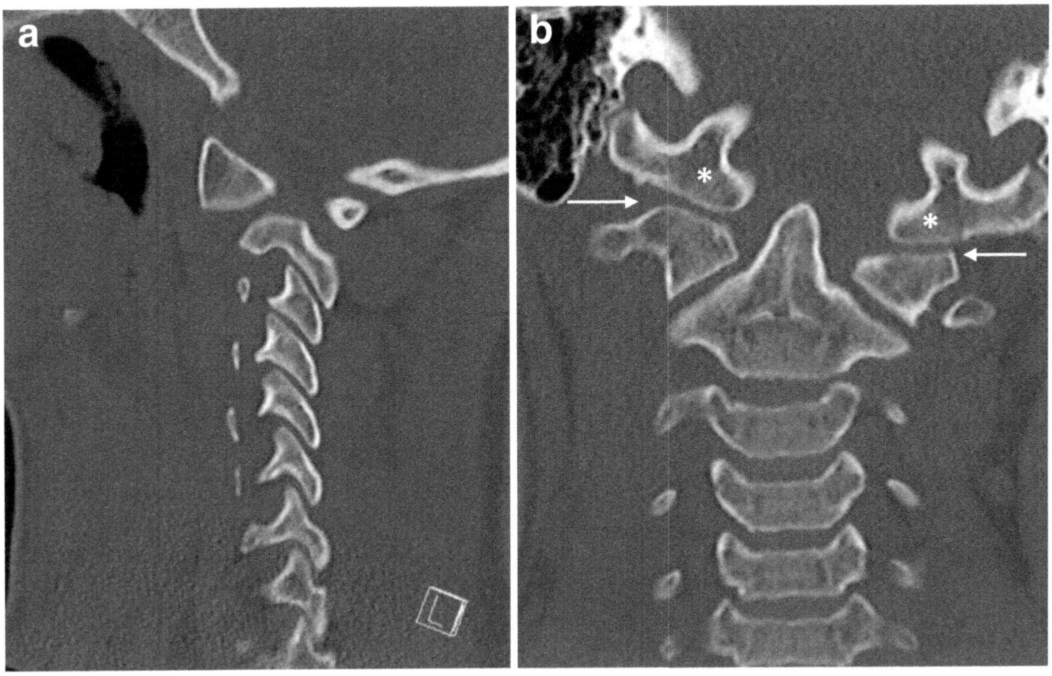

Fig. 16.1 Computed Tomography imaging of patient with Down Syndrome in both sagittal (**a**) and Coronal (**b**) views. Patients with Down Syndrome (DS) have a characteristic "rocker-bottom" shape of the atlanto-occipital joint with wide, flat occipital condyles (*) interfacing with a flat C1 superior articulating surface (arrow) which predisposes the joint to sliding and instability. This can be seen on a lateral CT reconstruction of the cervical spine. Care should be taken to not only evaluate for movement at the C1–2 joint but also movement between the occipital condyles (*) and C1 on dynamic imaging

moves with the anterior arch of C1. A dystopic os odontoideum describes an ossicle which is located towards the clivus and is fused to the basion. Both types are associated with instability [10]. These must be differentiated from an ossiculum terminale which is a failure of fusion of the terminal secondary ossification center of the tip of the odontoid and is only rarely associated with instability [11].

Os odontoideum is more commonly encountered in children with congenital conditions which result in skeletal dysplasia or connective tissue abnormalities including DS, Klippel-Feil syndrome, Morquio's disease, achondroplasia, and skeletal epiphyseal dysplasia [9]. There is frequently a remote history of trauma, although some hypothesize that the traumatic event may occur in utero. Patients typically present with occipitocervical or neck pain alone, myelopathy, cranial nerve/vascular dysfunction from basilar invagination, although it can also be found incidentally. The natural history is variable with many patients being asymptomatic prior to progressive neurologic decline or even precipitous catastrophic neurologic injury [12].

Cervical radiographs with AP, lateral, and open mouth views of the odontoid are frequently sufficient for the diagnosis of os odontoideum. Dynamic flexion/extension films should be obtained to assess for instability. CT may be useful to further delineate osseous abnormalities for surgical planning (Fig. 16.2). A post-traumatic os odontoideum is suggested by a well corticated ossicle separate from the odontoid body, as described above. A congenital etiology is suggested by a "jigsaw" sign with the odontoid process separated at the level of a persistent neurocentral synchondrosis below the superior articulating facets of C2 [13]. MRI is indicated for suspected neural compression. If there is concern for significant vascular compromise, vascular imaging may be useful.

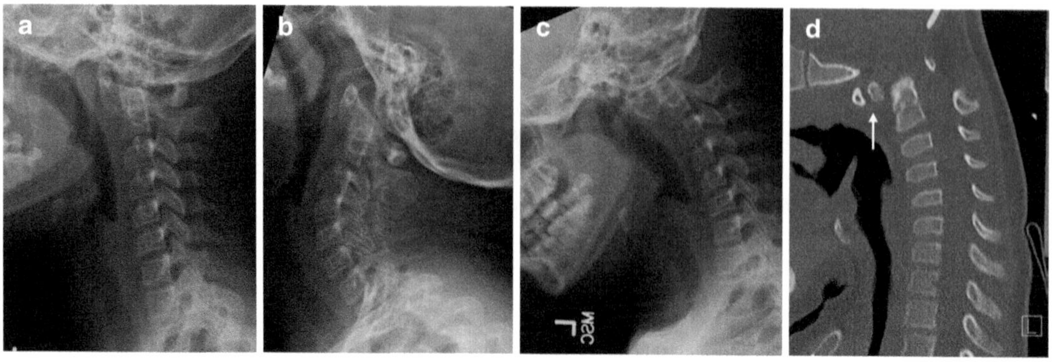

Fig. 16.2 Pt with Os Odontoidium noted on imaging. Cervical radiographs in the lateral position (**a**–**c**) are useful to evaluate cervical alignment. Dynamic flexion/extension films demonstrate instability with movement from 2 mm in neutral (**a**) and in extension (**b**) to 8 mm in flexion (**c**). CT is also helpful to better delineate osseous abnormalities with a well corticated ossicle (arrow, **d**)

Operative C1-2 fusion is recommended for management of os odontoideum because of the potential for instability and catastrophic neurologic injury [12]. An os odontoideum in normal anatomic alignment can be treated with C1-2 fusion using a combination of C1 lateral mass and C2 pars or pedicle screws or C1/2 transarticular screw fixation with or without posterior cabling. Because of the well-corticated nature of an os-odontoideum, an anterior odontoid screw which is used in select type 2 odontoid fractures is not recommend due to a high rate of fusion failure [14]. Patients with significant deformity of the CVJ should be reduced intraoperatively and may require more extensive instrumentation. If there is persistent anterior compression of the brainstem, spinal cord, or vasculature with a irreducible deformity, the patient should be assessed for an anterior decompression or odontoidectomy [9, 10]. Patients should be counseled against participation in sports prior to surgical correction and evidence of fusion. If an asymptomatic patient without radiographic evidence of instability declines surgery, he or she should be encouraged to have regular follow-up with flexion/extension radiographs to assess for the development of instability.

Subaxial Cervical Spine and Klippel-Feil Syndrome

Embryology and Anatomy

Forty-two somites formed during fourth week of gestation contribute to the formation of sclerotomes which will proceed to develop into the basicranium and axial skeleton. As discussed above, the first six sclerotomes contribute to the formation of the craniovertebral junction. The remaining 36 form the subaxial cervical and thoracolumbar, sacral spine and coccyx [15].

Subsequent somite development is divided into four parts: the membranous, chondrification, ossification, and term phases. During the membranous phase in the fifth week of gestation, a condensation of mesenchymal sclerotomal cells form a vertebral centrum. Each sclerotome is organized into a loosely cellular cranial and densely packed caudal portion with a hypocellular cleft known as the fissure of von Ebner. A process known as resegmentation then occurs in which the cranial portion of one sclerotome merges with the caudal portion of the sclerotome above to form the primitive vertebral body; the spinal nerve will emerge at the level of the loosely packed cranial portion. Cells from the fissure of Ebner migrate towards and encase the notochord to form the precursor to the vertebral disc [16].

Chondrification occurs during the sixth week of gestation with the formation of three paired centers: one pair forms the vertebral centrum which will surround the notochord and develop into the vertebral body, one pair forms ossification centers which will form the transverse processes and costal arches, and one pair forms the neural arch which will form the posterior elements [3]. During this phase, the notochord forms the nucleus pulposus of the future intervertebral disc and perinotochordal cells form the annulus of the disc. The anterior and posterior longitudinal ligaments also begin to form simultaneously [17].

Ossification begins during the eighth week of gestation and continues until after birth. As described above, there are three pairs of ossification centers per vertebrae with cartilaginous end plates cranial and caudal to each vertebral body [18, 19]. The anterior and posterior ossification centers are separated by the neurocentral synchondrosis which can be mistaken for a fracture in radiographs and the neural arch ossification centers are also separated by a spinous process synchondrosis; these are typically fused by age 8 [20]. The ring apophysis forms at the periphery of the vertebral endplate, begins to ossify in the early teens, and eventually fuses with the vertebral centrum later in adolescence [3, 21, 22].

Klippel-Feil Syndrome

Klippel-Feil syndrome (KFS) refers to the congenital fusion of cervical vertebrae secondary to failure of vertebral segmentation. The incidence is thought to be low, <1% [23, 24]. The Klippel-Feil triad describes a constellation of a short, webbed neck with a low hairline and limitation of neck range of motion. This triad is associated with scoliosis and rib abnormalities and a high, arched palate predisposing to deafness. Cardiovascular abnormalities are not uncommon [2]. There is a familial form of KFS with congenital fusion of C2 and C3 with other visceral abnormalities which has been mapped to chromosome 8 [25]. Genitourinary abnormalities are prevalent with KFS, as high as 64%, and patients found to have KFS should undergo renal ultrasound [26]. Sprengel deformity (congenital elevation of the scapula) is seen in up to 25% of patients [20].

Three types of KFS have been characterized. Type 1 is a congenital fusion of C2 and C3 with occipital assimilation of the atlas. Type 2 is a long cervical fusion sparing the CVJ. Type 3 describes two long fusion segments with an intervening normal disc space [27]. A functional classification system has also described two general cases: patients with congenital cervical fusion with a hypermobile segment are at increased risk for spinal cord injury, however, patients with congenital fusion and low mobility are predisposed to accelerated spondylosis and canal stenosis [28]. Chiari 1 malformation is frequently seen in conjunction with assimilation of the atlas and smaller posterior fossa volume [10].

The diagnosis of KFS is frequently made initially with cervical radiographs and complaints of neck pain, decreased range of motion, or neurologic symptoms [29]. Persistence of ossification centers in a young child can make the diagnosis difficult with radiographs alone at an early age. Flexion-extension radiographs should be obtained to assess for instability. With the presence of neurologic symptoms, MRI is indicated to delineate areas of neural compression—stenosis can occur at hypermobile segments or at the level of congenital fusions [30]. CT may be useful to define the bony anatomy, especially in the context of surgical planning.

There is a wide range of spinal abnormalities that can be seen in KFS, and each patient must be assessed individually. Surgery is indicated for patients presenting with neurologic decline or those with radiographic instability that may predispose them to neurologic injury. The integrity of the CVJ should be carefully examined, as patients may have concurrent CVJ hypermobility, Chiari malformation, or basilar invagination. Surgical goals are to decompress neural structures, stabilize instability, and restore normal alignment [10].

Developmental and Congenital Spinal Stenosis and Achondroplasia

Congenital and developmental spinal stenosis are terms that have often been used interchangeably, however, congenital stenosis refers specifically to narrowing of the spinal canal by congenital malformations and developmental stenosis refers to a genetic cause of stenosis with development over time [20]. In the absence of a readily identifiable genetic syndrome, a patient may be asymptomatic until presenting with some sort of injury (frequently hyperextension or axial loading) which results in transient neurologic injury [31].

Multiple skeletal dysplasias predispose a child to congenital or developmental stenosis or spinal abnormalities (*see* Table 16.1). Achondroplasia is relatively common, occurring in approximately 1/30,000 births secondary to a defect in the fibroblast growth receptor 3 (FGFR 3) gene [32]. In this condition, there is decreased growth at the neurocentral and spinous process synchondroses leading to narrowing of the sagittal and coronal diameter of the spinal canal with shortened pedicles and interpedicular distance. The lumbar spine of these patients tends to be hyperlordotic and patients frequently present with symptomatic lumbar stenosis (as many of 90% of patients with achondroplasia will have symptoms of lumbar stenosis in their lifetime) [20, 33]. These patients will also frequently have symptomatic Chiari malformations with sleep apnea, hypotonia, and developmental delay requiring suboccipital decompression [34].

The diagnosis of spinal stenosis is difficult with radiograph alone. The Pavlov ratio expresses the canal diameter as a ratio of vertebral body width to spinal canal width with a value <0.8 associated with transient neurapraxia in in football players [35]. MRI is necessary to assess compression of the neuraxis by elements of the spine. The levels

Table 16.1 Common skeletal dysplasias

Condition	Etiology	Musculoskeletal characteristics	Neurosurgical concerns
Achondroplasia [73]	FGFR-3 mutation resulting in decreased endochondral bone formation, but normal membraneous bone formation	Shortening of limbs, macrocephaly, frontal bossing, genu varum abnormalities, pelvic changes	Foramen magnum and spinal stenosis, hydrocephalus, thoracolumbar kyphosis
Down syndrome [74]	Trisomy 21	Rocker-bottom O-C1 joint, ligamentous laxity, hypotonia	Atlantoaxial and occipitocervical instability
Goldenhar syndrome [75, 76]	Disruption of the first and second branchial arches in utero	Hemifacial microsomia, epibulbar dermoid appendages, spinal defects	Vertebral hypoplasia, segmentation failure, vertebral formation failure
Spondyloepiphyseal dysplasia [77]	Abnormal growth of vertebrae and epiphysis, multiple etiologies, Type II collagen defects	Short-trunk dwarfism, shortened proximal/middle limbs, normal sized hands/feet	Odontoid hypoplasia, os odontoideum, atlantoaxial instability
Morquio syndrome [78]	Type IV mucopolysaccharidosis, inability to metabolize keratan sulfate	Short-trunk dwarfism, pectus carinatum, genus valgus, platyspondyly	Odontoid dysplasia, thoracolumbar kyphosis, scoliosis
Osteogenesis imperfecta [79]	Defect in type 1 collagen synthesis	Osteopenia, frequent fractures, and progressive skeletal deformities	Kyphosis, scoliosis, basilar invagination, compression fractures

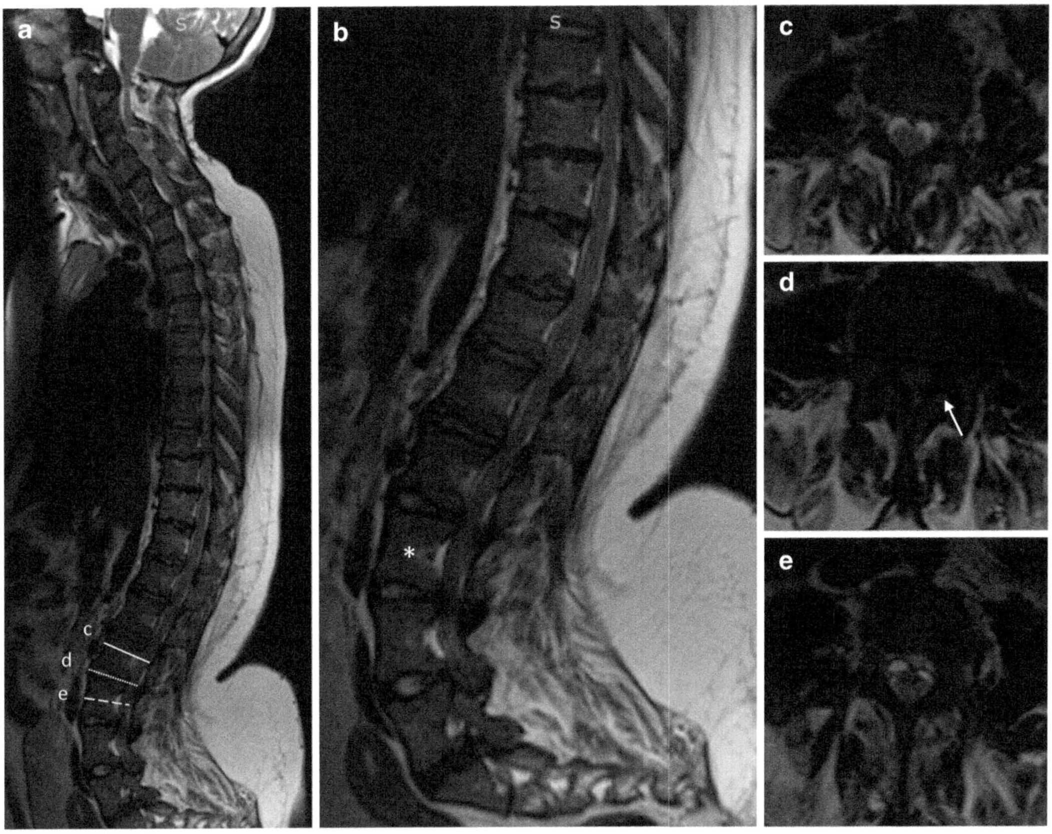

Fig. 16.3 MR imaging in this full length neuraxis T2-weighted sagittal (**a**) as well as sagittal (**b**) and axial (**c–e**) cuts of the lumbar spine demonstrate overt spinal stenosis throughout. This narrowing occurs due to premature fusion of the synchondrosis leading to a shortened interpedicular distance. This congenitally narrowed canal has further stenosis at the level of the discoligamentous complex (**d**) that lead to the characteristic finding of posterior scalloping along the vertebral body (*). This stenosis at the level of the disc and overgrowth of the posterior ligaments (arrow) and leads to loss of the cerebrospinal fluid (CSF) space at the level of the disc (dotted line) compared to just rostral (line) and caudal (dashed line). One concern for patients is an already stenotic canal can have further compromise by degenerative changes that can lead to symptomatic stenosis in patients as they age

studied should be guided by the patient's symptoms. Imaging of the entire neuraxis may be indicated in patients with certain skeletal dysplasias such as achondroplasia to assess for associated abnormalities such as Chiari malformation, hydrocephalus, or syrinx (Fig. 16.3).

Surgery is indicated for symptomatic patients with radiographic evidence of neural compression. The indications for spinal stabilization should be guided by pre-existing instability and iatrogenic instability caused by decompression as well as the need to correct any deformity. For cervical stenosis, laminectomy alone should be avoided for a patient with a kyphotic or neutral standing alignment and the patient should be assessed for fusion. Cervical laminoplasty is a motion-sparing procedure for idiopathic developmental stenosis which is can retain as much as 70% of the subaxial cervical spine motion [36].

Decompression of the neural elements, especially in the lumbar spine, can be challenging in patients with achondroplasia. The congenitally narrow canal places the facets near the spinous processes and facet hypertrophy can frequently hide the pars interarticularis requiring significant facet removal to adequately decompress the thecal sac. Hyperlordosis of the lumbar spine creates a deep working field, and prominent iliac crests can impede exposure of lower lumbar segments and make sacral screw placement more difficult. The presence of thoracolumbar kyphosis should trigger assessment for thoracolumbar fusion in a patient needing decompression for lumbar stenosis due to concerns for post-laminectomy kyphosis. These patients need to be monitored for post-decompressive instability [20].

Up to 80% of infants with achondroplasia will present with thoracolumbar kyphosis which is most noticeable when sitting and typically improves with age. Casting or bracing may be necessary if kyphosis persists past walking age; fusion may be necessary if the kyphosis is refractory to conservative measures by age 5 [37].

Transient Neurapraxia with Developmental Cervical Stenosis

Transient neurapraxia following trauma is not an uncommon neurosurgical complaint to reveal developmental cervical stenosis. This is described as a transient sensory or motor changes which recover completely without obvious bony or ligamentous abnormality [38]. Patients with symptomatic neurapraxia (e.g., central cord syndrome) and evidence of neural compression should be assessed for surgical decompression and/or stabilization. Guidelines have been developed for athletes who have sustained a cervical cord neurapraxia and returning to athletic activities: absolute contraindications for returning to play included cervical cord neurapraxia with MRI evidence of cord defect or edema and multiple episodes or episodes associated with ligamentous instability or symptoms lasting >36 h. Relative contraindications included a Pavlov ratio <0.8 with one episode of neurapraxia, neurapraxia with MRI evidence of disc disease or spondylosis, or neurapraxia with MRI evidence of cord compression. There was no contra-indication for return to play in patients with a single episode of cervical cord neurapraxia without the above conditions and a Pavlov ratio ≥0.8 [39]. Return to play guidelines have been further expanded and are detailed in Table 16.2 [40]. Patients can typically be cleared for return to normal activities

Table 16.2 Guidelines for return to play after transient cervical neurapraxia [40]

No contraindications to return to play
1. Healed C1 or C2 fracture treated non-operatively without instability
2. Single level Klippel-Feil abnormality (excluding O-C1) without instability or stenosis on MRI
3. Spina bifida occulta
4. Pavlov ratio <0.8 in asymptomatic individual
5. Healed, stable subaxial spine fracture without kyphotic deformity
6. Status-post single level anterior cervical discectomy and fusion with evidence of fusion
7. Two "stingers" in a single or multiple seasons
8. Single or multi-level posterior cervical foraminotomy
Relative contraindications to return to play
1. Absence of any absolute contraindication with appropriate counseling
2. History of transient quadriplegia or quadriparesthesia with full recovery and mild-to-moderate stenosis on MRI
3. Healed single-level posterior cervical fusion
4. Three or more "stingers" in a single season
5. Healed two level anterior or posterior cervical fusion
6. Occipital-C1 assimilation
Absolute contraindications to play
1. Cervical myelopathy in history or exam
2. Cervical cord abnormality on MRI
3. Prior C1-2 fusion
4. Radiographic evidence of asymptomatic ligamentous laxity
5. Radiographic evidence of C1-2 hypermobility
6. C1-2 rotatory fixation
7. Evidence of "spear tackler's spine"
8. Radiographic evidence of distraction/extension cervical spine injury
9. Multi-level Klippel-Feil abnormality
10. Radiographic evidence of basilar invagination
11. MRI evidence of Chiari malformation
12. >2 episodes of transient quadriplegia or quadriparasthesia
13. Healed subaxial cervical fracture with kyphosis or scoliosis
14. Evidence of spinal cord compression after healed fracture
15. Continued neck discomfort or evidence of neurologic deficit or decreased range of motion from baseline after any cervical spine injury
16. Symptomatic disc herniation
17. Three level cervical spine fusion

following thoracic or lumbar decompression and/or fusion if the patient is pain free and neurologically intact. Return to contact sports is not recommended after surgery at the cervicothoracic or thoracolumbar junction [41].

Pediatric Degenerative Disc Disease and Disc Herniation

Pediatric disc herniation and disc degeneration is rare compared to the adult population with an estimated incidence of 0.1–0.2%. It is seen more commonly in children older than 11 years [42]. Obesity, heavy lifting, and repetitive athletic activities have been thought to be risk factors, although a recent study found no association between sports participation and disc herniation [43, 44]. There are genetic predispositions to herniated discs which are not well characterized, as evidenced by an increased incidence in pediatric patients with a first-degree relative with low back pain and case reports of monozygotic twins with lumbar disc herniations [45, 46].

Herniated discs occur almost exclusively in the lumbar region in children. The fetal disc contains approximately 90% water and gradually becomes desiccated throughout life to approximately 60% as an adult. As described above, the annulus of the disc is well developed by 6-months-old and has reached full maturity by 10-years-old [17]. The disc is well-vascularized at birth, however, the vascular supply disappears with age and is typically gone by age 8 [43]. Disc herniation occurs secondary to an injury to the annulus which allows nuclear material to escape, usually during disc loading such as when flexing or twisting.

Most patients experience a painful initial event; however, back pain is uncommon with pediatric disc herniations compared to adults. Radicular pain is common. Most patients have a reproducible straight-leg-test sign and the majority demonstrate a positive crossed straight-leg-test. The pain is exacerbated in flexion or with Valsalva [47]. A thorough physical exam must be conducted on every patient, although neurologic dysfunction is less common in the pediatric patient compared to the adult.

Diagnosis is made with imaging. Radiographs are frequently unrevealing, but limitations in range of motion on flexion/extension have been reported—flexion is limited in up to 50% of patients with herniated discs [48]. MRI delineates the soft tissue anatomy of the spine and will most frequently reveal a central or paracentral disc herniation if present (Fig. 16.4). The most common symptomatic levels are L4/5 and L5/S1 [47]. Fractures of the ring apophysis may occur with disc herniation (in as high as 28% of pediatric disc herniations) and are associated with a higher rate of surgical intervention [49].

Similar to adult lumbar disc herniations, conservative management with rest and NSAIDs is first trialed for children with disc herniations in the absence of neurologic deficit. Bracing is not useful and may weaken axial musculature. Epidural steroid injections may be offered and provide symptomatic relief [47].

There is, however, evidence suggesting that pediatric patients do not respond as well as adults to nonsurgical management [50–52]. Discectomy is indicated for patients with refractory pain or progressive neurologic symptoms. The herniated disc fragment is typically more hydrated in the pediatric patient compared to the adult requiring removal of multiple small pieces rather than a single extruded fragment [51]. Bony fragments or a fractured apophyseal fragment may be present and require the use of an osteotome or burr to adequately decompress the nerve root or thecal sac [47]. Greater than 90% of pediatric patients will experience minimal to no pain at 1 year following surgery [53]. Fusion is not indicated for a simple herniated disc without associated deformity. Long-term recurrence of pain is not uncommon, and it has been estimated that 80% and 74% of patients undergoing discectomy will be able to avoid repeat surgery 10- and 20-years postoperatively, respectively [54].

Return to sports or activities which predisposed the patient to disc herniation may delay or impede the success of conservative management. If an initial trial of conservative management is successful, a gradual re-introduction of activity is reasonable. Recurrent pain preventing these activities may be an indication for surgery [51]. It has been suggested that gradual return to normal

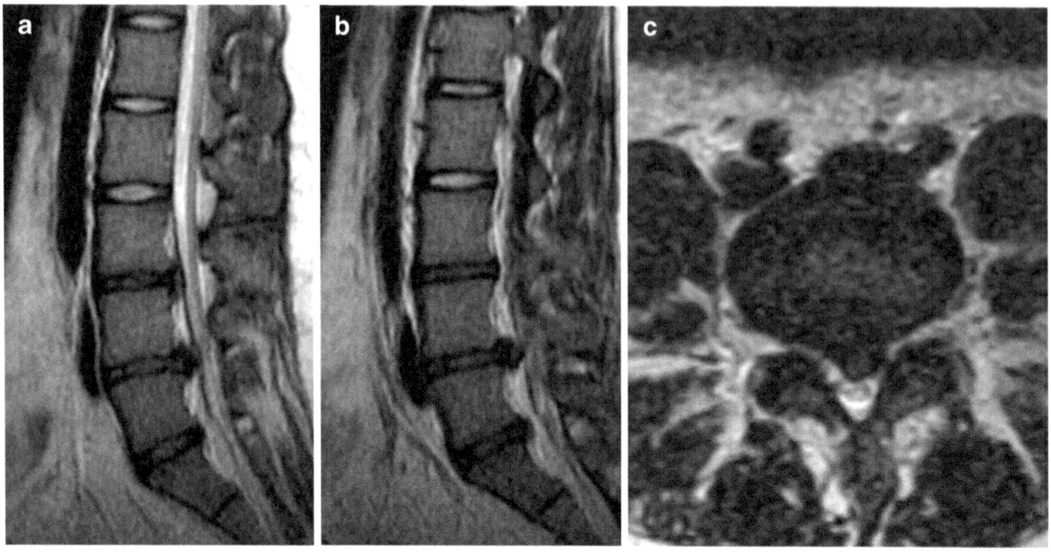

Fig. 16.4 MRI T2-weighted imaging in the sagittal and axial planes demonstrate a broad based disc herniation at L4–5 as well as degenerative disc disease at L3–4 and L5–1. Midline sagittal imaging (**a**) demonstrates extrusion and displacement of the posterior longitudinal ligament, and parasagittal imaging (**b**) shows the herniated disc as well. Axial imaging (**c**) shows the significant broad based herniation with encroachment upon the canal and compromise of the neuroforamina bilaterally with compression of both traversing nerve roots as well as the exiting L4 nerve root

play is acceptable with after recovery from single- or even multi-level discectomy [41].

Spondylolisthesis and Spondylolysis

Spondylolisthesis refers to displacement of one vertebral body on another. Spondylolysis refers to a defect in the pars interarticularis. Marchetti and Bartolozzi classified spondylolisthesis into developmental or acquired categories. Spondylolisthesis is thought to occur in 6–12% of the adult population [55]. Spondylolysis can be seen in up to 11% of young gymnasts and 20% of dancers presenting with low back pain, up to 30% of wrestlers, and 43% of wrestlers [56–58]. Spondylolisthesis is subcategorized into high dysplastic or low dysplastic, each with either spondylolysis or an elongated pars. Dysplastic elements can include the facets, elongated pars, or spina bifida at L5 or S1. High dysplastic spondylolisthesis is characterized by a vertical sacrum with doming, significant lumbosacral kyphosis, and a trapezoidal L5 with hypoplastic transverse processes. The low dysplastic type has a more normal lumbosacral junction without doming of the sacrum and a rectangular L5 vertebral body [59].

Acquired spondylolisthesis can be traumatic, post-surgical, pathologic, or degenerative [60]. The highest loads during flexion or extension are concentrated at the pars interarticularis at the lumbosacral junction [61]. Repetitive activity in an incompletely ossified spine predisposes this area of stress concentration to fatigue failure and fracture (spondylolysis). This disrupts the posterior bony elements, weakening the posterior tension band, and predisposing the spine to spondylolisthesis.

Back pain with or without radiculopathy is the most common presenting symptom for patients with spondylolisthesis, although many patients are asymptomatic. The back pain is usually mechanical in nature, worsening with standing and prolonged activity [59]. With higher grade spondylolistheses, the likelihood of radicular symptoms increases. Patients with a high-grade spondylolisthesis may exhibit increased lumbar lordosis with prominent abdomen and a heart-shaped buttocks.

Diagnosis of spondylolysis or spondylolisthesis is made with AP, lateral, and oblique standing radiographs of the lumbar spine, looking for defects in the typical "Scottie dog" appearance. The Meyerding grading system is frequently used to describe the severity of a spondylolisthesis: grade 0 has no displacement of one vertebral body on another, grade 1 has 0–25% displacement, grade 2 has 25–50%, grade 3 has 50–75%, grade 4 is 75–100%, and >100% is grade 5 or spondyloptosis. Flexion/extension radiographs demonstrate the stability of spondylolysis or spondylolisthesis. MRI is useful to assess the degree of neural compression and CT may be useful to further define the bony anatomy and pars defect which may have some prognostic value for the success of conservative management in spondylolysis [62]. Increased uptake on bone scanning may be seen in early lesions which correlates with increased T2 signal on MRI [63].

Spondylolysis is usually successfully treated conservatively with period of rest and physical therapy [64]. Early spondylolysis confirmed on bone scintigraphy or MRI has excellent healing potential and typically responds to bracing with a thoraco-lumbo-sacral orthosis for 3–6 months which reduces lumbar lordosis and removes stress from the loaded pars [62]. With spondylolisthesis, bracing is successful in alleviating pain is as many as 80% of patients with Meyerding grade 1, but less successful in higher grades [65]. Patients with painful grade 1 spondylolisthesis or spondylolysis can be allowed to return to normal activities after resolution of pain without restriction. With grade 2 spondylolisthesis, return to activity is allowed after resolution of symptoms while avoiding hyperextension activities which place stress on the pars [59]. Patients with spines which are still growing should be monitored with radiographs every 6–12 months to detect progression of the listhesis. Continued symptoms after 6 months of conservative treatment should be evaluated for surgery.

Surgical management of spondylolysis without spondylolisthesis typically involves direct pars repair with a pars screw. Contraindications to direct pars repair include dysplastic bony elements, segmental instability, spina bifida, and degenerated discs or facets at that level [59].

Surgery is recommended for patients with spondylolisthesis with persistent symptoms despite appropriate conservative management, Meyerding grade 3 or greater spondylolisthesis in an immature spine because of risk of progression, and with radiographic evidence of progression of the spondylolisthesis [59]. For Meyerding grade 1 or 2 spondylolisthesis, posterolateral fusion of the affected levels without reduction of the deformity with decompression of the neural elements as indicated is recommended [66–68].

Surgical management of higher-grade spondylolisthesis (greater than Meyerding grade 2) is challenging and optimal techniques remain controversial. Posterolateral fusion without reduction has shown high rates of nonunion. The primary goal of surgery should be to decompress neural elements and restore global sagittal balance of the spine. Achieving adequate fusion and restoring sagittal balance may include incorporating additional levels and the pelvis to a construct at the lumbosacral junction. Transdiscal fixation with pedicle screws through S1 pedicles and L5/S1 disc space terminating in the L5 vertebral body has been used successfully [59]. Reduction of the spondylolisthesis is controversial, may be associated with a high rate of neurologic injury, and may ultimately not be necessary to relieve the patient's symptoms [69]. Treatment of spondyloptosis is surgical and high risk requiring full or partial corpectomies, sacral dome osteotomies, posterior and frequently anterior column instrumentation and fusion, and frequently casting or bracing [70–72] (Fig. 16.5).

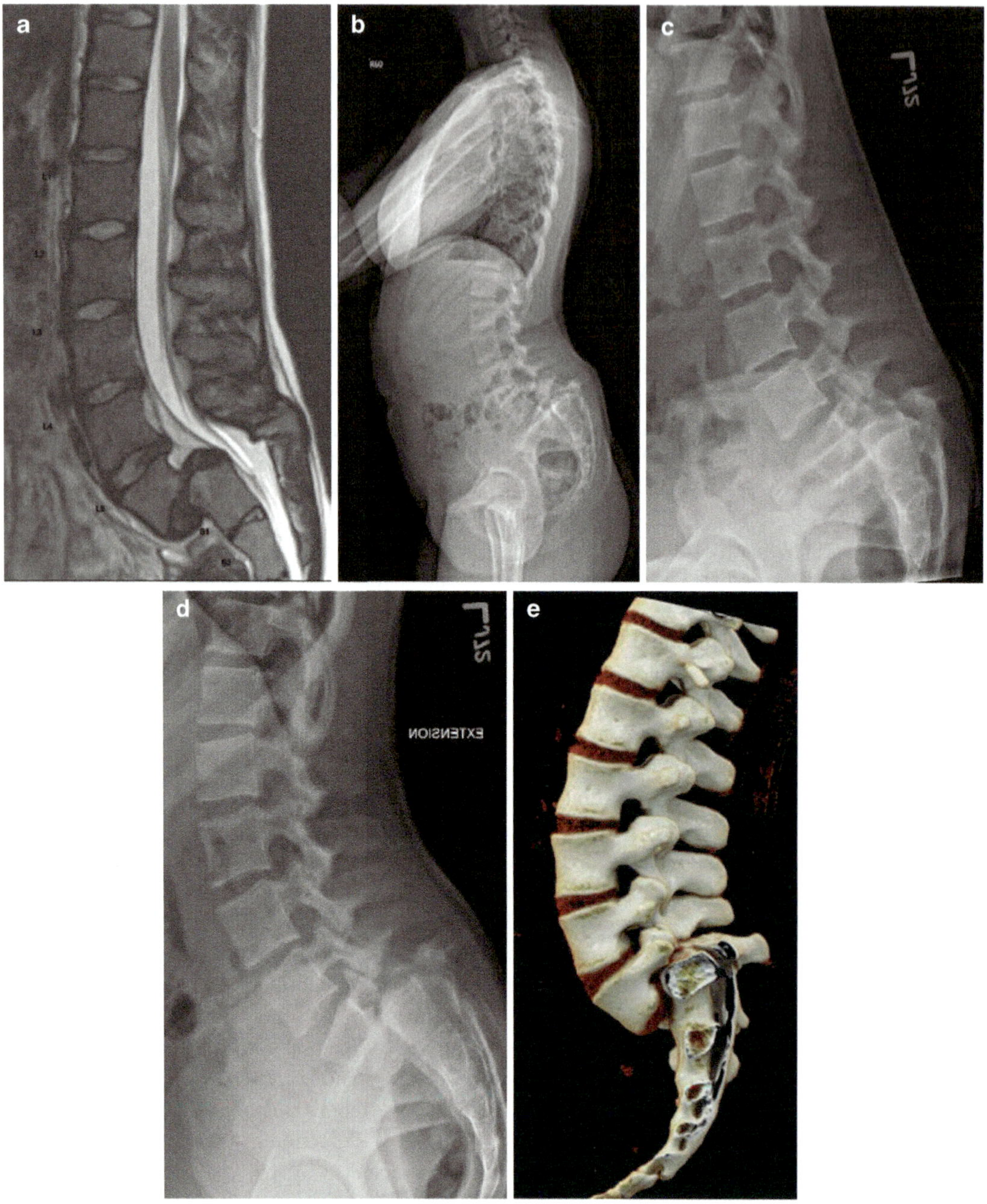

Fig. 16.5 Lateral MRI (**a**), standing x-rays (**b**), and flexion/extension x-rays (**c**, **d**) demonstrate a grade 4 spondylolisthesis with near total forward displacement of the L5 vertebral body in front of the sacrum. There is not significant movement of the body with dynamic imaging in flexion (**c**) or extension (**d**). CT can be helpful to better define the anatomy for surgical considerations. Three dimensional imaging (**e**) can be recreated to gain an overall sense of alignment as well

Conclusion

Compared to adult counterparts, pediatric musculoskeletal and spinal malformations requiring surgery are much less frequent. Management involves similar principles to that of adult patients: decompress symptomatic neural elements, stabilize unstable segments, and correct or prevent further deformity. Treatment requires knowledge of the natural history of a patient's condition and familiarity with a broad range of surgical techniques which must be adapted for the unique anatomy of pediatric patients. With increasing knowledge of conditions leading to these malformations and improved surgical technique, outcomes are continuing to improve for children affected by these disorders.

Questions

1. An 11-year-old with Down Syndrome presents to their pediatrician for a well child visit. She complaints of pain when bouncing on a trampoline. What is your next step?
   (a) MRI of the entire spine
   (b) Observation with serial x-rays
   (c) Clinical assessment in 6 months
   (d) AP and lateral cervical spine x-rays with dynamic x-rays
2. You are seeing a 15-year-old with achondroplasia. He has recently quit playing soccer as he cannot keep running during the length of the game. He claims his legs start burning towards the end of the game, but improve when he sits and rests. What is your most pressing clinical concern?
   (a) Worsening hydrocephalus
   (b) Foramen magnum stenosis
   (c) Tibial bowing
   (d) Thoracolumbar kyphosis with subsequent spinal stenosis
   (e) Leg length discrepancy
3. A 17-year-old with BMI of 37 presents with significant lower back pain that radiates to her right foot and is found to have a herniated disc at L5-S1. What is your next step?
   (a) Rest, Medrol dose pack, followed by physical therapy
   (b) L5-S1 discectomy
   (c) L5-S1 TLIF
   (d) L5-S1 ALIF
   (e) Bracing at least 18 h a day and physical therapy
4. A 16-year-old gymnast presents with acute back pain after practice that worsens with movement. What is the most likely finding on plain x-ray?
   (a) Degenerative changes throughout the lumbar spine
   (b) L4 compression fracture
   (c) Radiolucent defect of pars interarticularis
   (d) Desiccation of the disc space

Answers

1. (d)
2. (d)
3. (a)
4. (c)

References

1. Mackie EJ, Ahmed YA, Tatarczuch L, Chen KS, Mirams M. Endochondral ossification: how cartilage is converted into bone in the developing skeleton. Int J Biochem Cell Biol. 2008;40(1):46–62. https://doi.org/10.1016/j.biocel.2007.06.009.
2. Menezes AH. Craniocervical developmental anatomy and its implications. Childs Nerv Syst. 2008;24(10):1109–22. https://doi.org/10.1007/s00381-008-0600-1.
3. Dias M, Brockmeyer D. Anatomy, embryology, and normal and abnormal development of the craniovertebral junction and cervical spine. In: Advanced pediatric craniocervical surgery. Thieme Medical Publishers; 2006. p. 1–26.
4. Menezes A. Congenital and developmental anomalies of the craniovertebral junction. In: The craniovertebral junction: diagnosis, pathology, surgical techniques. Thieme Medical Publishers; 2011. p. 72–82.
5. Menezes AH. Evaluation and treatment of congenital and developmental anomalies of the cervical spine: invited submission from the Joint Section Meeting on Disorders of the Spine and Peripheral Nerves, March 2004. J Neurosurg Spine. 2004;1(2):188–97. https://doi.org/10.3171/spi.2004.1.2.0188.
6. White AA, Panjabi MM. The clinical biomechanics of the occipitoatlantoaxial complex. Orthop Clin North Am. 1978;9(4):867–78. https://doi.org/10.1016/S0030-5898(20)32199-4.
7. Bonadio WA. Cervical spine trauma in children: part I. General concepts, normal anatomy, radiographic

evaluation. Am J Emerg Med. 1993;11(2):158–65. https://doi.org/10.1016/0735-6757(93)90112-O.
8. Brockmeyer D. Down syndrome and craniovertebral instability. Pediatr Neurosurg. 1999;31(2):71–7. https://doi.org/10.1159/000028837.
9. Arvin B, Fournier-Gosselin MP, Fehlings MG. Os odontoideum. Neurosurgery. 2010;66(Suppl 3):A22–31. https://doi.org/10.1227/01.NEU.0000366113.15248.07.
10. Brockmeyer DL. Common pathological conditions of the pediatric craniovertebral junction and cervical spine. In: Advanced pediatric craniocervical surgery. Thieme Medical Publishers; 2006. p. 43–54.
11. Viswanathan A, Whitehead WE, Luerssen TG, Illner A, Jea A. "Orthotopic" ossiculum terminale persistens and atlantoaxial instability in a child less than 12 years of age: a case report and review of the literature. Cases J. 2009;2(1):8530. https://doi.org/10.4076/1757-1626-2-8530.
12. Rozzelle CJ, Aarabi B, Dhall SS, et al. Os odontoideum. Neurosurgery. 2013;72(Suppl 3):159–69. https://doi.org/10.1227/NEU.0b013e318276ee69.
13. Fagan Andrew B, Askin Geoffrey N, Earwaker John WS. The jigsaw sign. A reliable indicator of congenital aetiology in os odontoideum. Eur Spine J. 2004;13(4):295. https://doi.org/10.1007/s00586-004-0732-2.
14. Apfelbaum RI, Lonser RR, Veres R, Casey A. Direct anterior screw fixation for recent and remote odontoid fractures. Neurosurg Focus. 2000;8(6):1–10. https://doi.org/10.3171/foc.2000.8.6.3.
15. Gossler A, de Angelis MH. 6 Somitogenesis. In: Current topics in developmental biology. Vol. 38. Elsevier; 1997. p. 225–87. https://doi.org/10.1016/S0070-2153(08)60248-3.
16. Keynes RJ, Stern CD. Mechanisms of vertebrate segmentation. Development. 1988;103(3):413–29. https://doi.org/10.1242/dev.103.3.413.
17. Lawson LY, Harfe BD. Developmental mechanisms of intervertebral disc and vertebral column formation: mechanisms of intervertebral disc and vertebral column formation. Wiley Interdiscip Rev Dev Biol. 2017;6(6):e283. https://doi.org/10.1002/wdev.283.
18. Chandraraj S, Briggs CA. Multiple growth cartilages in the neural arch. Anat Rec. 1991;230(1):114–20. https://doi.org/10.1002/ar.1092300111.
19. Ford DM, McFadden KD, Bagnall KM. Sequence of ossification in human vertebral neural arch centers. Anat Rec. 1982;203(1):175–8. https://doi.org/10.1002/ar.1092030116.
20. Lee JY, Lim MR, Vaccaro AR. Congenital and developmental spinal stenosis. In: Surgery of the pediatric spine. Thieme Medical Publishers; 2008.
21. Costa L, de Reuver S, Kan L, et al. Ossification and fusion of the vertebral ring apophysis as an important part of spinal maturation. J Clin Med. 2021;10(15):3217. https://doi.org/10.3390/jcm10153217.
22. Adib O, Berthier E, Loisel D, Aubé C. Pediatric cervical spine in emergency: radiographic features of normal anatomy, variants and pitfalls. Skelet Radiol. 2016;45(12):1607–17. https://doi.org/10.1007/s00256-016-2481-9.
23. Brown MW, Templeton AW, Hodges FJ. The incidence of acquired and congenital fusions in the cervical spine. Am J Roentgenol Radium Therapy, Nucl Med. 1964;92:1255–9.
24. Guille JT, Sherk HH. Congenital osseous anomalies of the upper and lower cervical spine in children. J Bone Joint Surg Am. 2002;84(2):277–88. https://doi.org/10.2106/00004623-200202000-00017.
25. Clarke RA, Singh S, McKenzie H, Kearsley JH, Yip MY. Familial Klippel-Feil syndrome and paracentric inversion inv(8)(q22.2q23.3). Am J Hum Genet. 1995;57(6):1364–70.
26. Drvaric DM, Ruderman RJ, Conrad RW, Grossman H, Webster GD, Schmitt EW. Congenital scoliosis and urinary tract abnormalities: are intravenous pyelograms necessary? J Pediatr Orthop. 1987;7(4):441–3. https://doi.org/10.1097/01241398-198707000-00012.
27. Hensinger RN, Lang JE, MacEwen GD. Klippel-Feil syndrome; a constellation of associated anomalies. J Bone Joint Surg Am. 1974;56(6):1246–53.
28. Pizzutillo PD, Woods M, Nicholson L, MacEwen GD. Risk factors in Klippel-Feil syndrome. Spine. 1994;19(18):2110–6. https://doi.org/10.1097/00007632-199409150-00020.
29. Tracy MR, Dormans JP, Kusumi K. Klippel-Feil syndrome: clinical features and current understanding of etiology. Clin Orthop. 2004;424:183–90. https://doi.org/10.1097/01.blo.0000130267.49895.20.
30. Ritterbusch JF, McGinty LD, Spar J, Orrison WW. Magnetic resonance imaging for stenosis and subluxation in Klippel-Feil syndrome. Spine. 1991;16(10 Suppl):S539–41. https://doi.org/10.1097/00007632-199110001-00017.
31. Cantu RC. Cervical spine injuries in the athlete. Semin Neurol. 2000;20(2):173–8. https://doi.org/10.1055/s-2000-9825.
32. Muenke M, Schell U. Fibroblast-growth-factor receptor mutations in human skeletal disorders. Trends Genet. 1995;11(8):308–13. https://doi.org/10.1016/s0168-9525(00)89088-5.
33. Wynne-Davies R, Walsh WK, Gormley J. Achondroplasia and hypochondroplasia. Clinical variation and spinal stenosis. J Bone Joint Surg Br. 1981;63B(4):508–15. https://doi.org/10.1302/0301-620X.63B4.7298674.
34. Bianchi F, Benato A, Frassanito P, Tamburrini G, Massimi L. Functional and morphological changes in hypoplasic posterior fossa. Childs Nerv Syst. 2021;37(10):3093–104. https://doi.org/10.1007/s00381-021-05193-w.
35. Pavlov H, Torg JS, Robie B, Jahre C. Cervical spinal stenosis: determination with vertebral body ratio method. Radiology. 1987;164(3):771–5. https://doi.org/10.1148/radiology.164.3.3615879.
36. Shaffrey CI, Wiggins GC, Piccirilli CB, Young JN, Lovell LR. Modified open-door laminoplasty for treatment of neurological deficits in younger patients with congenital spinal stenosis: analy-

sis of clinical and radiographic data. J Neurosurg. 1999;90(2 Suppl):170–7. https://doi.org/10.3171/spi.1999.90.2.0170.
37. Tolo VT. Surgical treatment of kyphosis in achondroplasia. In: Human achondroplasia: a multidisciplinary approach. Plenum Press; 1988. p. 257–63.
38. Torg JS, Pavlov H, Genuario SE, et al. Neurapraxia of the cervical spinal cord with transient quadriplegia. J Bone Joint Surg Am. 1986;68(9):1354–70.
39. Torg JS, Guille JT, Jaffe S. Injuries to the cervical spine in American football players. J Bone Joint Surg Am. 2002;84(1):112–22. https://doi.org/10.2106/00004623-200201000-00017.
40. Vaccaro AR, Klein GR, Ciccoti M, et al. Return to play criteria for the athlete with cervical spine injuries resulting in stinger and transient quadriplegia/paresis. Spine J. 2002;2(5):351–6. https://doi.org/10.1016/s1529-9430(02)00202-4.
41. Burnett MG, Sonntag VKH. Return to contact sports after spinal surgery. Neurosurg Focus. 2006;21(4):1–3. https://doi.org/10.3171/foc.2006.21.4.6.
42. Martínez-Lage JF, Martínez-Robledo A, López F, Poza M. Disc protrusion in the child. Childs Nerv Syst. 1997;13(4):201–7. https://doi.org/10.1007/s003810050069.
43. Dafford K, Kim SH, Lee M, Kim D. Lumbar disk herniations. In: Surgery of the pediatric spine. Thieme Medical Publishers; 2008. p. 217–24.
44. Lepard JR, Zimmerman KD, Arynchyna AA, et al. Pediatric herniated lumbar disc: a population-based risk factor analysis. J Neurosurg Pediatr. 2020;25(3):311–8. https://doi.org/10.3171/2019.9.PEDS19167.
45. Varlotta GP, Brown MD, Kelsey JL, Golden AL. Familial predisposition for herniation of a lumbar disc in patients who are less than twenty-one years old. J Bone Joint Surg Am. 1991;73(1):124–8.
46. Obukhov SK, Hankenson L, Manka M, Mawk JR. Multilevel lumbar disc herniation in 12-year-old twins. Childs Nerv Syst. 1996;12(3):169–71. https://doi.org/10.1007/BF00266823.
47. Lavelle WF, Bianco A, Mason R, Betz RR, Albanese SA. Pediatric disk herniation. J Am Acad Orthop Surg. 2011;19(11):649–56. https://doi.org/10.5435/00124635-201111000-00001.
48. Kurihara A, Kataoka O. Lumbar disc herniation in children and adolescents. A review of 70 operated cases and their minimum 5-year follow-up studies. Spine. 1980;5(5):443–51.
49. Chang CH, Lee ZL, Chen WJ, Tan CF, Chen LH. Clinical significance of ring apophysis fracture in adolescent lumbar disc herniation. Spine. 2008;33(16):1750–4. https://doi.org/10.1097/BRS.0b013e31817d1d12.
50. Cahill KS, Dunn I, Gunnarsson T, Proctor MR. Lumbar microdiscectomy in pediatric patients: a large single-institution series. J Neurosurg Spine. 2010;12(2):165–70. https://doi.org/10.3171/2009.9.SPINE09756.
51. Slotkin JR, Mislow JMK, Day AL, Proctor MR. Pediatric disk disease. Neurosurg Clin N Am. 2007;18(4):659–67. https://doi.org/10.1016/j.nec.2007.08.001.
52. Ozgen S, Konya D, Toktas OZ, Dagcinar A, Ozek MM. Lumbar disc herniation in adolescence. Pediatr Neurosurg. 2007;43(2):77–81. https://doi.org/10.1159/000098377.
53. Kumar R, Kumar V, Das NK, Behari S, Mahapatra AK. Adolescent lumbar disc disease: findings and outcome. Childs Nerv Syst. 2007;23(11):1295–9. https://doi.org/10.1007/s00381-007-0370-1.
54. Papagelopoulos PJ, Shaughnessy WJ, Ebersold MJ, Bianco AJ, Quast LM. Long-term outcome of lumbar discectomy in children and adolescents sixteen years of age or younger. J Bone Joint Surg Am. 1998;80(5):689–98. https://doi.org/10.2106/00004623-199805000-00009.
55. Kalichman L, Kim DH, Li L, Guermazi A, Berkin V, Hunter DJ. Spondylolysis and spondylolisthesis: prevalence and association with low back pain in the adult community-based population. Spine. 2009;34(2):199–205. https://doi.org/10.1097/BRS.0b013e31818edcfd.
56. Teitz CC. Sports medicine concerns in dance and gymnastics. Clin Sports Med. 1983;2(3):571–93.
57. Rossi F, Dragoni S. Lumbar spondylolysis: occurrence in competitive athletes. Updated achievements in a series of 390 cases. J Sports Med Phys Fitness. 1990;30(4):450–2.
58. Jackson DW, Wiltse LL, Cirincoine RJ. Spondylolysis in the female gymnast. Clin Orthop. 1976;117:68–73.
59. Tsirikos AI, Garrido EG. Spondylolysis and spondylolisthesis in children and adolescents. J Bone Joint Surg Br. 2010;92-B(6):751–9. https://doi.org/10.1302/0301-620X.92B6.23014.
60. Gallagher B, Moatz B, Tortolani PJ. Classifications in spondylolisthesis. Semin Spine Surg. 2020;32(3):100802. https://doi.org/10.1016/j.semss.2020.100802.
61. Dietrich M, Kurowski P. The importance of mechanical factors in the etiology of spondylolysis: a model analysis of loads and stresses in human lumbar spine. Spine. 1985;10(6):532–42. https://doi.org/10.1097/00007632-198507000-00007.
62. Morita T, Ikata T, Katoh S, Miyake R. Lumbar spondylolysis in children and adolescents. J Bone Joint Surg Br. 1995;77(4):620–5.
63. van den Oever M, Merrick MV, Scott JH. Bone scintigraphy in symptomatic spondylolysis. J Bone Joint Surg Br. 1987;69(3):453–6. https://doi.org/10.1302/0301-620X.69B3.2953729.
64. Pizzutillo PD, Hummer CD. Nonoperative treatment for painful adolescent spondylolysis or spondylolisthesis. J Pediatr Orthop. 1989;9(5):538–40. https://doi.org/10.1097/01241398-198909010-00007.
65. Steiner ME, Micheli LJ. Treatment of symptomatic spondylolysis and spondylolisthesis with the modified Boston brace. Spine. 1985;10(10):937–43. https://doi.org/10.1097/00007632-198512000-00013.

66. Lenke LG, Bridwell KH, Bullis D, Betz RR, Baldus C, Schoenecker PL. Results of in situ fusion for isthmic spondylolisthesis. J Spinal Disord. 1992;5(4):433–42. https://doi.org/10.1097/00002517-199212000-00008.
67. Seitsalo S, Osterman K, Poussa M, Laurent LE. Spondylolisthesis in children under 12 years of age: long-term results of 56 patients treated conservatively or operatively. J Pediatr Orthop. 1988;8(5):516–21. https://doi.org/10.1097/01241398-198809000-00003.
68. Mac-Thiong JM, Labelle H. Spondylolysis and spondylolisthesis. In: Surgery of the pediatric spine. Thieme Medical Publishers; 2008.
69. Transfeldt EE, Mehbod AA. Evidence-based medicine analysis of isthmic spondylolisthesis treatment including reduction versus fusion in situ for high-grade slips. Spine. 2007;32(19 Suppl):S126–9. https://doi.org/10.1097/BRS.0b013e318145b353.
70. Ferris LR, Ho E, Leong JC. Lumbar spondyloptosis. A long term follow up of three cases. Int Orthop. 1990;14(2):139–43. https://doi.org/10.1007/BF00180118.
71. Gaines RW, Nichols WK. Treatment of spondyloptosis by two stage L5 vertebrectomy and reduction of L4 onto S1. Spine. 1985;10(7):680–6. https://doi.org/10.1097/00007632-198509000-00015.
72. Boachie-Adjei O, Do T, Rawlins BA. Partial lumbosacral kyphosis reduction, decompression, and posterior lumbosacral transfixation in high-grade isthmic spondylolisthesis: clinical and radiographic results in six patients. Spine. 2002;27(6):E161–8. https://doi.org/10.1097/00007632-200203150-00019.
73. Groves ML, Kashanian A, Danielpour M, Stadler JA. Neurosurgical evaluation and management of adults with achondroplasia. Neurosurg Clin N Am. 2022;33(1):25–35. https://doi.org/10.1016/j.nec.2021.09.011.
74. Hankinson TC, Anderson RCE. Craniovertebral junction abnormalities in Down syndrome. Neurosurgery. 2010;66(Suppl 3):A32–8. https://doi.org/10.1227/01.NEU.0000365803.22786.F0.
75. Anderson PJ, David DJ. Spinal anomalies in Goldenhar syndrome. Cleft Palate Craniofac J. 2005;42(5):477–80. https://doi.org/10.1597/04-142051r.1.
76. Bogusiak K, Puch A, Arkuszewski P. Goldenhar syndrome: current perspectives. World J Pediatr. 2017;13(5):405–15. https://doi.org/10.1007/s12519-017-0048-z.
77. Veeravagu A, Lad SP, Camara-Quintana JQ, Jiang B, Shuer L. Neurosurgical interventions for spondyloepiphyseal dysplasia congenita: clinical presentation and assessment of the literature. World Neurosurg. 2013;80(3–4):437.e1–8. https://doi.org/10.1016/j.wneu.2012.01.030.
78. Mikles M, Stanton RP. A review of Morquio syndrome. Am J Orthop (Belle Mead NJ). 1997;26(8):533–40.
79. Sasaki-Adams D, Kulkarni A, Rutka J, Dirks P, Taylor M, Drake JM. Neurosurgical implications of osteogenesis imperfecta in children: report of 4 cases. J Neurosurg Pediatr. 2008;1(3):229–36. https://doi.org/10.3171/PED/2008/1/3/229.

Traumatic Brain Injury 17

Timothy C. Gooldy and P. David Adelson

Abbreviations

CBF	Cerebral blood flow
CBV	Cerebral blood volume
$CMRO_2$	Cerebral metabolic rate for oxygen
CN	Cranial nerve
CPP	Cerebral perfusion pressure
CSF	Cerebrospinal fluid
CSW	Cerebral salt wasting
CT	Computed tomogram or computed tomography
CTA	Computed tomography angiography
CVP	Central venous pressure
EDH	Epidural hematoma
EEG	Electroencephalogram
EVD	External ventricular drain
FiO_2	Fraction of inspired oxygen
GCS	Glasgow Coma Scale
ICP	Intracranial pressure
ICU	Intensive care unit
INR	International normalized ratio
MAP	Mean arterial pressure
MRI	Magnetic resonance imaging
$PbrO_2$	Partial pressure of oxygen in brain tissue
PTS	Posttraumatic seizures
SCI	Spinal cord injury
SDH	Subdural hematoma
SIADH	Syndrome of inappropriate antidiuretic hormone
SpO_2	Peripheral oxygen saturation
TAI	Traumatic axonal injury
TBI	Traumatic brain injury

T. C. Gooldy
Department of Neurosurgery, Barrow Neurological Institute, St. Joseph's Hospital and Medical Center, Phoenix, AZ, USA
e-mail: timothy.gooldy@barrowbrainandspine.com

P. D. Adelson (✉)
Department of Neurosurgery, Rockefeller Neuroscience Institute, College of Medicine, West Virginia University, J. W. Ruby Memorial Hospital and Children's Hospital, Morgantown, WV, USA
e-mail: david.adelson@hsc.wvu.edu

Introduction

Worldwide, more than 50 million people of all ages experience a traumatic brain injury (TBI) each year, and it is estimated that about one-half of the world's population will have one or more TBIs over their lifetime [1]. Despite preventive education and improvements in neurocritical care, TBI remains a leading cause of injury-related morbidity and mortality, particularly among the pediatric population. This chapter addresses the fundamentals of neurosurgical care management specific to pediatric TBI, starting with the presentation of patients in the field and progressing through their hospital stay and beyond.

Pediatric neurotrauma has fundamental physiologic differences from neurotrauma in adults. Even within the pediatric population, the range

N. Shimony, G. Jallo (eds.), *Pediatric Neurosurgery Board Review*,
https://doi.org/10.1007/978-3-031-23687-7_17

of physiologic normative values varies widely across the age spectrum. This variation between patients of different ages is perhaps most relevant to managing intracranial pressure (ICP) and mean arterial pressure (MAP) in the neurosurgical and neurocritical care settings. Pathophysiology after TBI also differs between children and adults. Diffuse brain injury is more common in children and varies with age, whereas focal injury and extra-axial hematomas are less common. The pressure-volume relationships within the skull, metabolic responses to injury, and cerebral hemodynamics also differ in children and adults. All these factors have clinical implications for treating pediatric patients who have TBI. Furthermore, the technical aspects of operative management—anesthesia control, operative planning, blood volume management, and tissue handling—require special consideration in the pediatric population. Although it is beyond the scope of this chapter to cover the details of all the types of emergency operations performed in children, key principles common to the most important of these procedures are addressed.

Emergency Evaluation and Triage

With the high incidence of TBI in the pediatric population, neurosurgical providers must be familiar and comfortable with the triage and workup of these patients. Even neurosurgeons who are not generally involved or consulted until several steps into the process require this knowledge base.

In the field, standard emergency medical services protocols should be followed for a patient with a suspected TBI, starting with airway, breathing, and circulation [2]. Concomitant spinal cord injury (SCI) should be presumed until it can be ruled out. Emergency medical services personnel must convey important information about the trauma, including the type or mechanism, the degree of force, the position of the patient upon arrival, and the patient's initial level of consciousness. Intubation is generally performed either at the scene of the trauma or at the discretion of the trauma service on presentation. Possible skull base fractures should be considered as well.

Notification protocols between the trauma and neurosurgery services can help expedite the neurologic assessment of incoming patients with suspected TBI. Such notification should allow for an initial neurologic examination before the patient is sedated and paralytics are administered, which can confound the clinical picture. A basic Glasgow Coma Scale (GCS) assessment takes no more than a minute, and it provides an initial grading of the severity of the TBI [3]. This scale is a modified pediatric version of the GCS (*see* Table 17.1), which classifies head injuries by total points as mild (14–15 points), moderate (9–13 points), or severe (3–8 points). The Infant Face Scale can be used for patients too young for the GCS [4].

Table 17.1 Pediatric Glasgow Coma Scale[a]

Verbal		Eye		Motor	
Best response	Points	Best response	Points	Best response	Points
No verbal response	1	No eye opening	1	No motor response	1
Inconsolable, agitated	2	Eyes open to pain	2	Extension to pain	2
Inconsistently inconsolable, moaning	3	Eyes open to speech	3	Abnormal flexion to pain	3
Cries but consolable, abnormal interactions	4	Eyes open spontaneously	4	Infant withdraws from pain	4
Smiles, orients to sounds, follows objects	5			Infant withdraws from touch	5
				Infant moves spontaneously	6

[a]Data source: Durham et al. [4]

Intubation, Ventilation, and Circulation

Intubation

Rapid sequence intubation is the preferred method of securing the airway in children with suspected elevated ICP because it provides protection against the reflex responses to laryngoscopy and resultant increases in ICP. A comatose patient may still require pharmacologic agents for pretreatment, induction of anesthesia, and neuromuscular blockade. Problems associated with elevated ICP may be compounded by the techniques and medications used in airway management because these may further exacerbate an already elevated ICP. Hence, throughout the intubation procedure, attention should be focused on maintaining adequate cerebral perfusion with good blood pressure control and minimizing the risk of herniation. In practice, the position of the patient's body should be optimized before endotracheal intubation, and hypoventilation should be avoided. Keep the upper part of the body up, with the patient's head in the midline, until the patient must be laid flat to perform a direct laryngoscopy. During this phase, one should always assume concurrent SCI until it can be ruled out.

Anesthesia

Anesthesia should be induced using an agent that will not affect the maintenance of good cerebral perfusion (i.e., one that will not elevate ICP or decrease MAP). Common agents include etomidate, propofol, and thiopental (*see* Table 17.2 for recommended dose, onset, and duration).

Etomidate is a short-acting imidazole derivative that provides hypnosis with minimal hemodynamic effect. It is a good choice for patients with hypotension and suspected elevated ICP because it decreases cerebral blood flow (CBF) and ICP while it preserves cerebral perfusion pressure (CPP). Of note, etomidate may decrease the seizure threshold, which is a concern in children with an increased risk for posttraumatic seizures (PTS).

Propofol is an alternative induction agent with potent vasodilator and myocardial depressive actions such that hypotension can be expected. Hence, simultaneous vasopressor and fluid administration may be necessary to maintain CPP when using this induction agent. Propofol is used to reduce ICP and has anticonvulsant effects.

Thiopental decreases the cerebral metabolic rate for oxygen ($CMRO_2$), CBF, and ICP. However, this potent venodilator is also a negative inotrope with a strong tendency to cause hypotension and reduce cerebral perfusion. A smaller dose should be used in patients with suspected inadequate preload or hemodynamic compromise, especially in multitrauma situations.

Ketamine is an alternative induction agent for hypotensive patients with suspected increased ICP. Administration triggers a catecholamine surge that can increase blood pressure. A previous concern about using ketamine was that it

Table 17.2 Anesthesia agents

Agent	Dose, IV push	Pros	Cons	Onset of action	Duration of effect
Etomidate	0.3 mg/kg	Decreases CBF and ICP; preserves CPP	Lowers seizure threshold	30–60 s	3–5 min
Propofol	2 mg/kg	Lowers ICP; anticonvulsant	Hypotension	10–50 s	3–10 min
Thiopental	1–5 mg/kg	Decreases cerebral metabolic rate, CBF, and ICP	Hypotension and reduced CPP	30–60 s	3–50 min
Ketamine	2 mg/kg	Lowers ICP; increases MAP	May be contraindicated in normotensive or hypertensive patients	45–60 s	10–20 min

Abbreviations: *CBF* cerebral blood flow, *CPP* cerebral perfusion pressure, *ICP* intracranial pressure, *IV* intravenous, *MAP* mean arterial pressure may contribute to elevated ICP, but more recent reports suggest otherwise [5].

Neuromuscular Blockade

The two agents typically used to induce neuromuscular blockage—succinylcholine and rocuronium—are summarized in Table 17.3, which also lists their recommended dose, onset of action, and duration of effect. Succinylcholine is a depolarizing neuromuscular blocking agent that is the medication of choice for emergency endotracheal intubation of patients with a TBI and suspected elevated ICP. This drug has a rapid onset and a short duration of action. However, its administration should be avoided in patients with a suspected SCI, hyperkalemia, known neuromuscular disease, or a history of malignant hyperthermia. Its use in patients with eye injuries is controversial because of the risk of extrusion of intraocular contents. Alternatively, a nondepolarizing drug, such as rocuronium, can be used when the contraindications for succinylcholine are present.

Postintubation Procedures and Mechanical Ventilation

Immediately after endotracheal intubation, the fraction of inspired oxygen (FiO_2) can be reduced to 0.5, or the lowest fraction that achieves adequate oxygenation (saturated pulse oxygenation [SpO_2] >94%). The head of the patient's bed should be returned to the 30-degree position, and the patient's head should be kept midline to optimize perfusion and venous outflow.

A central venous line will have to be placed, but it should not involve moving the patient into the Trendelenburg position, turning the neck to the side, or compressing neck vessels. These maneuvers will lead to an increase in ICP and, possibly, to evolution to herniation. Instead, a large-bore brachial venous line or another alternative, such as an intraosseous line, may be required in the acute setting until ICP can be monitored and treated as needed.

The postintubation mechanical ventilation goals include normalization of oxygenation and pH to target levels (Box 17.1) and work-of-breathing:

- Normalization of oxygenation with the lowest FiO_2 to maintain SpO_2 > 94%: In some instances, positive end-expiratory pressure will be required. However, ICP must be monitored during the application of positive end-expiratory pressure in TBI patients because the associated increase in intrathoracic pressure may decrease venous return, resulting in ICP elevation.
- Normalization of ventilation to achieve pH 7.35–7.45, with $PaCO_2$ 35–45 mm Hg: The latter can be followed with exhaled CO_2 monitoring. Overventilation with large tidal volumes (>8 mL/kg) should be avoided to limit the risk of acute lung injury.
- Normalization of work-of-breathing and patient-ventilator synchrony: This normalization often requires avoiding agitation and awareness by using a paralytic agent and simultaneously using sedative analgesic medications. For pediatric patients, the use of a benzodiazepine-opiate combination or dexmedetomidine is preferable. Continuous propofol infusion is contraindicated in the younger pediatric population (<12 years) because the difference in metabolism compared to that of the adult population can result in metabolic acidosis and can increase the risk of propofol-infusion syndrome [6]. Pediatric patients older than 12 years would probably not be affected by a propofol infusion, but no defined age threshold has been reported in the literature.

Table 17.3 Neuromuscular blockades

Agent	Dose, IV push	Mechanism	Onset of action	Duration of effect
Succinylcholine	1.5–2.0 mg/kg	Depolarizing neuromuscular blockade	30–60 s	5–15 min
Rocuronium	1.2–1.4 mg/kg	Nondepolarizing neuromuscular blockade	45–60 s	47–70 min

Abbreviation: *IV* intravenous

Hyperventilation

Box 17.1 Therapeutic Ventilation Targets

- SpO_2: >94%
- pH: 7.35–7.45
- $PaCO_2$: 35–45 mm Hg

When life-threatening increased ICP and brain herniation are suspected, hyperventilation may be required temporarily until a computed tomogram (CT) can be obtained and definitive treatment can be provided to lower ICP (i.e., external ventricular drain [EVD], hematoma evacuation, decompressive craniectomy). Because prolonged hyperventilation can contribute to cerebral ischemia as a result of cerebral arterial vasoconstriction, hyperventilation should not be continued without brain oxygen monitoring. In these circumstances, the maximal cerebral vasoconstriction is achieved at a $PaCO_2$ of 20 mm Hg. Hyperventilation below this level is ineffective and may result in hypotension, which could further worsen cerebral hypoperfusion.

Circulation

As mentioned previously, the injured brain is susceptible to hypotension and inadequate perfusion, resulting in possible ischemia. A general guideline for the minimum appropriate MAP for children older than 1 year is the fifth percentile of systolic blood pressure for age or 70 mm Hg + (2× age in years).

All causes of hypotension should be considered and investigated. Cranial blood loss is usually not significant enough to alter hemodynamics, unless the patient is bleeding from the scalp or is an infant with a subgaleal hematoma. Cardiogenic shock from the injury itself can lead to presentation with hypotension and tachycardia, whereas a patient with neurogenic shock, usually from an SCI above the level of T4, will also present with hypotension but may lack compensatory tachycardia. Treatment generally consists of fluid resuscitation, but hypotonic concentrations should be avoided.

Detailed Neurologic Examination

The neurologic assessment of the pediatric patient is addressed in detail in Chap. 1. However, we present specific portions of the examination here that are relevant to the pediatric trauma patient.

Breathing Patterns

Several abnormal patterns of respiration have been observed in patients with severe TBI. These patterns may provide important localizing information (*see* Table 17.4).

Table 17.4 Abnormal breathing patterns related to localized traumatic brain injury

Abnormal breathing pattern	Location of injury
Posthyperventilation apnea	Forebrain damage
Cheyne-Stokes respiration or alternating phases of hyperpnea	Deep cerebral hemispheres or diencephalon
Hyperventilation or persistent rapid breathing	Rostral brainstem or tegmentum
Apneustic breathing (prolong sustained end-inspiratory pauses)	Mid to caudal pons
Cluster breathing (periodic respirations that are irregular in amplitude)	Lower pontine to high medulla
Ataxic respiration (random and irregular breathing)	Medulla

Ophthalmic Examination

Pupillary Evaluation

The pupillary light reflex consists of an afferent pathway through the optic nerve (cranial nerve [CN] II) and an efferent pathway that involves both sympathetic and parasympathetic fibers. Pupil size should be noted both before and after stimulation with light. Both direct and consensual reactions should also be noted. Any abnormal responses should prompt investigation into possible adverse effects of medications or poisons so as not to confound the actual neurologic examination findings (*see* Table 17.5).

Ipsilateral pupillary dilation without response to direct or consensual stimulation represents a compression of the parasympathetic fibers along the oculomotor nerve (CN III), often from transtentorial herniation. This reaction is generally considered to be an indication for emergency workup and intervention, including hyperventilation, hyperosmolar therapy, new imaging, and possible surgical intervention. Bilateral pupillary dilation represents bilateral CN III compression or severe global hypoxia-ischemia. Pinpoint pupils can be associated with pontine lesions or a response to some drugs (e.g., opiates). Ipsilateral pupillary constriction with ptosis and anhidrosis (Horner syndrome) may represent transtentorial herniation or damage to the sympathetic tracts at either the cervical level or the level of the hypothalamus. Hippus involves pupils that are fixed to light but still retain ciliospinal reflex, which is an accommodation response that can be seen in patients with injury to the midbrain.

Table 17.5 Mechanisms and pathologies related to abnormal pupillary reactions

Abnormal reaction	Mechanism	Possible pathology
Ipsilateral pupillary dilation	Compression of CN III parasympathetic fibers	Transtentorial herniation
Bilateral pupillary dilation	Bilateral CN III compression, severe global hypoxia-ischemia	Global brain swelling with bilateral transtentorial herniation, anoxic injury
Pinpoint pupils	Drug effect, disruption of sympathetic pupillary pathways	Opiate overdose, pontine lesion
Horner syndrome	Damage to sympathetic trunk	Transtentorial herniation, hypothalamic injury, cervical injury
Hippus	Response to accommodation	Midbrain injury

Abbreviation: CN III, cranial nerve III (oculomotor nerve)

Ocular Responses

Ocular motion generally cannot be evaluated in the unresponsive TBI patient, but the examiner should still note the position of the patient's eyes at rest. Dysconjugate or deviated eyes may indicate seizures or cortical injury. Spontaneous eye movements may include roving, ocular bobbing, nystagmus, increased blinking, lid retraction, and convergent or divergent spasms.

Brainstem reflexes may need to be evaluated, especially in cases when it is necessary to determine brain death or nonsurvivable injury. Testing for the oculocephalic reflex (doll's eyes) should be performed only if the cervical spine is known to be stable. Testing for the oculovestibular reflex (cold water calorics) can also be performed.

Fundus Examination

Retinal hemorrhages can represent nonaccidental trauma. Papilledema is a reliable sign of intracranial hypertension, but it may not present acutely in patients for the first 24–48 h [7]. Evaluation of the fundus may require the use of short-acting mydriatics. It is important to label the patient as having received these medications. In the comatose patient, dilating one eye at a time can avoid eliminating the ability to perform a pupillary examination.

Motor Examination

Prior to performing a stimulatory examination, the clinician should observe the patient for any spontaneous movements. Responses should be identified as unilateral, bilateral, spontaneous, or induced only with stimulation. Seizure activity should not be confused with a true motor response, which can be difficult to discern in infants and toddlers. Abnormal responses (posturing) to painful stimuli can be linked to the level of injury (Box 17.2). Before a peripheral stimulatory motor examination is performed, SCI or atlanto-occipital dislocation should be ruled out by applying supraorbital pain stimulation. Decorticate rigidity (flexor posturing) indicates impairment of or injury to the corticospinal pathways above the level of the red nucleus (cerebral hemispheres, internal capsule, rostral cerebral peduncle). Decerebrate rigidity (extensor posturing) indicates impairment or injury between the levels of the red nucleus and the vestibular nuclei (rostral midbrain to mid-pons).

Box 17.2 Interpreting Motor Examination Results

- Decorticate rigidity (flexor posturing): Represents impairment of or injury to the corticospinal pathways above the level of the red nucleus (cerebral hemispheres, internal capsule, rostral cerebral peduncle)
- Decerebrate rigidity (extensor posturing): Represents impairment or injury between the levels of the red nucleus and the vestibular nuclei (rostral midbrain to mid-pons)

Posttraumatic Seizures

Although generalized tonic-clonic seizures and myoclonic jerks are easily identified, PTS should be carefully noted. Close observation is especially important for infants, who may experience subclinical seizures. Infants may also present with cyanosis, chewing movements, or bicycling of the limbs in response to stimulation. Gaze deviations in infants can represent seizure activity in the contralateral frontal eye fields.

Trauma-Specific Evaluation

Additional examinations should be performed to assess the child for lacerations, depressions, swellings, and ecchymosis. Any of these findings should be investigated to evaluate for an underlying injury. Patients with skull-base fractures may present with ecchymosis of the retroauricular area (Battle sign) or the periorbital space (raccoon eyes). Additional signs of this type of fracture include otorrhea or rhinorrhea of blood or cerebrospinal fluid (CSF) and hemotympanum. Patients with facial fractures may present with instability of the facial bones and zygoma (i.e., Le Fort fracture) and facial step-off abnormalities (e.g., orbital rim fracture).

For infants with an unfused cranium, the clinician should measure the head circumference and palpate the fontanelles and sutures to identify any bulging or splaying of suture lines. These examinations are generally less sensitive to acute pathology, but they are more useful in chronic conditions of elevated ICP.

Head Injury Patterns and Mechanisms

Development and Head Injury Patterns

The stage of development of the skull, brain, and intracranial vasculature factors into the types of injuries seen in different pediatric age groups. The disproportionally large head and relatively weak neck muscles of the infant increase the risk of rotational and acceleration-deceleration injuries. The relatively softer cranial vault, anatomy of the dura, and rich vascular supply of the subarachnoid space all place young children at greater risk for intracranial injury and bleeding, even without a skull fracture. The high-water content and viscosity of the young brain also increase the risk for axonal injury. With maturation of the skull and brain, adult patterns of intracranial injury are seen. Pediatric patients with a thinner skull anatomy are more prone to skull fracture and epidural hematoma (EDH), whereas adult patients are more likely to present with subdural and intraparenchymal hemorrhages.

Blunt Force Injury

Blunt force injury occurs when the head comes into forcible contact with a flat, smooth surface. Common examples include injury from a fall when the patient is on an elevated surface, with the head striking the ground, or injury from a blow to the head made by a blunt object. The curvature of the skull at the point of impact generally deforms and flattens. The area of impact is spread over an area proportional to the deformation of the skull.

If a fracture has occurred, its direction and extent will be related to the thickness of the scalp, the elasticity of the bone, and any local weakness in the skull. Fracture lines develop as the skull deformity exceeds the limits of tolerance. In children, the unfused cranial sutures may be involved, producing a "bursting fracture" or diastasis of cranial sutures.

In addition to the direct injury caused by blunt force trauma, the cranium and its contents are subjected to significant deceleration forces during a fall or to acceleration forces when experiencing a blow. This deceleration or acceleration may result in parenchyma injury on both the ipsilateral and contralateral sides (coup-contrecoup injury).

Compression Injury

Compression injuries are rarer than other types of injuries. For example, a television falling from a stand can cause a crush injury. Severe instances of compression may occur without the injured child experiencing an initial loss of consciousness. Fractures often involve the foramina at the skull base and produce CN palsies when flattening forces are applied to the skull. The internal carotid artery may even be torn where it passes through the skull base, resulting in fatal hemorrhage or ischemia. Less severe cases may result in vessel dissection and resultant stroke. Side-to-side compression injuries cause fractures through the middle fossa across the sella turcica to the opposite side. In these cases, the pituitary gland and its stalk are at greater risk, potentially resulting in hypothalamic-pituitary dysfunction.

Sharp or Penetrating Injury

The area of impact and the extent of skull distortion are small in a sharp head injury. The injury may result in a scalp laceration, local depression, or fragmentation of the skull; tearing of the dura; and direct injury to the underlying brain. Examples of a sharp injury include an impact from a sharp object or a fall onto the corner of a table. In these cases, the area of impact is small; thus, the force is focal and not distributed throughout the rest of the skull. The effect on the underlying bone can be explosive, with fragments driven into the underlying brain. This bone fragmentation may result in underlying focal contusions or in hemorrhage arising from torn superficial vessels of the cortex.

Penetrating Blast Injury

Although penetrating injuries are less common than closed head injuries, penetrating craniocerebral injuries account for significant morbidity and mortality within the pediatric population. The extent of brain tissue damage and compromised vascular supply can lead to worsened secondary mechanisms of injury. Common neurosurgical techniques and principles apply to the management of these injuries, including evacuation of mass lesions, debridement of devitalized tissue, and decompression. In blast injuries, the pressure wave and forces applied to brain tissue can disrupt nerve connections and result in significant morbidity.

Types of Intracranial Injury

The 4 main pathologies in pediatric TBI and intracranial damage are (1) extra-axial hemorrhages, including EDHs and subdural hematomas (SDHs); (2) focal hemorrhagic and nonhemorrhagic lesions that involve the cortical gray matter; (3) diffuse traumatic axonal injury (TAI); and (4) secondary injury caused by edema, space-occupying hemorrhages, and ischemia.

Extra-Axial Hemorrhage

Epidural Hematoma

EDHs comprise 2–3% of all head injury hospital admissions for children, and they are more frequent with advancing age, peaking in the second decade of life [8]. In infants, EDHs are most often secondary to venous or bony bleeding rather than arterial bleeding. These venous EDHs often have delayed presentation because the infant has significant intracranial reserve from unfused sutures and open fontanelles until compensation is no longer possible. In older children and adults, EDHs tend to arise from arterial injuries. These patients may present with a classic loss of consciousness at the time of injury, followed by a lucid interval, then subsequent rapid deterioration with the increasing intracranial mass effect.

Subdural Hematoma

SDHs are a common problem in children, especially in those who experience abusive TBI. Their clinical presentation depends on the location and size of the hemorrhage and the presence of concurrent parenchymal injury. The mechanisms causing an acute SDH are more commonly associated with a TBI that results in immediate loss of consciousness and possible focal neurologic deficits (e.g., hemiparesis, pupillary abnormalities, seizures) at the time of injury. Chronic SDHs may represent repetitive, less severe trauma (e.g., shaken baby syndrome) that accumulates over time, with a less acute focal neurologic presentation. SDHs can be of venous or arterial origin but most often involve the cortical veins at their attachment to the dura and venous sinuses.

Focal Hemorrhagic and Nonhemorrhagic Lesions

Traumatic Intraparenchymal Hemorrhage

Traumatic intraparenchymal hematomas (i.e., contusions) are less common in children than in adults. These contusions most commonly involve the white matter of the frontal and temporal lobes, the body and splenium of the corpus callosum, and the corona radiata. Contusions in the cortex frequently involve the inferior, lateral, and anterior aspects of the frontal and temporal lobes; these lesions are believed to be the result of either direct impact or shearing between gray and white matter. Microhemorrhagic lesions are best visualized on susceptibility-weighted imaging.

Diffuse Traumatic Axonal Injury

Diffuse TAI results from shearing forces on areas of the brain that have different structural integrities, such as the boundaries between gray and white matter or the corpus callosum. The neuronal axons that cross multiple brain regions are particularly vulnerable. TAIs vary from small cortical foci to a more severe form of diffuse injury that is widespread and may include the brainstem.

CT imaging may show small focal hemorrhages, but it is often not sensitive enough to demonstrate underlying axonal damage. Magnetic resonance imaging (MRI) with susceptibility-weighted sequences is the preferred imaging modality for a suspected TAI. TAI grading is determined by the location of axonal injury (Box 17.3) [9]. Controversy exists over the prognostic value of this grading system, although it is generally agreed that unfavorable functional outcomes increase with higher grade.

Box 17.3 TAI Grading by Axonal Injury Location [9]

- Grade 1: Cerebral hemispheres
- Grade 2: Focal lesions in the corpus callosum in addition to diffuse hemispheric lesions
- Grade 3: Involvement of the brainstem in addition to the corpus callosum and hemispheres

Concussion (Mild TBI)

The term mild TBI is now being used interchangeably with concussion to reflect the serious nature of this injury despite minimal outward symptoms or signs at presentation. A mild TBI involves a complex physiologic process induced by mechanical forces applied to the head. These injuries are typically associated with normal neuroimaging findings, and the disruption in brain function is related to neurometabolic dysfunction rather than structural damage. Concussions may or may not include the loss of consciousness, and they result in a wide constellation of symptoms, including physical, cognitive, emotional, and sleep-related factors. The duration of symptoms is also variable, lasting from seconds to months or even years. Return to activity should proceed in a slow step-wise fashion, with a halt of progression if any symptoms return [10].

Historical grading systems have focused only on the length of acute symptoms and whether the injured person lost consciousness. Modern assessments have become far more extensive and nuanced, but their review is beyond the scope of this chapter.

Postconcussive syndrome describes continued symptoms that persist longer than a few weeks after the injury, and it is thought to be more common in patients with a history of multiple concussions. These persistent symptoms should prompt referral to the appropriate specialist (e.g., vestibular rehabilitation, sleep disorders, neuropsychology, psychotherapy, pain management).

Secondary Injury

Early-Phase Edema

During the early phase of posttraumatic injury in children, cerebral edema develops and peaks 24–72 h after injury [11]. Cerebral edema can be unilateral or bilateral, depending on the primary mechanism. Focal and global brain swelling can act as a mass, leading to shifts and herniation syndromes (*see* Table 17.6), sometimes without an increase in global ICP. These cases may require delayed surgical decompression, even if the initial offending insult (e.g., EDH, SDH) has already been addressed.

Posttraumatic Ischemia, Tissue Oxygenation, and Metabolism

After a traumatic head injury, CBF may be reduced and secondary insults such as hypotension and hypoxemia can have devastat-

Table 17.6 Mechanisms and symptoms related to herniation syndrome

Herniation syndrome	Mechanism	Signs and symptoms
Subfalcine and cingulate	One cerebral hemisphere is displaced under the falx cerebri across the midline, causing compression of the anterior circulation	Unilateral or bilateral weakness of lower extremities
Uncal (transtentorial)	Displacement of supratentorial structures inferiorly below the level of the tentorium cerebelli, causing distortion and compression of blood supply to infratentorial structures	Pupillary dilation, bradycardia
Foramen magnum (tonsillar herniation)	Downward herniation of the cerebellum, causing compression of the brainstem	Downbeat nystagmus, bradycardia, bradypnea, hypertension (Cushing triad)

ing effects. Brain swelling and accompanying intracranial hypertension can contribute to this secondary ischemia. Infants with severe TBI commonly have cerebral hypoperfusion, and a global CBF of <20 mL/100 g/min is associated with poor outcomes [12, 13]. After early posttraumatic hypoperfusion, CBF may actually increase to levels greater than metabolic demand, producing a state of hyperemia [14]. Alternatively, a phase of increased metabolism of glucose may accompany posttraumatic hypoperfusion. The increasing use of monitoring techniques that reflect the coupling between CBF and metabolism (e.g., microdialysis and oxygen probes) can provide important information that influences practice (e.g., blood pressure and ventilator settings).

Imaging

Indications for Imaging

The appropriateness of imaging techniques must be determined by the provider at an individual patient level. The American College of Radiology has published guidelines for the various imaging modalities for use in basic pediatric trauma situations, with helpful indications of relative radiation levels. Although these techniques can be a helpful resource, more detailed examination of their usage is beyond the scope of this review [15].

Radiation Concerns in the Developing Brain

The effect of ionizing radiation on the immature central nervous system is a concern in pediatric medicine. Ultimately, adequate imaging must be obtained to make informed medical and surgical decisions. With improved technology, effective imaging can usually be obtained with lower radiation levels through modifications in the processing algorithms.

Plain Radiographs

Plain skull films (radiographs) are rarely used today in pediatric trauma centers because their usefulness has been surpassed by CT, which provides soft tissue assessment and superior evaluation of bony structures. Plain radiographs are generally used only as part of a full skeletal survey to document child abuse.

Computed Tomography

For TBI cases, the noncontrast axial head CT is the initial imaging modality of choice in pediatric patients. National Emergency X-Radiography Utilization Study (NEXUS) criteria have been established for cranial CTs in pediatric patients (Box 17.4) [16, 17]. This imaging can be performed rapidly, and it provides immediate information regarding cranial injury, intra- and extra-axial hemorrhage, fractures, ventricular assessment, and ischemia to some degree. Imaging should extend to the craniocervical junction or below (when cervical trauma is suspected) to evaluate for atlanto-occipital dislocation, rotatory subluxation of C1 on C2, and other disruptions.

Box 17.4 NEXUS II Criteria for Cranial CT in Pediatric TBI [16, 17]

- Evidence of skull fracture
- Scalp hematoma
- Neurologic deficit
- Abnormal level of alertness (GCS <14) or decline in level of consciousness
- Abnormal behavior
- Persistent vomiting
- Coagulopathy
- Seizure
- Amnesia

The relative infrequency of anticoagulant use in the pediatric population decreases the risk of secondary or expanded hemorrhage [18]. Repeat CT is generally not indicated. Repeat radiation exposure can be avoided by considering repeat CT only in cases whose results would change their management or if other imaging modalities are not available or are inadequate.

CT Pan Scan

At some trauma centers, the use of wide field of view CT (so-called "*CT pan scan*") has increased; this imaging examines the head, cervical spine, abdomen, and pelvis. Although the decision to use CT pan scan is largely made at the discretion of the trauma service, a collaborative consensus and criteria should be established between departments to effectively identify the individual pediatric patients who require such extensive evaluation to avoid subjecting children to unnecessary radiation exposure.

Magnetic Resonance Imaging

In the acute setting, MRI is generally not indicated in pediatric trauma patients primarily because of time constraints and the potential need for sedation to ensure adequate image quality. MRI may also not provide the level of bony evaluation necessary in these cases.

In the postacute setting, MRI can be beneficial for evaluating more subtle parenchymal injury, the progression of hemorrhage, and soft tissue in cervical spine injuries without bony compromise. It is worth noting that, after the acute phase, certain implants and monitors, such as ICP sensors, electroencephalogram (EEG) leads, and cranial bolts, may have to be removed or adjusted prior to an MRI to prevent artifact and inducible radiofrequency heating.

The rapid-sequence MRI ("quick brain," "one-bang," "fast brain") can be useful in evaluating ventricular anatomy and the progression of hemorrhage. These sequences require less time than standard MRIs and may negate the need for sedation.

Ultrasound

Although CT remains the imaging standard for emergent diagnosis of both skull fractures and TBIs, good evidence suggests that point-of-care transcranial Doppler ultrasound can be used to evaluate pediatric patients with possible skull fractures. With minimal training, emergency providers can use this readily available tool to screen young patients with a high index of suspicion for skull fractures before subjecting them to CT and radiation exposure. Depending on the imaging criteria, ultrasound may be used in individual patients without a clear-cut skull fracture or TBI [19–22].

CT Angiography

CT angiography (CTA) is frequently used in adult patients with TBI, but providers are more hesitant to use it in pediatric patients because it is associated with significantly higher levels of radiation exposure than other imaging modalities. Specific criteria that are independent risk factors for blunt cerebrovascular injury warrant CTA imaging (Box 17.5) [23]. A prospective protocol can help ensure that the correct children get adequate imaging, while also defining those who are not likely to benefit.

Box 17.5 Risk Factors Warranting CTA [23]

- GCS <8
- Fracture of petrous temporal bone or fracture through the carotid canal
- Skull base fracture
- Focal neurologic deficit

Intensive Care Management of Pediatric TBI Patients

Although evidence-based literature on managing pediatric patients with TBIs in the intensive care unit (ICU) is scarce, aggressive treatment protocols specifically for children based on available evidence serve as the basis of consensus guidelines [24]. Additionally, the Approaches and Decisions for Acute Pediatric TBI Trial (ADAPT) [25–27], a comparative analysis trial with 1000 national and international pediatric patients, has provided emerging data, and there is an expectation of further development of these recommendations. Importantly, each patient should be evaluated and treated within the context of the relevant injury.

Physiologic Differences Between Pediatric and Adult Patients

The physiology of adult and pediatric patients is fundamentally different enough to warrant being noted and considered. Autoregulation is the ability to change or the mechanism of change in cerebrovascular resistance that maintains CBF over a range of increases and decreases in CPP. When the autoregulatory system is disrupted, then decreased CPP may go uncompensated, resulting in ischemia. Pediatric patients tend to have a lower autoregulatory reserve and may require a lower ICP target threshold to maintain adequate perfusion. In addition, MAP, CBF, and $CMRO_2$ all tend to be lower in pediatric patients [28].

Intracranial Hypertension

Secondary injury to the brain after severe TBI results from a cascade of events, including reduced perfusion, decreased oxygen and metabolite delivery, and decreased clearance of waste and toxins. Subsequent brain swelling from vasogenic and cytotoxic edema within the closed compartment of the skull leads to intracranial hypertension, which can further potentiate ischemia and herniation syndromes. ICP is measured to determine the level of swelling, intracranial volume, and direct pressure inside the cranium, and it is used to indirectly calculate CPP, with the target varying by age (Box 17.6) [29]. CPP results from the difference between MAP and mean ICP. Sustained levels of inadequate perfusion can result in cerebral ischemia.

Box 17.6 CPP Targets by Age [29]

- Adults (≥18 years): >50–60 mm Hg
- Children (6–17 years): >50 mm Hg
- Infants and young children (0–5 years): >40 mm Hg

Intracranial Monitoring Methods

Indications for intracranial monitoring in pediatric patients are controversial, but the general consensus is for ICP monitoring of any patient with severe TBI (GCS 3–8 after resuscitation) [29]. The most recent guidelines also provide a consensus algorithm for ICP management and include other pathways for monitoring pathology (e.g., CPP, brain oxygen, and herniation pathways).

Various devices and techniques can be used to monitor intracranial processes. Invasive ICP monitoring options include EVDs, intraparenchymal sensors, and lumbar drains. Noninvasive methods are also available, but these have not yet been shown to be of as high quality as direct measurements; these methods include tympanic-membrane displacement monitoring, serial retinal evaluation for optic sheath diameter, and serial imaging and clinical examination.

Advanced neuromonitoring methods may provide important clinical information other than ICP and CPP. These methods include brain tissue oxygenation monitors, EEG, transcranial Doppler, CBF velocity, and microdialysis. Unfortunately, although numerous technologies enable the measurement of the complex physiology of the brain after injury, these techniques are often underutilized.

Managing Elevated Intracranial Pressure

Baseline Care

Baseline care and evaluation are presumed in tiered recommendations. The baseline assumes that for a pediatric patient with severe TBI (GCS 3–8), successful endotracheal intubation and mechanical ventilation have been performed with a normocapnic target. Adequate analgesia and sedation are initiated to limit coughing and dyssynchronous patient-ventilator interactions. Elevation of the patient's head to 30° in the midline promotes venous return. Removal or loosening of the cervical collar limits venous compression in the neck. A baseline cranial CT determines the need for surgical intervention. An ICP monitor is placed for ICP and CPP management. Normothermia is maintained, with particular avoidance of hyperthermia. Specific physiologic parameters should be optimized with help from the ICU team (Box 17.7). Ventilation settings should be titrated to an SpO_2 of 90–100 mm Hg through adjustment of FiO_2. The minute ventilation rate should be adjusted for $PaCO_2$ of 35–40 mm Hg.

Fluid status and intravascular volume are monitored with central venous pressure (CVP), urine output, blood urea nitrogen, serum creatinine, and clinical examination. The target goal for CVP is 4–10 mm Hg [30]. Patients should receive maintenance fluids at an infusion rate of 75%, with a goal for urine output of >1 mL/kg/h. The general consensus is that younger patients should receive normal saline plus 5% dextrose to avoid severe hypoglycemia, whereas older patients should receive normal saline. Hypotonic fluids should be avoided. Glucose ranges should be 85–180 mg/dL. The hemoglobin minimum target is 7 g/dL, and transfusion should be initiated when levels fall below this level to avoid a decrease in oxygen-carrying capacity and potential ischemia.

Box 17.7 Therapeutic Target Ranges for Physiologic Parameters in Pediatric Patients [29]

- ICP: <20 mm Hg
- CPP: 40–50 mm Hg (based on age)
- SpO_2: 90–100 mm Hg
- $PaCO_2$: 35–40 mm Hg
- Temperature (normothermia): 35.5–37.7 °C
- CVP: 4–10 mm Hg
- Glucose: 85–160 mg/dL
- Hemoglobin: >7 g/dL

Consensus and Guidelines-Based Algorithm for First- and Second-Tier Therapies to Manage Elevated Intracranial Hypertension [24]

Tier 1

Tier 1 comprises four pathways: herniation, ICP control, CPP control, and brain oxygenation. Ideally, all four pathways should be monitored concurrently with efforts made to optimize each (*see* Fig. 17.1, Box 17.8).

Herniation Pathway

Practitioners should be familiar with the signs of the various herniation syndromes (*see* Table 17.6). Such familiarity enables quick action to temporize the patient and, if possible, to reverse the process until definitive interventions can be undertaken. Hallmark signs include pupillary dilation, hypertension, bradycardia, and new extensor posturing. New cranial imaging is necessary to evaluate for new or expanding surgical lesions. While the patient is being prepared for imaging, interventions should be undertaken to reverse herniation, if possible. These interventions include CSF drainage, hyperventilation

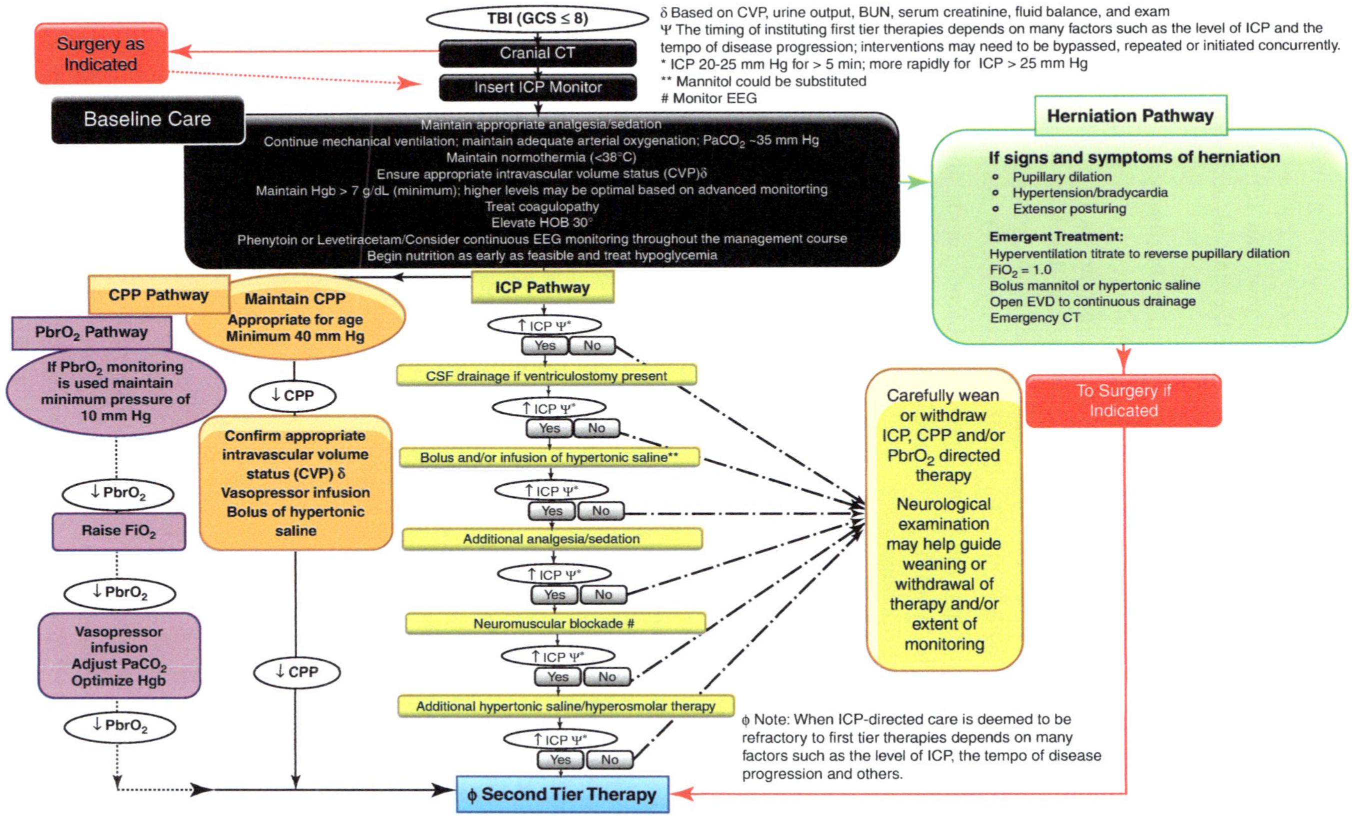

Fig. 17.1 Treatment algorithm for first-tier therapies to manage severe traumatic brain injury (TBI) in infants, children, and adolescents showing baseline care (*black*), intracranial pressure (ICP) pathway (*yellow*), herniation pathway (*green*), cerebral perfusion pressure (CPP) pathway (*orange*), and brain tissue partial pressure of oxygen ($PbrO_2$) pathway (*pink*). Solid lines represent the ICP and CPP pathways, reflecting their primary roles. Dotted lines represents the $PbrO_2$ pathway. Dotted and dashed line represents the weaning or withdrawal of various interventions. Although a linear approach is presented, variations in timing and combinations of pathways depend on the clinical context. The blue box represents refractory intracranial hypertension and the need for progression to second-tier therapy (*see* Fig. 17.2) *Used with permission from Wolters Kluwer Health Inc., Kochanek PM, Tasker RC, Bell MJ*, et al. *Management of pediatric severe traumatic brain injury: 2019 consensus and guidelines-based algorithm for first and second tier therapies. Pediatric Critical Care Medicine 2019;20(3):269–279.* https://journals.lww.com/pccmjournal/Fulltext/2019/03000/Management_of_Pediatric_Severe_Traumatic_Brain.8.aspx. *BUN* blood urea nitrogen, *CSF* cerebrospinal fluid, *CT* computed tomography, *CVP* central venous pressure, *EEG* electroencephalogram, *EVD* external ventricular drain, FiO_2 fraction of inspired oxygen, *GCS* Glasgow Coma Scale, *Hgb* hemoglobin, *HOB* head of bed, $PaCO_2$ partial pressure of carbon dioxide

with 100% FiO_2, and a bolus of hyperosmolar fluids.

Options for hyperosmolar therapy include boluses of mannitol (0.5–1.0 g/kg over 10 min) and 23.4% hypertonic saline (0.5 mL/kg, for a maximum dose of 30 mL). Of note, no evidence shows the superiority of either therapy for reversal of herniation.

An EVD is considered the first-line therapy for CSF drainage because it allows concurrent monitoring of ICP. Published reports describe lumbar drain placement and drainage when imaging shows open basal cisterns and a lack of significant mass or midline shift [31, 32]. Caution should be taken with the use of this modality because it can be troublesome and even dangerous in patients when the head of the bed has to be elevated. Excessive drainage, either intentional or inadvertent, can potentiate herniation.

ICP and CPP Pathways

ICP should be maintained below 20 mm Hg, with a need for intervention when an increase is sustained for 5 min. The CPP target should be 40–50 mm Hg (see Box 17.6 for targets by age), with infants at the lower end and adolescents at the upper end of the range.

Because MAP plays a direct role in ICP and CPP, blood pressure should be optimized. This optimization should be performed first by ensuring normovolemia before using vasopressors.

Although the ICP and CPP pathways are inherently correlated, different interventions can have mixed effects on each pathway. Part of the argument for multimodal monitoring is that different treatments might be applied in different physiologic milieus. For example, hypertonic saline administration will decrease ICP and improve CPP, but excessive fluid overload will drive up MAP and may have a detrimental effect. This effect can be particularly problematic in a patient who has luxury perfusion or vasogenic edema. In these instances, one might try mild hyperventilation rather than hypertonic saline, but this approach requires brain oxygen monitoring to check for ischemia. Sedation with fentanyl and barbiturates will decrease ICP, but it will also decrease CPP through cardiac suppression, also putting the patient at risk for ischemia.

Permissive intracranial hypertension is an alternative to initiation of the second-tier therapies that involves allowing mild intracranial hypertension (20–25 mm Hg) as long as CPP is maintained. Herniation can still occur if ICP is markedly elevated, even with adequate CPP.

Brain Oxygenation Pathway

Brain tissue partial pressure of oxygen ($PbrO_2$) should be maintained above 10 mm Hg [33, 34]. Any decrease below this level should prompt interventions, such as increasing the FiO_2, raising MAP, increasing $PaCO_2$ (to increase CBF), and optimizing blood hemoglobin to increase oxygen-carrying capacity.

Tier 2

Failure to control and adequately maintain ICP, CPP, and brain oxygenation should prompt progression to second-tier therapies (*see* Fig. 17.2, Box 17.8).

Repeat Imaging

If the patient is stable, additional cranial imaging should be considered to rule out new or expanded lesions that could be treated surgically. Some centers use portable CT scanners to limit the risks and time constraints of patient transport. New surgical lesions should be addressed operatively; otherwise, patients should continue with escalated medical management. Options for medical management include barbiturate infusion, moderate hypothermia, hyperventilation, advanced levels of hyperosmolar therapy, and advanced neuromonitoring.

Barbiturate Infusion

Dosing of the barbiturate pentobarbital should be 2–4 mg/kg/h, titrated to burst suppression, with the patient monitored by EEG. Pentobarbital suppresses $CMRO_2$ and alters vascular tone [35–38]. Its mechanism of action results in improved coupling of regional blood flow to metabolic demand, which increases brain oxygenation with

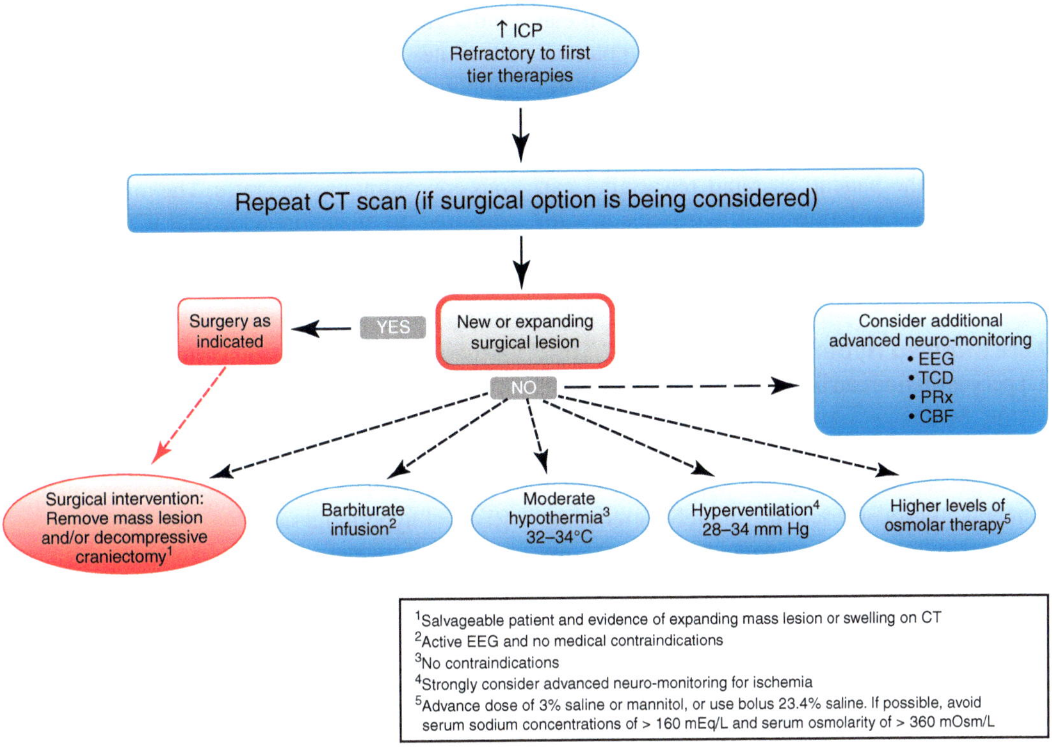

Fig. 17.2 Treatment algorithm for second-tier therapies to manage severe traumatic brain injury in infants, children, and adolescents. This second-tier therapy algorithm is linked to the first-tier therapy algorithm (*see* Fig. 17.1) and represents treatment options when tier 1 management is inadequate. These therapies can be applied alone, serially, or in combination. *Used with permission from Wolters Kluwer Health Inc., Kochanek PM, Tasker RC, Bell MJ,* et al. *Management of pediatric severe traumatic brain injury: 2019 consensus and guidelines-based algorithm for first and second tier therapies. Pediatric Critical Care Medicine 2019;20(3):269–279.* https://journals.lww.com/pccmjournal/Fulltext/2019/03000/Management_of_Pediatric_Severe_Traumatic_Brain.8.aspx. *CBF* cerebral blood flow, *CT* computed tomography, *EEG* electroencephalogram, *ICP* intracranial pressure, *PRx* pressure reactivity index, *TCD* transcranial Doppler ultrasonography

lower CBF and cerebral blood volume (CBV), that in turn results in decreased ICP. The $CMRO_2$ can be reduced by approximately 50%; any further reduction requires hypothermia.

Risks of this therapy include hypotension and hemodynamic compromise resulting in decreased CBF. Thus, close monitoring of volume status is required, including of CVP, arterial blood pressure, and MAP. Patients in a barbiturate coma often require vasopressors to maintain adequate CPP.

Late Moderate Hypothermia

Therapeutic hypothermia (<35 °C) has long been an area of investigation because of its role in decreasing cerebral metabolic demands, inflammation, lipid peroxidation, excitotoxicity, cell death, and acute seizures [39, 40]. Unfortunately, studies have failed to show further meaningful translation of prophylactic hypothermia to clinical benefit, with potential adverse effects including hypotension, pressor requirements, and poor outcomes [41–43].

Hypothermia decreases ICP in the short-term, but it does not provide a long-term benefit for control of ICP. These findings suggest a potential use in early refractory cases after the use of definitive interventions such as CSF drainage and decompression [41, 43, 44].

Although early or prophylactic hypothermia is not recommended over normothermia to improve overall outcomes [29], late moderate hypothermia can be applied in refractory cases. The target temperature is 34–35 °C [45], which can provide some neuroprotection with less potential for increased risk. Concurrent paralytics should be used to prevent shivering, which can elevate ICP. Special care should be observed when rewarming the patient, as rapid rewarming can result in rebound intracranial hypertension with adverse outcomes [46]. The suggested rewarming rate is 1 °C every 12–24 h [42].

Late Induced Hyperventilation

Hyperventilation can be considered in the delayed setting as a temporizing measure for reversal of herniation syndromes until more definitive interventions can be undertaken. Hypocapnia drives cerebral vasoconstriction, thereby reducing CBF and CBV and improving ICP. Despite the improvement in ICP, the decrease in CBF may lead to hypoperfusion and ischemia [12, 47]. When hyperventilation is used for a sustained period, brain oxygenation monitoring should be conducted to limit potential cerebral ischemia [13]. Maximal cerebral vasoconstriction is achieved at a $PaCO_2$ of 20 mm Hg, so hyperventilation below this level is ineffective and may result in hypotension, which will worsen cerebral hypoperfusion. Normal ranges for $PaCO_2$ are 35–45 mm Hg and should be decreased to 28–34 mm Hg when inducing late hyperventilation.

Hyperosmolar Therapy

Although mannitol is still used as a hyperosmolar therapy in the acute setting, most centers use hypertonic saline, which can be bolused and titrated to the required effect through continuous infusion. With either or both modalities, both sodium levels and osmolarity must be monitored. Target ranges for hyperosmolar therapy are a sodium level of 155–160 mmol/L and osmolarity of 320–340 mOsm/L [48, 49].

Since no hyperosmolar therapy is clearly superior, many centers use both mannitol and hypertonic saline concurrently because of the variations in their mechanisms of action. Compared to mannitol, hypertonic saline increases intravascular volume, whereas mannitol increases intravascular volume only transiently and can have a potent diuretic effect. Additionally, as mannitol pulls free water into the systemic circulation, it dilutes the sodium concentration. Thus, it is important to monitor both osmolarity and sodium concentrations.

Hypertonic saline can be administered in various concentrations and rates. The minimum dose required to maintain adequate ICP should be used. The mechanism relies on creating a concentration gradient across the blood-brain barrier to draw free water into the systemic circulation. A particular benefit of hypertonic saline is that it will maintain or increase intravascular volume, which is important because low-volume status increases the risk of hypoperfusion in a brain with possibly compromised autoregulation. Risks of hypertonic saline therapy include severe hypertonicity, defined as >170 mmol/L for longer than 72 h, which may lead to thrombocytopenia, deep vein thrombosis, renal failure, neutropenia, and acute respiratory distress syndrome [48].

Mannitol has different effects based on its two different mechanisms of action [50]. The initial effect is mediated through an immediate reduction in blood viscosity that lasts approximately 75 min. When autoregulation is intact, viscosity-mediated reflex vasoconstriction maintains a constant level of CBF and results in a reduction of CBV and ICP. Secondarily, mannitol acts through an osmotic mechanism, similar to that of hypertonic saline. The increase in osmolarity creates a concentration gradient, pulling free water into the systemic circulation. The onset is slightly slower, taking 15–30 min to have an effect, but it lasts as long as 6 h. Mannitol's reliance on an intact blood-brain barrier creates a risk of accumulation in injured areas of the brain, causing a paradoxical reversal in osmotic shift and increased focal swelling. This phenomenon may occur with prolonged administration of mannitol [51].

Mannitol is cleared renally via osmotic diuresis and elimination of free water, which requires urine output monitoring. When the patient has no urine response, a paradoxical decrease in sodium and osmolality can occur through intravascular dilution. The risk of renal failure increases with serum osmolality levels greater than 320 mOsm/L. The dosing and timing of mannitol administration can vary, with a bolus of 0.5–1.0 g/kg generally used for herniation reversal. Intermittent dosing of 0.25–1.0 g/kg every 6 h can be used to maintain ICP control.

Box 17.8 Therapeutic Targets and Dosing for Tier 1 and Tier 2

- ICP: <20 mm Hg
- CPP: 40–50 mm Hg (see Box 17.6 for targets by age)
- $PbrO_2$: >10 mm Hg
- Pentobarbital: 2–4 mg/kg/h (titrated to burst suppression)
- Late moderate hypothermia: 34–35 °C
- Rewarming: 1 °C every 12–24 h
- Normal $PaCO_2$: 35–45 mm Hg
- Hyperventilation $PaCO_2$: 28–34 mm Hg
- Sodium: 155–160 mmol/L
- Osmolarity: 320–340 mOsm/L
- Hypertonic saline (3%) bolus: 2–5 mL/kg (max 250 mL)
- Hypertonic saline (3%) infusion: 0.1–1.0 mL/kg/h
- Hypertonic saline (23.4%) bolus: 0.5 mL/kg (max 30 mL)
- Mannitol bolus: 0.5–1.0 g/kg (over 10 min)
- Intermittent mannitol: 0.25–1.0 g/kg (every 6 h)

Advanced Neuromonitoring

The following alternative methods of monitoring should be considered to optimize ICP, CPP, and $PbrO_2$ or to evaluate for underlying processes contributing to a refractory response to treatment or poor examination findings.

- Continuous EEG: This monitoring may be used to identify whether subclinical seizures are contributing to poor examination results or intracranial hypertension and to help titrate the dose of barbiturates.
- Transcranial Doppler and CBF velocity: Because subarachnoid hemorrhage is common after TBI, transcranial Doppler may help identify areas of regional ischemia due to vasospasm or autoregulatory dysfunction.
- Pressure reactivity index: This measure uses the ICP-to-blood pressure cross-correlation coefficient to help identify an optimal CPP level, depending on the patient's ability to autoregulate. Monitoring may help prevent cerebral hyperemia or ischemia. Although this measure provides a global assessment, the status of autoregulation may be regionally dependent.
- $PbrO_2$: Monitoring brain tissue oxygenation may help identify whether hyperventilation or autoregulation failure is producing ischemia.

Surgical Decompression

Surgical decompression is indicated for refractory ICP after tier 1 and tier 2 therapies have been exhausted. High-quality reports in the medical literature about surgical decompression in pediatric patients with TBIs and refractory ICPs are limited, but most findings have paralleled those of adults, with decompressive craniectomy resulting in lower mortality but higher rates of vegetative state [52–54].

Weaning of Therapies

When all monitored values have been normalized and stable for 12–24 h, interventions should be withdrawn in the reverse order of application.

Postacute Pathology

Posttraumatic Seizures and Anticonvulsants

PTS may precipitate adverse secondary events in the injured brain with elevations in ICP and blood pressure, as well as changes in oxygen delivery and metabolism. Younger children in particular have lower seizure thresholds [55], putting them at higher risk for PTS. EEG monitoring of young children should be considered to evaluate for subclinical seizures. Early PTS occurs at the time of injury or within 7 days and represents mechanisms of the primary injury that lower the seizure threshold. Late PTS occurs more than 7 days after injury and is related to neurobiological changes arising from secondary brain injury. Patients experiencing PTS have an increased risk of developing posttraumatic epilepsy [56], which is defined as recurrent seizures persisting past 7 days after an injury. The incidence of PTS in patients with TBI ranges from 12 to 19%, with infants having a 70 to 80% risk. PTS in infants may also be subclinical. Patients with suspected PTS should be monitored by EEG [57–60].

Risk Factors

The risk factors for PTS vary widely. Risk factors include the location of lesions (temporal and frontal lobes), cerebellar contusions, retained bone and metal fragments, depressed skull fractures, focal neurologic deficits, loss of consciousness, length of posttraumatic amnesia, EDH or SDH, penetrating injury, and younger age [55, 59, 61, 62].

Prophylaxis

Because of the high incidence of PTS in pediatric patients after a TBI, the prophylactic administration of anticonvulsants should be considered to prevent derangements in acute physiology and the development of chronic epilepsy. Studies have shown that treatment with prophylactic anticonvulsants can help prevent early PTS from progressing to late PTS and chronic PTS but with no benefit to prophylactic treatment beyond 7 days after a TBI [56].

Medication Options

The choice of prophylactic anticonvulsant should balance the protective and prophylactic efficacy of the medications against their adverse effects. Good options include levetiracetam (10 mg/kg every 12 h) and fosphenytoin (15 mg/kg loading dose followed by maintenance dosing of 2 mg/kg every 8 h). Historically, phenytoin has been used, but it requires hemodynamic monitoring during administration.

Continuous EEG

Continuous EEG should be considered when the patient's mental status is not explained by other factors (i.e., metabolic, ICP, infection) to evaluate for nonconvulsive seizures.

Temperature Management

Fever/Hyperthermia/Pyrexia

Maintenance of normothermia and avoidance of hyperthermia are important in the postacute setting to prevent poor outcomes [63, 64]. Hyperthermia, defined as >38 °C, should prompt investigation for another underlying pathology before being labeled neurogenic.

Meningitis

Although fever is usually the earliest sign of meningitis, this is not always the case. Early fever after TBI (>38.5 °C within 24 h) can be a result of dysautonomia related to the severity of the injury and can be expected particularly in patients with subarachnoid hemorrhage [64]. A fever higher than 39 °C should heighten concern for meningitis, especially in patients with concurrent skull fractures.

Extracranial causes of fever, such as chest infection, fat embolism, and wound infection, should be considered and investigated. Many patients with TBI may also have other bodily injuries that can precipitate infection and fever.

Before antibiotic treatment is initiated, cultures should be obtained to select the appropriate targeted treatment. Empiric treatment should cover streptococcus and staphylococcus. Normothermia should be maintained as needed with acetaminophen, hydration, and cooling blankets.

Malignant Cerebral Edema

Global or regional edema after TBI can progress to, or even present in, a delayed fashion. This process is driven by cytotoxic injury in response to traumatic blood and direct tissue injury. Additionally, vasogenic edema can develop as a loss of vascular autoregulation leads to hyperemia and subsequent mismatch of metabolism and CBF [65, 66]. As Jha et al. [67] noted in their review, some studies have shown an increased likelihood of vasogenic edema with subarachnoid hemorrhage. Treatment follows the same algorithm as that for elevated ICP. However, the use of the pressure reactivity index may help identify the optimal CPP for the current state of autoregulation.

Corticosteroids

Corticosteroids have been investigated for use in patients with TBI because of their ability to alter vascular permeability, decrease edema and CSF production, and reduce the production of free radicals [68–70]. However, few quality trials have evaluated the use of corticosteroids in children. The risks likely parallel those in the adult population, with increased rates of ventilator-associated pneumonia, longer ventilator dependence, and increased mortality [71, 72]. The use of corticosteroids is not suggested as a way to improve outcomes or reduce ICP. Children with known primary or secondary adrenal insufficiency should receive corticosteroid replacement therapy to avoid acute adrenal insufficiency [29].

Posttraumatic Hydrocephalus

Posttraumatic hydrocephalus develops as a form of communicating hydrocephalus, with patients usually presenting in the postacute stage of their hospitalization [9, 73, 74]. Proposed mechanisms include impaired CSF absorption at the arachnoid villi because of blood and other inflammatory agents, skull fractures with resultant meningitis, and decreased CSF outflow from increased dural sinus pressure. Treatment requires ventricular shunting.

Hypothalamic-Pituitary Dysfunction

During TBI, the hypothalamus, pituitary, and sellar anatomy are at risk either from direct injury (fracture lines may track down the skull base and through the sella turcica) and shear injury or from swelling and edema that compress the small hypophyseal vessels, resulting in ischemia. Injury to these regions with TBI can result in endocrinopathies with alterations leading to suboptimal hormonal regulation, particularly with cortisol and water homeostasis or later hypothalamic-pituitary-adrenal axis dysfunction [75, 76].

Cortisol

Patients with TBI should be monitored closely for adrenal insufficiency, which can be life-threatening. Signs of insufficiency include hypotension, hyponatremia, and hypoglycemia. These signs can be difficult to evaluate in posttraumatic patients concurrently receiving hyperosmolar therapy and blood pressure support.

Low basal cortisol levels, with subnormal responses to stress testing, should also raise concern for adrenal insufficiency. Patients with basal cortisol concentrations below 200 nmol/L should receive supplementation with hydrocortisone. In patients with levels of 200–400 nmol/L, replacement should be considered if their symptoms appear related to adrenal insufficiency.

Water Homeostasis

Posterior pituitary dysfunction can lead to failure in water homeostasis, resulting in either cranial (central) diabetes insipidus or syndrome of inappropriate antidiuretic hormone (SIADH). Posttraumatic patients may also experience cerebral salt wasting (CSW), so the patient's volume status should be evaluated carefully to differentiate CSW from SIADH and guide appropriate treatment. In most cases, water balance issues are usually transient and resolve within days to weeks after injury [75, 76].

Hyponatremia: SIADH vs CSW

Patients with SIADH or CSW will present with hyponatremia (serum sodium <130 mmol/L). The key differentiating factor is the patient's volume status. Hyponatremia is detrimental because it exacerbates cerebral swelling, elevates ICP, and may potentiate seizures.

SIADH results from the inappropriate and excessive release of antidiuretic hormone (vasopressin) from the hypothalamus. The excess vasopressin results in retained free water in the renal system, producing a diluting effect on systemic sodium concentrations and elevating volume status. Treatment consists of fluid restriction in the conscious patient and vaptans in the comatose patient.

CSW results from the inappropriate and excessive release of natriuretic peptides, leading to primary natriuresis and subsequent volume depletion. A secondary hormonal response occurs in the renin-angiotensin and arginine-vasopressin system. The overall effect results in hyponatremia (<135 mmol/L), brisk diuresis (>3 mL/kg/h), elevated urine sodium (>120 mmol/L), or elevated urine osmolality (>300 mOsm/L). The patient's volume status will be low, and treatment consists of volume and sodium replacement.

Hypernatremia: Diabetes Insipidus

The mechanism causing diabetes insipidus is the opposite of the mechanism causing SIADH. Hypothalamic or posterior pituitary injury results in the decreased release of the antidiuretic hormone, resulting in excessive loss of free water at the level of the kidneys. Patients develop hypernatremia and brisk dilute urine production. Treatment in the conscious patient involves drinking to thirst. In the comatose patient, hypotonic fluids or desmopressin can be used.

Other Hormones

The assessment of growth hormone, gonadal, and thyroid axes is not necessary during the acute phase, as no evidence suggests that replacement of these hormones in the deficient patient improves outcomes. However, the endocrine axes should be assessed in the post-ICU period at 3, 6, and 12 months after injury because abnormalities may persist in up to 25% of patients [77–81].

Venous Thromboembolism Prophylaxis

Venous thromboembolism is a concern in the posttraumatic pediatric patient, although it is less common in children than adults. Risk factors include older age, venous catheterization, non-accidental trauma, increased length of hospital stay, infection, orthopedic surgery, and cranial surgery [82]. The use and timing of pharmacologic prophylaxis must be balanced against the potential risk of expanded intracranial hemorrhage. One study showed increased efficacy of low-molecular-weight heparin compared to unfractionated heparin [83].

Nutrition

After TBI, an increase in metabolism requires increased caloric supply to support recovery. Particularly, pediatric patients already have high nutritional needs for their normal growth and development [84, 85]. Enteral nutrition is preferred over parenteral sources whenever possible because of the increased rates of infection and prolonged lengths of stay associated with parenteral nutrition [86]. Nutritional support should be initiated within 72 h after injury, with the goal of full nutritional replacement by day 7 [87]. No evidence supports the use of an immune-modulating diet [29]. No clinical benefit has been shown for tightly controlled glucose concentrations, which carry a risk of severe hypoglycemia and have been associated with harm to recovery [88, 89]. The recommended glucose range is 150–180 mg/day.

Fluids

The use of hypotonic (low-sodium) crystalloids has been associated with increased morbidity and mortality in children with TBI [90]. Conversely, the prolonged administration of hypertonic fluids should be used with caution, as they can lead to hyperchloremia and acidosis. Glucose-containing fluids can be considered in young children, for whom avoidance of severe hypoglycemia is necessary (Box 17.9).

Box 17.9 Maintenance Fluid Rate

4-2-1 Rule

- First 10 kg of weight: 4 mL/kg/h
- Second 10 kg of weight: Add 2 mL/kg/h
- Each kg >20 kg of weight: 1 mL/kg/h

Surgical Management of Pediatric Neurotrauma

Preoperative Considerations

Treatment of coagulopathy should be performed before inserting intracranial monitors or performing other operative interventions. At an international normalized ratio (INR) of ≤1.6, bleeding complications are infrequent with intracranial monitors, and the use of fresh-frozen plasma to reduce INR below this level is not recommended [91]. For craniotomy or craniectomy, treatment of coagulopathy should ideally address active bleeding and be titrated to thromboelastometry. Over-resuscitating with plasma to normalize INR may actually worsen coagulopathy, producing fibrinolysis shutdown and poor outcomes [92, 93]. Coagulation factor goals are shown in Box 17.10.

Box 17.10 Coagulation Factor Goals

- INR: 1.2
- Platelets: 100,000 per mcL
- Partial thromboplastin time: >36 s

Anesthesia Considerations

The endotracheal tube should be secured appropriately because manipulation of the head during surgery may dislodge it from optimal placement. Smooth induction of anesthesia is critical to prevent any physiologic responses that may increase ICP. Blood pressure should also be optimized to prevent increased ICP and bleeding during surgery. Adequate intravenous access should be placed before surgery in preparation for possible transfusion. Preoperative mannitol or hypertonic saline administration should be considered, especially in patients with diffuse posttraumatic edema.

Surgical Preparation

During positioning, the head of the patient should be elevated to promote venous return, and spinal precautions should be observed. Planning the surgical incision requires consideration of possible open fontanels and suture lines.

Intraoperative Considerations

Tissue should be handled as delicately as possible because of the thinner and more friable nature of the pediatric scalp, especially in infants. Meticulous hemostasis is essential at all points during surgery because pediatric patients have less total blood volume and cannot tolerate the volume of blood loss typical of an adult patient (Box 17.11).

Box 17.11 Estimated Total Blood Volume by Age

- Premature infant: 100 mL/kg
- Full-term infant: 80 mL/kg
- 1–12 months old: 75 mL/kg
- >1 year old: 70 mL/kg

The use of subgaleal drains varies and largely depends on the preference of the surgeon. With appropriate hemostasis at the time of closure, drains generally do not have to stay in longer than 24 h after surgery, and output beyond this time likely represents CSF rather than postoperative bleeding.

Decompressive Craniectomy

Removal of a large bone flap may be indicated in cases of persistent swelling after mass lesion evacuation or after failure of tiered medical therapies for refractory intracranial hypertension. Care should be taken to preserve the pericranium when opening for potential use in sealing off violated sinuses, although these may be undeveloped in the young child. Techniques vary and again depend on the particular pathology and surgeon preference. Bone may be removed either unilaterally or bilaterally, with or without subtemporal decompression. Dural management also varies, ranging from no manipulation to simple scoring to wide opening with expansile or onlay duraplasty.

Most commonly, the craniectomy bone flap is stored in a freezer for future replacement. However, a subcutaneous abdominal pocket is an option if a freezer is not available or if the patient will require cranioplasty at another medical location and there is not an appropriate method for the transportation of biologic materials. Of note, abdominal pocket storage can be difficult in smaller children.

Cranial Reconstruction

The timing of cranioplasty is variable. It can be performed at any time after swelling and ICP have normalized enough to facilitate easy replacement. An autologous bone flap is preferable, but alternatives include other autologous sources (contralateral split-thickness, rib) as well as synthetic materials such as titanium mesh or custom-printed implants [94].

Nonoperative Skull Fractures

Closed fractures can be managed conservatively unless a significant deformity is present. In pediatric patients, CSF pulsations will often remodel the fracture and push the deformity back out. Patients should still be followed for the potential development of a leptomeningeal cyst ("growing skull fracture"), which results from dural laceration and herniation of leptomeninges and brain parenchyma. Over time, CSF pulsations can force continued herniation, resulting in growth and nonunion of the fracture.

Open fractures, if nonoperative, should be thoroughly cleaned and closed. Patients with wounds without concern for significant contamination should receive only a short course of oral prophylactic antibiotics (first-generation cephalosporin for 1–3 days). Grossly contaminated wounds, including animal bites, warrant broader and longer antibiotic coverage.

Prognostication

Prognostication in pediatric patients with TBI is difficult because high-quality evidence is lacking. Among several image grading systems, the Marshall CT classification has been shown to correlate with Glasgow Outcome Scale scores and has been validated in the pediatric population [95]. The Marshall CT classification is based on criteria of midline shift, patency of basal cisterns, and presence of high or mixed density lesions (contusions and hemorrhages) (*see* Table 17.7) [96].

Table 17.7 Marshall CT classification[a]

Classification	Characteristic(s)
I: Diffuse injury (no visible pathology)	• No visible intracranial pathology
II: Diffuse injury	• Midline shift: 0–5 mm • Basal cisterns: remain visible • High or mixed density lesions: <25 cm^3
III: Diffuse injury (swelling)	• Midline shift: 0–5 mm • Basal cisterns: compressed or completely effaced • High or mixed density lesions: >25 cm^3
IV: Diffuse injury (shift)	• Midline shift: >5 mm • Basal cisterns: compressed or effaced • High or mixed density lesions: >25 cm^3
V: Evacuated mass lesion	• Any lesion evacuated surgically
VI: Nonevacuated mass lesion	• High or mixed density lesions: >25 cm^3 • Not surgically evacuated

Abbreviation: *CT* computed tomography
[a]Data source: Maas et al. [96]

Managing Discussions

Because prognosis in children is often difficult, any discussions of fatality, prognostication, and withdrawal of care should be carried out using a multidisciplinary approach. The neurosurgical staff, intensivists, trauma staff, and religious and/or spiritual counselors, as indicated by family beliefs, should all be involved.

Lethal and Fatal Injuries

Unfortunately, in some instances, a child sustains a lethal head injury, and the intensive intervention and care previously described in this chapter are not appropriate. The injury patterns in these patients are similar to those seen in fatal adult injuries [97]. A postresuscitated child with a GCS score of 3 and bilateral fixed and dilated pupils (not due to medication) fits into this category. The protocols and methods by which trauma care providers assess and determine these cases are usually established by regional and local health systems. They generally include formal brain death testing and may include adjuvant testing, such as perfusion scans, CT angiograms, and EEG.

Long-Term Sequelae and Outcomes

Long-term outcomes for pediatric TBI patients are still not well understood and vary by population. Previous studies have been small and of limited quality. The recently concluded Approaches and Decisions for Acute Pediatric TBI Trial (ADAPT) may provide further insight into management and outcome. This significant public health issue for the pediatric population clearly requires improved study and resources to further improve outcomes.

Example Practice Questions

Questions:

1. Which of the following represents a potential primary mechanism of injury for TBI?
   (a) Apoptosis
   (b) Excitotoxicity
   (c) Hypoxia
   (d) Motor vehicle collision
2. Which of the following represents a secondary insult for TBI?
   (a) Apoptosis
   (b) Excitotoxicity
   (c) Hypoxia
   (d) Motor vehicle collision
3. Which of the following represents a secondary mechanism of injury for TBI?
   (a) Hypotension
   (b) Excitotoxicity
   (c) Hypoxia
   (d) Motor vehicle collision
4. According to the Pediatric Guidelines, ICP monitoring is indicated for patients with:
   (a) A GCS score of 3–8
   (b) Mild-to-moderate TBI in a conscious patient with a mass lesion
   (c) Both
   (d) Neither

5. According to the Pediatric Guidelines, hyperventilation ($PaCO_2 < 30$ mm Hg) is indicated for patients after severe TBI:
   (a) Prophylactically during the first 24 h
   (b) For brief periods after neurologic deterioration
   (c) Both
   (d) Neither
6. According to the Pediatric Guidelines, patients with intracranial hypertension can be treated with hypertonic saline:
   (a) Initially, with a load of 25 mg/kg and then up to 100 mg/kg every 4–6 h
   (b) Initially with a load of 0.25 mg/kg and then up to 1.0 mg/kg every 4–6 h
   (c) For a serum osmolality of up to 315–320 mOsm/L
   (d) For a serum osmolality of up to 355–360 mOsm/L
7. According to the literature, moderate hypothermia for 24 or 48 h in pediatric patients with severe TBI:
   (a) Is indicated as a first-tier therapy
   (b) Has a lower mortality but higher morbidity
   (c) Is not indicated as a way to lower mortality
   (d) Has a higher mortality but lower morbidity

Answers

1. d
2. c
3. b
4. c
5. b
6. d
7. c

Acknowledgments We thank the staff of Neuroscience Publications at Barrow Neurological Institute for assistance with manuscript preparation.

Disclosures Dr. Adelson is a consultant for Medtronic, PLC. No other authors have any conflicts of interest for this work.

Financial Support None.

References

1. Dewan MC, Mummareddy N, Wellons JC 3rd, Bonfield CM. Epidemiology of global pediatric traumatic brain injury: qualitative review. World Neurosurg. 2016;91:497–509.e491. https://doi.org/10.1016/j.wneu.2016.03.045.
2. Gaither JB, Spaite DW, Bobrow BJ, Keim SM, Barnhart BJ, Chikani V, Sherrill D, Denninghoff KR, Mullins T, Adelson PD, Rice AD, Viscusi C, Hu C. Effect of implementing the out-of-hospital traumatic brain injury treatment guidelines: the Excellence in Prehospital Injury Care for Children Study (EPIC4Kids). Ann Emerg Med. 2021;77(2):139–53. https://doi.org/10.1016/j.annemergmed.2020.09.435.
3. Teasdale G, Jennett B. Assessment of coma and impaired consciousness. A practical scale. Lancet. 1974;2(7872):81–4. https://doi.org/10.1016/s0140-6736(74)91639-0.
4. Durham SR, Clancy RR, Leuthardt E, Sun P, Kamerling S, Dominguez T, Duhaime AC. CHOP Infant Coma Scale ("Infant Face Scale"): a novel coma scale for children less than two years of age. J Neurotrauma. 2000;17(9):729–37. https://doi.org/10.1089/neu.2000.17.729.
5. Gregers MCT, Mikkelsen S, Lindvig KP, Brøchner AC. Ketamine as an anesthetic for patients with acute brain injury: a systematic review. Neurocrit Care. 2020;33(1):273–82. https://doi.org/10.1007/s12028-020-00975-7.
6. Hemphill S, McMenamin L, Bellamy MC, Hopkins PM. Propofol infusion syndrome: a structured literature review and analysis of published case reports. Br J Anaesth. 2019;122(4):448–59. https://doi.org/10.1016/j.bja.2018.12.025.
7. Nazir S, O'Brien M, Qureshi NH, Slape L, Green TJ, Phillips PH. Sensitivity of papilledema as a sign of shunt failure in children. J AAPOS. 2009;13(1):63–6. https://doi.org/10.1016/j.jaapos.2008.08.003.
8. Parslow RC, Morris KP, Tasker RC, Forsyth RJ, Hawley CA. Epidemiology of traumatic brain injury in children receiving intensive care in the UK. Arch Dis Child. 2005;90(11):1182–7. https://doi.org/10.1136/adc.2005.072405.
9. Adams JH, Doyle D, Ford I, Gennarelli TA, Graham DI, McLellan DR. Diffuse axonal injury in head injury: definition, diagnosis and grading. Histopathology. 1989;15(1):49–59. https://doi.org/10.1111/j.1365-2559.1989.tb03040.x.
10. Centers for Disease Control and Prevention. HEADS UP: responding to a concussion and action plan. 2019. https://www.cdc.gov/headsup/basics/concussion_respondingto.html. Accessed 1 Dec 2021.
11. Venkatasubramanian C, Mlynash M, Finley-Caulfield A, Eyngorn I, Kalimuthu R, Snider RW, Wijman CA. Natural history of perihematomal edema after intracerebral hemorrhage measured by serial magnetic resonance imaging. Stroke. 2011;42(1):73–80. https://doi.org/10.1161/strokeaha.110.590646.

12. Adelson PD, Srinivas R, Chang Y, Bell M, Kochanek PM. Cerebrovascular response in children following severe traumatic brain injury. Childs Nerv Syst. 2011;27(9):1465–76. https://doi.org/10.1007/s00381-011-1476-z.
13. Adelson PD, Clyde B, Kochanek PM, Wisniewski SR, Marion DW, Yonas H. Cerebrovascular response in infants and young children following severe traumatic brain injury: a preliminary report. Pediatr Neurosurg. 1997;26(4):200–7. https://doi.org/10.1159/000121192.
14. Kochanek PM, Clark RS, Ruppel RA, Adelson PD, Bell MJ, Whalen MJ, Robertson CL, Satchell MA, Seidberg NA, Marion DW, Jenkins LW. Biochemical, cellular, and molecular mechanisms in the evolution of secondary damage after severe traumatic brain injury in infants and children: lessons learned from the bedside. Pediatr Crit Care Med. 2000;1(1):4–19. https://doi.org/10.1097/00130478-200007000-00003.
15. American College of Radiology. ACR appropriateness criteria head trauma: child. 2019. https://acsearch.acr.org/docs/3083021/Narrative/. Accessed 1 Dec 2021.
16. Gupta M, Mower WR, Rodriguez RM, Hendey GW. Validation of the pediatric NEXUS II head computed tomography decision instrument for selective imaging of pediatric patients with blunt head trauma. Acad Emerg Med. 2018;25(7):729–37. https://doi.org/10.1111/acem.13431.
17. Oman JA, Cooper RJ, Holmes JF, Viccellio P, Nyce A, Ross SE, Hoffman JR, Mower WR. Performance of a decision rule to predict need for computed tomography among children with blunt head trauma. Pediatrics. 2006;117(2):e238–46. https://doi.org/10.1542/peds.2005-1063.
18. Rivas JJ, Lobato RD, Sarabia R, Cordobés F, Cabrera A, Gomez P. Extradural hematoma: analysis of factors influencing the courses of 161 patients. Neurosurgery. 1988;23(1):44–51. https://doi.org/10.1227/00006123-198807000-00010.
19. Parri N, Crosby BJ, Mills L, Soucy Z, Musolino AM, Da Dalt L, Cirilli A, Grisotto L, Kuppermann N. Point-of-care ultrasound for the diagnosis of skull fractures in children younger than two years of age. J Pediatr. 2018;196:230–236.e2. https://doi.org/10.1016/j.jpeds.2017.12.057.
20. Rabiner JE, Friedman LM, Khine H, Avner JR, Tsung JW. Accuracy of point-of-care ultrasound for diagnosis of skull fractures in children. Pediatrics. 2013;131(6):e1757–64. https://doi.org/10.1542/peds.2012-3921.
21. Parri N, Crosby BJ, Glass C, Mannelli F, Sforzi I, Schiavone R, Ban KM. Ability of emergency ultrasonography to detect pediatric skull fractures: a prospective, observational study. J Emerg Med. 2013;44(1):135–41. https://doi.org/10.1016/j.jemermed.2012.02.038.
22. Weinberg ER, Tunik MG, Tsung JW. Accuracy of clinician-performed point-of-care ultrasound for the diagnosis of fractures in children and young adults. Injury. 2010;41(8):862–8. https://doi.org/10.1016/j.injury.2010.04.020.
23. Ravindra VM, Riva-Cambrin J, Sivakumar W, Metzger RR, Bollo RJ. Risk factors for traumatic blunt cerebrovascular injury diagnosed by computed tomography angiography in the pediatric population: a retrospective cohort study. J Neurosurg Pediatr. 2015;15(6):599–606. https://doi.org/10.3171/2014.11.Peds14397.
24. Kochanek PM, Tasker RC, Carney N, Totten AM, Adelson PD, Selden NR, Davis-O'Reilly C, Hart EL, Bell MJ, Bratton SL, Grant GA, Kissoon N, Reuter-Rice KE, Vavilala MS, Wainwright MS. Guidelines for the management of pediatric severe traumatic brain injury, third edition: update of the brain trauma foundation guidelines, executive summary. Neurosurgery. 2019;84(6):1169–78. https://doi.org/10.1093/neuros/nyz051.
25. Bell MJ, Adelson PD, Hutchison JS, Kochanek PM, Tasker RC, Vavilala MS, Beers SR, Fabio A, Kelsey SF, Wisniewski SR. Differences in medical therapy goals for children with severe traumatic brain injury-an international study. Pediatr Crit Care Med. 2013;14(8):811–8. https://doi.org/10.1097/PCC.0b013e3182975e2f.
26. Bell MJ, Adelson PD, Wisniewski SR. Challenges and opportunities for pediatric severe TBI-review of the evidence and exploring a way forward. Childs Nerv Syst. 2017;33(10):1663–7. https://doi.org/10.1007/s00381-017-3530-y.
27. Kurz JE, Poloyac SM, Abend NS, Fabio A, Bell MJ, Wainwright MS. Variation in anticonvulsant selection and electroencephalographic monitoring following severe traumatic brain injury in children-understanding resource availability in sites participating in a comparative effectiveness study. Pediatr Crit Care Med. 2016;17(7):649–57. https://doi.org/10.1097/pcc.0000000000000765.
28. Vavilala MS, Lee LA, Lam AM. The lower limit of cerebral autoregulation in children during sevoflurane anesthesia. J Neurosurg Anesthesiol. 2003;15(4):307–12. https://doi.org/10.1097/00008506-200310000-00003.
29. Kochanek PM, Tasker RC, Carney N, Totten AM, Adelson PD, Selden NR, Davis-O'Reilly C, Hart EL, Bell MJ, Bratton SL, Grant GA, Kissoon N, Reuter-Rice KE, Vavilala MS, Wainwright MS. Guidelines for the management of pediatric severe traumatic brain injury, third edition: update of the brain trauma foundation guidelines. Pediatr Crit Care Med. 2019;20(3S Suppl 1):S1–s82. https://doi.org/10.1097/pcc.0000000000001735.
30. Kapapa T, König K, Pfister U, Sasse M, Woischneck D, Heissler H, Rickels E. Head trauma in children, part 2: course and discharge with outcome. J Child Neurol. 2010;25(3):274–83. https://doi.org/10.1177/0883073809332699.
31. Tuettenberg J, Czabanka M, Horn P, Woitzik J, Barth M, Thomé C, Vajkoczy P, Schmiedek P, Muench E. Clinical evaluation of the safety and efficacy of lumbar cerebrospinal fluid drainage for the treatment of refractory increased intracranial pressure.

J Neurosurg. 2009;110(6):1200–8. https://doi.org/10.3171/2008.10.Jns08293.
32. Levy DI, Rekate HL, Cherny WB, Manwaring K, Moss SD, Baldwin HZ. Controlled lumbar drainage in pediatric head injury. J Neurosurg. 1995;83(3):453–60. https://doi.org/10.3171/jns.1995.83.3.0453.
33. Figaji AA, Zwane E, Graham Fieggen A, Argent AC, Le Roux PD, Peter JC. The effect of increased inspired fraction of oxygen on brain tissue oxygen tension in children with severe traumatic brain injury. Neurocrit Care. 2010;12(3):430–7. https://doi.org/10.1007/s12028-010-9344-3.
34. Figaji AA, Zwane E, Thompson C, Fieggen AG, Argent AC, Le Roux PD, Peter JC. Brain tissue oxygen tension monitoring in pediatric severe traumatic brain injury. Part 1: relationship with outcome. Childs Nerv Syst. 2009;25(10):1325–33. https://doi.org/10.1007/s00381-009-0822-x.
35. Chen HI, Malhotra NR, Oddo M, Heuer GG, Levine JM, LeRoux PD. Barbiturate infusion for intractable intracranial hypertension and its effect on brain oxygenation. Neurosurgery. 2008;63(5):880–886; discussion 886–7. https://doi.org/10.1227/01.Neu.0000327882.10629.06.
36. Piatt JH Jr, Schiff SJ. High dose barbiturate therapy in neurosurgery and intensive care. Neurosurgery. 1984;15(3):427–44. https://doi.org/10.1227/00006123-198409000-00023.
37. Kassell NF, Hitchon PW, Gerk MK, Sokoll MD, Hill TR. Alterations in cerebral blood flow, oxygen metabolism, and electrical activity produced by high dose sodium thiopental. Neurosurgery. 1980;7(6):598–603. https://doi.org/10.1227/00006123-198012000-00011.
38. Demopoulos HB, Flamm ES, Pietronigro DD, Seligman ML. The free radical pathology and the microcirculation in the major central nervous system disorders. Acta Physiol Scand Suppl. 1980;492:91–119.
39. Dietrich WD, Bramlett HM. The evidence for hypothermia as a neuroprotectant in traumatic brain injury. Neurotherapeutics. 2010;7(1):43–50. https://doi.org/10.1016/j.nurt.2009.10.015.
40. Polderman KH. Application of therapeutic hypothermia in the ICU: opportunities and pitfalls of a promising treatment modality. Part 1: indications and evidence. Intensive Care Med. 2004;30(4):556–75. https://doi.org/10.1007/s00134-003-2152-x.
41. Beca J, McSharry B, Erickson S, Yung M, Schibler A, Slater A, Wilkins B, Singhal A, Williams G, Sherring C, Butt W. Hypothermia for traumatic brain injury in children—a phase II randomized controlled trial. Crit Care Med. 2015;43(7):1458–66. https://doi.org/10.1097/ccm.0000000000000947.
42. Adelson PD, Wisniewski SR, Beca J, Brown SD, Bell M, Muizelaar JP, Okada P, Beers SR, Balasubramani GK, Hirtz D. Comparison of hypothermia and normothermia after severe traumatic brain injury in children (Cool Kids): a phase 3, randomised controlled trial. Lancet Neurol. 2013;12(6):546–53. https://doi.org/10.1016/s1474-4422(13)70077-2.
43. Adelson PD, Ragheb J, Kanev P, Brockmeyer D, Beers SR, Brown SD, Cassidy LD, Chang Y, Levin H. Phase II clinical trial of moderate hypothermia after severe traumatic brain injury in children. Neurosurgery. 2005;56(4):740–754; discussion 740–54. https://doi.org/10.1227/01.neu.0000156471.50726.26.
44. Hutchison JS, Ward RE, Lacroix J, Hébert PC, Barnes MA, Bohn DJ, Dirks PB, Doucette S, Fergusson D, Gottesman R, Joffe AR, Kirpalani HM, Meyer PG, Morris KP, Moher D, Singh RN, Skippen PW. Hypothermia therapy after traumatic brain injury in children. N Engl J Med. 2008;358(23):2447–56. https://doi.org/10.1056/NEJMoa0706930.
45. Stippler M, Ortiz V, Adelson PD, Chang YF, Tyler-Kabara EC, Wisniewski SR, Fink EL, Kochanek PM, Brown SD, Bell MJ. Brain tissue oxygen monitoring after severe traumatic brain injury in children: relationship to outcome and association with other clinical parameters. J Neurosurg Pediatr. 2012;10(5):383–91. https://doi.org/10.3171/2012.8.Peds12165.
46. Salonia R, Empey PE, Poloyac SM, Wisniewski SR, Klamerus M, Ozawa H, Wagner AK, Ruppel R, Bell MJ, Feldman K, Adelson PD, Clark RS, Kochanek PM. Endothelin-1 is increased in cerebrospinal fluid and associated with unfavorable outcomes in children after severe traumatic brain injury. J Neurotrauma. 2010;27(10):1819–25. https://doi.org/10.1089/neu.2010.1402.
47. Skippen P, Seear M, Poskitt K, Kestle J, Cochrane D, Annich G, Handel J. Effect of hyperventilation on regional cerebral blood flow in head-injured children. Crit Care Med. 1997;25(8):1402–9. https://doi.org/10.1097/00003246-199708000-00031.
48. Gonda DD, Meltzer HS, Crawford JR, Hilfiker ML, Shellington DK, Peterson BM, Levy ML. Complications associated with prolonged hypertonic saline therapy in children with elevated intracranial pressure. Pediatr Crit Care Med. 2013;14(6):610–20. https://doi.org/10.1097/PCC.0b013e318291772b.
49. Peterson B, Khanna S, Fisher B, Marshall L. Prolonged hypernatremia controls elevated intracranial pressure in head-injured pediatric patients. Crit Care Med. 2000;28(4):1136–43. https://doi.org/10.1097/00003246-200004000-00037.
50. Shawkat H, Westwood M-M, Mortimer A. Mannitol: a review of its clinical uses. Contin Educ Anaesth Crit Care Pain. 2012;12(2):82–5. https://doi.org/10.1093/bjaceaccp/mkr063.
51. Boone MD, Oren-Grinberg A, Robinson TM, Chen CC, Kasper EM. Mannitol or hypertonic saline in the setting of traumatic brain injury: what have we learned? Surg Neurol Int. 2015;6:177. https://doi.org/10.4103/2152-7806.170248.
52. Cooper DJ, Rosenfeld JV, Murray L, Arabi YM, Davies AR, D'Urso P, Kossmann T, Ponsford J, Seppelt I, Reilly P, Wolfe R. Decompressive craniectomy in diffuse traumatic brain injury. N Engl J Med. 2011;364(16):1493–502. https://doi.org/10.1056/NEJMoa1102077.

53. Hutchinson PJ, Kolias AG, Timofeev IS, Corteen EA, Czosnyka M, Timothy J, Anderson I, Bulters DO, Belli A, Eynon CA, Wadley J, Mendelow AD, Mitchell PM, Wilson MH, Critchley G, Sahuquillo J, Unterberg A, Servadei F, Teasdale GM, Pickard JD, Menon DK, Murray GD, Kirkpatrick PJ. Trial of decompressive craniectomy for traumatic intracranial hypertension. N Engl J Med. 2016;375(12):1119–30. https://doi.org/10.1056/NEJMoa1605215.
54. Taylor A, Butt W, Rosenfeld J, Shann F, Ditchfield M, Lewis E, Klug G, Wallace D, Henning R, Tibballs J. A randomized trial of very early decompressive craniectomy in children with traumatic brain injury and sustained intracranial hypertension. Childs Nerv Syst. 2001;17(3):154–62. https://doi.org/10.1007/s003810000410.
55. Holmes GL. Effects of seizures on brain development: lessons from the laboratory. Pediatr Neurol. 2005;33(1):1–11. https://doi.org/10.1016/j.pediatrneurol.2004.12.003.
56. Pingue V, Mele C, Nardone A. Post-traumatic seizures and antiepileptic therapy as predictors of the functional outcome in patients with traumatic brain injury. Sci Rep. 2021;11(1):4708. https://doi.org/10.1038/s41598-021-84203-y.
57. Chiaretti A, De Benedictis R, Polidori G, Piastra M, Iannelli A, Di Rocco C. Early post-traumatic seizures in children with head injury. Childs Nerv Syst. 2000;16(12):862–6. https://doi.org/10.1007/s003810000368.
58. Arango JI, Deibert CP, Brown D, Bell M, Dvorchik I, Adelson PD. Posttraumatic seizures in children with severe traumatic brain injury. Childs Nerv Syst. 2012;28(11):1925–9. https://doi.org/10.1007/s00381-012-1863-0.
59. Liesemer K, Bratton SL, Zebrack CM, Brockmeyer D, Statler KD. Early post-traumatic seizures in moderate to severe pediatric traumatic brain injury: rates, risk factors, and clinical features. J Neurotrauma. 2011;28(5):755–62. https://doi.org/10.1089/neu.2010.1518.
60. Bennett KS, DeWitt PE, Harlaar N, Bennett TD. Seizures in children with severe traumatic brain injury. Pediatr Crit Care Med. 2017;18(1):54–63. https://doi.org/10.1097/pcc.0000000000000948.
61. Herman ST, Abend NS, Bleck TP, Chapman KE, Drislane FW, Emerson RG, Gerard EE, Hahn CD, Husain AM, Kaplan PW, LaRoche SM, Nuwer MR, Quigg M, Riviello JJ, Schmitt SE, Simmons LA, Tsuchida TN, Hirsch LJ. Consensus statement on continuous EEG in critically ill adults and children, part I: indications. J Clin Neurophysiol. 2015;32(2):87–95. https://doi.org/10.1097/wnp.0000000000000166.
62. Yablon SA. Posttraumatic seizures. Arch Phys Med Rehabil. 1993;74(9):983–1001.
63. Sakurai A, Atkins CM, Alonso OF, Bramlett HM, Dietrich WD. Mild hyperthermia worsens the neuropathological damage associated with mild traumatic brain injury in rats. J Neurotrauma. 2012;29(2):313–21. https://doi.org/10.1089/neu.2011.2152.
64. Natale JE, Joseph JG, Helfaer MA, Shaffner DH. Early hyperthermia after traumatic brain injury in children: risk factors, influence on length of stay, and effect on short-term neurologic status. Crit Care Med. 2000;28(7):2608–15. https://doi.org/10.1097/00003246-200007000-00071.
65. Chen KH, Lee CP, Yang YH, Yang YH, Chen CM, Lu ML, Lee YC, Chen VC. Incidence of hydrocephalus in traumatic brain injury: a nationwide population-based cohort study. Medicine (Baltimore). 2019;98(42):e17568. https://doi.org/10.1097/md.0000000000017568.
66. Lang DA, Teasdale GM, Macpherson P, Lawrence A. Diffuse brain swelling after head injury: more often malignant in adults than children? J Neurosurg. 1994;80(4):675–80. https://doi.org/10.3171/jns.1994.80.4.0675.
67. Jha RM, Kochanek PM, Simard JM. Pathophysiology and treatment of cerebral edema in traumatic brain injury. Neuropharmacology. 2019;145(Pt B):230–46. https://doi.org/10.1016/j.neuropharm.2018.08.004.
68. Maxwell RE, Long DM, French LA. The effects of glucosteroids on experimental cold-induced brain edema. Gross morphological alterations and vascular permeability changes. J Neurosurg. 1971;34(4):477–87. https://doi.org/10.3171/jns.1971.34.4.0477.
69. Pappius HM, McCann WP. Effects of steroids on cerebral edema in cats. Arch Neurol. 1969;20(2):207–16. https://doi.org/10.1001/archneur.1969.00480080107013.
70. Weiss MH, Nulsen FE. The effect of glucocorticoids on CSF flow in dogs. J Neurosurg. 1970;32(4):452–8. https://doi.org/10.3171/jns.1970.32.4.0452.
71. Annane D, Pastores SM, Rochwerg B, Arlt W, Balk RA, Beishuizen A, Briegel J, Carcillo J, Christ-Crain M, Cooper MS, Marik PE, Umberto Meduri G, Olsen KM, Rodgers S, Russell JA, Van den Berghe G. Guidelines for the diagnosis and management of critical illness-related corticosteroid insufficiency (CIRCI) in critically ill patients (Part I): Society of Critical Care Medicine (SCCM) and European Society of Intensive Care Medicine (ESICM) 2017. Intensive Care Med. 2017;43(12):1751–63. https://doi.org/10.1007/s00134-017-4919-5.
72. Edwards P, Arango M, Balica L, Cottingham R, El-Sayed H, Farrell B, Fernandes J, Gogichaisvili T, Golden N, Hartzenberg B, Husain M, Ulloa MI, Jerbi Z, Khamis H, Komolafe E, Laloë V, Lomas G, Ludwig S, Mazairac G, Muñoz Sanchéz Mde L, Nasi L, Olldashi F, Plunkett P, Roberts I, Sandercock P, Shakur H, Soler C, Stocker R, Svoboda P, Trenkler S, Venkataramana NK, Wasserberg J, Yates D, Yutthakasemsunt S. Final results of MRC CRASH, a randomised placebo-controlled trial of intravenous corticosteroid in adults with head injury-outcomes at 6 months. Lancet. 2005;365(9475):1957–9. https://doi.org/10.1016/s0140-6736(05)66552-x.
73. Bontke CF, Boake C. Traumatic brain injury rehabilitation. Neurosurg Clin N Am. 1991;2(2):473–82.

74. Portnoy HD, Chopp M, Branch C, Shannon MB. Cerebrospinal fluid pulse waveform as an indicator of cerebral autoregulation. J Neurosurg. 1982;56(5):666–78. https://doi.org/10.3171/jns.1982.56.5.0666.
75. Ortiz JB, Sukhina A, Balkan B, Harootunian G, Adelson PD, Lewis KS, Oatman O, Subbian V, Rowe RK, Lifshitz J. Epidemiology of pediatric traumatic brain injury and hypothalamic-pituitary disorders in Arizona. Front Neurol. 2019;10:1410. https://doi.org/10.3389/fneur.2019.01410.
76. Srinivas R, Brown SD, Chang YF, Garcia-Fillion P, Adelson PD. Endocrine function in children acutely following severe traumatic brain injury. Childs Nerv Syst. 2010;26(5):647–53. https://doi.org/10.1007/s00381-009-1038-9.
77. Ulutabanca H, Hatipoglu N, Tanriverdi F, Gökoglu A, Keskin M, Selcuklu A, Kurtoglu S, Kelestimur F. Prospective investigation of anterior pituitary function in the acute phase and 12 months after pediatric traumatic brain injury. Childs Nerv Syst. 2014;30(6):1021–8. https://doi.org/10.1007/s00381-013-2334-y.
78. Personnier C, Crosnier H, Meyer P, Chevignard M, Flechtner I, Boddaert N, Breton S, Mignot C, Dassa Y, Souberbielle JC, Piketty M, Laborde K, Jais JP, Viaud M, Puget S, Sainte-Rose C, Polak M. Prevalence of pituitary dysfunction after severe traumatic brain injury in children and adolescents: a large prospective study. J Clin Endocrinol Metab. 2014;99(6):2052–60. https://doi.org/10.1210/jc.2013-4129.
79. Norwood KW, Deboer MD, Gurka MJ, Kuperminc MN, Rogol AD, Blackman JA, Wamstad JB, Buck ML, Patrick PD. Traumatic brain injury in children and adolescents: surveillance for pituitary dysfunction. Clin Pediatr (Phila). 2010;49(11):1044–9. https://doi.org/10.1177/0009922810376234.
80. Khadr SN, Crofton PM, Jones PA, Wardhaugh B, Roach J, Drake AJ, Minns RA, Kelnar CJ. Evaluation of pituitary function after traumatic brain injury in childhood. Clin Endocrinol (Oxf). 2010;73(5):637–43. https://doi.org/10.1111/j.1365-2265.2010.03857.x.
81. Casano-Sancho P, Suárez L, Ibáñez L, García-Fructuoso G, Medina J, Febrer A. Pituitary dysfunction after traumatic brain injury in children: is there a need for ongoing endocrine assessment? Clin Endocrinol (Oxf). 2013;79(6):853–8. https://doi.org/10.1111/cen.12237.
82. Harris DA, Lam S. Venous thromboembolism in the setting of pediatric traumatic brain injury. J Neurosurg Pediatr. 2014;13(4):448–55. https://doi.org/10.3171/2014.1.Peds13479.
83. van Erp IA, Gaitanidis A, El Moheb M, Kaafarani HMA, Saillant N, Duhaime AC, Mendoza AE. Low-molecular-weight heparin versus unfractionated heparin in pediatric traumatic brain injury. J Neurosurg Pediatr. 2021;27:469–74. https://doi.org/10.3171/2020.9.Peds20615.
84. Mtaweh H, Smith R, Kochanek PM, Wisniewski SR, Fabio A, Vavilala MS, Adelson PD, Toney NA, Bell MJ. Energy expenditure in children after severe traumatic brain injury. Pediatr Crit Care Med. 2014;15(3):242–9. https://doi.org/10.1097/pcc.0000000000000041.
85. Malakouti A, Sookplung P, Siriussawakul A, Philip S, Bailey N, Brown M, Farver K, Zimmerman JJ, Bell MJ, Vavilala MS. Nutrition support and deficiencies in children with severe traumatic brain injury. Pediatr Crit Care Med. 2012;13(1):e18–24. https://doi.org/10.1097/PCC.0b013e31820aba1f.
86. Fivez T, Kerklaan D, Mesotten D, Verbruggen S, Wouters PJ, Vanhorebeek I, Debaveye Y, Vlasselaers D, Desmet L, Casaer MP, Garcia Guerra G, Hanot J, Joffe A, Tibboel D, Joosten K, Van den Berghe G. Early versus late parenteral nutrition in critically ill children. N Engl J Med. 2016;374(12):1111–22. https://doi.org/10.1056/NEJMoa1514762.
87. Taha AA, Badr L, Westlake C, Dee V, Mudit M, Tiras KL. Effect of early nutritional support on intensive care unit length of stay and neurological status at discharge in children with severe traumatic brain injury. J Neurosci Nurs. 2011;43(6):291–7. https://doi.org/10.1097/JNN.0b013e318234e9b2.
88. Jacobi J, Bircher N, Krinsley J, Agus M, Braithwaite SS, Deutschman C, Freire AX, Geehan D, Kohl B, Nasraway SA, Rigby M, Sands K, Schallom L, Taylor B, Umpierrez G, Mazuski J, Schunemann H. Guidelines for the use of an insulin infusion for the management of hyperglycemia in critically ill patients. Crit Care Med. 2012;40(12):3251–76. https://doi.org/10.1097/CCM.0b013e3182653269.
89. Agus MS, Wypij D, Hirshberg EL, Srinivasan V, Faustino EV, Luckett PM, Alexander JL, Asaro LA, Curley MA, Steil GM, Nadkarni VM. Tight glycemic control in critically ill children. N Engl J Med. 2017;376(8):729–41. https://doi.org/10.1056/NEJMoa1612348.
90. Feld LG, Neuspiel DR, Foster BA, Leu MG, Garber MD, Austin K, Basu RK, Conway EE Jr, Fehr JJ, Hawkins C, Kaplan RL, Rowe EV, Waseem M, Moritz ML. Clinical practice guideline: maintenance intravenous fluids in children. Pediatrics. 2018;142(6):e20183083. https://doi.org/10.1542/peds.2018-3083.
91. Davis JW, Davis IC, Bennink LD, Hysell SE, Curtis BV, Kaups KL, Bilello JF. Placement of intracranial pressure monitors: are "normal" coagulation parameters necessary? J Trauma. 2004;57(6):1173–7. https://doi.org/10.1097/01.ta.0000151257.79108.fb.
92. Leeper CM, Neal MD, Billiar TR, Sperry JL, Gaines BA. Overresuscitation with plasma is associated with sustained fibrinolysis shutdown and death in pediatric traumatic brain injury. J Trauma Acute Care Surg. 2018;85(1):12–7. https://doi.org/10.1097/ta.0000000000001836.
93. Desgranges FP, Javouhey E, Mottolese C, Migeon A, Szathmari A, Baudin F, de Queiroz M, Cogniat B, Chassard D. Intraoperative blood loss during decompressive craniectomy for intractable intracranial hypertension after severe traumatic brain injury in children. Childs Nerv Syst. 2014;30(8):1393–8. https://doi.org/10.1007/s00381-014-2417-4.

94. Iaccarino C, Kolias A, Adelson PD, Rubiano AM, Viaroli E, Buki A, Cinalli G, Fountas K, Khan T, Signoretti S, Waran V, Adeleye AO, Amorim R, Bertuccio A, Cama A, Chesnut RM, De Bonis P, Estraneo A, Figaji A, Florian SI, Formisano R, Frassanito P, Gatos C, Germanò A, Giussani C, Hossain I, Kasprzak P, La Porta F, Lindner D, Maas AIR, Paiva W, Palma P, Park KB, Peretta P, Pompucci A, Posti J, Sengupta SK, Sinha A, Sinha V, Stefini R, Talamonti G, Tasiou A, Zona G, Zucchelli M, Hutchinson PJ, Servadei F. Consensus statement from the international consensus meeting on post-traumatic cranioplasty. Acta Neurochir (Wien). 2021;163(2):423–40. https://doi.org/10.1007/s00701-020-04663-5.
95. Liesemer K, Riva-Cambrin J, Bennett KS, Bratton SL, Tran H, Metzger RR, Bennett TD. Use of Rotterdam CT scores for mortality risk stratification in children with traumatic brain injury. Pediatr Crit Care Med. 2014;15(6):554–62. https://doi.org/10.1097/pcc.0000000000000150.
96. Maas AI, Hukkelhoven CW, Marshall LF, Steyerberg EW. Prediction of outcome in traumatic brain injury with computed tomographic characteristics: a comparison between the computed tomographic classification and combinations of computed tomographic predictors. Neurosurgery. 2005;57(6):1173–1182; discussion 1173–82. https://doi.org/10.1227/01.neu.0000186013.63046.6b.
97. Graham DI, Ford I, Adams JH, Doyle D, Lawrence AE, McLellan DR, Ng HK. Fatal head injury in children. J Clin Pathol. 1989;42(1):18–22. https://doi.org/10.1136/jcp.42.1.18.

18 Traumatic Spine Injury

Jeffrey Nadel, John A. Heflin,
Douglas L. Brockmeyer, and Rajiv R. Iyer

Cervical Spine Trauma

Epidemiology

Pediatric cervical spine trauma is relatively common and has the potential to be debilitating and costly to children and families. In children, approximately 60–80% of all traumatic vertebral column injuries affect the cervical spine, despite cervical trauma being the primary reason for hospital admission in only 2% of pediatric trauma cases [1–13]. The overall incidence of pediatric spinal injury is approximately 1–2 per 100,000 [2, 5, 7, 8, 14], increasing with age and varying with race [5] and geography [7]. Unsurprisingly, there is also bimodal seasonal variation with more injuries observed between June and September and December and January, coinciding with breaks from schooling [15, 16].

The mean age of those suffering from pediatric cervical spine injuries is approximately 9.5–10.5 years old [1, 2, 11, 12]. However, given the changes in spinal biomechanics throughout the aging process, certain types of cervical spinal injuries are more common in particular age groups. Specifically, in children under 4 years old, there is a higher incidence of craniocervical junction (CCJ) and upper cervical spine injuries (C1–C4), with the incidence of lower cervical spine injuries (C5–C7) increasing with age [1–7, 9–15, 17, 18]. It is hypothesized that this trend occurs due to the timing of maturation of the CCJ relative to the sub-axial spine, as well as the proportionally large head size in the infantile and early childhood period which contributes to a higher fulcrum level of flexion forces [19].

The etiology of pediatric cervical spine injury varies by age. In all-comers, the most-frequent cause of pediatric cervical spine injury is motor vehicle collisions, representing upwards of 70% of all injuries sustained [1–7, 9–12, 14, 15, 17, 18]. Ground-level falls and falls from low height are more-prevalent in infants and toddlers; whereas with adolescence, motor vehicle collisions and sports-related injuries account for most cervical spine injuries [1, 2, 9–11, 15].

There is also a sex predilection in pediatric cervical spine injury, with males more-frequently affected than females. In early childhood, the male-to-female ratio is approximately 1.3:1; whereas in late adolescence, the ratio elevates to nearly 2.5:1 [1–3, 5, 11, 12, 14, 17–19]. In early childhood, the primary mechanisms of cervical spine trauma include falls, passengers in motor vehicle collisions, and automobile-pedestrian accidents. These causes tend not to stratify between males

J. Nadel · D. L. Brockmeyer · R. R. Iyer (✉)
Department of Neurosurgery, University of Utah School of Medicine, Salt Lake City, UT, USA
e-mail: Douglas.Brockmeyer@hsc.utah.edu; rri2105@cumc.columbia.edu

J. A. Heflin
Department of Orthopedic Surgery, University of Utah School of Medicine, Salt Lake City, UT, USA

N. Shimony, G. Jallo (eds.), *Pediatric Neurosurgery Board Review*,
https://doi.org/10.1007/978-3-031-23687-7_18

and females. However, with increasing age, the etiology of trauma shifts to motor vehicle collisions with the child as driver and sports-related injuries. Generally, males are more likely to participate in aggressive contact sports or engage in risky driving practices, thus potentially leading to cervical spine injury [1–3, 5, 11, 12, 14, 17–19].

Cervical Spinal Biomechanics and Stabilizing Structures

Understanding the biomechanics of the CCJ and sub-axial cervical spine is essential to fully appreciate how the osseous and ligamentous structures provide stability in these regions. The CCJ is distinct from the sub-axial spine due to its wide range of motion, bony geometry, lack of intervertebral discs, and the unique facet morphology in this region. The occipal-C1 articulation primarily allows for flexion and extension of the head and neck and is responsible for approximately 50% of this motion. Due to the shape and orientation with which the C1 lateral mass cradles the occipital condyle, as well as the tight atlanto-occipital joint capsule, rotation and lateral bending occur minimally at this level [20–24]. The C1–C2 articulation, in turn, provides approximately 50% of the rotation of the cervical spine. The odontoid process is held against the C1 ring by the transverse ligament, thereby creating a fixed post around which the head can rotate. For the first 10° of rotation, C1 and C2 rotate together in a coupled fashion. However, beyond 10°, they uncouple and C1 continues to rotate around the fixed odontoid. There is minimal contribution to flexion-extension or lateral bending at this level [20–24]. The sub-axial cervical spine, from C3 to C7, is responsible for the remaining contribution to flexion-extension, rotation, and lateral bending.

The primary structures stabilizing the occipital-C1 joint are the atlanto-occipital capsular ligaments [25–29]. This has been demonstrated by finite element analysis; their disruption alone is sufficient to create atlanto-occipital instability [25–29]. The tectorial membrane—the cranial extension of the posterior longitudinal ligament, provides minimal stability to the occipital-C1 articulation. It is rare for the tectorial membrane to be disrupted in trauma without concomitant injury to the capsular ligaments.

The C1–C2 articulation is a more complex. The primary stabilizing structures include the odontoid process, the transverse ligament, and C1–C2 capsular ligaments with adjunctive support from the apical ligament of the odontoid process and alar ligaments. The odontoid process of C2 is a peg-shaped protrusion of the C2 vertebral body through the C1 ring and adds bony integrity to the articulation. It prevents anterior-posterior translation at the C1–C2 level, and its absence or injury creates C1–C2 instability. The transverse ligament is a cruciate structure that inserts onto the medial tubercles of the C1 lateral masses and holds the odontoid process against the posterior wall of the ventral arch of C1. This allows for neck rotation to occur while resisting flexion. The C1–C2 capsular ligaments are the ligamentous structures covering the joint between the C1 lateral mass and C2 superior facet. The apical and alar ligaments confer a small amount of additional stability to the C1–2 joint. The apical ligament inserts on the tip of the odontoid process and projects to the basion. It assists with preventing anterior-posterior translation at the C1–C2 joint. The alar ligaments are paired structures that insert on the odontoid process and project to the lateral walls of the foramen magnum. With rotation, one loosens while the other tightens and, in this manner, they serve as additional protection from excessive rotation around the odontoid process.

Imaging and Pediatric Cervical Spine Clearance

Historically, there has been much debate over the appropriate means of clearing pediatric cervical collars once traumatic cervical spine injury has been ruled out. The primary imaging modalities used in pediatric cervical spine trauma include static or dynamic plain radiographs, CT imaging, or magnetic resonance imaging (MRI) [13]. Plain radiographs are employed more-frequently in pediatric patients due to the lower dose of radiation delivered. Static radiographs are useful for detecting overt osseous abnormalities and understanding a patient's stationary alignment. Dynamic radiographs, performed by comparing imaging in the flexed and extension positions, are highly valuable in the determination of the presence of cervical instability as they demonstrate whether listhesis or abnormal spinal alignment occurs with motion. Dynamic radiographs should only be performed if the patient is neurologically intact, may be difficult due to complete in the early post-trauma period due to neck pain or stiffness [13]. CT imaging provides more detailed visualization of bony anatomy and therefore may detect osseous injuries not appreciated on plain radiographs. The benefit of routine CT over plain radiography in children under 10 years is limited since most cervical spine injuries in this age group are ligamentous rather than osseous [13]. MRI is the best modality to assess the integrity of soft-tissue structures such as the stabilizing ligaments, intervertebral discs, surrounding paraspinal musculature, or the presence of a compressive hematoma. MRI for injury evaluation and clearance of the cervical spine is appropriate if the child is obtunded, intubated, or unable to cooperate with dynamic radiographs. It is also a useful adjunctive tool if radiographs or CT are equivocal [13, 30–32].

In the setting of pediatric trauma, the decision of whether to image the cervical spine requires balancing the pre-test probability of an injury with judicious use of radiation in children. A major decision-making aid for whether post-traumatic imaging of the cervical spine is indicated are the National Emergency X-Ray Utilization Study (NEXUS) criteria. The NEXUS criteria are a group of validated criteria that help to guide appropriate post-trauma cervical spine imaging. Trauma patients that do not require cervical spine imaging must meet all of the following criteria: (a) alert and clinically stable; (b) without focal neurologic deficit; (c) no alteration in level of consciousness at the time of exam; (d) no known consumption of intoxicating agents; (e) no midline spinal tenderness; and (f) no distracting injury (i.e., other significant injury that is painful enough to distract the patient from spinal pain). If a patient is does not meet any of the above criteria, then cervical spine imaging with X-Rays (XRs) or computed tomography (CT) is indicated. The NEXUS criteria are 99.6% sensitive (95% CI: 98.6–100%) for ruling out cervical spine injury [33–35].

A number of projects advocated for use of screening radiographs following trauma [36–39]. If the child had abnormal screening radiographs, was non-communicative or ≤3 years old, did not meet NEXUS criteria, or had an abnormal neurological examination, then a neurosurgical consultation was obtained. However, if a patient had normal screening radiographs, was communicative and >3 years old, met NEXUS criteria, had a normal neurological examination, and had normal flexion-extension XRs, then non-neurosurgical personnel were able to successfully clear cervical collars without evidence of missed or delayed injuries. This body of literature led to the recent publication of a consensus statement and clinical algorithm from the Pediatric Cervical Spine Clearance Working Group that has been increasingly adopted [40]. Figure 18.1 demonstrates the algorithm as outlined by the consensus statement. The protocol divides patients into categories based on presenting Glasgow Coma Score (GCS). Depending on severity of the GCS decline, different imaging options are recommended, and spinal consultation is determined based on the results of the initial screening imaging obtained. Currently, children with a GCS <8 undergo MRI for final cervical spine clearance, but ongoing research is investigating the role of a negative CT scan alone in clearing the cervical spine in the pediatric population.

Patterns of Pediatric Cervical Spine Injury, Radiographic Correlates of Instability, and Surgical Management

The traumatic forces exerted onto the cervical spine create distinct patterns of injury at the occiput-C1 articulation, C1–C2 articulation, and in the sub-axial spine. The most common force

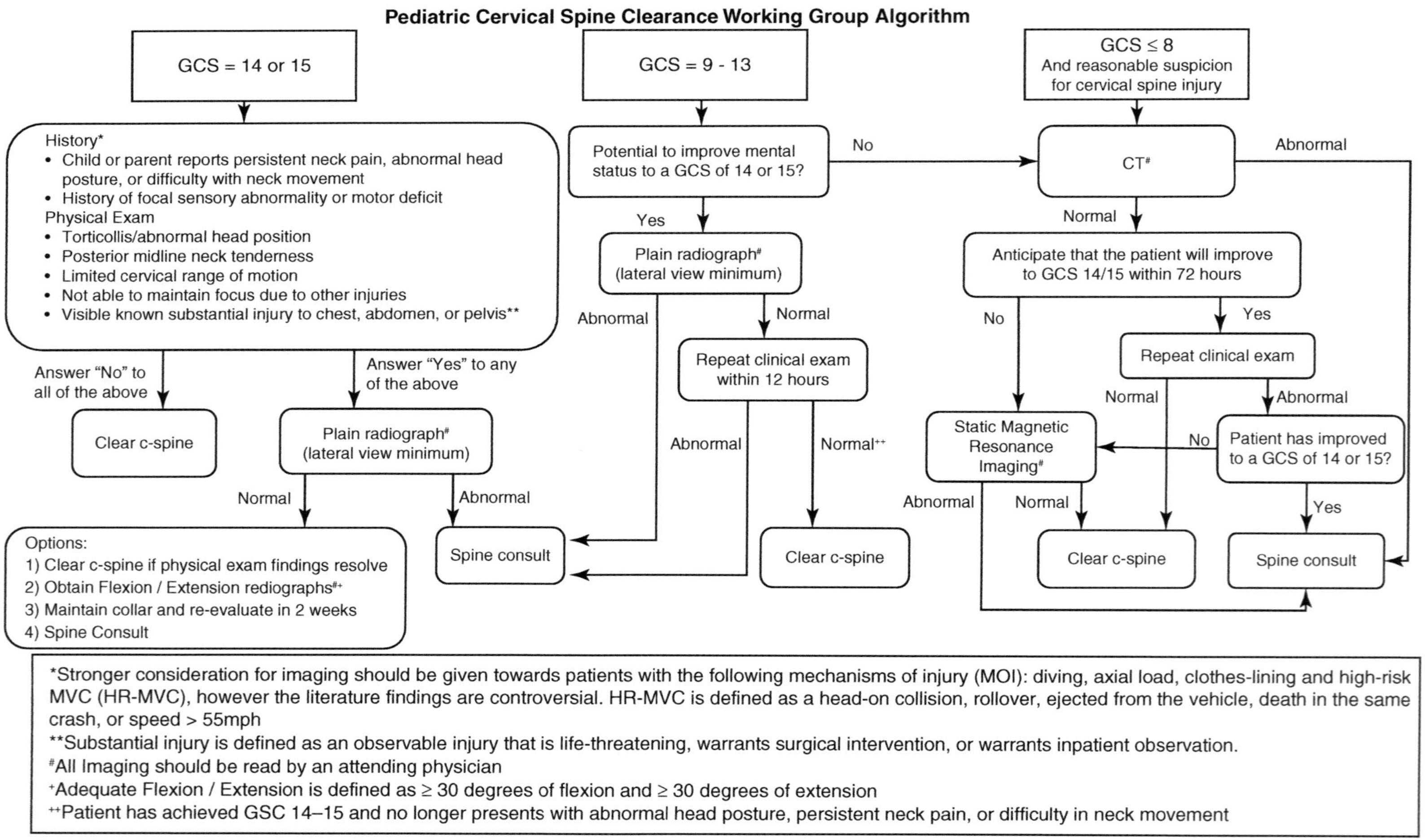

Fig. 18.1 Pediatric Cervical Spine Clearance Working Group clinical algorithm for clearance of cervical collars (from Herman M et al., JBJS 2019)

vectors causing injury include compression, flexion, extension, and rotation [41–43].

Injuries to the Occiput-C1 Junction

The most common patterns of injury at the occiput-C1 junction include occipital condyle fractures, C1 fractures, and atlanto-occipital dissociation (AOD). Occipital condyle fractures are relatively common injuries that are most-often identified on baseline radiographs or CT obtained after trauma. They infrequently present with lower cranial nerve deficits and may be associated with persistent neck pain. Anderson and Montesano created a classification system to categorize the most-common patterns of condylar injury [44]. A Type I occipital condyle fracture is a comminuted fracture of the condyle without injury to the alar ligaments or skull base. It is generally secondary to axial compressive forces and considered to be stable. A Type 2 occipital condyle fracture is a linear fracture of the skull base that extends into the occipital condyle. It is also considered to be a stable lesion, although may be unstable if the fracture is diastatic and thus separates the condyle from the occipital bone. A Type 3 fracture is an avulsion fracture of the occipital condyle at the insertion point of the alar ligament. This type of fracture may be unstable. Guidelines generally suggest conservative treatment for occipital condyle fractures with at least 3 months of rigid cervical orthoses or halo-vest immobilization [41, 45].

C1 fractures most commonly occur with compressive or axial loading forces. They can manifest as isolated fractures of either the anterior arch or posterior arch, involve both the anterior and posterior arch simultaneously (known as a Jefferson fracture), or involve the unilateral or bilateral C1 lateral mass [46]. C1 fractures themselves are usually not associated with neurological morbidity. In children, given that the C1 ring is often not completely formed, it is possible for a Jefferson fracture to manifest as a disruption at a synchondrosis or an ossification center. It is essential to determine the integrity of the transverse ligament when assessing C1 fractures. Radiographically, this can be done by measuring the atlanto-dental interval (ADI), employing the Rule of Spence, or visualizing transverse ligamentous injury on MRI. The ADI is the distance between the posterior aspect of the anterior arch of C1 and the anterior aspect of the odontoid process on lateral radiographs. In children, the normal value is <5 mm. Values greater than 5 mm suggest injury to the transverse ligament and possibly the alar and apical ligaments. The Rule of Spence assesses lateral displacement of the lateral masses. On open-mouth odontoid view radiographs, the offset distance between the C1 lateral mass and the C2 articular surface is measured bilaterally. If the sum of the distances from each side is greater than 7 mm, it suggests that the C1 lateral masses have pathologically migrated off the C2 articular surface and thus the transverse ligament is injured. In appropriate situations, MRI may also be obtained in the setting of C1 fractures, allowing for visualization of the integrity of the transverse ligament. C1 fractures with an intact transverse ligament are best treated conservatively with rigid cervical orthosis or halo vest therapy for at least 3 months. Conversely, fractures in the setting of a disrupted transverse ligament are unstable and unlikely to heal with external bracing alone and may require stabilization [21, 42, 43, 46].

One of the most severe and morbid injuries of the pediatric CCJ is atlanto-occipital dislocation (AOD), where there is instability and dissociation between the occiput and atlas (*see* Fig. 18.2). Given the high likelihood of associated neurological morbidity associated with AOD, including possible brainstem involvement, early detection is critical and a high index of suspicion with severe mechanisms of injury is imperative. There are several radiographic findings that suggest AOD. For historical purposes, the original criteria for determining occipital-C1 instability was the Basion-dental interval (BDI), which is the measurement between the tip of the odontoid process and the basion on a mid-sagittal image [47]. The upper limit of normal in children is 10–12.5 mm, which is larger than the accepted normal value of 5 mm in adults due to incomplete ossification of the tip of the odontoid is young children. Over time, new measurements emerged to better evaluate AOD given how the BDI differs among

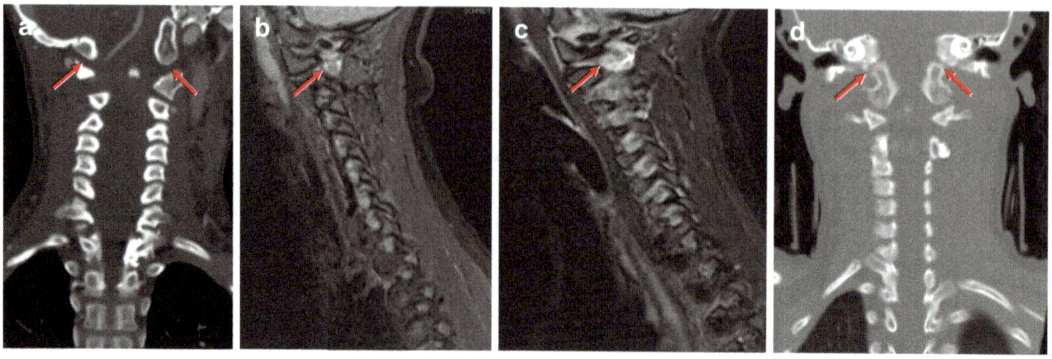

Fig. 18.2 Patient with radiographic evidence of atlanto-occipital dissociation. Panel A: CT C-Spine demonstrating asymmetric gapping of the left occipital condyle-C1 joint compared to the right. Panels B and C: MRI C-Spine with sagittal T1 STIR sequence demonstrating bilateral capsular ligamentous injury on sagittal T1 STIR imaging. Panel D: Post-operative CT C-Spine demonstrating interval improvement in asymmetric gapping of the occipital condyle-C1 joints bilaterally following occiput to C2 instrumentation and fusion

children of different ages. Another radiographic measurement is the Basion-Axial Interval (BAI), which is the distance between the basion and a line extending cranially from the posterior aspect of the odontoid process [48]. In children, the BAI generally does not exceed 12 mm. The Powers Ratio is the measured ratio between a line drawn from the basion to the posterior ring of C1 and a line drawn from the opisthion to the anterior arch of C1 [49]. A ratio over 1 is suspicious for AOD.

Currently, the most common measurement used in the radiographic determination of AOD is the occipital condyle-C1 interval (CCI) as measured on high resolution CT due to its high sensitivity and specificity [50–54]. In early studies, it was demonstrated that a normal CCI in children was 1.28 ± 0.26 mm. Recent studies validating these results suggest that a CCI ≥ 4 mm meets criteria for AOD [50–54]. In the presence of AOD, emergent surgical management is indicated with a posterior fusion, many times from the occiput to the high cervical spine. Prior to surgical intervention, strict cervical spine immobilization is essential. Placing a patient in traction in the presence of AOD is contraindicated in most cases.

Injuries to C2

Osseous injuries to C2 also occur in children. Examples of these fractures include traumatic spondylolisthesis of C2, also known as Hangman's fractures, and odontoid process fractures [41–43]. Hangman's fractures most-commonly occur due to fractures through the bilateral pars of C2 and are the result of hyperextension injuries. The primary classification scheme of these fractures was originally described by Effendi et al. and modified by Levine and Edwards [55, 56]. The Effendi Classification and Levine and Edwards Classification both rely on measurement of the amount of anterior-posterior translation of C2 as well as the kyphotic angulation of the injury. Type 1 Hangman's fractures are minimally displaced fractures with <3 mm of anterior-posterior translation, no angulation, and an intact C2–3 disc. These are considered stable injuries and the treatment of choice is usually external orthosis. Type 2 Hangman's fractures are displaced fractures with >3 mm of anterior-posterior translation but 10 degrees of angulation or less. In these situations, the C2–3 disc and posterior longitudinal ligament are often disrupted, and the fracture line is typically vertical. These fractures are generally unstable, requiring halo immobilization or surgical fixation in many cases. Type 2a Hangman's fractures are those with minimal or no anterior-posterior translation but with significant angulation greater than 10°. The fracture line is usually horizontal or oblique in orientation. Similar to Type 2 Hangman's fractures, Type 2a fractures are unstable and require halo or surgical immobilization. Type 3 Hangman's fractures are Type

2 fractures that also present with bilateral facet joint dislocation. These fractures are rare and involve a distraction mechanism. Given the joint dislocation, treatment for these injuries is surgical reduction and fixation. In patient's requiring surgical treatment or in those who fail a trial of external bracing, C2–3 anterior cervical discectomy and fusion could be considered, in addition to posterior instrumentation above and below the fracture.

Odontoid fractures were first classified according to Anderson and D'Alonzo, where the divided odontoid fractures into three primary types [57]. Type I odontoid fractures traverse the tip of the odontoid process and are generally considered stable fractures. Type II odontoid fractures cross through the base of the odontoid and have been shown to be unstable fractures that usually require surgical treatment (*see* Fig. 18.3). Type III odontoid fractures cross through the body of C2 and most often do not require surgery. Surgical stabilization of Type II odontoid fractures can be accomplished with C1–C2 posterior spinal instrumentation and fusion. An anterior approach to odontoid fractures with odontoid screw placement is also possible, but certain challenges to this approach include the steep trajectory required, the need for biplanar fluoroscopy, and other possible adverse effects such as post-operative dysphagia. Furthermore, placement of an odontoid screw requires the appropriate fracture morphology and an intact transverse ligament. In young children, when the odontoid process has not entirely ossified, patients may present with dentocentral synchondrosis disruption and subluxation, which is the equivalent injury to an odontoid fracture in a young child. Finally, odontoid fractures in children must be differentiated from os odontoideum, in which the rostral portion of the odontoid process fails to fuse with the remaining C2 vertebral body, in which osseous margins are corticated.

Injuries to the Sub-Axial Cervical Spine

Sub-axial cervical spine injuries can be purely osseous or osseoligamentous injuries. Assessing stability of the sub-axial cervical spine injuries can be performed by assessing the extent of angulation or listhesis at injured levels, as well as uncovering of the facet joints posteriorly. In children under 8 years old, it can be normal to have sagittal displacement of up to 4.5 mm. In

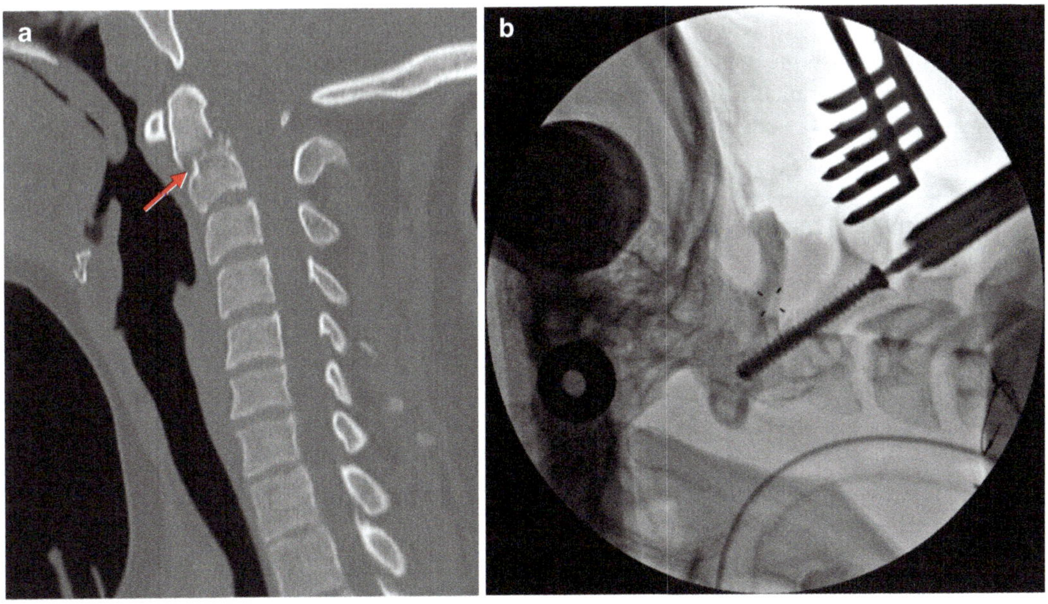

Fig. 18.3 Panel A: Mid-sagittal CT C-Spine demonstrating a Type II occipital condyle fracture. Panel B: Intra-operative fluoroscopy demonstrating trajectory and placement of transarticular screw

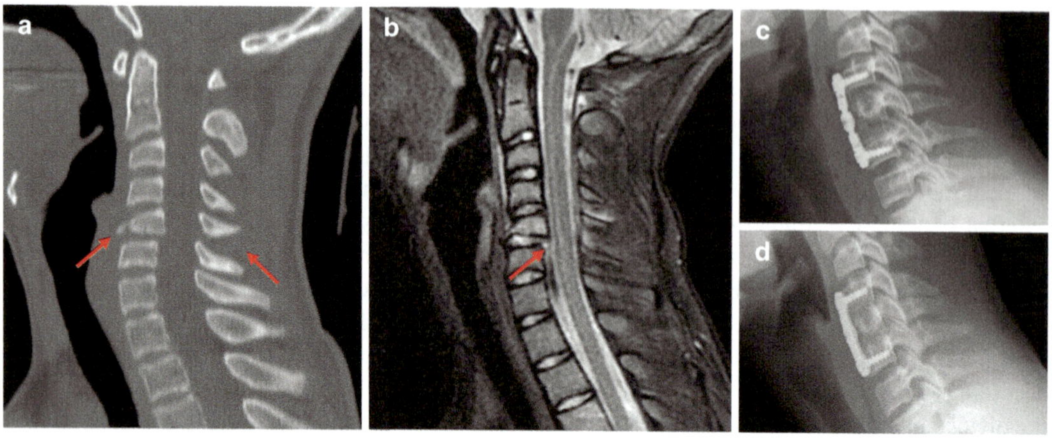

Fig. 18.4 Panel A: Mid-sagittal CT C-Spine showing a C5 burst fracture with mild vertebral body retropulsion and interspinous splaying. Panel B: Mid-sagittal MRI T1 STIR sequence demonstrating traumatic disruption of the posterior longitudinal ligament. Panel C: Immediate post-operative imaging demonstrating the instrumentation construct. Panel D: Post-operative imaging 3 months after surgery demonstrating interval bony fusion of the segment

children over 8 years old, the upper limit of sagittal displacement is 3.5 mm [18, 42, 43, 58]. In terms of angulation, the threshold for possible instability is more than 7 degrees of angulation between two adjacent levels. For children with 7–11 degrees of angulation and no neurological deficit, consideration of flexion-extension films should be performed [18, 42, 43, 58]. In the setting of sub-axial spinal instability, anterior or posterior surgical approaches may be considered, depending on the disrupted spinal components, degree of spinal deformity, and patient-specific anatomy (*see* Fig. 18.4).

Thoracolumbar Trauma

Introduction and Epidemiology

Traumatic injury of the thoracolumbar spine in children occurs far less frequently than that of the cervical spine. Unique biomechanical properties of the pediatric spine contribute to this distribution, for example, the relatively large head in children make them prone to flexion injuries, predisposing children to cervical injuries higher in the subaxial spine and craniocervical junction [11]. Thoracolumbar trauma in children begin to resemble adult patterns of injury around 8–9 years of life, when the osseoligamentous structures of the spine become similar to that of an adult. The young pediatric spine features more ligamentous laxity than that of adults, facet joints are less developed and more horizontally oriented, and bony structures continue to grow and ossify at various centers including a central body ossification center, as well as two neurocentral ossification centers connecting the anterior and posterior elements. Structural spinal stability in the thoracolumbar spine of children is more reliant on ligamentous structures, but the natural laxity of these soft tissue components can lead to spinal cord injury without radiographic abnormality (SCIWORA), which may also be referred to as a transient neuropraxia, or spinal cord concussion.

Thoracolumbar spine trauma is not surprisingly more common during the summer months and winter breaks when children are away from school. The reported incidence of thoracolumbar fractures in children has been reported around 0.07% annually, also the true incidence may be higher as many children with minor injuries may not undergo imaging if medical attention is not sought out [59]. Common causes of injury include motor vehicle accidents (MVAs), falls, and sports-related injuries [11, 60, 61]. The majority of these injuries are seen in the adolescent population, although injury in younger children is also possible [62]. A higher prevalence of spinal injuries has also been shown in children of lower socioeconomic status [63]. The spine service at a busy pediatric institution will often be faced with treatment and management decisions for thoracolumbar trauma, which vary from conservative management with observation or bracing, to open fracture reduction and instrumented surgical stabilization.

Imaging

Radiographic evaluation of a child with a suspected thoracolumbar injury is variable and without as formally established criteria or study as compared to cervical spine trauma, and thus some inconsistency exists across institutions. For children who are neurologically intact, AP and lateral plain radiographs are mostly sufficient to detect clinically relevant osseous thoracolumbar spine injuries. Completion of standing spine films may also be considered when trying to establish a baseline for a patient in whom future alignment issues may arise due to the injury, and provides evaluation of a patient's global spinal alignment. If a significant fracture or alignment concern is noted on plain radiography, further characterization may be appropriate with CT or MRI. In some circumstances, for example, a child who is intubated, has a neurological deficit, or experienced a high impact mechanism of injury (such as high-speed motor vehicle accident), upfront CT imaging of the thoracolumbar spine is often part of the general trauma diagnostic work up without antecedent XRs. Even in situations when dedicated pan-spine CT was not performed, spinal reconstructions of abdominopelvic imaging can often be performed if necessary. MRI also plays an important role in characterizing thoracolumbar spinal injuries as it avoids ionizing radiation and provides a higher level of detail with regard to ligamentous structures, the spinal cord and other neural elements, the intervertebral discs, and in the detection of hematoma formation.

Injury Classifications

In the early 1960s, Holdsworth described a two-column model for spinal injuries and categorized injuries in terms of mechanism, with flexion, flexion/rotation, extension and compression injuries resulting in fracture, dislocation, or fracture-dislocation of the spine [64]. Later, Denis provided insight by introducing the three-column model of spine injuries, introducing the middle column, which is comprised of the posterior vertebral body, posterior longitudinal ligament and posterior anulus fibrosis [65]. Magerl in 1994 further expounded on these systems by creating a classification scheme based on the fundamental pathomorphology of the injury, separating them into injuries of compression, distraction, and torsion [66].

More recently, the thoracolumbar injury classification system (TLICS) combined an understanding of fracture morphology, the posterior ligamentous complex (PLC; comprised of the supraspinous ligament, interspinous ligament, ligamentum flavum and facet capsules), as well as the neurological status of the patient, to provide a numerically weighted tool based on these factors that provides guidance for the management of patients with thoracolumbar injuries (*see* Table 18.1) [67]. An additional system that is widely used is the AOSpine TL spine injury classification, which employs the Magerl fracture morphological classification as well as neurological status in the evaluation of thoracolumbar spinal injuries. Both systems are widely utilized, and in addition, have both been found to be valid and reliable for the classification and management of thoracolumbar injuries in children [68–71].

Specific Pathology

Compression Fractures

The most common thoracolumbar spine fractures in children are compression fractures, which typically result from axial loading injuries or flexion forces on the spine, which specifically involve

Table 18.1 Thoracolumbar Injury Classification System (TLICS). Score 0–3 predicts no need for surgery. Score > 4 predicts need for surgery. Score = 4 is intermediate and surgeons preference

Injury category	Point value
Injury morphology	
Compression	1
Burst	2
Translation or rotation	3
Distraction	4
Posterior Ligamentous Complex (PLC) status	
Intact	0
Injury suspected or indeterminate	2
Injured	3
Neurologic status	
Intact	0
Nerve root involvement	2
Spinal Cord or conus medullaris injury	
Incomplete	3
Complete	2
Cauda equina syndrome	3

the anterior column alone and result in varying degrees of decreased vertebral body height. Because these bony fractures involve the anterior column in isolation, they are not typically considered to be unstable. In children, mild compression fractures (less than 20% height loss) can be difficult to discern from normal physiological wedging that is seen in the growing spine [72]. In fact, one study demonstrated that anterior vertebral body height loss up to 11% was observed in 95% of normal children undergoing CT imaging [73]. The skeletally immature spines in children also feature more convex endplates that eventually evolve into the more concave adult pattern, which predisposes to a somewhat wedged appearance early in life and can be useful in identifying changes from this norm that are more suggestive of a fracture [74]. Compression fractures and physiologic wedging can be difficult to distinguish on plain radiographs alone, although CT imaging is often unnecessary in cases involving thoracolumbar compression fractures in isolation, thus demonstrating the importance of understanding a patient's clinical status and history of trauma in distinguishing these phenomena. Nonetheless, if performed, CT imaging allows for closer inspection of the endplate disruptions that are indicative of fracture.

Importantly, masqueraders of compression fractures can include incompletely ossified ring apophyses, or Schmorl's nodes, which appear as endplate irregularities but are not induced by trauma. Hence, clinical history is important for the diagnosis of compression fracture, and evaluation of a child with back pain following an injury can serve as important evidence for a compression fracture as opposed to such alternative phenomena. Finally, it is important to note that abnormal vertebral shape can also occur in children with underlying bone diseases or chronic steroid use.

Most compression fractures in children are managed conservatively with observation, pain relief with analgesics, anti-inflammatories, and muscle relaxants. Bracing can be a useful adjunct for children with significant pain with mobilization. The natural presence of the rib cage and its articulations with the spine make the thoracic spine less mobile than the cervical and lumbar regions, providing some degree of internal support without a brace. Severe compression fractures with significant deformity may require surgical intervention, and a more severe injury is also more likely to be accompanied by ligamentous injury that could contribute to the deformity.

While practice patterns are variable, some practitioners will simply follow children with compression fractures clinically, while others may elect to perform repeat imaging with plain films (regional or global standing films). Repeat imaging at a clinical interval can ensure that the fracture is not contributing to a new deformity, as the presence of significant vertebral wedging can lead to a kyphotic deformity across a spinal segment.

Burst Fractures

Burst fractures of the pediatric spine involve the posterior aspect of the vertebral body and can be classified based on single end plate involvement (incomplete burst), or both superior and inferior endplate involvement (complete burst). Often, these injuries occur at the thoracolumbar junction, where the more rigid thoracic spine, owing to its chest wall articulations, transitions into the more mobile lumbar spine. Often, posterior cortex involvement can lead to fracture fragment retropulsion into the spinal canal, which can lead to spinal cord or conus medullaris compression or radiculopathy due to neuroforaminal narrowing, and even cauda equina compression. Varying amounts of fracture comminution may also be present.

Management of burst fractures is quite heterogeneous, with practice patterns varying across institutions and surgeons. Several factors should be considered, including the presence/absence of a kyphotic deformity, the patient's neurological status, the degree of comminution, neural canal compromise, posterior ligamentous complex integrity, and the ability of the patient to support themselves in an erect posture and to ambulate (with or without a brace). All these factors must be considered when deciding on operative or nonoperative management of these injuries.

CT and MRI are both useful imaging studies to evaluate burst fractures in sufficient detail. With these injuries, MRI is particularly useful in determining the extent of injury to the posterior ligamentous complex and obtaining an MRI has been shown to change management in up to 25% cases that may have originally been managed nonoperatively [75, 76].

In patients who are neurologically intact without overtly unstable injuries, conservative management of burst fractures is an option if pain can be adequately controlled to the point where mobilization can occur with or without bracing. While the TLICS score aids in the decision for surgical or nonsurgical intervention, borderline operative/nonoperative burst fracture cases will be frequently encountered, especially in neurologically intact patients with a suspected but not overtly injured posterior ligamentous complex (TLICS score of 4, surgeon's choice of intervention). Studies comparing outcomes of nonoperative versus operative treatment of thoracolumbar fractures have had varying results and have been mainly conducted in the adult population, with some demonstrating more favorable outcomes with operative treatment [77, 78], others showing the ultimate superiority of nonoperative treatment [79], and others with more equivocal results [80]. While there is no universally accepted set of criteria for burst fractures guiding the decision for surgical intervention in children and adolescents, the multitude of factors listed above, the treating surgeon's determination of the likelihood of a fracture to heal, the ability of a child to ambulate and return to normal activities quickly, and the possible predisposition to a kyphotic deformity are all factors that should be considered.

If the nonoperative treatment approach is employed, the use of a brace for burst fractures is controversial, with little literature in the pediatric population to either recommend or avoid its use. A randomized trial by Bailey and colleagues [81] evaluated skeletally mature patients aged 16–60 years with less than 35° kyphosis across a thoracolumbar burst fracture, randomizing patients to receiving a thoracolumbosacral orthosis (TLSO) or no orthosis, and demonstrated that hospital length of stay was similar, and that quality of life measures were similar at 3 months post-injury. This evidence would suggest equivalency in clinical improvement with or without brace use for thoracolumbar burst fractures in neurologically intact adult patients. As stated by the Congress of Neurological Surgeons thoracolumbar trauma guidelines, the decision to use a brace is therefore left to the discretion of the treating physician [82].

Surgical approaches for burst fractures include posterior-based constructs (*see* Fig. 18.5), anterior reconstruction with corpectomy and cage/plating, as well as combined approaches. A fair amount of heterogeneity exists on these approaches, including more specific surgical aspects such as the number of instrumented levels needed for adequate stabilization, the need for arthrodesis versus percutaneous instrumentation without arthrodesis, the removal of such instrumentation once healing is adequate, and the role of instrumentation of the fractured level itself. Ultimately, evidence has suggested that there is no biomechanical advantage of any single approach or construct type for these injuries [83]. Furthermore, the need for decompression may vary from case to case, which on a spectrum may involve a laminectomy at the affected level,

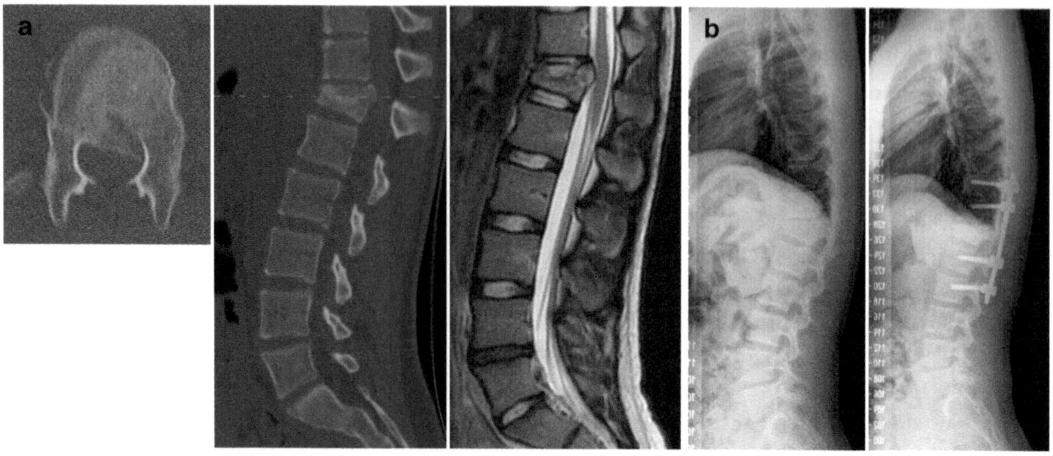

Fig. 18.5 Surgical approaches for burst fractures. Panel A: Axial and sagittal CT and sagittal T2 MRI demonstrating a T12 burst fracture with retropulsion of a fragment into the spinal canal. Panel B: Pre-operative and post-operative XR images demonstrating the posterior-based construct for surgical stabilization

transpedicular decompression for fracture fragment reduction from a posterior approach, or a retropleural/retroperitoneal approach for corpectomy and anterior column restoration. For cases in which the posterior longitudinal ligament is intact, anterior/middle column longitudinal forces with ligamentotaxis (compressive forces on a posterior-based pedicle screw construct) can lead to fracture fragment reduction without the need for ventral decompression.

Ultimately, if applying evidence from the adult population to children, there is a lack of data suggesting superior clinical outcomes with either an anterior, posterior, or combined approach, as summarized by a recently synthesized thoracolumbar trauma guidelines [84].

Flexion Distraction/Translational Injuries

Severe flexion or rotational forces to the pediatric spine can lead to injuries affecting all three columns of the thoracolumbar spine, which can be associated with significant neurological compromise due to spinal cord injury. These can include spinal dislocation injuries in which facets joints may be perched or jumped (*see* Fig. 18.6), with or without subluxation of the anterior vertebral bodies. Other three column injuries include bony or ligamentous chance fractures which can occur with seat-belt injuries, rendering the spine unstable. For severe mechanisms of traumatic injury, such as high-speed motor vehicles collisions, falls from height, and others, a high index of suspicion for a significant traumatic spine injury should be maintained until ruled out [85]. The use of CT and MRI is helpful in characterizing the osseoligamentous involvement for such injuries. The majority of these cases will require operative intervention for fracture reduction or spinal realignment, instrumented stabilization and arthrodesis, and decompression.

Ring Apophyseal Fractures

In the immature spine, the ring apophysis is present at the vertebral endplates and contributes to spinal growth. This cartilaginous structure ossifies around 6 years of life, and fuses around adulthood [86]. The ring apophysis is biomechanically weak, and repeated stresses or trauma can lead to a ring apophyseal fracture, which is often associated with a disc herniation at the same level (*see* Fig. 18.7) [72, 87]. Repeated shear stress can lead to this phenomenon, and CT is a useful adjunct to MRI when evaluating a child or adolescent with radiculopathy and a disc herniation, as a bony "limbus" can be detected with CT and would appear as a small bony ridge or fragment that is avulsed from the posterior corner of the vertebral body. Importantly, ring apophyseal fractures can be concurrently present in up to 25–30% of ado-

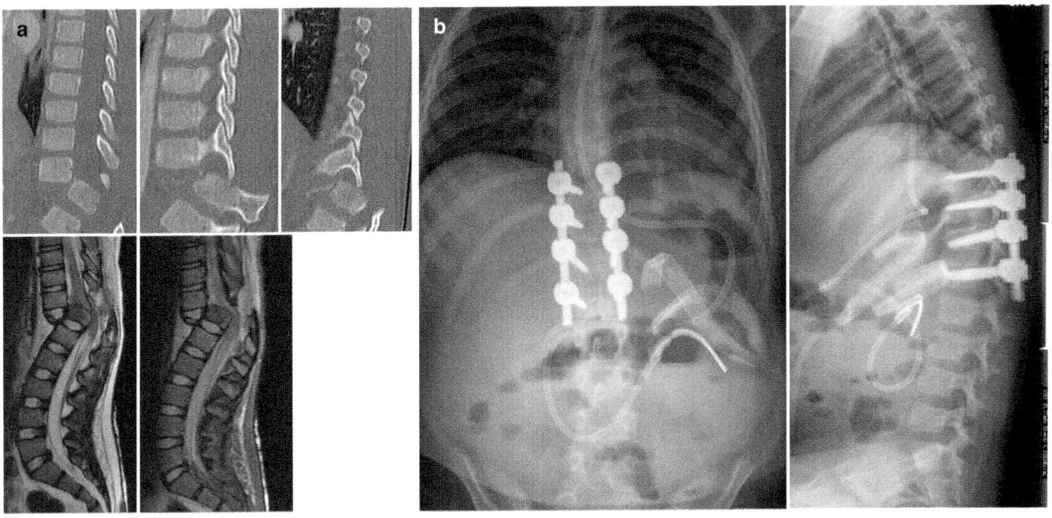

Fig. 18.6 Flexion-distraction and spinal dislocation injuries. Panel A: Sagittal CT and sagittal MRI images demonstrating severe flexion-distraction injuries leading to spinal dislocation and complete disruption of the spinal canal. Panel B: Post-operative XR images demonstrating posterior fixation after flexion-distraction injuries

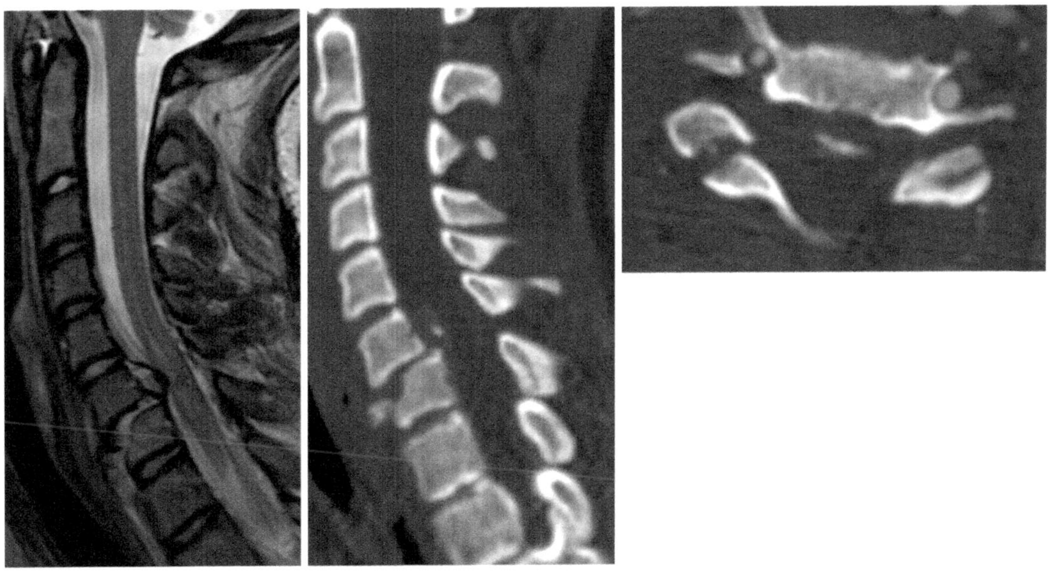

Fig. 18.7 Adolescent girl evaluated after a motor vehicle collision found to have a flexion distraction injury with a large disc herniation at C6–7. On sagittal and axial CT imaging, calcification is seen along with the disc herniation consistent with a ring apophyseal fracture into the spinal canal. The patient underwent emergent decompression and stabilization in the acute setting

lescents who are found to have a disc herniation [86]. However, ring apophyseal fractures in isolation are frequently missed, and should be ruled out as a possible etiology for radiculopathy in adolescents. Back pain may also be present as this likely represents more of a chronic disorder involving repeated shear stress, and associated Modic endplate changes have also been shown to occur in associated with apophyseal ring fractures [88]. However, acute fracture is also possible with significant trauma. Surgical treatment may be necessary with laminectomy and decompression, which can result in good functional outcomes [89]. More controversy exists on the necessity of removal of the bone fragment associated with the ring apophyseal fracture, with satisfactory outcomes being reported with either approach [90]. However, as ring apophyseal fractures frequently occur concurrently with disc herniation, removal of the bony fragment may play an important role in symptom resolution for patients with treated disc herniations with persistent pain and radiculopathy.

Conclusion

Pediatric spine trauma is relatively common and carries unique considerations in comparison to that in the adult population with respect to biomechanics, bony/ligamentous anatomy, imaging, and clinical management. An awareness of the nuances associated with the growing, immature spine, as well as careful clinical and imaging evaluation can lead to early detection and effective treatment of these injuries.

Questions

1. The cervical spine comprises what percentage of all traumatic vertebral column injuries?
   (a) 2–5%
   (b) 10–20%
   (c) 40–50%
   (d) 60–80%
2. The thoracolumbar Injury Classification System score of ___ predicts need for surgery
   (a) 1
   (b) 2
   (c) 3
   (d) 4
3. Which time of injury suggests a three column injury of the thoracolumbar spine
   (a) Flexion/distraction
   (b) Compression
   (c) Burst fracture
   (d) Ring apophyseal fracture

Answers

1. (d)
2. (d)
3. (a)

References

1. Brown RL, Brunn MA, Garcia VF. Cervical spine injuries in children: a review of 103 patients treated consecutively at a level 1 pediatric trauma center. J Pediatr Surg. 2001;36(8):1107–14. https://doi.org/10.1053/jpsu.2001.25665.
2. Kokoska ER, Keller MS, Rallo MC, Weber TR. Characteristics of pediatric cervical spine injuries. J Pediatr Surg. 2001;36(1):100–5. https://doi.org/10.1053/jpsu.2001.20022.
3. Mohseni S, Talving P, Branco BC, et al. Effect of age on cervical spine injury in pediatric population: a National Trauma Data Bank review. J Pediatr Surg. 2011;46(9):1771–6. https://doi.org/10.1016/j.jpedsurg.2011.03.007.
4. Beckmann NM, Chinapuvvula NR, Zhang X, West OC. Epidemiology and imaging classification of pediatric cervical spine injuries: 12-year experience at a level 1 trauma center. AJR Am J Roentgenol. 2020;214(6):1359–68. https://doi.org/10.2214/AJR.19.22095.
5. Vitale MG, Goss JM, Matsumoto H, Roye DPJ. Epidemiology of pediatric spinal cord injury in the United States: years 1997 and 2000. J Pediatr Orthop. 2006;26(6):745–9. https://doi.org/10.1097/01.bpo.0000235400.49536.83.
6. Chaudhry AS, Prince J, Sorrentino C, et al. Identification of risk factors for cervical spine injury from pediatric trauma registry. Pediatr Neurosurg. 2016;51(4):167–74. https://doi.org/10.1159/000444192.
7. Shin JI, Lee NJ, Cho SK. Pediatric cervical spine and spinal cord injury: a National Database Study. Spine. 2016;41(4):283–92. https://doi.org/10.1097/BRS.0000000000001176.
8. Kim W, Ahn N, Ata A, Adamo MA, Entezami P, Edwards M. Pediatric cervical spine injury in the United States: defining the burden of injury, need for operative intervention, and disparities in imaging across trauma centers. J Pediatr Surg. 2021;56(2):293–6. https://doi.org/10.1016/j.jpedsurg.2020.05.009.
9. Givens TG, Polley KA, Smith GF, Hardin WD. Pediatric cervical spine injury: a three-year experience. J Trauma Acute Care Surg. 1996;41(2):310–4.
10. Carreon LY, Glassman SD, Campbell MJ. Pediatric spine fractures: a review of 137 hospital admissions. Clin Spine Surg. 2004;17(6):477–82. https://doi.org/10.1097/01.bsd.0000132290.50455.99.
11. Cirak B, Ziegfeld S, Knight VM, Chang D, Avellino AM, Paidas CN. Spinal injuries in children. J Pediatr Surg. 2004;39(4):607–12. https://doi.org/10.1016/j.jpedsurg.2003.12.011.
12. Lykissas M, Gkiatas I, Spiliotis A, Papadopoulos D. Trends in pediatric cervical spine injuries in the United States in a 10-year period. J Orthop Surg (Hong Kong). 2019;27(1):2309499019834734. https://doi.org/10.1177/2309499019834734.

13. McCall T, Fassett D, Brockmeyer D. Cervical spine trauma in children: a review. Neurosurg Focus. 2006;20(2):1–8. https://doi.org/10.3171/foc.2006.20.2.6.
14. Hamilton MG, Mylks ST. Pediatric spinal injury: review of 174 hospital admissions. J Neurosurg. 1992;77(5):700–4. https://doi.org/10.3171/jns.1992.77.5.0700.
15. Hill SA, Miller CA, Kosnik EJ, Hunt WE. Pediatric neck injuries: a clinical study. J Neurosurg. 1984;60(4):700–6. https://doi.org/10.3171/jns.1984.60.4.0700.
16. Ramgopal S, Dunnick J, Siripong N, Conti KA, Gaines BA, Zuckerbraun NS. Seasonal, weather, and temporal factors in the prediction of admission to a pediatric trauma center. World J Surg. 2019;43(9):2211–7. https://doi.org/10.1007/s00268-019-05029-4.
17. Hadley MN, Zabramski JM, Browner CM, Rekate H, Sonntag VKH. Pediatric spinal trauma: review of 122 cases of spinal cord and vertebral column injuries. J Neurosurg. 1988;68(1):18–24. https://doi.org/10.3171/jns.1988.68.1.0018.
18. Osenbach RK, Menezes AH. Spinal cord injury without radiographic abnormality in children. Pediatr Neurosci. 1989;15(4):168–174; discussion 175. https://doi.org/10.1159/000120464.
19. Albright AL, Pollack IF, Adelson PF. Principles and practice of pediatric neurosurgery. 3rd ed. Thieme; 2015. https://www.thieme.in/principles-and-practice-of-pediatric-neurosurgery. Accessed 20 Feb 2022.
20. Bogduk N, Mercer S. Biomechanics of the cervical spine. I: normal kinematics. Clin Biomech (Bristol, Avon). 2000;15(9):633–48. https://doi.org/10.1016/s0268-0033(00)00034-6.
21. Swartz EE, Floyd RT, Cendoma M. Cervical spine functional anatomy and the biomechanics of injury due to compressive loading. J Athl Train. 2005;40(3):155–61.
22. Dvorak J. Rotation of the cervical spine by using computerized-tomography (CT). Spine (Phila Pa 1976). 1988;13(5):595–7.
23. Panjabi M, Dvorak J, Duranceau J, et al. Three-dimensional movements of the upper cervical spine. Spine (Phila Pa 1976). 1988;13(7):726–30. https://doi.org/10.1097/00007632-198807000-00003.
24. The physiology of the joints. Vol. 3. The trunk and the vertebral column. Postgrad Med J. 1975;51(599):682–3.
25. Astin JH, Wilkerson CG, Dailey AT, Ellis BJ, Brockmeyer DL. Finite element modeling to compare craniocervical motion in two age-matched pediatric patients without or with Down syndrome: implications for the role of bony geometry in craniocervical junction instability. J Neurosurg Pediatr. 2020;27(2):218–24. https://doi.org/10.3171/2020.6.PEDS20453.
26. Finley SM, Astin JH, Joyce E, Dailey AT, Brockmeyer DL, Ellis BJ. FEBio finite element model of a pediatric cervical spine. J Neurosurg Pediatr. 2021;29(2):218–24. https://doi.org/10.3171/2021.7.PEDS21276.
27. Herron MR, Park J, Dailey AT, Brockmeyer DL, Ellis BJ. Febio finite element models of the human cervical spine. J Biomech. 2020;113:110077. https://doi.org/10.1016/j.jbiomech.2020.110077.
28. Phuntsok R, Ellis BJ, Herron MR, Provost CW, Dailey AT, Brockmeyer DL. The occipitoatlantal capsular ligaments are the primary stabilizers of the occipitoatlantal joint in the craniocervical junction: a finite element analysis. J Neurosurg Spine. 2019;30(5):593–601. https://doi.org/10.3171/2018.10.SPINE181102.
29. Phuntsok R, Mazur MD, Ellis BJ, Ravindra VM, Brockmeyer DL. Development and initial evaluation of a finite element model of the pediatric craniocervical junction. J Neurosurg Pediatr. 2016;17(4):497–503. https://doi.org/10.3171/2015.8.PEDS15334.
30. Kanwar R, Delasobera BE, Hudson K, Frohna W. Emergency department evaluation and treatment of cervical spine injuries. Emerg Med Clin North Am. 2015;33(2):241–82. https://doi.org/10.1016/j.emc.2014.12.002.
31. McAllister AS, Nagaraj U, Radhakrishnan R. Emergent imaging of pediatric cervical spine trauma. Radiographics. 2019;39(4):1126–42. https://doi.org/10.1148/rg.2019180100.
32. Wang MX, Beckmann NM. Imaging of pediatric cervical spine trauma. Emerg Radiol. 2021;28(1):127–41. https://doi.org/10.1007/s10140-020-01813-1.
33. Hoffman JR, Wolfson AB, Todd K, Mower WR. Selective cervical spine radiography in blunt trauma: methodology of the National Emergency X-Radiography Utilization Study (NEXUS). Ann Emerg Med. 1998;32(4):461–9. https://doi.org/10.1016/s0196-0644(98)70176-3.
34. Stiell IG, Clement CM, McKnight RD, et al. The Canadian C-spine rule versus the NEXUS low-risk criteria in patients with trauma. N Engl J Med. 2003;349(26):2510–8. https://doi.org/10.1056/NEJMoa031375.
35. Hoffman JR, Mower WR, Wolfson AB, Todd KH, Zucker MI. Validity of a set of clinical criteria to rule out injury to the cervical spine in patients with blunt trauma. National Emergency X-Radiography Utilization Study Group. N Engl J Med. 2000;343(2):94–9. https://doi.org/10.1056/NEJM200007133430203.
36. Anderson RCE, Scaife ER, Fenton SJ, Kan P, Hansen KW, Brockmeyer DL. Cervical spine clearance after trauma in children. J Neurosurg Pediatr. 2006;105(5):361–4. https://doi.org/10.3171/ped.2006.105.5.361.
37. Anderson RCE, Kan P, Hansen KW, Brockmeyer DL. Cervical spine clearance after trauma in children. Neurosurg Focus. 2006;20(2):1–4. https://doi.org/10.3171/foc.2006.20.2.4.
38. Anderson RCE, Kan P, Vanaman M, et al. Utility of a cervical spine clearance protocol after trauma in children between 0 and 3 years of age: clinical article. J Neurosurg Pediatr. 2010;5(3):292–6. https://doi.org/10.3171/2009.10.PEDS09159.
39. Brockmeyer DL, Ragel BT, Kestle JRW. The pediatric cervical spine instability study. A pilot study assessing the prognostic value of four imaging modalities

in clearing the cervical spine for children with severe traumatic injuries. Childs Nerv Syst. 2012;28(5):699–705. https://doi.org/10.1007/s00381-012-1696-x.
40. Herman MJ, Brown KO, Sponseller PD, et al. Pediatric cervical spine clearance: a consensus statement and algorithm from the pediatric cervical spine clearance working group. JBJS. 2019;101(1):e1. https://doi.org/10.2106/JBJS.18.00217.
41. Joaquim AF, Patel AA. Craniocervical traumatic injuries: evaluation and surgical decision making. Global Spine J. 2011;1(1):37–42. https://doi.org/10.1055/s--0031-1296055.
42. Copley PC, Tilliridou V, Kirby A, Jones J, Kandasamy J. Management of cervical spine trauma in children. Eur J Trauma Emerg Surg. 2019;45(5):777–89. https://doi.org/10.1007/s00068-018-0992-x.
43. Jones TM, Anderson PA, Noonan KJ. Pediatric cervical spine trauma. J Am Acad Orthop Surg. 2011;19(10):600–11.
44. Anderson PA, Montesano PX. Morphology and treatment of occipital condyle fractures. Spine (Phila Pa 1976). 1988;13(7):731–6. https://doi.org/10.1097/00007632-198807000-00004.
45. Momjian S, Dehdashti AR, Kehrli P, May D, Rilliet B. Occipital condyle fractures in children. PNE. 2003;38(5):265–70. https://doi.org/10.1159/000069825.
46. Kim D, Viswanathan VK, Menger RP. C1 fractures. In: StatPearls. StatPearls Publishing; 2022. http://www.ncbi.nlm.nih.gov/books/NBK534091/. Accessed 28 Mar 2022.
47. Wholey MH, Bruwer AJ, Baker HL. The lateral roentgenogram of the neck; with comments on the atlanto-odontoid-basion relationship. Radiology. 1958;71(3):350–6. https://doi.org/10.1148/71.3.350.
48. Harris JH, Carson GC, Wagner LK, Kerr N. Radiologic diagnosis of traumatic occipitovertebral dissociation: 2. Comparison of three methods of detecting occipitovertebral relationships on lateral radiographs of supine subjects. AJR Am J Roentgenol. 1994;162(4):887–92. https://doi.org/10.2214/ajr.162.4.8141013.
49. Powers B, Miller MD, Kramer RS, Martinez S, Gehweiler JA. Traumatic anterior atlanto-occipital dislocation. Neurosurgery. 1979;4(1):12–7. https://doi.org/10.1227/00006123-197901000-00004.
50. Pang D, Nemzek WR, Zovickian J. Atlanto-occipital dislocation: part 1—normal occipital condyle-C1 interval in 89 children. Neurosurgery. 2007;61(3):514–521; discussion 521. https://doi.org/10.1227/01.NEU.0000290897.77448.1F.
51. Pang D, Nemzek WR, Zovickian J. Atlanto-occipital dislocation—part 2: the clinical use of (occipital) condyle-C1 interval, comparison with other diagnostic methods, and the manifestation, management, and outcome of atlanto-occipital dislocation in children. Neurosurgery. 2007;61(5):995–1015; discussion 1015. https://doi.org/10.1227/01.neu.0000303196.87672.78.
52. Theodore N, Aarabi B, Dhall SS, et al. The diagnosis and management of traumatic atlanto-occipital dislocation injuries. Neurosurgery. 2013;72(Suppl 2):114–26. https://doi.org/10.1227/NEU.0b013e31827765e0.
53. Martinez-Del-Campo E, Kalb S, Soriano-Baron H, et al. Computed tomography parameters for atlantooccipital dislocation in adult patients: the occipital condyle-C1 interval. J Neurosurg Spine. 2016;24(4):535–45. https://doi.org/10.3171/2015.6.SPINE15226.
54. Walters BC, Hadley MN, Hurlbert RJ, et al. Guidelines for the management of acute cervical spine and spinal cord injuries: 2013 update. Neurosurgery. 2013;60(CN_suppl_1):82–91. https://doi.org/10.1227/01.neu.0000430319.32247.7f.
55. Effendi B, Roy D, Cornish B, Dussault RG, Laurin CA. Fractures of the ring of the axis. A classification based on the analysis of 131 cases. J Bone Joint Surg Br. 1981;63-B(3):319–27. https://doi.org/10.1302/0301-620X.63B3.7263741.
56. Levine AM, Edwards CC. The management of traumatic spondylolisthesis of the axis. J Bone Joint Surg Am. 1985;67(2):217–26.
57. Anderson LD, D'Alonzo RT. Fractures of the odontoid process of the axis. J Bone Joint Surg Am. 1974;56(8):1663–74.
58. Pang D, Sun P. Pediatric vertebral column and spinal cord injuries. In: Youmans neurological surgery. 5th ed. Vol. 3. W.B. Saunders; 2004. p. 3515–57.
59. Karlsson MK, Magnus KK, Moller A, et al. A modeling capacity of vertebral fractures exists during growth: an up-to-47-year follow-up. Spine (Phila Pa 1976). 2003;28(18):2087–92. https://doi.org/10.1097/01.BRS.0000084680.76654.B1.
60. Kim C, Vassilyadi M, Forbes JK, Moroz NWP, Camacho A, Moroz PJ. Traumatic spinal injuries in children at a single level 1 pediatric trauma centre: report of a 23-year experience. Can J Surg. 2016;59(3):205–12. https://doi.org/10.1503/cjs.014515.
61. Babu RA, Arimappamagan A, Pruthi N, et al. Pediatric thoracolumbar spinal injuries: the etiology and clinical spectrum of an uncommon entity in childhood. Neurol India. 2017;65(3):546–50. https://doi.org/10.4103/neuroindia.NI_1243_15.
62. Dogan S, Safavi-Abbasi S, Theodore N, et al. Thoracolumbar and sacral spinal injuries in children and adolescents: a review of 89 cases. J Neurosurg Pediatr. 2007;106(6):426–33. https://doi.org/10.3171/ped.2007.106.6.426.
63. Piatt J. Principles of system design not realized for pediatric craniospinal trauma care in the United States. J Neurosurg Pediatr. 2018;22(1):9–17. https://doi.org/10.3171/2018.1.PEDS17625.
64. Holdsworth FW. Fractures, dislocations, and fracture-dislocations of the spine. J Bone Joint Surg Am. 1963;45-B(1):6–20. https://doi.org/10.1302/0301-620X.45B1.6.
65. Denis F. The three column spine and its significance in the classification of acute thoracolumbar spinal

injuries. Spine (Phila Pa 1976). 1983;8(8):817–31. https://doi.org/10.1097/00007632-198311000-00003.
66. Magerl F, Aebi M, Gertzbein SD, Harms J, Nazarian S. A comprehensive classification of thoracic and lumbar injuries. Eur Spine J. 1994;3(4):184–201. https://doi.org/10.1007/BF02221591.
67. Vaccaro AR, Lehman RA, Hurlbert RJ, et al. A new classification of thoracolumbar injuries: the importance of injury morphology, the integrity of the posterior ligamentous complex, and neurologic status. Spine (Phila Pa 1976). 2005;30(20):2325–33. https://doi.org/10.1097/01.brs.0000182986.43345.cb.
68. Sellin JN, Steele WJ, Simpson L, et al. Multicenter retrospective evaluation of the validity of the Thoracolumbar Injury Classification and Severity Score system in children. J Neurosurg Pediatr. 2016;18(2):164–70. https://doi.org/10.3171/2016.1.PEDS15663.
69. Mo AZ, Miller PE, Troy MJ, Rademacher ES, Hedequist DJ. The AOSpine thoracolumbar spine injury classification system: a comparative study with the thoracolumbar injury classification system and severity score in children. OTA Int. 2019;2(4):e036. https://doi.org/10.1097/OI9.0000000000000036.
70. Dauleac C, Mottolese C, Beuriat PA, Szathmari A, Di Rocco F. Superiority of thoracolumbar injury classification and severity score (TLICS) over AOSpine thoracolumbar spine injury classification for the surgical management decision of traumatic spine injury in the pediatric population. Eur Spine J. 2021;30(10):3036–42. https://doi.org/10.1007/s00586-020-06681-4.
71. Dawkins RL, Miller JH, Menacho ST, et al. Thoracolumbar injury classification and severity score in children: a validity study. Neurosurgery. 2019;84(6):E362–7. https://doi.org/10.1093/neuros/nyy408.
72. Sayama C, Chen T, Trost G, Jea A. A review of pediatric lumbar spine trauma. Neurosurg Focus. 2014;37(1):E6. https://doi.org/10.3171/2014.5.FOCUS1490.
73. Gaca AM, Barnhart HX, Bisset GS. Evaluation of wedging of lower thoracic and upper lumbar vertebral bodies in the pediatric population. Am J Roentgenol. 2010;194(2):516–20. https://doi.org/10.2214/AJR.09.3065.
74. Jaremko JL, Siminoski K, Firth GB, et al. Common normal variants of pediatric vertebral development that mimic fractures: a pictorial review from a national longitudinal bone health study. Pediatr Radiol. 2015;45(4):593–605. https://doi.org/10.1007/s00247-014-3210-y.
75. Winklhofer S, Thekkumthala-Sommer M, Schmidt D, et al. Magnetic resonance imaging frequently changes classification of acute traumatic thoracolumbar spine injuries. Skelet Radiol. 2013;42(6):779–86. https://doi.org/10.1007/s00256-012-1551-x.
76. Qureshi S, Dhall SS, Anderson PA, et al. Congress of neurological surgeons systematic review and evidence-based guidelines on the evaluation and treatment of patients with thoracolumbar spine trauma: radiological evaluation. Neurosurgery. 2019;84(1):E28. https://doi.org/10.1093/neuros/nyy373.
77. Siebenga J, Leferink VJM, Segers MJM, et al. Treatment of traumatic thoracolumbar spine fractures: a multicenter prospective randomized study of operative versus nonsurgical treatment. Spine (Phila Pa 1976). 2006;31(25):2881–90. https://doi.org/10.1097/01.brs.0000247804.91869.1e.
78. Landi A, Marotta N, Mancarella C, Meluzio MC, Pietrantonio A, Delfini R. Percutaneous short fixation vs conservative treatment: comparative analysis of clinical and radiological outcome for A.3 burst fractures of thoraco-lumbar junction and lumbar spine. Eur Spine J. 2014;23(Suppl 6):671–6. https://doi.org/10.1007/s00586-014-3554-x.
79. Wood KB, Li W, Lebl DR, Lebl DS, Ploumis A. Management of thoracolumbar spine fractures. Spine J. 2014;14(1):145–64. https://doi.org/10.1016/j.spinee.2012.10.041.
80. Shen WJ, Liu TJ, Shen YS. Nonoperative treatment versus posterior fixation for thoracolumbar junction burst fractures without neurologic deficit. Spine (Phila Pa 1976). 2001;26(9):1038–45. https://doi.org/10.1097/00007632-200105010-00010.
81. Bailey CS, Urquhart JC, Dvorak MF, et al. Orthosis versus no orthosis for the treatment of thoracolumbar burst fractures without neurologic injury: a multicenter prospective randomized equivalence trial. Spine J. 2014;14(11):2557–64. https://doi.org/10.1016/j.spinee.2013.10.017.
82. Hoh DJ, Qureshi S, Anderson PA, et al. Congress of neurological surgeons systematic review and evidence-based guidelines on the evaluation and treatment of patients with thoracolumbar spine trauma: nonoperative care. Neurosurgery. 2019;84(1):E46–9. https://doi.org/10.1093/neuros/nyy369.
83. Bartanusz V, Harris J, Moldavsky M, Cai Y, Bucklen B. Short segment spinal instrumentation with index vertebra pedicle screw placement for pathologies involving the anterior and middle vertebral column is as effective as long segment stabilization with cage reconstruction: a biomechanical study. Spine (Phila Pa 1976). 2015;40(22):1729–36. https://doi.org/10.1097/BRS.0000000000001130.
84. Anderson PA, Raksin PB, Arnold PM, et al. Congress of neurological surgeons systematic review and evidence-based guidelines on the evaluation and treatment of patients with thoracolumbar spine trauma: surgical approaches. Neurosurgery. 2019;84(1):E56. https://doi.org/10.1093/neuros/nyy363.
85. Andras LM, Skaggs KF, Badkoobehi H, Choi PD, Skaggs DL. Chance fractures in the pediatric population are often misdiagnosed. J Pediatr Orthop. 2019;39(5):222–5. https://doi.org/10.1097/BPO.0000000000000925.
86. Chang CH, Lee ZL, Chen WJ, Tan CF, Chen LH. Clinical significance of ring apophysis fracture

in adolescent lumbar disc herniation. Spine (Phila Pa 1976). 2008;33(16):1750–4. https://doi.org/10.1097/BRS.0b013e31817d1d12.
87. Sairyo K, Goel VK, Masuda A, et al. Three dimensional finite element analysis of the pediatric lumbar spine. Part II: biomechanical change as the initiating factor for pediatric isthmic spondylolisthesis at the growth plate. Eur Spine J. 2006;15(6):930–5. https://doi.org/10.1007/s00586-005-1033-0.
88. Manabe H, Sakai T, Omichi Y, et al. Role of growth plate (apophyseal ring fracture) in causing modic type changes in pediatric low back pain patients. Eur Spine J. 2021;30(9):2565–9. https://doi.org/10.1007/s00586-021-06885-2.
89. Thomas JG, Boatey J, Brayton A, Jea A. Neurogenic claudication associated with posterior vertebral rim fractures in children. J Neurosurg Pediatr. 2012;10(3):241–5. https://doi.org/10.3171/2012.5.PEDS1247.
90. Wu X, Ma W, Du H, Gurung K. A review of current treatment of lumbar posterior ring apophysis fracture with lumbar disc herniation. Eur Spine J. 2013;22(3):475–88. https://doi.org/10.1007/s00586-012-2580-9.

Central Nervous System Infections and Their Management

19

Nathan K. Leclair and David S. Hersh

Introduction

Infection of the central nervous system (CNS) can have devastating consequences for patients of all age groups. Despite the presence of the blood-brain barrier, common pathogens (i.e., bacteria and viruses) infiltrate the CNS through a variety of routes. Fungi, parasites, and amoeba are rarer causes of CNS infections but nonetheless can lead to fulminant disease. Here, we summarize the major etiologies, clinical presentations, and treatment strategies for CNS infections in the pediatric population. The diagnosis and treatment of CNS infections requires a multi-disciplinary approach that often includes both surgical and medical management.

N. K. Leclair
School of Medicine, University of Connecticut, Farmington, CT, USA
e-mail: nleclair@uchc.edu

D. S. Hersh (✉)
Division of Neurosurgery, Connecticut Children's, Hartford, CT, USA

Department of Surgery, UConn School of Medicine, Farmington, CT, USA
e-mail: Dhersh@connecticutchildrens.org

Bacterial and Viral Meningitis

Inflammation of the meninges, or meningitis, can have complex and varying presentations in the pediatric population. Causative organisms vary based on age and geographic location of the patient.

Bacterial Meningitis

As a result of vaccination campaigns, the incidence of bacterial meningitis has declined among all age groups except infants under 2 months [1]. However, even with treatment the case fatality rate approaches 7% [1], and survivors can have significant neurological morbidity. Causative organisms vary by age and are summarized in Table 19.1. Infections of the meninges can occur via hematogenous spread, penetrating trauma, spread of an adjacent head and neck infection (e.g., sinusitis or mastoiditis), or seeding of an implanted device (e.g., CSF shunt). Congenital dermal sinuses can also result in recurrent episodes of bacterial meningitis due to a persistent communication between the CNS and the external environment [2, 3].

Neonates and infants with bacterial meningitis present with irritability, poor feeding, lethargy, and poor tone [4, 5]. Older children typically present with general signs of acute infection (fever, nausea, vomiting), neck stiffness, altered

N. Shimony, G. Jallo (eds.), *Pediatric Neurosurgery Board Review*,
https://doi.org/10.1007/978-3-031-23687-7_19

Table 19.1 Features of bacterial meningitis

Causative organism	Age range	Associations	Antibiotic regimen
Streptococcus pneumoniae	All ages	Most common cause overall in children and adults	Ceftriaxone or cefotaxime, consider penicillin if sensitive
Group B Streptococci	Neonates and infants		Penicillin G or Ampicillin
Neisseria meningitidis	Older children	Outbreaks in close quarters (e.g., colleges)	Ceftriaxone or cefotaxime
Listeria monocytogenes	Neonates and infants		Ampicillin plus gentamicin
Staphylococcus aureus		Associated with surgical site infections	Vancomycin
Gram-negative bacilli	Neonates and infants		Ceftriaxone or cefotaxime plus gentamicin Meropenem (alternative to cephalosporin)
Haemophilus influenzae		Decreased in rate since vaccination	Ceftriaxone or cefotaxime

mental status, and photophobia. Symptoms can occur with rapid onset (<24 h) or have a subacute course; those with rapidly progressing symptoms tend to have worse outcomes [6]. Seizures are relatively common, occurring in up to one third of children [7] and up to one half of all neonates presenting with bacterial meningitis [5, 8, 9]. On physical exam, a bulging fontanelle, papilledema, and altered mental status can be seen in a quarter of patients secondary to an increase in intracranial pressure, and can be accompanied by the Cushing triad (hypertension, bradycardia, and respiratory depression) [5]. Nuchal rigidity, indicative of meningeal irritation, is a more common finding in older children, and may be accompanied by the Kernig and Brudzinski signs [4, 10]. The sensitivity and specificity of the Kernig's sign is 52.6% and 77.5%, respectively, Brudzinski's sign 51.4% and 95%, and nuchal rigidity 64.5% and 53.5% [11].

CSF studies demonstrate an elevated protein concentration, decreased glucose level, elevated lactate, elevated ferritin, pleocytosis with an elevated neutrophil count on the differential, and organisms on a Gram stain [12, 13]. Additionally, CSF PCR testing can be used to identify causative organisms [12]. CSF and blood cultures should be obtained to identify the causative organism and antibiotic sensitivities. Negative cultures should be interpreted with caution in the context of empiric antibiotics, as sterilization of the CSF can occur rapidly after antibiotic administration [14].

Antibiotics should be given empirically for suspected bacterial meningitis. First line therapy includes ampicillin and gentamicin for neonates, and vancomycin and ceftriaxone for children older than 1 month [4, 15]. These "broad spectrum antibiotics" can be narrowed to more specific agents once the pathogen is identified and sensitivity testing has been completed (*see* Table 19.1). The bacterial meningitis score (BMS) can be used to identify patients at high or low risk for bacterial causes of meningitis [16], and can help guide the use of empiric antibiotics while awaiting cultures.

A serious complication of bacterial meningitis is post-infectious hydrocephalus (PIH). PIH accounts for approximately 40% of new cases of hydrocephalus annually, with a higher rate in developing countries [17, 18]. Pyogenic inflammation can lead to the development of fibrous adhesions that obstruct CSF flow and may result in multi-loculated hydrocephalus [19]. Surgical treatment involves CSF diversion via a CSF shunt or endoscopic third ventriculostomy (ETV). PIH is typically associated with lower rates of ETV success compared to other etiologies of hydrocephalus [18, 20, 21], although neuroendoscopy may play a role in fenestrating multi-loculated compartments.

Viral Meningitis

Viruses that are associated with viral meningitis are summarized in Table 19.2. Viral meningitis typically has a less severe clinical course compared to acute bacterial meningitis. Infants less than 6 months of age have the highest incidence [22], and present with fever, irritability, poor feeding, and other nonspecific symptoms. Older children present with nonspecific symptoms as well as nuchal rigidity and photophobia. Systemic findings associated with specific viral infections can also help differentiate viral from bacterial meningitis (*see* Table 19.2).

CSF studies also help differentiate bacterial from viral and fungal meningitis (*see* Table 19.3) [12]. In the setting of viral meningitis, CSF pleocytosis may be present, although to a lesser extent than in bacterial meningitis, and is characterized by a lymphocyte predominance. CSF glucose and protein

Table 19.2 Viral causes of meningitis and encephalitis

Virus	Specific viruses	Associated findings	Notes
Enterovirus	• Poliovirus • Coxsackie virus • Echovirus • Parechovirus	• Exanthema • Hand-foot-mouth disease	
Herpes viruses	• HSV-1 • HSV-2 • EBV • CMV • HHV6	• Herpetic gingivostomatitis (HSV-1) • HSV keratitis	Neonatal transmission (HSV-2)
Arboviruses	• St Louis encephalitis virus • La Crosse encephalitis virus • West Nile virus • Eastern equine encephalitis virus • Western equine encephalitis virus • Powassan virus		Vector-borne illnesses spread by mosquito and tick bites
HIV		• Neurodevelopmental delay • Secondary opportunistic infections	Neonatal transmission from mother to child
Influenza		• Flu-like prodrome	
Lymphocytic Choriomeningitis Virus (LCMV)		Biphasic presentation: 1. General febrile illness followed by recovery 2. Progression to CNS involvement manifesting as meningitis or encephalitis	
Mumps		• Parotitis	
Rabies		• Encephalomyelitis, anxiety, nightmares, hallucinations, insomnia	

Table 19.3 CSF studies in the setting of meningitis

Microbe	Protein content	Glucose	Pleocytosis	Other
Bacterial	High	Low	Neutrophilia	High lactate and ferritin
Viral	Normal to slightly elevated	Normal to slightly low	Lymphocytosis	Viral PCR of CSF
Fungal	High	Low	Neutrophilia	Beta-D glucan positive
Tuberculosis	High	Low	Lymphocytosis	High adenosine deaminase, acid fast bacilli

concentrations can be normal or subtly decreased and increased, respectively. Viral RT-PCR testing should be performed to identify the causal pathogen.

Viral meningitis has a self-limiting course and therefore treatment is supportive. Cases that occur in the context of HIV are treated with anti-retroviral therapy. In cases where the clinical exam and laboratory studies cannot rule out bacterial meningitis, empiric antibiotics should be administered until the cultures are finalized.

Viral Encephalitis

Encephalitis is defined as diffuse inflammation of the brain parenchyma. The most common cause of encephalitis is a viral infection, which can lead to a primary encephalitis in which the virus directly infects brain tissue, or a post-infectious encephalitis whereby a viral infection induces an autoimmune response involving the brain. Other classifications of primary CNS parenchymal infections include rhombencephalitis (brainstem), myelitis (spinal cord), radiculitis (nerve root), and meningoencephalitis (meninges and brain). The diagnosis is usually made clinically and supported by imaging studies as well as CSF viral PCR or next generation sequencing [23].

Etiology

Herpes viruses are the most common viruses to cause a primary viral encephalitis. These include herpes simplex virus 1 and 2 (HSV-1 and HSV-2), cytomegalovirus (CMV), Epstein-Barr virus (EBV), human herpes virus 6, and varicella-zoster virus (VZV). HSV-induced encephalitis is typically caused by HSV-1, except in neonates in whom HSV-2 can be passed from the mother to child [24, 25]. HSV tends to migrate along the olfactory or trigeminal nerves [26], and therefore has a predilection for inducing a focal encephalitis localized to the medial temporal lobe and inferior frontal lobes [24]. White matter changes in these regions can be visualized on MRI [23, 27, 28]. CMV encephalitis, on the other hand, is extremely rare and is typically associated with immunocompromised patients [29]. Pediatric cases of encephalitis caused by VZV [30] or EBV [31] are rare, as well.

Enteroviruses, including coxsackieviruses, polioviruses, and echoviruses, are a major cause of viral encephalitis in children [32–34]. Enterovirus infections have a strong seasonality, with summer and fall months associated with an increased risk of infection [35]. Infections are classically associated with hand, foot, and mouth disease. Enterovirus infections, particularly with Enterovirus A71, have led to large scale outbreaks of encephalitis in Asia [36].

Arboviruses are another important cause of primary infectious encephalitis [37]. These tend to follow unique geographic distributions. Transmission occurs through arthropod bites, including fleas, ticks, and mosquitoes.

Clinical Presentation and Diagnosis

Children present with fever, altered mental status, seizures, and focal neurological signs depending on the localization of the encephalitis [34]. Additional clinical findings can point to specific viral causes such as concurrent hand, foot, and mouth disease in patients with an enterovirus infection. Abnormal MRI and electroencephalogram findings are common, and CSF analysis generally demonstrates a pleocytosis [34]. Changes on MRI FLAIR sequences are sensitive but not specific for viral encephalitis [38]. CSF PCR can also be used to identify the causative virus [39]. However, false negative PCRs can occur, especially early in the disease course [40, 41].

Treatment

Treatment of viral encephalitis is mainly supportive. For patients with suspected viral encephalitis, empiric treatment with intravenous acyclovir should be initiated immediately [23, 42, 43]. Public health measures, including vaccination campaigns and arthropod control, have decreased the overall incidence of viral encephalitis. In severe cases, intractably elevated intracranial pressure has been treated with decompressive craniectomy to prevent brain herniation [44–46].

Tuberculosis, Parasitic, and Fungal Infections

Tuberculosis, parasitic, and fungal infections of the CNS are less common but should still be on the differential for patients presenting clinically with signs of CNS infection.

CNS Tuberculosis

CNS tuberculosis (TB) is rare, occurring in approximately 1–2% of patients with active TB, but nevertheless carries a high fatality rate [47] and is of particular concern in immunocompromised patients, such as those with HIV [48]. CNS infections occur after a primary infection in the lung seeds the bloodstream. TB infections involving the CNS present with three main patterns: intracranial granulomas, meningitis, and spinal arachnoiditis [47]. Granulomatous foci may form in the brain, meninges, and surrounding tissues, and produce TB meningitis when they rupture into the subarachnoid space [47]. TB meningitis typically has a subacute presentation, beginning with a prodromal phase of nonspecific signs of infection followed by signs of meningeal irritation ~1–3 weeks later, and culminating in a paralytic phase characterized by multiple neurological deficits, seizures, hemiparesis, and coma [47, 49]. Seizures are a common finding in children [50]. Cranial nerve palsies can be found in a quarter of patients, with the abducens nerve being the most common cranial nerve involved [49, 51, 52]. Severe complications of TB meningitis include vision loss from exudative compression of the optic nerve, obstructive hydrocephalus due to ventricular entrapment by TB tubercles, and ischemia secondary to inflammation or exudative entrapment of cerebral vessels. Radiographically, close to half of all patients with TB meningitis demonstrate ring-enhancing tuberculomas on MRI [53]. Spinal arachnoiditis is a less common presentation of CNS TB that involves inflammation of the arachnoid, resulting in subacute symptoms that may include radicular pain, paresthesias, motor dysfunction, and incontinence [54].

CSF studies typically demonstrate low CSF glucose levels, an elevated protein content, and a lymphocytic pleocytosis [49]. CSF smears demonstrate acid-fast bacilli in up to 50% of patients [55]; large volumes of CSF and prolonged monitoring (greater than 1 month) are typically required to detect acid fast bacilli in culture. PCR tests demonstrate a sensitivity of 68% and specificity of 95% [56]. Adenosine deaminase has also been used as a specific marker for TB meningitis but has a low sensitivity [57, 58]. Treatment of CNS tuberculosis in children consists of 2 months of a four-drug regimen with isoniazid, rifampin, pyrazinamide and either ethionamide or streptomycin. Ethambutol is not indicated for treatment in children due to a high risk of optic neuritis. Following this 2-month intensive treatment phase, patients are administered isoniazid and rifampin for 7–10 months [59]. Neurosurgical intervention may be required in patients with ventricular entrapment and resulting hydrocephalus.

Pott's disease (tuberculous spondylitis) is an important complication of primary TB, as well. Pott's disease involves osteomyelitis that most commonly affects the upper lumber and lower thoracic region, leading to vertebral body collapse and spinal kyphosis (Gibbus deformity) [60]. Spinal deformity and adjacent cold abscesses can lead to spinal cord compression and neurological deficits [60]. Treatment includes the same long-term TB antibiotic treatment regimen described above, as well as deformity correction for severe cases [61].

Neurocysticercosis

Neurocysticercosis is an infection of the CNS by the tapeworm *Taenia solium*. Infections are endemic in developing nations [62]. Pigs serve as the intermediate host; when raw or undercooked pork containing cysticerci is ingested by humans, the tapeworm attaches to the intestine, resulting in taeniasis. Eggs are shed in human feces into the environment, and when contaminated food or water is ingested, the oncospheres hatch, move through the intestinal wall and enter the bloodstream, migrating to the CNS and other organs where they undergo further maturation into cysticerci [63, 64]. Patients with intraparenchymal cysts commonly present with seizures [62, 63, 65]. Extraparenchymal cysts can arise in the basal subarachnoid cisterns and sylvian fissure, where they can produce significant mass effect and hydrocephalus; as a result they are associated with a worse overall prognosis and carry a higher mortality rate [62, 65]. Basal subarachnoid neurocysticercosis, or racemose neurocysticercosis, has a predilection for continued proliferation, eventually leading to arachnoiditis and fibrosis [65].

Diagnostic criteria include direct visualization of parasites by fundoscopy, evidence of cystic lesion(s) with an internal scolex on neuroimaging, and histopathologic demonstration of the parasite [66]. Treatment includes antiparasitics, such as albendazole or praziquantel, in addition to corticosteroids and antiepileptics [67]. When severe, diffuse cerebral edema is present, antiparasitics should not be used as they can exacerbate the inflammatory reaction. In such cases, initial treatment should be limited to corticosteroids [67]. Cases of extraparenchymal neurocysticercosis often require surgical management for treatment of the resulting mass effect and/or hydrocephalus [67].

Toxoplasmosis

Toxoplasmosis is one of the neonatal TORCH infections (Toxoplasmosis, Other [syphilis, varicella-zoster, parvovirus B19], Rubella, Cytomegalovirus, and Herpes). Congenital toxoplasmosis has a prevalence of 10–33 cases per 100,000 live births in the United States [68]. Congenital toxoplasmosis is responsible for significant perinatal morbidity and is caused by transplacental transmission of the *Toxoplasma gondii* parasite following a primary infection of the mother [68]. Primary infections are associated with eating undercooked meat contaminated with Toxoplasma cysts and exposure to cat feces [69]. Congenital toxoplasmosis is classically associated with a triad of chorioretinitis, intracranial calcifications, and hydrocephalus [70]. Treatment of congenital toxoplasmosis consists of a 12 month regimen of pyrimethamine, sulfadiazine, and folic acid [70].

Amebic Encephalitis

Amebic encephalitis is almost uniformly fatal [71–73]. The three most common species of ameba that infect the human CNS are *Naegleria fowleri, Acanthamoeba*, and *Balamuthia mandrillaris*. These infections are classically associated with exposure to freshwater lakes and ponds during the summer months [72].

Naegleria fowleri produces a rapidly fatal necrotizing primary amebic encephalitis [72–75]. Due to the fulminant nature of the disease, rapid diagnosis is required. The clinical presentation is similar to that of bacterial meningitis and includes fever, headache, photophobia, seizures, altered mental status, and focal neurological deficits. CSF studies also mimic bacterial meningitis with a neutrophil dominant pleocytosis, low glucose, and elevated protein. Ameba can be seen upon microscopic evaluation of the CSF [73]. Standard treatment guidelines are lacking, but successful treatment of primary amebic encephalitis has been reported with miltefosine [76], as well as a combination of amphotericin B, fluconazole, and rifampin [77].

Acanthamoeba and *Balamuthia mandrillaris* can cause disseminated disease in other organs along with a granulomatous amebic encephalitis that is characterized by a prolonged subacute/chronic meningitis [78]. Granulomatous amebic encephalitis is an opportunistic infection occurring mainly in immunocompromised populations [78]. The diagnosis is often made post-mortem and consists of the identification of ameba trophozoites and cysts on histology [78]. Acanthamoeba species also characteristically cause keratitis, while *Balamuthia mandrillaris* causes a characteristic face lesion that often precedes CNS involvement [78].

Fungal Infections

Fungal infections of the CNS are rare and typically occur in immunocompromised patients. Fungal pathogens are the cause of meningitis in less than 1% of cases [79]. Fungal meningitis typically follows a chronic course. A travel history is important, as fungal infections are endemic in some areas of the United States [80]. For example, histoplasmosis and blastomycosis infections occur in the Midwest and South, and coccidiomycosis in the West [80, 81]. The diagnosis can be supported by the identification of beta-D-glucan, a component of the fungal cell wall, in the CSF [82, 83].

Abscesses and Empyemas

Pott's Puffy Tumor

Pott's puffy tumor refers to a specific subset of cranial infections that includes an osteomyelitis of the frontal bone and a subperiosteal abscess, with overlying edema of the forehead [84]. Imaging studies demonstrate bony resorption, bone edema, and a periosteal reaction [85]. Treatment requires surgical drainage and antibiotic treatment [86]. Empiric therapy usually includes vancomycin and a third-generation cephalosporin; antibiotics can be tailored to individual organisms following culture and susceptibility testing.

Epidural Abscess

Epidural abscesses are infections involving the space between the dura and the overlying bone. Intracranially, they most commonly result from direct extension of an adjacent head and neck infection involving the mastoid, paranasal sinuses, orbit, and skull. Intracranial epidural abscesses can also occur following a craniotomy or a penetrating trauma. Spinal epidural abscesses, on the other hand, typically result from hematogenous spread. The most common etiologies include *Streptococcus* and *Staphylococcus* species [87, 88].

Patients typically present with fever, headache, neck pain, and mental status changes [87]. Radiologically, intracranial epidural abscesses have a convex shape and do not cross the cranial sutures. On MRI, epidural abscesses restrict diffusion, are hyperintense on T2-weighted sequences, and are peripherally contrast-enhancing. Dural thickening and enhancement may be present as well [87, 89]. Similarly, on CT epidural abscesses demonstrate peripheral enhancement with a center that is iso- or hypodense (*see* Fig. 19.1).

Surgical drainage of the abscess is typically required, followed by administration of empiric broad spectrum antibiotics such as a combination of vancomycin, a third generation cephalosporin, and metronidazole [87]. When associated with an adjacent sinus infection, drainage of the impacted sinuses by an otolaryngologist is also typically required [90].

Subdural Empyema

Subdural empyemas involve the space between the dura and the arachnoid. Underlying etiologies are similar to those that cause epidural abscesses and bacterial meningitis [87, 90, 91].

Patients present with a similar clinical picture as bacterial meningitis. Seizures are a common presenting symptom [91, 92]. Contrast enhanced MRI demonstrates a crescentic shape with an enhancing rim and diffusion restriction. Subdural empyemas can lead to severe complications including brain abscesses and venous sinus thrombosis [93]. As a result, early detection and treatment is critical [94–96]. The treatment of subdural empyemas consists of both antibiotics and emergent surgical drainage [97]. Although options include a craniotomy or a burr hole washout, craniotomies have been shown to be more effective and are associated with lower rates of re-operation [98].

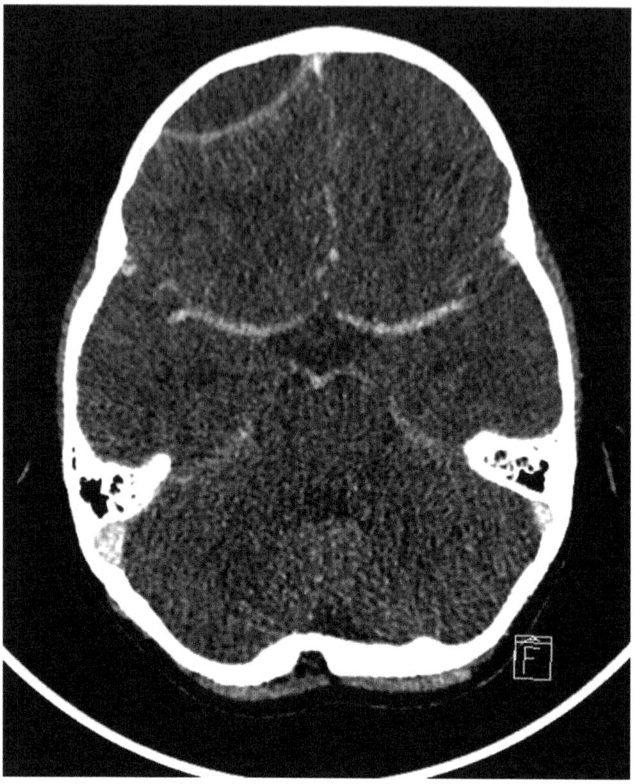

Fig. 19.1 CT scan of an intracranial epidural abscess in a pediatric patient with sinusitis. Right frontal epidural abscess with characteristic rim enhancement. Note that the epidural abscess does not cross the suture lines

Intraparenchymal Brain Abscess

Intracerebral abscesses are focal areas of infection involving the brain parenchyma. They can arise from direct extension of an adjacent primary source (e.g., sinusitis, otitis/mastoiditis, or meningitis). Alternatively, cerebral abscesses can be seeded via hematogenous spread [87], and may be seen as a complication of dental infections. Particularly, congenital heart defects that allow bypass of the pulmonary circulation may facilitate the spread of septic emboli from distant sites [99, 100].

The most common causative organisms are *Streptococci*, *Staphylococcus aureus*, and *Enterobacteriaceae* [101]. Fungal infections are more common causes of brain abscesses in immunocompromised patients [102, 103]. Brain abscesses that occur following a neurosurgical procedure are often caused by skin flora including *Staphylococcus aureus* and *Streptococcus epidermidis* [102].

Patients present with fever, altered mental status, headaches, and focal neurological deficits that depend on the location of the abscess [87, 102]. Treatment includes aspiration or surgical excision of the abscess and empiric antibiotic administration consisting of vancomycin, a third or fourth generation cephalosporin, and metronidazole [104]. The primary goals of surgery are to confirm the diagnosis, obtain purulent material to facilitate the identification of the organism and guide antibiotic treatment, and reduce the mass effect of the abscess [105]. Historically, needle aspiration has been advocated to accomplish these goals, particularly for deep abscesses [106]. Alternatively, complete surgical excision of the abscess is typically performed in the setting of multi-loculated abscesses, traumatic abscesses, fungal abscesses, or when the abscess has not responded to an initial aspiration. Primary excision of the abscess has been associated with a lower rate of recurrence, a shorter duration of antibiotic treatment, and a shorter hospital stay

[107]; however, it also carries increased risk to the adjacent tissue.

Special Considerations

Shunt Infections

Etiology

Cerebrospinal fluid (CSF) shunts divert CSF to other sites in the body and allow for decompression of the ventricular system in patients with hydrocephalus. These include ventriculoperitoneal, ventriculoatrial, and ventriculopleural shunts. Infections remain a significant complication of ventricular shunts, with an incidence of approximately 4–16% [108–112]. The vast majority of shunt infections occur early after initial placement or revision, typically within the first 6 months [110, 113], and are caused by the direct spread of normal skin flora. The most commonly involved pathogen is coagulase-negative staphylococcus (*Staphylococcus epidermidis*), accounting for approximately half of all cases, followed by *Staphylococcus aureus* [114]. Propionibacterium acnes is a rare cause of shunt infection and difficult to diagnose as it requires prolonged culturing (approximately 2 weeks) [115]. Late shunt infections occurring more than 1 year after surgery are less frequent, with an annual incidence of 0.28% in shunted pediatric patients, often presenting in the context of bowel perforation, a ruptured appendix, or peritonitis [116]. Sources of inoculation for late shunt infections include direct spread from a peritoneal infection, hematogenous spread, and traumatic exposure of the shunt [116].

Risk Factors

Multiple risks factors have been associated with shunt infections. Younger age at shunt placement is significantly associated with a heightened risk of infection [109, 111–113], as well as a previous history of shunt infection, use of a neuroendoscope, and multiple shunt-related procedures [109, 112]. Placement of a gastrostomy tube has been studied as a potential risk factor for ventriculoperitoneal shunt infection [117–119]. Recommendation vary, but a meta-analysis indicated a lower risk of infection in patients receiving a gastrostomy tube after ventriculoperitoneal shunt placement [120]. Waiting 7–10 days between percutaneous endoscopic gastrostomy (PEG) placement and shunt placement was recommended.

Prevention

Recently, antibiotic-coated shunts (clindamycin and rifampin) have been employed in an effort to reduce infection rates. Some studies have shown that antibiotic-coated shunts decrease the overall incidence of shunt infections from 6% in conventional shunts to 2% in antibiotic-coated shunts [121, 122]. The Hydrocephalus Clinical Research Network has also been instrumental in developing perioperative protocols to minimize the risk of shunt infection. Proposed practices include a formal hand scrub, double gloving, and the use of post-operative intravenous cefazolin [123].

Furthermore, antibiotic prophylaxis is typically administered to patients with a ventriculoatrial shunt who are undergoing a dental procedure, as these can potentially cause hematogenous seeding of the shunt hardware [124]. Antibiotic prophylaxis for dental procedures is no longer routinely used for patients with ventriculoperitoneal shunts.

Clinical Presentation

Patients typically present within 6 months of shunt placement or revision [111, 114], with signs of acute systemic infection including fever. Local signs of shunt infection include poor wound healing and drainage at the incision site. Additionally, shunt infection should be suspected in patients that demonstrate erythema and tenderness along the shunt tract (*see* Fig. 19.2a). Patients may experience abdominal pain secondary to peritoneal inflammation at the distal end of the shunt [125, 126]. Indolent distal infections can precipitate the formation of an abdominal pseudocyst—an abdominal CSF collection surrounded by a fibrous inflammatory capsule—leading to abdominal pain and distension as the primary presenting symptom [127].

Several important complications should be considered when a patient presents with a shunt

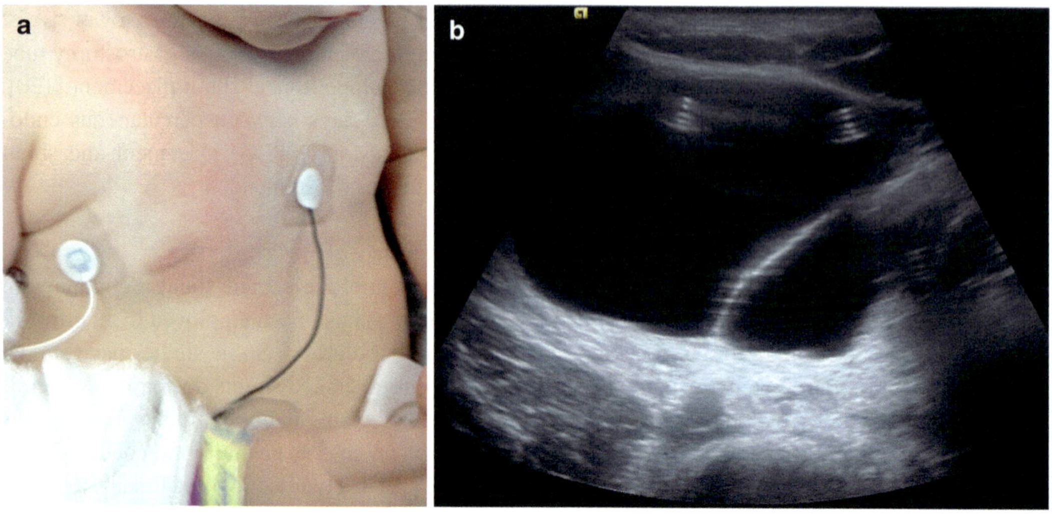

Fig. 19.2 Distal ventriculoperitoneal shunt infection. (**a**) Pediatric patient presenting with erythema along the shunt tract and abdominal tenderness. (**b**) Abdominal ultrasound demonstrates an abdominal pseudocyst surrounding the tip of the shunt catheter

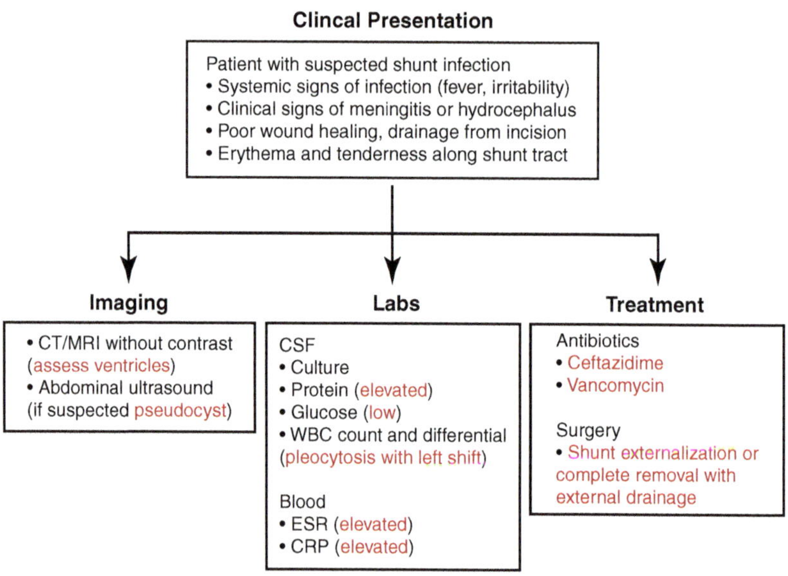

Fig. 19.3 Diagnostic findings and treatment of pediatric CSF shunt infections

infection. Ventriculoatrial shunt infections can lead to life threatening infective endocarditis [128, 129], as well as nephritis (frequently associated with *Staphylococcus epidermidis*) [130, 131]. Similarly, ventriculopleural shunt infections can lead to pleural effusions and/or empyemas [132]. Proximal spread of an infection can cause meningitis/ventriculitis [133].

Diagnosis

The diagnosis of CSF shunt infections typically relies on a combination of history, exam, serum inflammatory markers and CSF studies (*see* Fig. 19.3). Serum tests that indicate an acute infection include leukocytosis with a left shift on the differential, an elevated C-reactive protein, and an elevated erythrocyte sedimentation rate.

The C-reactive protein level may be a more reliable early predictor of infection as the erythrocyte sedimentation rate remains elevated for a longer period of time after surgery [134]. CSF cultures can reveal the causative organism, and sensitivities are important for antibiotic selection. CSF studies will typically demonstrate a pleocytosis (especially neutrophilia [135] and eosinophilia [136]), an elevated protein, decreased glucose, elevated procalcitonin, and elevated lactate levels [137, 138]. Blood cultures, especially in the context of ventriculoatrial shunts, are critical to evaluate for septicemia and isolate microbes.

Imaging studies may demonstrate signs of ventriculitis due to proximal spread of the infection, including enhancement of the ependymal wall as well as diffusion restricting debris in the ventricles [139]. Abdominal imaging is indicated in patients with a ventriculoperitoneal shunt who present with abdominal pain and/or distension, as the presence of an abdominal pseudocyst is pathognomonic for a distal shunt infection (*see* Fig. 19.2b). Abdominal ultrasound is often performed as a first line screening tool, while a CT of the abdomen can be used as a confirmatory study.

Treatment

Bacterial colonization of the shunt results in the formation of biofilms that limit antibiotic penetration and typically require removal of the shunt [140, 141]. Therefore, successful treatment of shunt infections typically requires removal of the shunt and administration of systemic antibiotics. Initial antibiotic coverage should be broad and usually includes vancomycin and a third generation cephalosporin for coverage of gram-negative organisms [139]. Antibiotic selection can be tailored to the causative organism once cultures and sensitivities are obtained. Antibiotic treatment is generally intravenous but can be delivered intrathecally if intravenous administration is unsuccessful or a highly drug resistant organism is suspected.

Shunt removal with external drainage and administration of antibiotics is considered the most effective paradigm for clearing a shunt infection [142]. If the shunt infection is localized to the distal component of the shunt, then externalization of the distal catheter and administration of antibiotics may be sufficient. In 2014, the Pediatric Hydrocephalus Systematic Review and Evidence-Based Guidelines Task Force concluded, "Supplementation of antibiotic treatment with partial (externalization) or complete shunt hardware removal are options in the management of CSF shunt infection. There is insufficient evidence to recommend either shunt externalization or complete shunt removal as the preferred surgical strategy for the management of CSF shunt infection. Therefore, clinical judgment is required" [143]. More recently, a prospective observational cohort study by the Hydrocephalus Clinical Research Network found that while the surgical approach (total shunt removal with external drain placement vs. distal shunt externalization) was not statistically associated with reinfection risk, surgical approaches other than total shunt removal were associated with a higher hazard of reinfection [144]. Further studies are needed to develop a standardized approach.

Once the CSF cultures remain negative and the CSF profile normalizes, at least 48 h of antibiotics are recommended prior to reinternalization of the shunt in the setting of coagulase-negative *Staphylococci* or *P. acnes* infections. Alternatively, in the setting of an abnormal CSF profile, at least 7 days of antibiotics are recommended prior to reinternalization. Finally, in the setting of *Staphylococcus aureus* or gram-negative bacilli infections, at least 10 days of antibiotics (following sterilization of the CSF) are recommended prior to reinternalization [139].

Trauma

Penetrating Injuries

Penetrating head trauma has been associated with an infection rate as high as 7% in large patient cohorts [145–147]. Particularly, the retention of foreign bodies is associated with a higher risk of infection, most commonly due to *Staphylococcus aureus* or *Staphylococcus epidermidis*. Preoperative imaging studies are paramount for visualizing the foreign body and any secondary injuries, although care must be taken to ascertain the presence of any metal within the foreign body prior to obtaining an MRI. Antibiotic management is variable, with only 64% of patients receiving prophylactic antibiotics; of those, 39% received a single dose of antibiotics [148, 149]. These studies have shown similar infection rates with or without the use of antibiotic prophylaxis.

Open Depressed Skull Fractures

Open skull fractures are associated with an infection rate of up to 10% [150]. Early washout is recommended to reduce the risk of infection (4.6% when debridement was performed within 48 h versus 36% when surgery was delayed by more than 48 h) [151]. Per the Guidelines for the Surgical Management of Traumatic Brain Injury, fragment elevation and reconstruction should be performed in most cases, and replacement of the primary bone fragment is an option when there is no evidence of wound infection [150, 152–154]. Nonoperative management can be considered in cases where "there is no clinical or radiographic evidence of dural penetration, significant intracranial hematoma, depression greater than 1 cm, frontal sinus involvement, gross cosmetic deformity, wound infection, pneumocephalus, or gross wound contamination" [150]. Antibiotic prophylaxis should be considered, although practices vary widely among centers [155].

Neurological Implications of COVID-19

The COVID-19 pandemic has introduced a new infection that has implications for the CNS. While primarily causing a respiratory syndrome, there is evidence for direct infection of the nervous system in humans [156], and there are several neurological complications related to SARS-CoV-2 infections. Anosmia associated with SARS-CoV-2 infection has been correlated with damage to the olfactory bulbs on MRI [157, 158]. Notably, anosmia is typically transient, and full recovery has been demonstrated in 96% of patients at 12 month follow up [159]. Alternatively, encephalitis is a potential complication among critically ill COVID-19 patients, occurring in 8.7% of hospitalized patients [160]. Abnormalities on MRI are common in such patients, and include signal abnormalities in the medial temporal lobe, multifocal white matter hyperintensities, and microhemorrhages [161].

COVID-19 patients are at a slightly elevated risk for several cerebrovascular issues including venous sinus thrombosis [162] and ischemic stroke [163, 164], which can present in pediatric patients [165]. It should be noted that COVID-19 severity is associated with increasing age, but that pediatric patients can still present with neurological complications; it remains too early to assess the long-term impact on neurocognitive development in children [166].

Conclusions

CNS infections are an important source of morbidity and mortality in pediatric patients. They include a diverse group of pathologies, with various clinical presentations, diagnostic strategies, and treatment paradigms. Many CNS infections can cause fulminant disease resulting in permanent disability or death, and require a multidisciplinary approach to both medical and surgical treatment.

Review Questions and Answers

1. A 2-week old infant was brought to the pediatrician due to irritability and fevers. He was admitted to the hospital with a fever of 101°F. CSF studies revealed an elevated protein, low glucose, and an elevated white blood cell count with a neutrophil predominance. CSF gram stain demonstrated gram positive rods. What is the most appropriate antibiotic regimen?
   (a) Penicillin G
   (b) Ceftriaxone
   (c) Ampicillin + gentamicin
   (d) Vancomycin

2. A 10-year-old boy suffered a seizure while on vacation with his family at a lake house. He presented to the ER with headache and altered mental status. Despite supportive care, the patient died 2 days later. What is the most likely causative organism?
   (a) *Naegleria fowleri*
   (b) *Streptococcus pneumoniae*
   (c) *Neisseria meningitidis*
   (d) *Powassan virus*
3. A child who underwent a ventriculoperitoneal shunt placement 3 months ago presents with headache and fever. On physical exam, his surgical incision is well healed; however, he is noted to have erythema along the shunt tract. An abdominal ultrasound reveals a cystic structure at the tip of the shunt. What is the most appropriate treatment strategy?
   (a) Externalization of the shunt and antibiotic treatment
   (b) Antibiotics only
   (c) Complete shunt removal and immediate replacement with a new shunt
   (d) Drainage of abdominal cyst alone

Answer Keys

1. c
2. a
3. a

References

1. Thigpen MC, Whitney CG, Messonnier NE, et al. Bacterial meningitis in the United States, 1998-2007. N Engl J Med. 2011;364(21):2016–25.
2. Masri A, Alassaf A, Khuri-Bulos N, Zaq I, Hadidy A, Bakri FG. Recurrent meningitis in children: etiologies, outcome, and lessons to learn. Childs Nerv Syst. 2018;34(8):1541–7.
3. Andiran N, Coskun T, Ozaydin E, Secmeer G. Recurrent meningitis associated with congenital paravertebral dermal sinus tract. Turk J Pediatr. 1998;40(1):121–5.
4. Swanson D. Meningitis. Pediatr Rev. 2015;36(12):514–24; quiz 525–6.
5. Pong A, Bradley JS. Bacterial meningitis and the newborn infant. Infect Dis Clin North Am. 1999;13(3):711–33, viii.
6. Kilpi T, Anttila M, Kallio MJ, Peltola H. Severity of childhood bacterial meningitis and duration of illness before diagnosis. Lancet. 1991;338(8764):406–9.
7. Briand C, Levy C, Baumie F, et al. Outcomes of bacterial meningitis in children. Med Mal Infect. 2016;46(4):177–87.
8. Gaschignard J, Levy C, Romain O, et al. Neonatal bacterial meningitis: 444 cases in 7 years. Pediatr Infect Dis J. 2011;30(3):212–7.
9. Chang CJ, Chang HW, Chang WN, et al. Seizures complicating infantile and childhood bacterial meningitis. Pediatr Neurol. 2004;31(3):165–71.
10. Curtis S, Stobart K, Vandermeer B, Simel DL, Klassen T. Clinical features suggestive of meningitis in children: a systematic review of prospective data. Pediatrics. 2010;126(5):952–60.
11. Bilavsky E, Leibovitz E, Elkon-Tamir E, Fruchtman Y, Ifergan G, Greenberg D. The diagnostic accuracy of the 'classic meningeal signs' in children with suspected bacterial meningitis. Eur J Emerg Med. 2013;20(5):361–3.
12. Sanaei Dashti A, Alizadeh S, Karimi A, Khalifeh M, Shoja SA. Diagnostic value of lactate, procalcitonin, ferritin, serum-C-reactive protein, and other biomarkers in bacterial and viral meningitis: a cross-sectional study. Medicine (Baltimore). 2017;96(35):e7637.
13. Domingues RB, Fernandes GBP, Leite F, Senne C. Performance of lactate in discriminating bacterial meningitis from enteroviral meningitis. Rev Inst Med Trop Sao Paulo. 2019;61:e24.
14. Kanegaye JT, Soliemanzadeh P, Bradley JS. Lumbar puncture in pediatric bacterial meningitis: defining the time interval for recovery of cerebrospinal fluid pathogens after parenteral antibiotic pretreatment. Pediatrics. 2001;108(5):1169–74.
15. van de Beek D, Cabellos C, Dzupova O, et al. ESCMID guideline: diagnosis and treatment of acute bacterial meningitis. Clin Microbiol Infect. 2016;22(Suppl 3):S37–62.
16. Nigrovic LE, Kuppermann N, Macias CG, et al. Clinical prediction rule for identifying children with cerebrospinal fluid pleocytosis at very low risk of bacterial meningitis. JAMA. 2007;297(1):52–60.
17. Dewan MC, Rattani A, Mekary R, et al. Global hydrocephalus epidemiology and incidence: systematic review and meta-analysis. J Neurosurg. 2018:1–15.
18. Warf BC. Hydrocephalus in Uganda: the predominance of infectious origin and primary management with endoscopic third ventriculostomy. J Neurosurg. 2005;102(1 Suppl):1–15.
19. Chatterjee S, Chatterjee U. Overview of post-infective hydrocephalus. Childs Nerv Syst. 2011;27(10):1693–8.
20. Kulkarni AV, Drake JM, Kestle JR, et al. Predicting who will benefit from endoscopic third ventriculostomy compared with shunt insertion in childhood hydrocephalus using the ETV Success Score. J Neurosurg Pediatr. 2010;6(4):310–5.

21. Warf BC, Dagi AR, Kaaya BN, Schiff SJ. Five-year survival and outcome of treatment for postinfectious hydrocephalus in Ugandan infants. J Neurosurg Pediatr. 2011;8(5):502–8.
22. Hviid A, Melbye M. The epidemiology of viral meningitis hospitalization in childhood. Epidemiology. 2007;18(6):695–701.
23. Tyler KL. Acute viral encephalitis. N Engl J Med. 2018;379(6):557–66.
24. Venkatesan A, Murphy OC. Viral encephalitis. Neurol Clin. 2018;36(4):705–24.
25. Kimberlin DW. Herpes simplex virus infections of the newborn. Semin Perinatol. 2007;31(1):19–25.
26. Bradshaw MJ, Venkatesan A. Herpes simplex virus-1 encephalitis in adults: pathophysiology, diagnosis, and management. Neurotherapeutics. 2016;13(3):493–508.
27. Granerod J, Davies NWS, Mukonoweshuro W, et al. Neuroimaging in encephalitis: analysis of imaging findings and interobserver agreement. Clin Radiol. 2016;71(10):1050–8.
28. Chow FC, Glaser CA, Sheriff H, et al. Use of clinical and neuroimaging characteristics to distinguish temporal lobe herpes simplex encephalitis from its mimics. Clin Infect Dis. 2015;60(9):1377–83.
29. Rafailidis PI, Mourtzoukou EG, Varbobitis IC, Falagas ME. Severe cytomegalovirus infection in apparently immunocompetent patients: a systematic review. Virol J. 2008;5:47.
30. Kennedy PG, Mogensen TH. Determinants of neurological syndromes caused by varicella zoster virus (VZV). J Neurovirol. 2020;26(4):482–95.
31. Dunmire SK, Hogquist KA, Balfour HH. Infectious mononucleosis. Curr Top Microbiol Immunol. 2015;390(Pt 1):211–40.
32. Koskiniemi M, Korppi M, Mustonen K, et al. Epidemiology of encephalitis in children. A prospective multicentre study. Eur J Pediatr. 1997;156(7):541–5.
33. Messacar K, Fischer M, Dominguez SR, Tyler KL, Abzug MJ. Encephalitis in US Children. Infect Dis Clin North Am. 2018;32(1):145–62.
34. Britton PN, Dale RC, Blyth CC, et al. Causes and clinical features of childhood encephalitis: a multicenter, prospective cohort study. Clin Infect Dis. 2020;70(12):2517–26.
35. Khetsuriani N, Lamonte-Fowlkes A, Oberst S, Pallansch MA, Centers for Disease Control and Prevention. Enterovirus surveillance—United States, 1970–2005. MMWR Surveill Summ. 2006;55(8):1–20.
36. Fujimoto T. [Hand-foot-and-mouth disease, aseptic meningitis, and encephalitis caused by enterovirus]. Brain Nerve. 2018;70(2):121–31.
37. Rust RS. Human arboviral encephalitis. Semin Pediatr Neurol. 2012;19(3):130–51.
38. Misra UK, Kalita J, Phadke RV, et al. Usefulness of various MRI sequences in the diagnosis of viral encephalitis. Acta Trop. 2010;116(3):206–11.
39. Wang L, Chen F, You D, et al. Development and validation of a multiplex-PCR based assay for the detection of 18 pathogens in the cerebrospinal fluid of hospitalized children with viral encephalitis. J Virol Methods. 2020;277:113804.
40. Tyler KL. Update on herpes simplex encephalitis. Rev Neurol Dis. 2004;1(4):169–78.
41. Denes E, Labach C, Durox H, et al. Intrathecal synthesis of specific antibodies as a marker of herpes simplex encephalitis in patients with negative PCR. Swiss Med Wkly. 2010;140:w13107.
42. Whitley RJ, Alford CA, Hirsch MS, et al. Vidarabine versus acyclovir therapy in herpes simplex encephalitis. N Engl J Med. 1986;314(3):144–9.
43. Tunkel AR, Glaser CA, Bloch KC, et al. The management of encephalitis: clinical practice guidelines by the Infectious Diseases Society of America. Clin Infect Dis. 2008;47(3):303–27.
44. Jouan Y, Grammatico-Guillon L, Espitalier F, Cazals X, Francois P, Guillon A. Long-term outcome of severe herpes simplex encephalitis: a population-based observational study. Crit Care. 2015;19:345.
45. Hasan A, AlSarraf L. Decompressive craniectomy in case of herpes encephalitis. Childs Nerv Syst. 2020;36(3):457–8.
46. Todeschi J, Gubian A, Wirth T, Coca HA, Proust F, Cebula H. Multimodal management of severe herpes simplex virus encephalitis: a case report and literature review. Neurochirurgie. 2018;64(3):183–9.
47. Leonard JM. Central nervous system tuberculosis. Microbiol Spectr. 2017;5(2).
48. Marais S, Pepper DJ, Schutz C, Wilkinson RJ, Meintjes G. Presentation and outcome of tuberculous meningitis in a high HIV prevalence setting. PLoS One. 2011;6(5):e20077.
49. Pehlivanoglu F, Yasar KK, Sengoz G. Tuberculous meningitis in adults: a review of 160 cases. ScientificWorldJournal. 2012;2012:169028.
50. Daniel BD, Grace GA, Natrajan M. Tuberculous meningitis in children: clinical management & outcome. Indian J Med Res. 2019;150(2):117–30.
51. Ramzan A, Nayil K, Asimi R, Wani A, Makhdoomi R, Jain A. Childhood tubercular meningitis: an institutional experience and analysis of predictors of outcome. Pediatr Neurol. 2013;48(1):30–5.
52. Sharma P, Garg RK, Verma R, Singh MK, Shukla R. Incidence, predictors and prognostic value of cranial nerve involvement in patients with tuberculous meningitis: a retrospective evaluation. Eur J Intern Med. 2011;22(3):289–95.
53. Wasay M, Farooq S, Khowaja ZA, et al. Cerebral infarction and tuberculoma in central nervous system tuberculosis: frequency and prognostic implications. J Neurol Neurosurg Psychiatry. 2014;85(11):1260–4.
54. Garg RK, Malhotra HS, Gupta R. Spinal cord involvement in tuberculous meningitis. Spinal Cord. 2015;53(9):649–57.
55. Thwaites GE, Chau TT, Farrar JJ. Improving the bacteriological diagnosis of tuberculous meningitis. J Clin Microbiol. 2004;42(1):378–9.
56. Pormohammad A, Nasiri MJ, McHugh TD, Riahi SM, Bahr NC. A systematic review and meta-analysis of

the diagnostic accuracy of nucleic acid amplification tests for tuberculous meningitis. J Clin Microbiol. 2019;57(6):e01113–8.
57. Solari L, Soto A, Agapito JC, et al. The validity of cerebrospinal fluid parameters for the diagnosis of tuberculous meningitis. Int J Infect Dis. 2013;17(12):e1111–5.
58. Erdem H, Ozturk-Engin D, Elaldi N, et al. The microbiological diagnosis of tuberculous meningitis: results of Haydarpasa-1 study. Clin Microbiol Infect. 2014;20(10):O600–8.
59. Nahid P, Dorman SE, Alipanah N, et al. Official American Thoracic Society/Centers for Disease Control and Prevention/Infectious Diseases Society of America clinical practice guidelines: treatment of drug-susceptible tuberculosis. Clin Infect Dis. 2016;63(7):e147–95.
60. Khanna K, Sabharwal S. Spinal tuberculosis: a comprehensive review for the modern spine surgeon. Spine J. 2019;19(11):1858–70.
61. Nussbaum ES, Rockswold GL, Bergman TA, Erickson DL, Seljeskog EL. Spinal tuberculosis: a diagnostic and management challenge. J Neurosurg. 1995;83(2):243–7.
62. Garcia HH, Nash TE, Del Brutto OH. Clinical symptoms, diagnosis, and treatment of neurocysticercosis. Lancet Neurol. 2014;13(12):1202–15.
63. Gripper LB, Welburn SC. Neurocysticercosis infection and disease—a review. Acta Trop. 2017;166: 218–24.
64. Coyle CM, Mahanty S, Zunt JR, et al. Neurocysticercosis: neglected but not forgotten. PLoS Negl Trop Dis. 2012;6(5):e1500.
65. Nash TE, Garcia HH. Diagnosis and treatment of neurocysticercosis. Nat Rev Neurol. 2011;7(10):584–94.
66. Del Brutto OH, Rajshekhar V, White AC Jr, et al. Proposed diagnostic criteria for neurocysticercosis. Neurology. 2001;57(2):177–83.
67. White AC Jr, Coyle CM, Rajshekhar V, et al. Diagnosis and treatment of neurocysticercosis: 2017 clinical practice guidelines by the Infectious Diseases Society of America (IDSA) and the American Society of Tropical Medicine and Hygiene (ASTMH). Clin Infect Dis. 2018;66(8):e49–75.
68. Neu N, Duchon J, Zachariah P. TORCH infections. Clin Perinatol. 2015;42(1):77–103, viii.
69. McAuley JB. Congenital toxoplasmosis. J Pediatr Infect Dis Soc. 2014;3(Suppl 1):S30–5.
70. Maldonado YA, Read JS, Committee on Infectious Diseases. Diagnosis, treatment, and prevention of congenital toxoplasmosis in the United States. Pediatrics. 2017;139(2):e20163860.
71. Pana A, Vijayan V, Anilkumar AC. Amebic meningoencephalitis. In: StatPearls. Treasure Island; 2021.
72. Yoder JS, Eddy BA, Visvesvara GS, Capewell L, Beach MJ. The epidemiology of primary amoebic meningoencephalitis in the USA, 1962-2008. Epidemiol Infect. 2010;138(7):968–75.
73. Capewell LG, Harris AM, Yoder JS, et al. Diagnosis, clinical course, and treatment of primary amoebic meningoencephalitis in the United States, 1937-2013. J Pediatr Infect Dis Soc. 2015;4(4):e68–75.
74. Visvesvara GS. Infections with free-living amebae. Handb Clin Neurol. 2013;114:153–68.
75. Pugh JJ, Levy RA. Naegleria fowleri: diagnosis, pathophysiology of brain inflammation, and antimicrobial treatments. ACS Chem Neurosci. 2016;7(9):1178–9.
76. Linam WM, Ahmed M, Cope JR, et al. Successful treatment of an adolescent with Naegleria fowleri primary amebic meningoencephalitis. Pediatrics. 2015;135(3):e744–8.
77. Vargas-Zepeda J, Gomez-Alcala AV, Vasquez-Morales JA, Licea-Amaya L, De Jonckheere JF, Lares-Villa F. Successful treatment of Naegleria fowleri meningoencephalitis by using intravenous amphotericin B, fluconazole and rifampicin. Arch Med Res. 2005;36(1):83–6.
78. Visvesvara GS, Moura H, Schuster FL. Pathogenic and opportunistic free-living amoebae: Acanthamoeba spp., Balamuthia mandrillaris, Naegleria fowleri, and Sappinia diploidea. FEMS Immunol Med Microbiol. 2007;50(1):1–26.
79. Hasbun R, Wootton SH, Rosenthal N, et al. Epidemiology of meningitis and encephalitis in infants and children in the United States, 2011-2014. Pediatr Infect Dis J. 2019;38(1):37–41.
80. Baddley JW, Winthrop KL, Patkar NM, et al. Geographic distribution of endemic fungal infections among older persons, United States. Emerg Infect Dis. 2011;17(9):1664–9.
81. Chu JH, Feudtner C, Heydon K, Walsh TJ, Zaoutis TE. Hospitalizations for endemic mycoses: a population-based national study. Clin Infect Dis. 2006;42(6):822–5.
82. Lyons JL, Roos KL, Marr KA, et al. Cerebrospinal fluid (1,3)-beta-D-glucan detection as an aid for diagnosis of iatrogenic fungal meningitis. J Clin Microbiol. 2013;51(4):1285–7.
83. Litvintseva AP, Lindsley MD, Gade L, et al. Utility of (1-3)-beta-D-glucan testing for diagnostics and monitoring response to treatment during the multistate outbreak of fungal meningitis and other infections. Clin Infect Dis. 2014;58(5):622–30.
84. Koltsidopoulos P, Papageorgiou E, Skoulakis C. Pott's puffy tumor in children: a review of the literature. Laryngoscope. 2020;130(1):225–31.
85. Lee YJ, Sadigh S, Mankad K, Kapse N, Rajeswaran G. The imaging of osteomyelitis. Quant Imaging Med Surg. 2016;6(2):184–98.
86. Bernard L, Dinh A, Ghout I, et al. Antibiotic treatment for 6 weeks versus 12 weeks in patients with pyogenic vertebral osteomyelitis: an open-label, non-inferiority, randomised, controlled trial. Lancet. 2015;385(9971):875–82.
87. Bonfield CM, Sharma J, Dobson S. Pediatric intracranial abscesses. J Infect. 2015;71(Suppl 1):S42–6.
88. Hlavin ML, Kaminski HJ, Fenstermaker RA, White RJ. Intracranial suppuration: a modern decade of postoperative subdural empyema and epidural

abscess. Neurosurgery. 1994;34(6):974–80; discussion 980–1.
89. Foerster BR, Thurnher MM, Malani PN, Petrou M, Carets-Zumelzu F, Sundgren PC. Intracranial infections: clinical and imaging characteristics. Acta Radiol. 2007;48(8):875–93.
90. Lundy P, Kaufman C, Garcia D, Partington MD, Grabb PA. Intracranial subdural empyemas and epidural abscesses in children. J Neurosurg Pediatr. 2019;24(1):14–21.
91. Banerjee AD, Pandey P, Devi BI, Sampath S, Chandramouli BA. Pediatric supratentorial subdural empyemas: a retrospective analysis of 65 cases. Pediatr Neurosurg. 2009;45(1):11–8.
92. De Bonis P, Anile C, Pompucci A, Labonia M, Lucantoni C, Mangiola A. Cranial and spinal subdural empyema. Br J Neurosurg. 2009;23(3):335–40.
93. Muzumdar D, Biyani N, Deopujari C. Subdural empyema in children. Childs Nerv Syst. 2018;34(10):1881–7.
94. Mauser HW, Van Houwelingen HC, Tulleken CA. Factors affecting the outcome in subdural empyema. J Neurol Neurosurg Psychiatry. 1987;50(9):1136–41.
95. Liu ZH, Chen NY, Tu PH, Lee ST, Wu CT. The treatment and outcome of postmeningitic subdural empyema in infants. J Neurosurg Pediatr. 2010;6(1):38–42.
96. Konar S, Gohil D, Shukla D, et al. Predictors of outcome of subdural empyema in children. Neurosurg Focus. 2019;47(2):E17.
97. French H, Schaefer N, Keijzers G, Barison D, Olson S. Intracranial subdural empyema: a 10-year case series. Ochsner J. 2014;14(2):188–94.
98. Nathoo N, Nadvi SS, Gouws E, van Dellen JR. Craniotomy improves outcomes for cranial subdural empyemas: computed tomography-era experience with 699 patients. Neurosurgery. 2001;49(4):872–7; discussion 877–8.
99. Udayakumaran S, Onyia CU, Kumar RK. Forgotten? Not yet. Cardiogenic brain abscess in children: a case series-based review. World Neurosurg. 2017;107:124–9.
100. Goodkin HP, Harper MB, Pomeroy SL. Intracerebral abscess in children: historical trends at Children's Hospital Boston. Pediatrics. 2004;113(6):1765–70.
101. Brook I. Microbiology and treatment of brain abscess. J Clin Neurosci. 2017;38:8–12.
102. Brouwer MC, Tunkel AR, McKhann GM 2nd, van de Beek D. Brain abscess. N Engl J Med. 2014;371(5):447–56.
103. Baddley JW, Salzman D, Pappas PG. Fungal brain abscess in transplant recipients: epidemiologic, microbiologic, and clinical features. Clin Transplant. 2002;16(6):419–24.
104. Mameli C, Genoni T, Madia C, Doneda C, Penagini F, Zuccotti G. Brain abscess in pediatric age: a review. Childs Nerv Syst. 2019;35(7):1117–28.
105. Infection in Neurosurgery Working Party of the British Society for Antimicrobial Chemotherapy. The rational use of antibiotics in the treatment of brain abscess. Br J Neurosurg. 2000;14(6):525–30.
106. Hall WA, Truwit CL. The surgical management of infections involving the cerebrum. Neurosurgery. 2008;62(Suppl 2):519–30; discussion 530–1.
107. Zhai Y, Wei X, Chen R, Guo Z, Raj Singh R, Zhang Y. Surgical outcome of encapsulated brain abscess in superficial non-eloquent area: a systematic review. Br J Neurosurg. 2016;30(1):29–34.
108. Pan P. Outcome analysis of ventriculoperitoneal shunt surgery in pediatric hydrocephalus. J Pediatr Neurosci. 2018;13(2):176–81.
109. Erps A, Roth J, Constantini S, Lerner-Geva L, Grisaru-Soen G. Risk factors and epidemiology of pediatric ventriculoperitoneal shunt infection. Pediatr Int. 2018;60(12):1056–61.
110. Choux M, Genitori L, Lang D, Lena G. Shunt implantation: reducing the incidence of shunt infection. J Neurosurg. 1992;77(6):875–80.
111. Vinchon M, Dhellemmes P. Cerebrospinal fluid shunt infection: risk factors and long-term follow-up. Childs Nerv Syst. 2006;22(7):692–7.
112. McGirt MJ, Zaas A, Fuchs HE, George TM, Kaye K, Sexton DJ. Risk factors for pediatric ventriculoperitoneal shunt infection and predictors of infectious pathogens. Clin Infect Dis. 2003;36(7):858–62.
113. Lee JK, Seok JY, Lee JH, et al. Incidence and risk factors of ventriculoperitoneal shunt infections in children: a study of 333 consecutive shunts in 6 years. J Korean Med Sci. 2012;27(12):1563–8.
114. Yakut N, Soysal A, Kepenekli Kadayifci E, et al. Ventriculoperitoneal shunt infections and re-infections in children: a multicentre retrospective study. Br J Neurosurg. 2018;32(2):196–200.
115. Portillo ME, Corvec S, Borens O, Trampuz A. Propionibacterium acnes: an underestimated pathogen in implant-associated infections. Biomed Res Int. 2013;2013:804391.
116. Vinchon M, Lemaitre MP, Vallee L, Dhellemmes P. Late shunt infection: incidence, pathogenesis, and therapeutic implications. Neuropediatrics. 2002;33(4):169–73.
117. Al-Holou WN, Wilson TJ, Ali ZS, et al. Gastrostomy tube placement increases the risk of ventriculoperitoneal shunt infection: a multiinstitutional study. J Neurosurg. 2018:1–6.
118. Gerges C, Wijesekera O, Herring E, et al. Evaluation of risk of gastrostomy and ventriculoperitoneal shunt placement in Pediatric patients: a systematic review of the literature. World Neurosurg. 2021;152:180–188.e1.
119. Tyler K, Leon SM, Lowe S, et al. Risk of ventriculoperitoneal shunt infection with coexisting percutaneous endoscopic gastrostomy tube and associated factors. Heliyon. 2020;6(3):e03523.
120. Oterdoom LH, Marinus Oterdoom DL, Ket JCF, van Dijk JMC, Scholten P. Systematic review of ventricular peritoneal shunt and percutaneous endoscopic

gastrostomy: a safe combination. J Neurosurg. 2017;127(4):899–904.
121. Mallucci CL, Jenkinson MD, Conroy EJ, et al. Antibiotic or silver versus standard ventriculoperitoneal shunts (BASICS): a multicentre, single-blinded, randomised trial and economic evaluation. Lancet. 2019;394(10208):1530–9.
122. Gutierrez-Gonzalez R, Boto GR, Fernandez-Perez C, del Prado N. Protective effect of rifampicin and clindamycin impregnated devices against Staphylococcus spp. infection after cerebrospinal fluid diversion procedures. BMC Neurol. 2010; 10:93.
123. Kestle JR, Holubkov R, Douglas Cochrane D, et al. A new Hydrocephalus Clinical Research Network protocol to reduce cerebrospinal fluid shunt infection. J Neurosurg Pediatr. 2016;17(4):391–6.
124. Antibiotic prophylaxis for dental patients at risk for infection. Pediatr Dent. 2018;40(6):386–91.
125. Wang KW, Chang WN, Shih TY, et al. Infection of cerebrospinal fluid shunts: causative pathogens, clinical features, and outcomes. Jpn J Infect Dis. 2004;57(2):44–8.
126. Kaestner S, Fraij A, Fass J, Deinsberger W. Ventriculoperitoneal shunt infections cause acute abdomen and peritonitis: a case series. J Surg Res. 2020;248:153–8.
127. Gaskill SJ, Marlin AE. Pseudocysts of the abdomen associated with ventriculoperitoneal shunts: a report of twelve cases and a review of the literature. Pediatr Neurosci. 1989;15(1):23–6; discussion 26–7.
128. Sun R, Warwick R, Harrisson S, Bandla N. Infective endocarditis as a complication of longstanding ventriculoatrial (VA) shunt: the importance of suspicion and early investigation in patients with VA shunt and pyrexia of unknown origin. BMJ Case Rep. 2021;14(1):e237161.
129. Burstrom G, Andresen M, Bartek J Jr, Fytagoridis A. Subacute bacterial endocarditis and subsequent shunt nephritis from ventriculoatrial shunting 14 years after shunt implantation. BMJ Case Rep. 2014;2014:bcr2014204655.
130. Gmeiner M, Wagner H, van Ouwerkerk WJR, et al. Long-term outcomes in ventriculoatrial shunt surgery in patients with pediatric hydrocephalus: retrospective single-center study. World Neurosurg. 2020;138:e112–8.
131. Hanak BW, Bonow RH, Harris CA, Browd SR. Cerebrospinal fluid shunting complications in children. Pediatr Neurosurg. 2017;52(6):381–400.
132. Iosif G, Fleischman J, Chitkara R. Empyema due to ventriculopleural shunt. Chest. 1991;99(6):1538–9.
133. Brook I. Meningitis and shunt infection caused by anaerobic bacteria in children. Pediatr Neurol. 2002;26(2):99–105.
134. Al-Jabi Y, El-Shawarby A. Value of C-reactive protein after neurosurgery: a prospective study. Br J Neurosurg. 2010;24(6):653–9.
135. Lan CC, Wong TT, Chen SJ, Liang ML, Tang RB. Early diagnosis of ventriculoperitoneal shunt infections and malfunctions in children with hydrocephalus. J Microbiol Immunol Infect. 2003;36(1):47–50.
136. McClinton D, Carraccio C, Englander R. Predictors of ventriculoperitoneal shunt pathology. Pediatr Infect Dis J. 2001;20(6):593–7.
137. Li Y, Zhang G, Ma R, et al. The diagnostic value of cerebrospinal fluids procalcitonin and lactate for the differential diagnosis of post-neurosurgical bacterial meningitis and aseptic meningitis. Clin Biochem. 2015;48(1–2):50–4.
138. Grille P, Verga F, Biestro A. Diagnosis of ventriculostomy-related infection: is cerebrospinal fluid lactate measurement a useful tool? J Clin Neurosci. 2017;45:243–7.
139. Tunkel AR, Hasbun R, Bhimraj A, et al. 2017 Infectious Diseases Society of America's clinical practice guidelines for healthcare-associated ventriculitis and meningitis. Clin Infect Dis. 2017;64(6):e34–65.
140. Gutierrez-Murgas Y, Snowden JN. Ventricular shunt infections: immunopathogenesis and clinical management. J Neuroimmunol. 2014;276(1–2):1–8.
141. Stevens NT, Greene CM, O'Gara JP, et al. Ventriculoperitoneal shunt-related infections caused by Staphylococcus epidermidis: pathogenesis and implications for treatment. Br J Neurosurg. 2012;26(6):792–7.
142. Schreffler RT, Schreffler AJ, Wittler RR. Treatment of cerebrospinal fluid shunt infections: a decision analysis. Pediatr Infect Dis J. 2002;21(7):632–6.
143. Tamber MS, Klimo P Jr, Mazzola CA, Flannery AM, Pediatric Hydrocephalus Systematic Review and Evidence-Based Guidelines Task Force. Pediatric hydrocephalus: systematic literature review and evidence-based guidelines. Part 8: management of cerebrospinal fluid shunt infection. J Neurosurg Pediatr. 2014;14(Suppl 1):60–71.
144. Simon TD, Kronman MP, Whitlock KB, et al. Reinfection after treatment of first cerebrospinal fluid shunt infection: a prospective observational cohort study. J Neurosurg Pediatr. 2018;21(4):346–58.
145. Harmon LA, Haase DJ, Kufera JA, et al. Infection after penetrating brain injury—an Eastern Association for the Surgery of Trauma multicenter study oral presentation at the 32nd annual meeting of the Eastern Association for the Surgery of Trauma, January 15-19, 2019, in Austin, Texas. J Trauma Acute Care Surg. 2019;87(1):61–7.
146. Bizhan A, Mossop C, Aarabi JA. Surgical management of civilian gunshot wounds to the head. Handb Clin Neurol. 2015;127:181–93.
147. Antibiotic prophylaxis for penetrating brain injury. J Trauma. 2001;51(2 Suppl):S34–40.
148. Marut D, Shammassian B, McKenzie C, Adamski J, Traeger J. Evaluation of prophylactic antibiotics in penetrating brain injuries at an academic level 1 trauma center. Clin Neurol Neurosurg. 2020;193:105777.

149. Sunshine K, Penuela M, Defta D, et al. Antibiotic prophylaxis in penetrating brain injury: a systematic review of the literature. Neurosurgery. 2020;67(Suppl 1).
150. Bullock MR, Chesnut R, Ghajar J, et al. Surgical management of depressed cranial fractures. Neurosurgery. 2006;58(3 Suppl):S56–60; discussion Si–iv.
151. Jennett B, Miller JD. Infection after depressed fracture of skull. Implications for management of nonmissile injuries. J Neurosurg. 1972;36(3):333–9.
152. Wylen EL, Willis BK, Nanda A. Infection rate with replacement of bone fragment in compound depressed skull fractures. Surg Neurol. 1999;51(4):452–7.
153. Bonfield CM, Naran S, Adetayo OA, Pollack IF, Losee JE. Pediatric skull fractures: the need for surgical intervention, characteristics, complications, and outcomes. J Neurosurg Pediatr. 2014;14(2):205–11.
154. Oktay K, Guzel E, Unal E, Yilmaz T, Okten AI, Guzel A. Outcome of primary bone fragment replacement in pediatric patients with depressed skull fracture. Pediatr Neurosurg. 2019;54(1):28–35.
155. McFall C, Beier AD, Hayward K, et al. Contemporary management of pediatric open skull fractures: a multicenter pediatric trauma center study. J Neurosurg Pediatr. 2021;27:1–5.
156. Meinhardt J, Radke J, Dittmayer C, et al. Olfactory transmucosal SARS-CoV-2 invasion as a port of central nervous system entry in individuals with COVID-19. Nat Neurosci. 2021;24(2):168–75.
157. Laurendon T, Radulesco T, Mugnier J, et al. Bilateral transient olfactory bulb edema during COVID-19-related anosmia. Neurology. 2020;95(5):224–5.
158. Lin E, Lantos JE, Strauss SB, et al. Brain imaging of patients with COVID-19: findings at an academic institution during the height of the outbreak in New York City. AJNR Am J Neuroradiol. 2020;41(11):2001–8.
159. Renaud M, Thibault C, Le Normand F, et al. Clinical outcomes for patients with anosmia 1 year after COVID-19 diagnosis. JAMA Netw Open. 2021;4(6):e2115352.
160. Shah VA, Nalleballe K, Zaghlouleh ME, Onteddu S. Acute encephalopathy is associated with worse outcomes in COVID-19 patients. Brain Behav Immun Health. 2020;8:100136.
161. Kremer S, Lersy F, de Seze J, et al. Brain MRI findings in severe COVID-19: a retrospective observational study. Radiology. 2020;297(2):E242–51.
162. Baldini T, Asioli GM, Romoli M, et al. Cerebral venous thrombosis and severe acute respiratory syndrome coronavirus-2 infection: a systematic review and meta-analysis. Eur J Neurol. 2021;28(10):3478–90.
163. Merkler AE, Parikh NS, Mir S, et al. Risk of ischemic stroke in patients with coronavirus disease 2019 (COVID-19) vs patients with influenza. JAMA Neurol. 2020;77:1366.
164. Khandelwal P, Al-Mufti F, Tiwari A, et al. Incidence, characteristics and outcomes of large vessel stroke in COVID-19 cohort: an international multicenter study. Neurosurgery. 2021;89(1):E35–41.
165. Coronado Munoz A, Tasayco J, Morales W, et al. High incidence of stroke and mortality in pediatric critical care patients with COVID-19 in Peru. Pediatr Res. 2022;91(7):1730–4.
166. Lin JE, Asfour A, Sewell TB, et al. Neurological issues in children with COVID-19. Neurosci Lett. 2021;743:135567.

Pediatric Spinal Deformity

20

Joanna E. Gernsback and Andrew Jea

Pediatric spinal deformity includes scoliosis and kyphosis. Scoliosis is defined as a coronal plane deformity greater than 10°, and can be congenital, neuromuscular, or idiopathic. Thoracic kyphosis is a sagittal plane deformity of greater than 50°, with a normal thoracic kyphosis being 20–40°. Cervical and lumbar kyphosis is defined as any loss in the normal lordosis of these regions of the spine. The goals of treatment for spinal deformity are a balanced spine, prevention of further deformity, management of pain, and curve correction. Children and adolescents typically present with curve progression and cosmetic issues, while adults present with pain and neurologic abnormalities.

Scoliosis

Congenital Scoliosis

Congenital scoliosis is typically due to bony anomalies (e.g., hemivertebra), which leads to unbalanced spinal growth [1, 2]. The incidence of congenital scoliosis is unknown. The familial incidence is 1–5%, with a slight male predominance [3–5]. Congenital scoliosis appears to be due to sporadic genetic and environmental factors, but the exact etiology is unknown [6, 7].

Vertebral anomalies can be failures of formation (type I deformity) or failures of segmentation (type II deformity); the two types can coexist (type III deformity). Failures of formation include wedged vertebrae with intact pedicles and hemivertebrae with a unilateral pedicle. These have asymmetric growth potential and lead to spinal deformity over time. Hemivertebrae can be fully segmented, semisegmented, nonsegmented, or incarcerated (*see* Fig. 20.1), with fully segmented hemivertebrae having the highest rates of progression, 1–3° a year [3]. Failures of segmentation include a unilateral bar (partial segmentation anomaly) and block vertebrae (complete segmentation anomaly). These also have asymmetric growth potentials, more pronounced in the unilateral bar (average 6° a year) [3]. Congenital spinal anomalies can be seen with Jeune's Syndrome, Jarcho-Levin Syndrome, Klippel-Feil Syndrome, Alagille Syndrome, and VATER/VACTERL syndrome (Vertebral anomalies, Anorectal malformations, Cardiovascular anomalies, Tracheoesophageal fistula, Esophageal atresia, Renal anomalies, Limb defects) [8].

Congenital scoliosis patients may present with rapid curve progression during periods of growth. The potential for deformity and the natural history depends on the specific anomalies and their location. A unilateral bar with contralateral

J. E. Gernsback · A. Jea (✉)
Department of Neurosurgery, University of Oklahoma Health Sciences Center, Oklahoma City, OK, USA
e-mail: Joanna-Gernsback@ouhsc.edu; Andrew-Jea@ouhsc.edu

N. Shimony, G. Jallo (eds.), *Pediatric Neurosurgery Board Review*,
https://doi.org/10.1007/978-3-031-23687-7_20

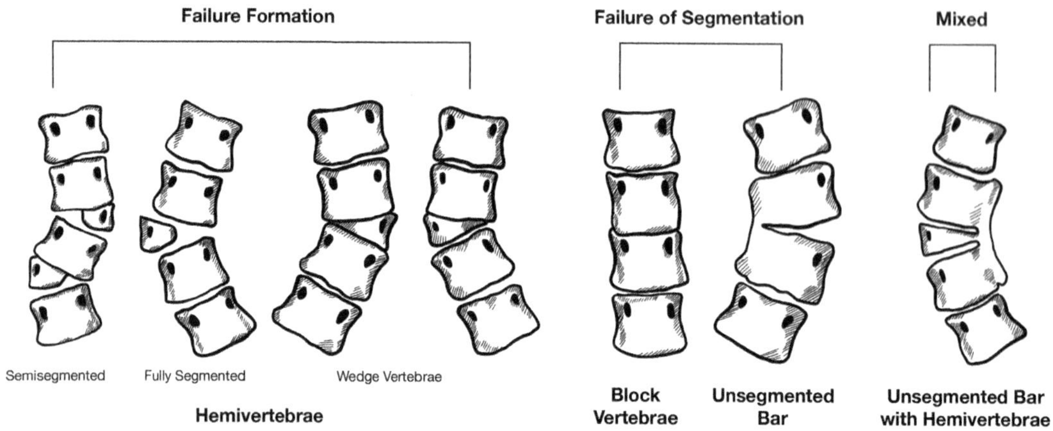

Fig. 20.1 Classification scheme of the various presentations of hemivertebrae [27]

hemivertebra is the most likely to progress, followed a unilateral unsegmented bar, then hemivertebra, wedge vertebra, and block vertebra. A unilateral bar progresses in the first 5 years and again during adolescence. Hemivertebrae and mixed anomalies progress slowly, then peak in adolescence. Location also matters, with thoracolumbar anomalies being the most likely to progress [3]. Overall, 70% of congenital scoliosis patients will progress.

Neuromuscular Scoliosis

Neuromuscular scoliosis is classified based on the underlying disorder: neurologic (e.g., cerebral palsy, spinal dysraphism) or muscular (e.g., muscular dystrophy) [9]. The incidence of scoliosis in patients with cerebral palsy ranges from 15 to 80% [10–12]. In patients with spinal dysraphism (e.g., myelomeningocele), the incidence of scoliosis is 40–50%. The type of spinal muscular atrophy (SMA) influences the incidence of scoliosis, which ranges from 30 to 100% [13–15]. Scoliosis in Duchenne Muscular Dystrophy (DMD) ranges from 50 to 75% [16, 17].

The pathogenesis of neuromuscular scoliosis includes trunk muscle weakness or paralysis and hypertonia. The spinal deformity is induced by the asymmetric control of the paraspinal musculature. Classic neuromuscular scoliosis includes a long, unbalanced thoracolumbar curve creating pelvic obliquity. This can make wheelchair positioning difficult (most patients are nonambulatory) and can cause pressure sores. The severe deformity can cause skin breakdown at the convexity, with skin maceration and infection at the concavity. A direct correlation between deformity size and decubitus ulcers has been noted [18]. Neuromuscular patients may present with rapidly progressive curves, and the risk of progression does not stop with skeletal maturity.

Idiopathic Scoliosis

Idiopathic scoliosis is the most common cause of spinal deformity, making up about 80% of scoliosis. It can present at any age, but most commonly is adolescent, presenting from 10 to 18. Adolescent idiopathic scoliosis (AIS) presents after age 10, and has an overall prevalence of 0.47–5.2%. The female to male ratio increases with age and curve size, up to 10:1. The underlying cause of AIS is unknown, although there are contributions from intrinsic genetic factors and extrinsic environmental factors [19]. Most patients have a positive family history. A meta-analysis of twin concordance demonstrated 73% for monozygotic twins and 36% for dizygotic twins [20]. Most AIS cases are detected during a sports physical, and present with a painless deformity. Asymmetry of the shoulders, waist, or rib cage may be noted.

Evaluation

The history includes age, birth history, neuromuscular disease or congenital syndrome, developmental milestones, family history, assessment of physiologic maturity, ambulatory status, foot shape, and pain. Physical exam should include strength, tone, range of motion with flexion contracture evaluation, walking ability and autonomy. The Adam's forward bend test (*see* Fig. 20.2) is when the patient bends forward at the waist and the examiner evaluates for symmetry. A scoliometer (*see* Fig. 20.3) can be placed on the back to estimate the curve and rotation. These are useful initial adjuncts to guide the need for radiographic studies. A scoliometry measurement of 7° correlates to a 20-degree curve.

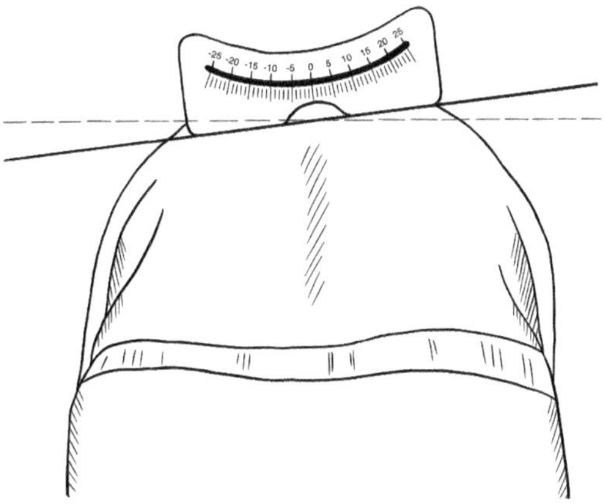

Fig. 20.3 Scoliometer. The inclination angle measured by scoliometer will help determine which patients may need radiography [29]

Fig. 20.2 Adam's forward bend test. (Left) As the patient bends over, the examiner looks from behind and from the side, horizontally along the contour of the back. (Right) A rotational deformity known as a rib hump (arrow) can be easily identified [28]

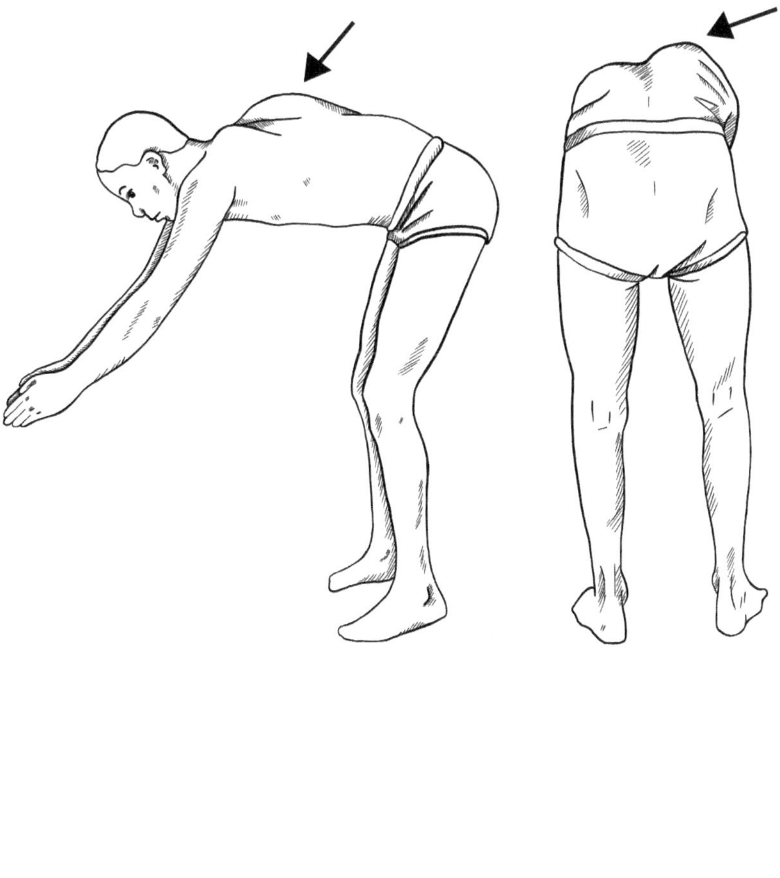

Imaging

Scoliosis x-rays are upright, long-cassette PA and lateral views of the entire spine. They are performed standing (sitting in a non-ambulatory patient). Lateral bending views can be included to assess the flexibility of the curve and may be useful for surgical planning, but are not needed routinely. MRIs of the spine should be completed in neuromuscular and congenital scoliosis, as well as in idiopathic cases with red flags (levoconvex curve, male gender, young age, rapid progression, significant pain, kyphosis), to rule out underlying causes, such as Chiari I malformation, syrinx, tumor, or spinal cord tethering. CTs are completed in complex cases for better visualization of the deformity, and occasionally for preoperative planning.

Scoliosis is diagnosed with a Cobb angle of at least 10°. The Cobb angle (*see* Fig. 20.4) is

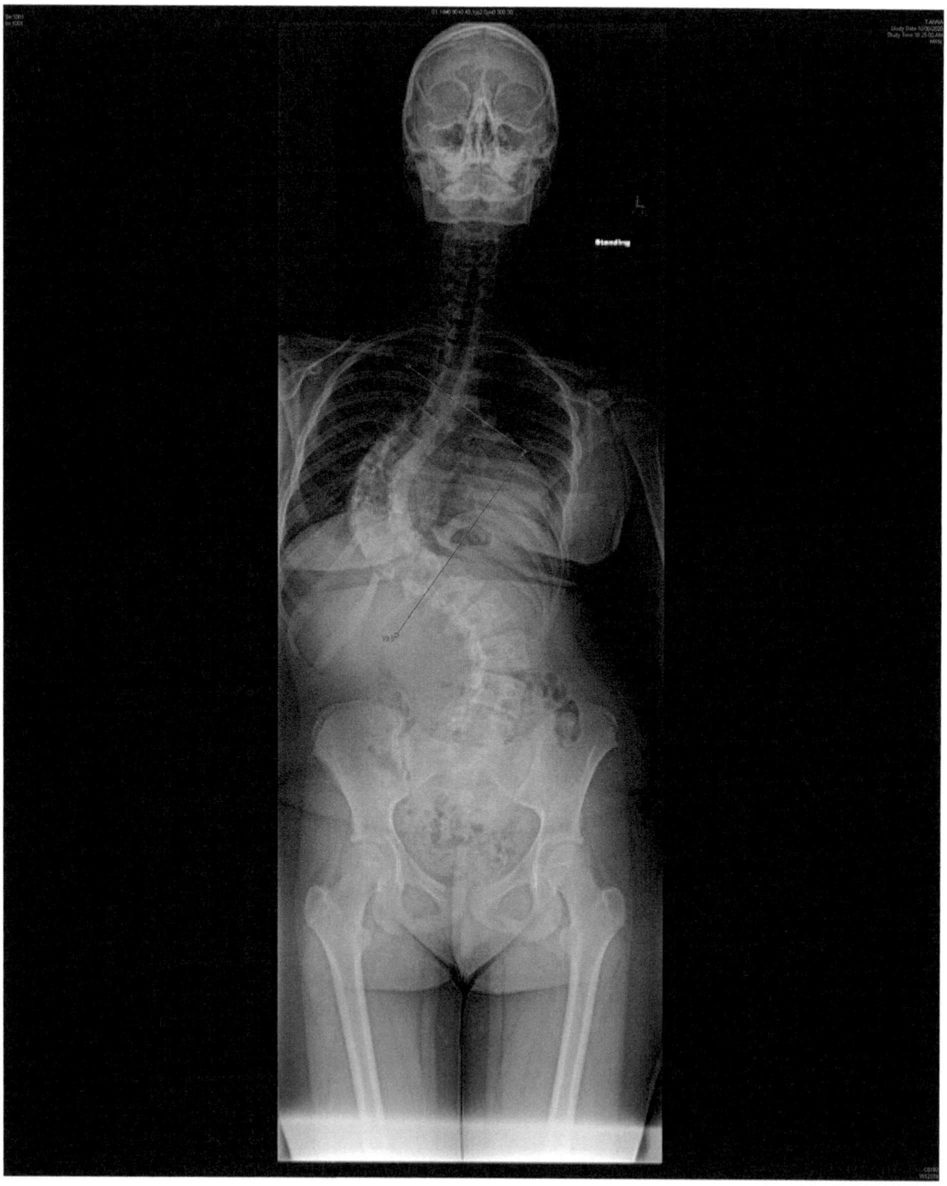

Fig. 20.4 The Cobb method of measuring the degree of scoliosis. The physician chooses the most tilted vertebrae above and below the apex of the curve. The angle between intersecting lines drawn perpendicular to the top of the superior vertebrae and the bottom of the inferior vertebrae is the Cobb angle (here, 62°) [28]

the angle formed by the intersection of a line drawn from the superior end plate of the superior end vertebra and the inferior end plate of the inferior end vertebra. The end vertebra is the vertebra most tilted from the horizontal apical vertebra. The apical vertebra is the vertebra or disc space deviated the farthest from the center of the vertebral column. Stable vertebrae are the most proximal vertebrae that are most closely bisected by the central sacral vertical line. Neutral vertebrae are those that are rotationally neutral, the spinous process is equidistant between the pedicles on PA x-rays. Coronal balance is determined by alignment of the C7 plumb line to the central sacral vertical line. Sagittal balance is determined by the C7 plumb line to the posterior-superior corner of S1. The Risser grade (*see* Fig. 20.5), which measures bony fusion of the iliac apophysis, can also be evaluated on scoliosis x-rays. Lower Risser grades are more likely to progress.

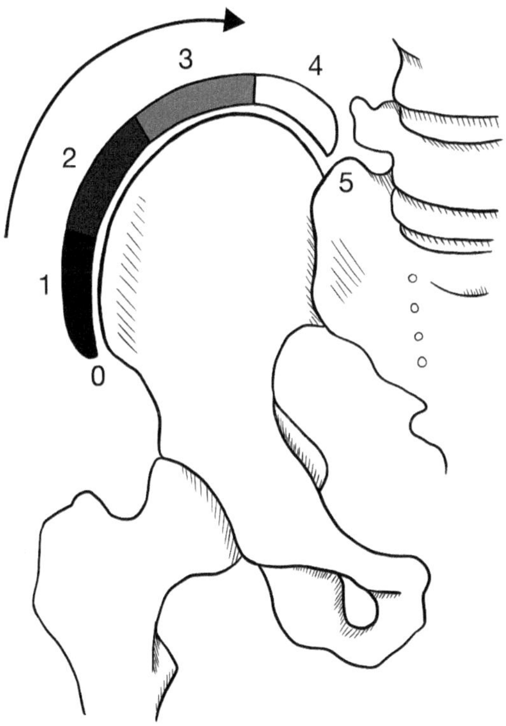

Fig. 20.5 Risser grades zero to 5. Grading is based on the degree of bony fusion of the iliac apophysis, from grade zero (no ossification) to grade 5 (complete bony fusion) [28]

Treatment

Treatment will depend on the cause and degree of deformity. Conservative treatment, including bracing or serial casting, typically does not prevent progression in congenital scoliosis, but may slow progression, and help with sitting balance and ventilation. With neuromuscular scoliosis, conservative measures are typically a bridge to surgery when the patient is more skeletally mature. Countering asymmetric posture with molded wheelchair adjustments can be used early on. Brace therapy can be utilized carefully, with frequent monitoring for pressure ulcers and skin integrity. For AIS, observation with serial x-rays is adequate for curves from 10 to 20°. A detorsional scoliosis brace is utilized for curves from 20 to 40°. The Bracing in Adolescent Scoliosis Trial (BRAIST) demonstrated that longer hours of brace usage were associated with greater benefit [21], thus most recommendations for bracing in the AIS population are for at least 18 h a day.

Surgery for congenital scoliosis is to slow or halt curve progression and restore spinal alignment. The goal of surgery for neuromuscular scoliosis is to correct the spinal deformity and pelvic obliquity, thus aligning the pelvic and scapular belts, thus maintaining a comfortable upright posture. Surgery in AIS is reserved for curves greater than 40–50°. The goal of surgery is to stop curve progression, restore physiologic alignment, and obtain an acceptable cosmetic result. It has been shown to reduce pain, improve self-image, improve function, and improve activity levels [22].

Surgery includes both arthrodesis and nonfusion options. Posterior arthrodesis with pedicle screws is typically the surgery of choice and is the most versatile. Extending the instrumentation from T2 to the pelvis is frequently necessary in neuromuscular cases, which are associated with pelvic obliquity. Congenital scoliosis may require osteotomies or hemivertebrectomies to correct the deformity. Anterior surgery can be utilized in select cases, possibly with the ability to spare levels, however worsened pulmonary function tests have been reported for thoracotomy cases. A limited apical fusion is occasionally performed on a severe curve to slow progression while waiting for the child to reach skeletal maturity. Fusionless surgery attempts to guide the growth of a curve. This can be done with growing rods, with posterior distraction along the concavity of the spine, in which the rods are lengthened over time, either with additional surgery or magnetically (e.g., MAGEC rods). Growth guidance systems, such as the Shilla technique and Luque Trolley rods, use vertebral fixation implants that freely slide along the rods, allowing for passive migration with growth. These procedures have about a 15% rate of rod breakage. Vertebral body stapling and tethering are growth-modulating techniques designed for skeletally immature patients, which will slow growth along the convexity of the curve.

Complications can present during surgery, in the immediate postoperative period, or in a delayed fashion. Neurologic injury is the main surgical risk, which is increased with kyphosis, excessive correction, and sublaminar wires. The risk of paraplegia is 1:1000 for AIS surgery. Neurologic monitoring with somatosensory-evoked potentials and motor-evoked potentials is the standard of care, with a drop in amplitude greater than 50% being a neurologic event. If this happens, check for technical problems, check the blood pressure and elevate if low, check the hemoglobin and transfuse if needed, lessen or reverse the correction, do a wake-up test, and potentially remove the instrumentation if the spine is stable. Infection occurs in 1–2% of AIS cases, and typically presents as late pain. The incision frequently looks normal. Cutibacterium acnes is the most common delayed infection organism.

Pseudoarthrosis occurs in 1–2% of AIS cases, and can present as late pain, progression of deformity, or hardware failure. An asymptomatic pseudoarthrosis can be observed. The crankshaft phenomenon is seen in skeletally immature patients undergoing a posterior spinal fusion. It is a rotation deformity caused by continued anterior growth with a posterior spinal fusion. It can be avoided by performing anterior-posterior surgery in very young patients. Short stature can also occur after fusion surgery in young children. Superior mesenteric artery (SMA) syndrome is a rare complication caused by compression of the third portion of the duodenum from narrowing between the SMA and the aorta. This presents with bowel obstruction symptoms in the first week after surgery, and is associated with electrolyte abnormalities, nausea, bilious vomiting, and weight loss. Risk factors include height less than 50th percentile, weight less than 25th percentile, and sagittal kyphosis. It is managed with a nasogastric tube and intravenous fluids.

Kyphosis

Scheuermann kyphosis (SK) is the most common cause of kyphosis in the pediatric population. The prevalence is 1–8% [23]. It is usually diagnosed between 11 and 17, with a possible male predominance. Twin studies demonstrate a genetic predisposition, but the underlying cause is unknown [24]. The pathophysiology appears to be a disorganized growth plate, with increased growth in the posterior vertebral body as compared to the anterior vertebral body.

There are two types of SK. Type I is thoracic only, with an apex most commonly around T7-8. Type II is an adult variant, involving the thoracolumbar spine [25], with scoliosis present in 88%. Curvature is measured using a Cobb angle on lateral x-rays, and is typically sharp, angulated, and rigid.

Pain tends to occur during the teenage years, in 50–75% of patients. Pain may be centered in the lower back due to compensatory (but pathologic) hyperlordosis in the lumbar spine. Younger patients are more likely to have pain, and only about 25% will have pain after skeletal maturity. Pain is rare is the curve is less than 50–60°. Teenagers may also present with cosmetic deformity, which can be mistaken for slouching. Postural kyphosis is typically less than 60°, however, and corrects with trunk extension. The mainstay of evaluation is standing scoliosis x-rays and a thorough neurologic exam. MRI can be considered to look for other anomalies if indicated. Sørenson defined SK as kyphosis in the sagittal plane greater than 40°, wedging of at least 5° in three successive vertebrae, with vertebral endplate irregularities. Associated radiographic findings include Schmorl's nodes, anterior narrowing of the disc space, scoliosis in 25%, and spondylolysis in 50% [26], possibly due to increased lumbar lordosis compensating for increased thoracic kyphosis.

Bracing (Milwaukee or TLSO brace most commonly) may be considered for skeletally immature patients with a mild to moderate curve, i.e., Type I SK with a 40 to 50-degree curve, Type II with a curve under 55°. The brace is worn 23 h a day for 1–2 years. Bracing will correct 40–50% of the kyphosis. NSAIDs and physical therapy are the mainstays of treatment for associated pain.

Surgery

Surgery is indicated when the curve is over 70–80° or progressive, loss of sagittal balance, for significant cosmetic deformity, progressive pain, and for neurologic deficit (rare). The ideal surgery is unknown, a posterior fusion with multiple osteotomies, such as Smith-Petersen, Ponte, and three-column osteotomies, is commonly accepted.

Many types of osteotomies are available. A Smith-Peterson osteotomy involves removing the posterior elements, including the facets, laminae, and posterior ligaments. This shortens the posterior column to allow manual extension. This gives a correction of 10–15°, although there is a potential loss of correction. The Ponte osteotomy is a variation that removes both the superior and inferior facets. This osteotomy is frequently utilized for AIS and Scheuermann's kyphosis. A more involved osteotomy is the pedicle subtraction osteotomy, which involves removing not only the posterior elements, but also a V-shaped wedge of vertebral body, thus shortening the middle column as well. This allows 30–40° of correction at a single level, but is more difficult to perform and caries a higher risk of complications. This is usually used for short angular deformities or severe positive sagittal imbalance. A vertebral column resection involves removing an entire vertebral body along with posterior elements and adjacent disc spaces, and is most useful for severe, fixed trunk translation, congenital kyphosis or hemivertebra excision. This is the most difficult variety of osteotomy, with the highest rates of neurologic complications.

It is recommended to limit the correction to 50% of the original curve to avoid spinal cord traction injury. The risk of spinal cord injury is highest in surgery for kyphosis compared to other spinal deformities. Lumbar hyperlordosis will usually self-correct. Fusion typically runs from the top of the kyphosis to the level below the first lordotic disc on lateral x-ray. The fusion should be balanced, and a plumb line from C7 should include the middle of the last fused vertebra.

Anesthesia is an important aspect of deformity surgery. Typically, a total intravenous anesthetic (TIVA) regimen is needed, so as not to interfere with neuromonitoring. Anesthetic gas cannot be used as it interferes with somatosensory evoked potentials, and muscle relaxers cannot be used as they interfere with motor evoked potentials. Additionally, blood loss is a major concern and transfusions are common. Administration of tranexemic acid (Lysteda or TXA) or aminocaproic acid (Amicar) may be utilized to decrease blood loss. Intraoperative salvage with a cell saver can be used to counter the blood loss as well. One should expect to need a packed red blood cell transfusion, and fresh frozen plasma and platelets should also be available.

Questions

1. You are seeing an otherwise healthy 13-year-old female with a 32-degree dextroconvex curve. She is Risser grade 3. What is your next step?
   (a) MRI of the entire spine
   (b) Observation with serial x-rays
   (c) Night bracing
   (d) Bracing at least 18 h a day
   (e) Posterior spinal fusion
   (f) Fusionless surgery
2. You are seeing an otherwise healthy 8-year-old female with an 18-degree dextroconvex curve. She is Risser grade 0. What is your next step?

(a) MRI of the entire spine
(b) Observation with serial x-rays
(c) Night bracing
(d) Bracing at least 18 h a day
(e) Posterior spinal fusion
(f) Fusionless surgery

3. You are seeing an otherwise healthy 14-year-old male with a 55-degree kyphosis that decreases to 40° when he stands up straight. He is Risser grade 4. What is your next step?
(a) Reassurance
(b) MRI of the entire spine
(c) Observation with serial x-rays
(d) Night bracing
(e) Bracing at least 18 h a day
(f) Posterior spinal fusion

Answers: 1-d; 2-a; 3-a

References

1. Cunin V. Early-onset scoliosis: current treatment. Orthop Traumatol Surg Res. 2015;101(1 Suppl):S109–18.
2. Odent T, Ilharreborde B, Miladi L, et al. Fusionless surgery in early-onset scoliosis. Orthop Traumatol Surg Res. 2015;101(6 Suppl):S281–8.
3. Shahcheraghi GH, Hobbi MH. Patterns and progression in congenital scoliosis. J Pediatr Orthop. 1999;19(6):766–75.
4. Purkiss SB, Driscoll B, Cole WG, Alman B. Idiopathic scoliosis in families of children with congenital scoliosis. Clin Orthop Relat Res. 2002;401:27–31.
5. Winter RB. Congenital scoliosis. Orthop Clin North Am. 1988;19(2):395–408.
6. Farley FA, Loder RT, Nolan BT, et al. Mouse model for thoracic congenital scoliosis. J Pediatr Orthop. 2001;21(4):537–40.
7. Imaizumi K, Masuno M, Ishii T, Kuroki Y, Okuzumi N, Nakamura Y. Congenital scoliosis (hemivertebra) associated with de novo balanced reciprocal translocation, 46,XX,t(13;17)(q34;p11.2). Am J Med Genet. 1997;73(3):244–6.
8. Williams BA, Matsumoto H, McCalla DJ, et al. Development and initial validation of the Classification of Early-Onset Scoliosis (C-EOS). J Bone Joint Surg Am. 2014;96(16):1359–67.
9. Vialle R, Thevenin-Lemoine C, Mary P. Neuromuscular scoliosis. Orthop Traumatol Surg Res. 2013;99(1 Suppl):S124–39.
10. Madigan RR, Wallace SL. Scoliosis in the institutionalized cerebral palsy population. Spine (Phila Pa 1976). 1981;6(6):583–90.
11. Balmer GA, MacEwen GD. The incidence and treatment of scoliosis in cerebral palsy. J Bone Joint Surg Br. 1970;52(1):134–7.
12. Koop SE. Scoliosis in cerebral palsy. Dev Med Child Neurol. 2009;51(Suppl 4):92–8.
13. Rodillo E, Marini ML, Heckmatt JZ, Dubowitz V. Scoliosis in spinal muscular atrophy: review of 63 cases. J Child Neurol. 1989;4(2):118–23.
14. Bono R, Inverno M, Botteon G, et al. Prospective study of gross motor development in children with SMA type II. Ital J Neurol Sci. 1995;16(4):223–30.
15. Evans GA, Drennan JC, Russman BS. Functional classification and orthopaedic management of spinal muscular atrophy. J Bone Joint Surg Br. 1981;63B(4):516–22.
16. Brooke MH, Fenichel GM, Griggs RC, et al. Duchenne muscular dystrophy: patterns of clinical progression and effects of supportive therapy. Neurology. 1989;39(4):475–81.
17. Robin GC. Scoliosis in Duchenne muscular dystrophy. Isr J Med Sci. 1977;13(2):203–6.
18. Majd ME, Muldowny DS, Holt RT. Natural history of scoliosis in the institutionalized adult cerebral palsy population. Spine (Phila Pa 1976). 1997;22(13):1461–6.
19. Kouwenhoven JW, Castelein RM. The pathogenesis of adolescent idiopathic scoliosis: review of the literature. Spine (Phila Pa 1976). 2008;33(26):2898–908.
20. Weinstein SL, Dolan LA, Cheng JC, Danielsson A, Morcuende JA. Adolescent idiopathic scoliosis. Lancet. 2008;371(9623):1527–37.
21. Weinstein SL, Dolan LA, Wright JG, Dobbs MB. Effects of bracing in adolescents with idiopathic scoliosis. N Engl J Med. 2013;369(16):1512–21.
22. Merola AA, Haher TR, Brkaric M, et al. A multicenter study of the outcomes of the surgical treatment of adolescent idiopathic scoliosis using the Scoliosis Research Society (SRS) outcome instrument. Spine (Phila Pa 1976). 2002;27(18):2046–51.
23. Ali RM, Green DW, Patel TC. Scheuermann's kyphosis. Curr Opin Pediatr. 1999;11(1):70–5.
24. Damborg F, Engell V, Andersen M, Kyvik KO, Thomsen K. Prevalence, concordance, and heritability of Scheuermann kyphosis based on a study of twins. J Bone Joint Surg Am. 2006;88(10):2133–6.

25. Blumenthal SL, Roach J, Herring JA. Lumbar Scheuermann's. A clinical series and classification. Spine (Phila Pa 1976). 1987;12(9):929–32.
26. Ogilvie JW, Sherman J. Spondylolysis in Scheuermann's disease. Spine (Phila Pa 1976). 1987;12(3):251–3.
27. Johal J, Loukas M, Fisahn C, Chapman JR, Oskouian RJ, Tubbs RS. Hemivertebrae: a comprehensive review of embryology, imaging, classification, and management. Childs Nerv Syst. 2016;32(11):2105–9.
28. Reamy BV, Slakey JB. Adolescent idiopathic scoliosis: review and current concepts. Am Fam Physician. 2001;64(1):111–6.
29. Horne JP, Flannery R, Usman S. Adolescent idiopathic scoliosis: diagnosis and management. Am Fam Physician. 2014;89(3):193–8.

Index

N. Shimony, G. Jallo (eds.), *Pediatric Neurosurgery Board Review*,
https://doi.org/10.1007/978-3-031-23687-7

D

E

F

G

T

W

Z

GPSR Compliance

The European Union's (EU) General Product Safety Regulation (GPSR) is a set of rules that requires consumer products to be safe and our obligations to ensure this.

If you have any concerns about our products, you can contact us on ProductSafety@springernature.com

In case Publisher is established outside the EU, the EU authorized representative is:

Springer Nature Customer Service Center GmbH
Europaplatz 3
69115 Heidelberg, Germany

Batch number: 10732817

Printed by Printforce, the Netherlands